"This is an outstanding, engaging text that does an excellent job in describing contemporary developments in the field (e.g., COVID-19, opioid crisis, gut microbiome) as well as providing rigorous coverage of classic studies. It is scholarly but fresh and provides many helpful tips for improving public health. The international and multicultural focus will especially appeal to today's students."

Eric Benotsch, Associate Professor,
Virginia Commonwealth University

The Psychology of Health and Illness

The Psychology of Health and Illness is a thoroughly updated version of Leslie Frazier's previous textbook on health psychology, which provides an engaging and contemporary approach to understanding health psychology from a truly international perspective. Combining both biopsychosocial and lifespan developmental perspectives, the book integrates core theory, research, and practice on global and cross-cultural health issues. It includes thoughtful and deliberately inclusive coverage of marginalized groups, especially BIPOC, LGBTQ+, and other underrepresented groups, designed to raise diversity and racial consciousness in a globally integrative way.

Alongside classic health psychology concepts, the author introduces students to cutting-edge scientific and medical topics such as epigenetics, the gut microbiome, and the nonmedical use of prescription drugs. The book also focuses on global public health and health disparities and promotes a strengths-based approach to health, rather than a deficits-based approach. It includes a wide range of pedagogical features including real-world applications, engaging anecdotes and case studies, opportunities for self-reflection, and numerous text boxes.

This is essential reading for undergraduate students on Health Psychology courses as well as those in related fields such as nursing and the allied health professions.

Leslie Frazier is the principal investigator and leader of the Health & Development Lab (HDL) in the Department of Psychology at Florida International University. She works with scholarly collaborators from around the world, community partners, graduate students, and undergraduate students. A developmental health psychologist, Dr. Frazier is interested in the intersections among psychosocial factors and identity/sense of self within the contexts of health and chronic illness in emerging adulthood and later life. Her research, funded by the Mental Research Institute, focuses on how psychosocial, sociocultural, and interpersonal factors impact our perceptions of ourselves, our health, and our well-being. Dr. Frazier and her team are currently investigating the factors that promote identity in people with disability, and the risk and resilience factors related to eating disorders in midlife menopausal women.

The Psychology of Health and Illness

A Multicultural Perspective

Leslie Frazier

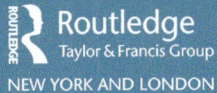

Routledge
Taylor & Francis Group
NEW YORK AND LONDON

Designed cover image: getty images via Aprison Photography

First published 2025
by Routledge
605 Third Avenue, New York, NY 10158

and by Routledge
4 Park Square, Milton Park, Abingdon, Oxon, OX14 4RN

Routledge is an imprint of the Taylor & Francis Group, an informa business

ISBN: 9781032643052 (hbk)
ISBN: 9781032639819 (pbk)
ISBN: 9781032643090 (ebk)

DOI: 10.4324/9781032643090

Typeset in Giovanni
by KnowledgeWorks Global Ltd.

Access the Instructor and Student Resources: www.routledge.com/9781032643052

Dedication

To Jack Frazier, fair winds and following seas, I miss you so much.

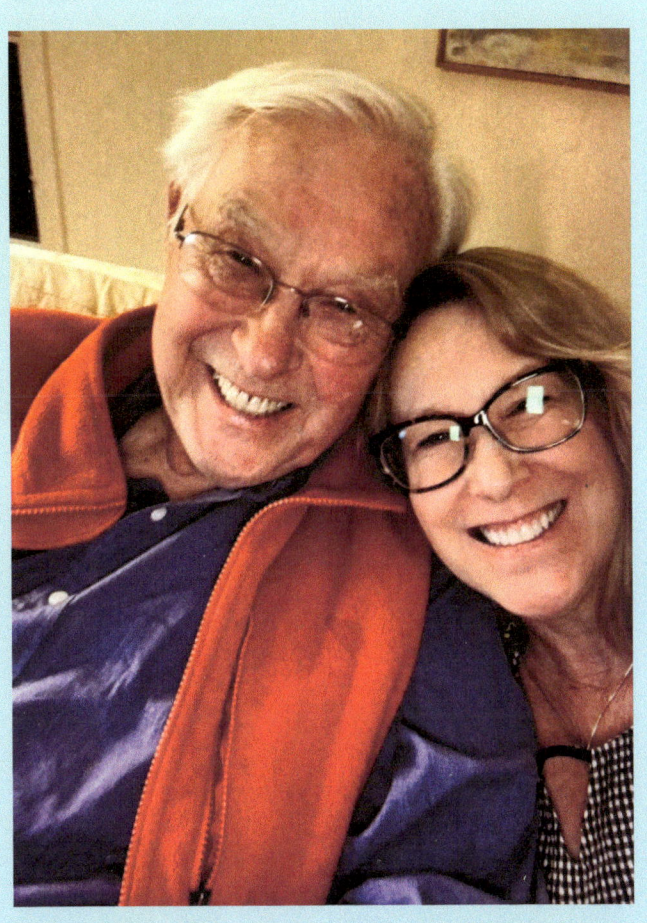

Contents

Preface to *The Psychology of Health and Illness: A Multicultural Perspective*

Shortly after I arrived at Florida International University, I developed the undergraduate survey course in health psychology. Even for me, with all my research and teaching experience, it came as a revelation. Probably no other psychology course touches on the lives of so many—including, I quickly found, every one of my students. It covers not only acute and chronic illness but also day-to-day stress, coping, and well-being. A course in health psychology must have a firm grounding in innovative and pioneering research, and for many students, it will provide their first introduction to how psychologists gather information on health and illness. It will introduce them to the biology of health and illness, as well as to models of behavior and behavioral change. Yet it also speaks to human stories, across the lifespan and around the world. Students will recognize those stories as their families, their friends, and their own.

In my health psychology course, I teach students to see health as more than just the absence of disease and help them recognize health disparities and the role of culture, gender identity, and age on health, both globally and within the United States. With the global public health issues facing the world today, health psychology and understanding the factors that influence people's perceptions of health, illness, and wellness have never been more profoundly important. In this textbook we tackle some of the current and recent historical global issues (i.e., the COVID-19 pandemic, natural disasters, war, climate change, global connectedness through technology) and how they impact our health and well-being. Health issues are everywhere, from headlines in the news to images on social media, from the political stage to the decisions we make every day. These issues can make a critical difference in how students choose health care for themselves, and whether they adopt health-enhancing behaviors for the rest of their lives, and whether they may choose a career in a health-related profession in the future. No wonder the course is so popular, and not just with students who major in psychology and allied health fields—all students can learn something that resonates with their lives. Since developing the undergraduate survey course, I have also developed a senior laboratory course in experimental health psychology, a senior seminar in the psychology of eating, graduate seminars, and a fully online version of the survey course. My appreciation of the scope and relevance of health psychology has only grown. So, too, has my need for a text that would address the full range of topics and speak directly to students and the world we live in today.

Issues of health change every day. Think about the opioid crisis, the global COVID-19 pandemic, and the controversy over vaccinations in the United States. Consider climate change, wars, immigration, and poverty. Globally, health and health disparities are important all around the world. Today's students need to be critical consumers of information in order to live healthier and happier lives. *The Psychology of Health and Illness: A Multicultural Perspective* incorporates the most recent developments in science, medicine, and society, and presents these issues in a way that is interesting, engaging, and valuable to students.

About This Text

The Psychology of Health and Illness: A Multicultural Perspective is a primary textbook for undergraduate courses. Drawing on the content I first wrote for a textbook on health psychology published by Worth, this book is a thoroughly updated version. It integrates the biopsychosocial and lifespan developmental perspectives and covers leading, innovative scientific and medical topics in ways that students can understand. It goes beyond mainstream textbooks in significant ways, building on traditional topics to aid student understanding, interest, and learning.

First, I provide a global and cross-cultural perspective. Many students approach health psychology with a nationalistic and ethnocentric view of health and illness. An important goal for this textbook is thus to introduce a global and cross-cultural perspective. It is my job to get students interested and to provide them with a well-rounded perspective, including health disparities within the United States and around the world.

Second, I take a developmental approach. There is a dynamic and reciprocal relationship between development and health across the lifespan; therefore, a developmental approach is necessary for understanding any health issue within its developmental context. My own research has focused on developmental health issues across adulthood, including health literacy, body image, weight-related concerns, and risks for eating disorders in emerging adulthood and midlife. I have

also studied how older adults cope with age-related transitions—including being diagnosed with a chronic illness or becoming a caregiver for a chronically ill loved one. This approach has special relevance to students, too, no matter where they are in the lifespan.

Since students often enter this course with a layperson's knowledge of health and illness, I **address misconceptions that they may have prior to taking this course.** Anyone teaching the health psychology course knows well the battle to lay aside preconceived notions that are not always grounded in science or actual medical practice. As a professor and now a textbook author, I feel that my most important goal is to emphasize that health psychology is a science and that its theories are grounded in science. I hope to convey how a foundation in science helps us make more informed decisions in our own lives.

I also emphasize that health psychology is directly relevant to each student's personal experience. Many students may have little background in biology, physiology, or, indeed, science. The medical and biological aspects of health psychology are challenging for them. My goal in writing this textbook is to convey this material in ways that are understandable and relatable for students. Students need to understand theory and research methods, but they thrive on **practical examples and applications.** *The Psychology of Health and Illness: A Multicultural Perspective* illustrates core theories with relevant and timely examples from a variety of nations, cultures, and ethnic groups. These examples help put a student's experience in a larger global health context. I also involve the student directly in these issues through engaging case studies and thought-provoking questions.

The field of health psychology is changing, and *The Psychology of Health and Illness: A Multicultural Perspective* reflects these changes. In this textbook, we seek to understand how diversity influences health psychology. This understanding is important because our personal and collective health is important to all of us, regardless of our diverse backgrounds, but also because our diversity, our racial, ethnic, gender, sexual, socioeconomic, religious, cultural, and national identities influence our health and wellness. As such, health psychology today must be foundationally grounded in an appreciation of **diversity**. Similarly, this textbook considers the importance of **intersectionality** because all of us are influenced by multiple social categories that interact to affect our lives. This textbook is designed to cultivate **cultural competency**, based on the belief that health disparities arise from social factors that lead to inequities and that health care should be diversity-affirming and strengths-based. Psychological research, research, and practice in health psychology, and this textbook aspire to the goal of creating **equity and inclusion**. My experience as a person who has an intersectional identity as a woman with disability, who has lived with cultural insensitivity, stigma, discrimination, and difficulties advocating for the accommodations that I am legally supposed to have—these experiences have shaped my perceptions, understanding, and appreciation for the need to present health psychology from a diverse perspective. Another outgrowth of this perspective is the commitment to using **person-first language**. Consistent with the American Psychological Association, in this textbook, we use person-first language to emphasize the person and not the disability or chronic condition—for example, I am a person with disability, not a disabled person. This applies to groups of people as well.

Content and Organization

Most textbooks in health psychology include similar content and follow a similar sequence. I do not deviate much from this format because it is a successful one. However, some improvements can make the wealth of material more contemporary, more easily accessible to students, and easier to absorb. This textbook integrates engaging applications, current case studies and examples, clear and thorough explanations, and a student-friendly tone. The text presents the implications of positive and negative health behaviors on a student's life.

The Biopsychosocial Perspective I include a chapter on health services and systems, a chapter on achieving emotional health and well-being, and the future of health psychology, including the implications of the biopsychosocial perspective. Yet the biopsychosocial perspective will be apparent in every other chapter as well.

The Global and Cross-Cultural Perspective This perspective extends to health around the world and to people of different races, ethnicities, socioeconomic status, genders, sexual orientations, and abilities. For example, Chapter 6 includes a full section on global and national health disparities in the context of stress. Chapter 7, in turn, discusses the role of culture in coping with stress, including the influences of religion, collectivism and individualism, and ethnic identity. The global perspective appears in every chapter.

The Developmental Approach I highlight the interplay among biopsychosocial and developmental influences, with relevant examples and empirical data, in every chapter. For example, Chapter 3 illustrates how health habits formed in childhood influence health outcomes later in life. Chapter 5 illuminates some of the developmental forces that make adolescence a window of vulnerability for risky health behaviors. Chapter 6 opens with the role of stress in the life of a college student and ends with the understanding of how acute and chronic stress have shaped every aspect of this student's life. In Chapter 12, we explore the differences in how patients and loved ones cope with the trajectory of life and death, including whether or not the death is off-time.

Addressing Misconceptions Like all of us, students are exposed to a wealth of misinformation delivered by the media, their families and friends, and their social networks. I have tried to counter common misconceptions throughout the text. Chapter 13, in particular, explores how misconceptions on the part of both patients and healthcare providers can have a negative impact on health.

Integrated Systems and Processes Rather than having a separate chapter on the systems of the body, the bodily systems, and physiological processes are described and explained when a health condition is presented. In this way, physiology provides a context for better understanding, while health conditions and health psychology provide a better motivation for difficult concepts in physiology. This holistic presentation represents a truly biopsychosocial approach to understanding health.

Chronic and Terminal Illnesses I combine chronic and terminal illnesses into one chapter (Chapter 12). This makes sense because chronic illness, unfortunately, often ends in a terminal phase. I believe that learning how patients experience this trajectory is important for understanding adjustment and quality of life at any point along the continuum.

Health-Enhancing and Health-Compromising Behaviors I dedicate separate chapters to these two types of behaviors (Chapters 4 and 5). Although some texts devote a single chapter to these topics, I have found that this division helps students better recognize poor choices and understand behavioral change. The division is also useful because there are different theoretical underpinnings for health-enhancing and health-compromising behaviors. The distinction helps them grasp the importance of a healthy lifestyle. However, these chapters can still be covered in the usual number of lectures.

Health Care Utilization and Alternatives I present the use of health services, patient–practitioner interactions, and alternative and complementary medicine in a single chapter (Chapter 13) because these topics are interrelated. I've brought these topics up to date, outlined contemporary and interactive scientific models, and presented the most relevant and important information. Alternatives to traditional Western medicine are also presented.

Health and Well-Being I include a unique chapter on health and well-being (Chapter 14). There, I focus on quality of life, life satisfaction, resilience, and the meaning that can be derived within the context of health challenges.

Weight and Eating Disorders Given the obesity epidemic, there is a whole chapter dedicated to understanding the factors that lead to unhealthy weight and eating patterns. There is also an alarming rise in eating disorders worldwide, and it is clear that these disorders are now affecting many previously unstudied and underrepresented minority groups. In this textbook, I dedicate a whole chapter to understanding weight and eating disorders and the factors that influence them.

Diversity and Health Disparities Throughout the text, I include theory, research, and evidence pertaining to U.S. and global health disparities, including gender-specific, LGBTQ, racial/ethnic, and socioeconomic issues. Health disparities, in fact, are addressed in every chapter.

The field of health psychology is constantly changing, and reviewers have helped me considerably in incorporating current trends and research. Their feedback and suggestions have been very helpful and have made the third edition a stronger textbook. When necessary, I discuss older ideas, historically relevant models, and classic experiments. Science is cumulative, after all. But my focus is on where science is now and where it is going in the future.

Pedagogical Approach

The goal of *The Psychology of Health and Illness: A Multicultural Perspective* is to capture students' interest and to provide them with a background in scientific principles in the field of health psychology. My aim is to integrate a developmental and cultural perspective into the traditional biopsychosocial model to expand understanding. The textbook is an informative, readable, current, and student-friendly learning aid. The emphases of this textbook make health psychology clearly relevant to a student's experience. These include its integration of global, cross-cultural, socioeconomic, multiethnic, age, developmental, and gender health issues. Together, they provide the broadest possible context for understanding health and illness, using the most up-to-date findings in models and treatment. I hope to inspire students to think critically and to become involved in health science, advocacy, service provision, public policy, and an informed discourse on health.

Pedagogical Tools

In this text, unique pedagogical tools help student learning as well. These tools underscore the text's emphases, engage the student, and promote critical thinking.

Within each chapter, thought-provoking issues drawn from the World Health Organization, Centers for Disease Control and Prevention, and other international health organizations highlight our current understanding of health and wellness. Chapters open with learning outcomes and personal profiles and then present information and content that address the questions that these case studies raise. Two types of boxes highlight current topics and issues in health psychology, while section-ending critical-thinking questions reinforce student learning. Throughout, students are encouraged to think about what they are learning in the context of their own experiences.

Chapter-Opening Vignettes Each chapter opens with a vignette that connects the chapter content to a real-life experience or human interest story. The chapter then makes explicit the issues raised. Every chapter also returns to the stories later, briefly but more than once, to ask how the vignette illustrates the material at hand and how that material applies.

Learning Outcomes These goals appear at the beginning of each chapter to help students preview the material and to guide their learning.

Thinking About Health These open-ended questions are the capstone of each major section, encouraging critical thinking. They ask students to think about what they have learned and relate it to what they have studied before and to their personal experiences. Of course, these questions also facilitate immediate review.

Around the World This box feature reinforces the emphases on different societal, economic, and cultural contexts. It presents theory, research, health crises, and cases from different parts of the world. This feature also uses global comparisons to point to similarities and differences, including health disparities, between groups. Examples include the HIV/AIDS crisis in sub-Saharan Africa, Blue Zones, and varying experiences of pain in different countries. Each of these boxes ends with a critical-thinking question.

In the News These boxed news stories add examples from current events to show the relevance, currency, and applications of health psychology. They draw on the popular media to highlight health issues that have had a significant impact on health outcomes and our scientific understanding. Examples include the dangers of vaping, hospital-acquired infections, and PTSD related to social media. Each of these boxes also ends with a critical-thinking question.

Chapter Summaries These summaries allow students to assess their understanding of the chapter. This feature reinforces the major points, helps students review the content, and allows them to see the bigger picture.

Key Terms and Glossary Key terms are boldfaced in the body of the text and listed at the end of each chapter. An end-of-book glossary allows students to quickly look up the important terms.

Infographics and Other Artwork I use figures and tables as necessary to illustrate important concepts, the results of studies, and available data. Of particular value are the frequent infographics. I also include photos and, when appropriate, cartoons to help illustrate certain important points.

CHAPTER 1

An Introduction to Health Psychology

Learning Outcomes

After reading this chapter, you should be able to:

- **Define** *health* and describe what the field of health psychology studies.
- **Describe** how epidemiology influences what we know about health.
- **Outline** the biopsychosocial model.
- **Explain** the importance of understanding health disparities.
- **Outline** how historical factors have changed conceptions of health and illness over time.
- **Explain** how the lifespan developmental perspective illuminates factors that influence health and illness.
- **Describe** the various global and cross-cultural influences on health and illness.

Sade was having a terrific year. Her research on eating disorders was flourishing and gaining national attention. She was mentoring slews of students in her laboratory. She and her partner had just bought a home and welcomed a puppy into their lives. Sade was doing it all with grace and enthusiasm. Then, at the age of 43, just back from an amazing vacation in Italy, she was diagnosed with Stage 3 cervical cancer (**Photo 1.1**).

Although she had kept up with her regular gynecological appointments, she had attributed some of the symptoms to her diet and recent life changes. When she got the result of an abnormal pap test, she thought for sure it was a mistake, so she asked the doctor to take another sample. These tests were followed by an MRI that showed a 2-centimeter tumor in her cervix. "To say that I was shocked by the news is a total understatement,"

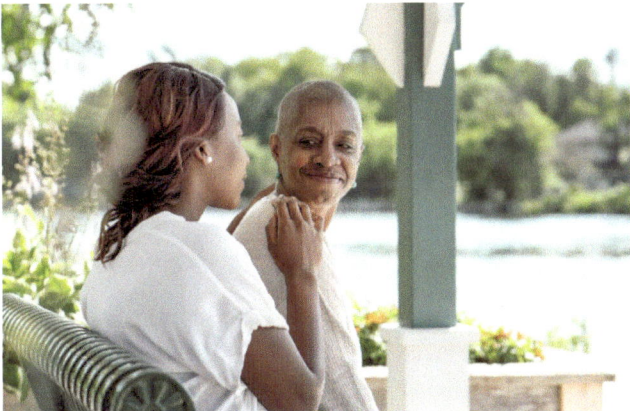

Photo 1.1

DOI: 10.4324/9781032643090-1

says Sade. She had no family history of the disease and had always been in good health. The diagnosis would prove to be the greatest test of her will thus far.

Sade became an advocate for cervical cancer—her own and others. She educated herself about her cancer and became active in her treatment planning, reframing the experience positively: Her diagnosis was not "a death sentence," but, rather, a challenge "to live a better life for as long as I can." With the support of her partner, family, and friends, Sade was courageous while undergoing surgery to remove the tumor, chemotherapy, radiation, and other supportive therapies. Even so, she never stopped being concerned for others. She continued to engage in life, advise her students, and help others through her eating disorders research, excelling in all areas of her life while coping with cervical cancer.

Since January 2023, Sade has been cancer-free. But that has not changed her commitment to improving her health and encouraging others to do the same. Cervical cancer is related to contracting human papillomavirus (HPV). Although it was not available when she was growing up, there are now vaccinations to prevent against HPV. She has been giving talks and raising awareness and funding to get parents to vaccinate their children and to provide support for people who do not have the financial means to undergo cervical cancer screening and treatment. And she continues to pursue her passions for painting and travel and focuses on enjoying each moment with her partner and puppy.

There is no good time to be ill, that's for sure. Yet, "having to take this journey with cervical cancer has taught me that I am a lot stronger than I thought I was," Sade says. Although she thinks about the possibility of a recurrence of cancer, she believes that the experience has changed her perspective on life for the better. She believes that her life "is exactly where it is supposed to be," and that helping others is one of the best ways of coping with her own cancer fears.

Sade's diagnosis was unexpected, but her story is typical, and it conveys many of the aspects of health and illness that we will discuss in this book. Her story shows the importance of health psychology in dealing with the onset and progression of disease as well as the psychosocial impact of living with illness. It points to the relationships between health, behavior, and social factors—what we will describe often as the *biopsychosocial model*. It illustrates how our perspective on health psychology changes over the course of a lifetime, what psychologists call a developmental perspective. Imagine that you are in a similar situation to Sade's. Think about the personal, psychological, social, cultural, and economic resources that she had at hand to help her find her way. What are your resources? How will learning about health psychology help you make the right decisions about your health and your family's health?

This chapter introduces health psychology. We examine what led to changing patterns of health and illness over time and what gave rise to the field. We then fast-forward to cutting-edge approaches to understanding the psychological factors that influence health and illness today.

What is Health Psychology?

Health psychology is focused on the psychological and behavioral aspects of physical and mental health. Health psychologists look at each of these aspects separately and consider how these aspects intersect. First, though, we need to define something more basic: health.

Defining Health

Health is difficult to define because it encompasses so many things. Is a fit, middle-aged person with a potentially debilitating condition healthy? Is an active, young person with a chronic=disease, like Sade, healthy? Who, then, is unhealthy? Is it someone with a dreadful cold or someone with a mild but persistent illness? Are you healthy? What makes you say *yes* or *no*?

For many years, practitioners believed that health is the absence of disease: You are healthy as long as you are not ill. In this view, Sade might not be considered healthy. Now, however, we take into account the complex and interrelated factors that influence health and how health is experienced. According to the World Health Organization (WHO), an agency within the United Nations, "Health … is not merely the absence of disease or infirmity" (WHO, 1946). Rather, **health** is a state of optimal well-being. That includes physical, mental, and social well-being (WHO, 1946).

Note first that health is the positive, desired state of being—the ideal against which other states are compared. Second, health is not just a physical state, it also involves the interplay among biological, psychological, and social processes. Finally, health occurs along a continuum, as seen in **Figure 1.1**, from disease or death to an optimal state of feeling well (Ryan & Travis, 1981).

In this **illness–wellness continuum**, moving from the center toward the left means that health is becoming worse, and treatment is needed. Moving to the right of the center means that our awareness, our education, and our activities

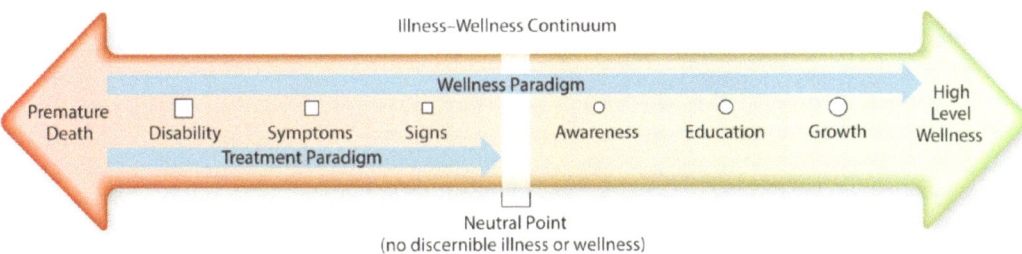

Figure 1.1 Illness–wellness continuum information.

Source: From Ryan and Travis (1981)

are promoting greater health and well-being. Where might Sade fall along this continuum? Where do you fall? To answer, we need to be aware of all aspects of health and the many factors that influence how we think about health. As we see next, that is the aim of health psychology.

The Missions of Health Psychology

Health psychology is devoted to understanding the psychological influences on what it means to be healthy, how and why we become ill, and how we cope with illness. More specifically, **health psychology** is the field of study focused on understanding the biological, psychological, and social influences on health and illness with the aims of promoting health, preventing illness, and improving health care systems and policies. Although aspects of health have always been central to psychology (Wallston, 1996), health psychology is a relatively young field. In 1978, the American Psychological Association recognized it as a new division, with four missions (Matarazzo, 1979):

1. To promote and maintain health
2. To prevent and treat illness
3. To identify the causes of health and illness
4. To analyze and improve the health care system

Let's consider each of these in turn (**Photo 1.2**).

Promoting and maintaining health is at the heart of **preventive medicine**, or efforts to maintain well-being and offset disease. Preventative medicine seeks to determine why some people are able to stay healthy while others become ill. We can then identify those at risk and educate them so that they can choose healthy behaviors. For example, simply getting a good night's sleep (for most of us, at least seven hours) is one of the best ways to stay healthy. Just six nights in a row of disrupted or poor sleep may lead to changes in metabolism and levels of *hormones*, the chemicals that regulate our bodies. It can increase stress and lessen our tolerance for pain and put us at risk for obesity, cardiovascular, and neurodegenerative diseases like Alzheimer's disease (Beck et al., 2023; Doufas, Panagiotou, & Ioannidis, 2012; Fan et al., 2020; Gao & Scullin, 2023; Hale et al., 2020; Kundermann, Spernal, Huber, Krieg, & Lautenbacher, 2004; Nguyen et al., 2018; Smith, Edwards, McCann, & Haythornthwaite, 2007; Xie et al., 2013).

As a college student, you are probably already aware of the effects of sleep loss. Young adults are particularly vulnerable to the effects of chronic sleep loss, which can have a significant impact on

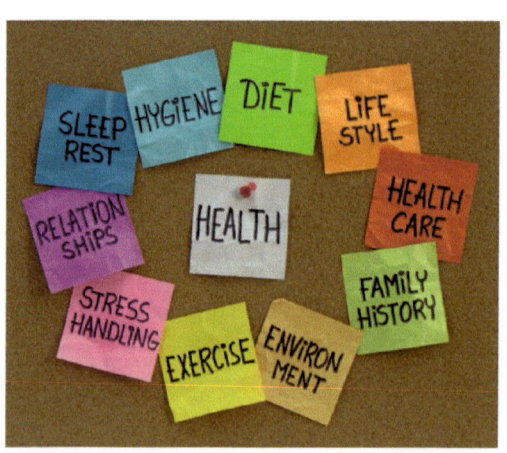

Photo 1.2   Health is affected by a number of factors, including your family history, lifestyle, and environment.

academic performance (Bermudez et al., 2022; Nguyen et al., 2018; Zitting et al., 2018). Sleep on this: Sleep researcher Dr. Michael Scullin taught a course on sleep at Baylor University and offered his students extra credit if they averaged ≥ 8 hours of sleep during the week of final exams. Students who opted into the challenge were monitored using a wearable sensor. On average most of the students slept around 8.5 hours most days—which is great for college students! Even more compelling was that those students who slept more performed better in the final exam than those students who slept less than 8 hours or did not participate in the challenge (Scullin, 2019). "If you provide a really strong incentive, people will change their behavior," Dr. Scullin has said. Hopefully, this information alone is enough to convince you to think about your sleep behaviors. More broadly, Dr. Scullin's quote illustrates one of the most important goals of health psychology: figuring out how to motivate people to change their behavior for better health (in Chapter 3, we will take a deeper look at this issue).

Sleep debt is also problematic in older adults facing **chronic disorders** (Frey et al., 2012; Gao & Scullin, 2023; Spiegel, Laproult, & Van Cauter, 1999), or disorders that persist or even worsen over time. Once these disorders develop, they may never go away, and they often require life changes. **Acute disorders**, in contrast, have an abrupt onset and short duration. The patient soon dies or gets better. (We return to chronic disorders later in this chapter and in Chapter 11.)

Think again about Sade, who was facing cancer. For years, her genetic profile, her stable family environment, her socioeconomic status, her education, and her lifestyle allowed her to enjoy good health. She was active, kept a balanced diet, and had a close-knit social network. As it turns out, all of those practices proved important to her well-being after she became ill as well.

That brings us to our second mission: to prevent and treat illness. Once again, health psychologists are concerned with identifying people who may be at risk and the psychological factors that contribute to risk. Additionally, we seek to understand how diagnosis and treatment affect patients differently so that we can better assist with recovery.

Our third mission is to identify the biological, cognitive, behavioral, and social factors that put people at risk. **Etiology** refers to the causes of a disease. More broadly, the field of **epidemiology** considers the factors that are correlated with, or occur most often with, the disease. It looks for patterns in the frequency and distribution of diseases within populations. Epidemiology informs etiology. For example, thanks to epidemiological research, we know that worldwide there have been 764,474,387 confirmed cases and 6,915,286 deaths due to the COVID-19 virus since the pandemic began (WHO, 2023a). It is likely that every person reading this, no matter where they are in the world, will know at least one person whose family was personally affected by COVID-19. Looking at the factors that put people at risk for COVID-19, evidence shows that older people and those with compromised immune systems are at greatest risk. We also know that human contact with an infected person elevates risk. There is a great deal of research coming out daily that focuses on the psychological factors that influence the perception of risk, behavioral risk-taking, and the impact that being ill with this virus can have on one's life. Throughout this book, we will examine that data, so that like health psychologists we can make informed, evidence-based choices to protect our own health and the health of those we care about. Health psychology helps to identify risk factors, and those who are at risk, with the aim of offsetting risk and reducing the burden of disease. After identifying those at risk for an illness, health psychologists can provide the education to change risky behaviors and prevent disease.

Our fourth and last mission turns to health policy. Health psychologists analyze the health care system at the local, state, national, and global levels. They ask how changes in the delivery of health care could improve the lives of patients, such as in the context of the opioid crisis in the United States. Each day, more than 136 people in the United States die after overdosing on opioids like fentanyl. The opioid crisis has resulted in many lives lost, for example, 103,550 people died in a 12-month period ending in November 2022 (Ahmad & Cisewski, 2023). **Figure 1.2** shows the drastic and alarming increase in different kinds of opioid-related deaths **(Photo 1.3)**.

In response to the opioid crisis, the U.S. Department of Health and Human Services (HHS) has prioritized improving access to treatment and recovery services, promoting the use of overdose-reversing drugs, strengthening

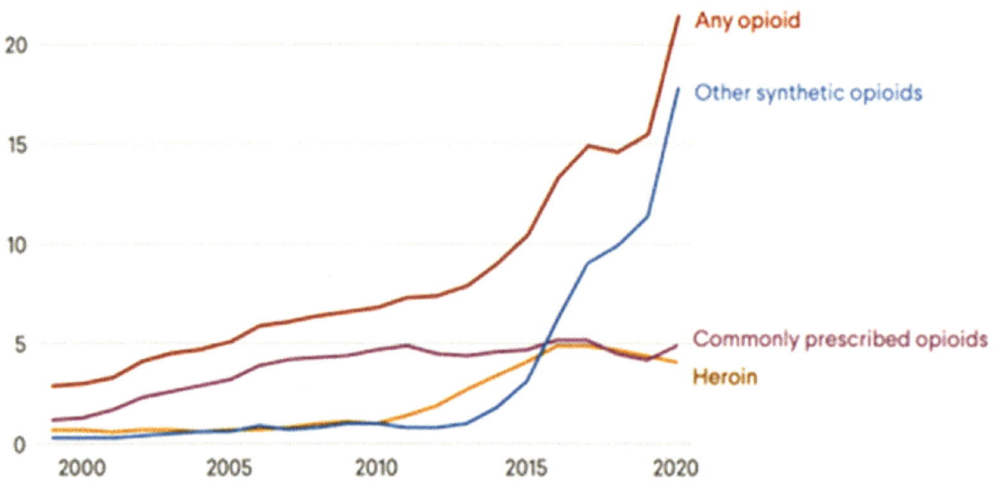

Opioid Overdose Deaths Have Risen Sharply

U.S. overdose deaths involving opioids per 100,000 people by type of opioid involved

Notes: Overdose deaths can involve multiple drugs. "Commonly prescribed opioids" includes natural and semisynthetic opioids and methadone. "Other synthetic opioids" includes synthetic opioid analgesics and excludes methadone.

COUNCIL on
FOREIGN
RELATIONS

Figure 1.2   Opioid overdose deaths on the rise.

Source: CDC

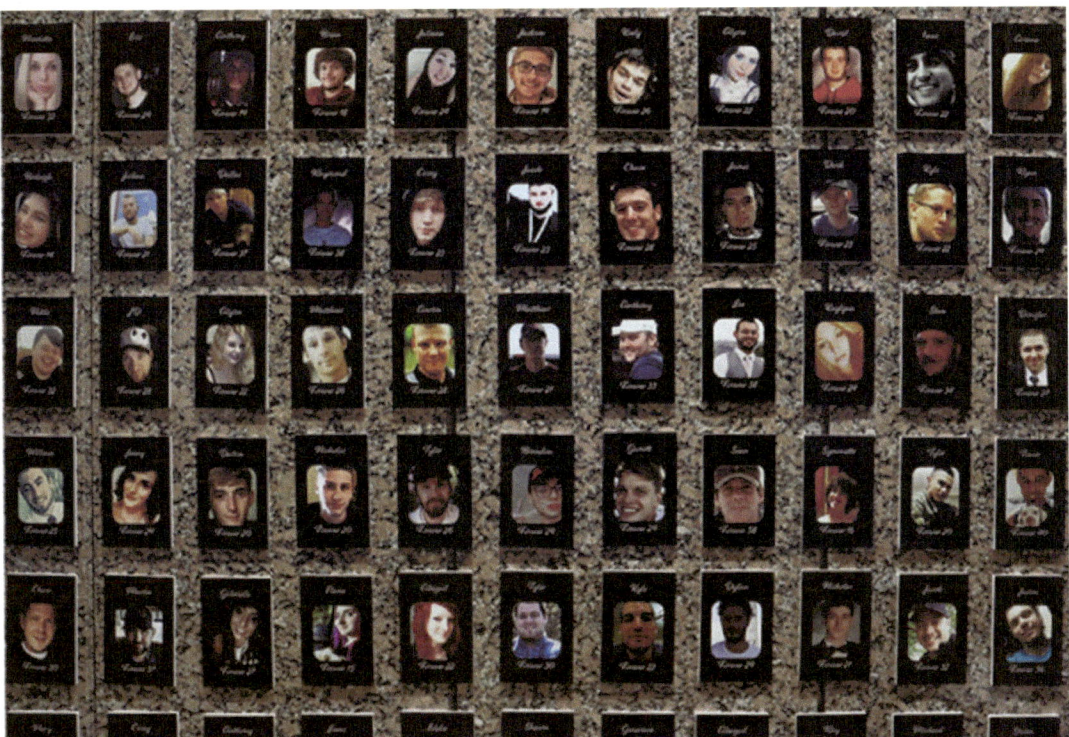

Photo 1.3   Photos of fentanyl victims shown at the U.S. Drug Enforcement Administration Headquarters.

Source: Alex Wong/Getty Images

public health surveillance, providing financial support for research on pain and addiction, and advancing health care practices for pain management. Similarly, the U.S. National Institutes of Health (NIH) is promoting scientific research on safe, effective, and nonaddictive strategies to manage pain, as well as prevention and intervention strategies that can save lives and support addiction recovery. The health policies of the HHS and NIH are driven in part by research and advocacy done by health psychologists. This goes to show the integral role that health psychology plays in improving people's lives.

Globally, there are many health policy priorities, top among them is long COVID-19 for which more research is badly needed to help find preventative measures and effective treatments for those whose lives are affected (Hanson et al., 2022). The impact of wars, natural disasters, food scarcity, and the COVID-19 pandemic has created a global mental health crisis. Making mental health a priority is important because mental disorders are one of the leading causes of disability worldwide (GBD 2019 Mental Disorders Collaborators, 2022). A related global health priority is the ongoing loss of healthcare workers, many of whom experience high rates of burn-out, fatigue, and health problems

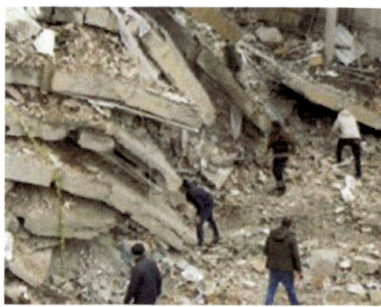
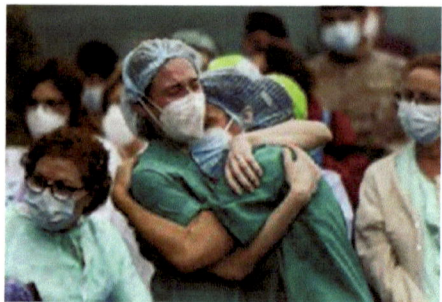

Photo 1.4   (a) The earthquake in Turkey in 2023. (b) Health care workers in the COVID-19 pandemic.

Source: (a) Altan Adem/AFP Getty Images; (b) World Economic Forum

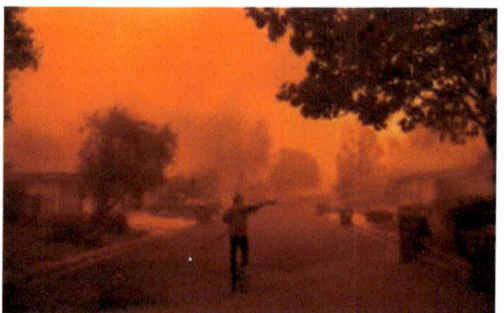

Photo 1.5   The impact of climate change for health.

Source: Wally Skalij/Los Angeles Times via Getty Images

of their own. According to the World Economic Forum (2023a), there is a shortage of healthcare workers in many regions globally. Climate change is another important health policy. It is already impacting the health and well-being of millions of people all over the globe, and this this global crisis is worsening. Poverty, weak healthcare systems, and the aging of the population are other major health policy issues facing the world today. All of these issues will be considered in the chapters to come [**Photos 1.4**(a and b) and **1.5**].

The field of health psychology may be relatively young, but it is growing rapidly, and you can easily see why. Every human being experiences good health and bad, and our thoughts, personality, and behaviors all influence our experiences. The psychological aspect of health psychology sets it apart from the fields of medicine, medical anthropology, sociology, and other disciplines concerned with wellness and disorders. Yet the guiding theory of healthy psychology recognizes and embraces them all, as we see next.

Thinking About Health

■ What does health mean to you? What factors influence your actual health and your perceived health?

■ Have you ever had an acute illness? Do you have a chronic condition? How does the timeline of the illness affect your life?

■ Can you apply the four goals of health psychology to your own life?

Around *the* World

A Little Soap and Water

Comparing preventive care in the United States and around the world can be as complicated as statistics and laboratory work. It can involve comparing entire populations and individual genes. Yet sometimes it can be as simple as washing your hands.

Stephen Luby traveled to Karachi, Pakistan, in the late 1990s to work with the Centers for Disease Control and Prevention. The job must have seemed overwhelming. Health problems in the Karachi slums included rampant intestinal illnesses, respiratory illnesses, and other infections. Through perseverance and ingenuity, Dr. Luby found a partner in Proctor & Gamble. He convinced the consumer products giant to give him a grant to study the impact of hand washing and to supply the soap. (Safeguard soap, to be precise.)

Dr. Luby set up what scientists call a clinical trial (we look in depth at research methods in Chapter 2). He randomly selected neighborhoods in which to give out soap, and he educated people on proper hand washing. Later, the researchers compared the illness rates in children in these neighborhoods with the rates in children in 11 other neighborhoods (not given soap) over a full year. (As we see in Chapter 2, the other neighborhoods composed what is called a control group.) The results were nothing short of astounding. Diarrheal illness fell by 52% for children in neighborhoods that received soap and education, as compared to others. Respiratory illness such as pneumonia fell by 48% and bacterial infections such as impetigo and skin infections fell by 35% (Gawande, 2009; Luby et al., 2005). All it took was solid research—and a little soap and water.

The Biopsychosocial Model

A good physician treats the disease; a great physician treats the patient who has the disease.

(William Osler, 1904)

The **biopsychosocial model**, as seen in **Figure 1.3**, highlights the role of biological, psychological, and social processes in health (Brody, 2014; Engel, 1977, 1980; Kazarian & Evans, 2001). It considers the interactions between these processes, as well as the entire experience of health and illness, and it is at the heart of health psychology.

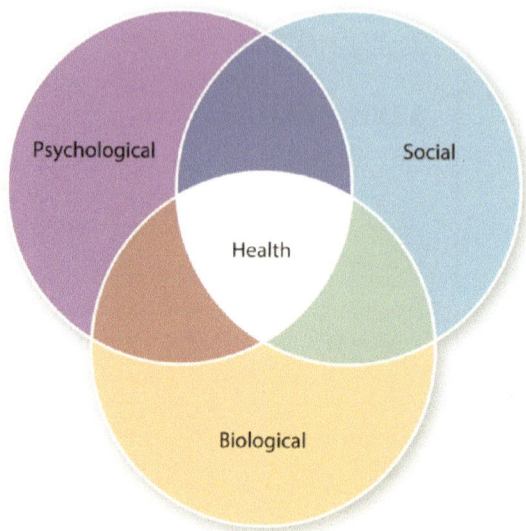

Figure 1.3   The biopsychosocial model of health.

Three Perspectives

Think back to Sade at the start of this chapter. Is she healthy? Most of us would say yes and no. Although her cancer is in remission, Sade has a serious, potentially debilitating, and life-threatening disease. She has experienced stress and discomfort. Yet she is outgoing, engaged in her family and her work, her cancer advocacy, and motivated to make the most of her life. What, then, are the factors that influence her experience of her health? The biopsychosocial model asks for the fullest possible picture.

Sade comes from an optimal background for health and wellness. Genetically and biologically, she has few risks. From a psychological perspective, we see that she is well-educated, has a good career and a close family, and enjoys new challenges. She is also self-aware and has strong coping skills. Finally, from a sociological perspective, she has the resources to obtain good information, treatment, and care.

Compare her with Alyanna Mohommad, a 6-year-old girl from Mogadishu, Somalia. Her mother recently died of malaria, and she is now one of the staggering number of orphans in her country. With more than 6.6 million people (1.8 million who are children) are facing crisis, food insecurity, and are in desperate need of humanitarian assistance, the odds are stacked against her (FSNAU-FEWSNET Technical Release, 2023). Her country is one of the poorest and most violent places on earth. In her short lifetime, Alyanna has witnessed civil war, terrorism, droughts and floods, and devastating famine. She currently lives in an orphanage, where there is a shortage of food, clothing, and health care. She has taken to scavenging food scraps from the streets, putting her at even greater risk of infection. She is severely malnourished, has recurring bouts of malaria, and, given her situation, is at high risk for gender-based violence and human trafficking. Although the life expectancy for women in Somalia is 58 years, Alyanna will probably not reach puberty.

From a biopsychosocial point of view, Alyanna is vulnerable at each level. Her physical condition is serious, and psychologically she is at a disadvantage because of her lack of loving and supportive caregivers and her fears of hunger and violence. On a social level, she has limited resources to cope with or change her situation. War, famine, poverty, natural disasters, and the lack of basic sanitation, education, and health care all affect her health.

Biological, psychological, and social factors make up the fabric of all of our lives, just as they do for Sade and Alyanna. As we shall see again and again, health psychology encompasses these factors.

Systems theory

The biopsychosocial model is grounded in systems theory. **Systems theory** conceptualizes something (the human body or society, for example) as a *system* governed by many different factors. A change in any level of the system can influence many other levels. In the same way, health psychologists look at how biological, psychological, and social factors come together to govern our health. Sade's cancer began with tiny changes in her cells and organs, but before long it affected her mind, her behavior, and her health care. In turn, her behavior and her health care were essential to her dealing successfully with pain and disease (**Photo 1.6**).

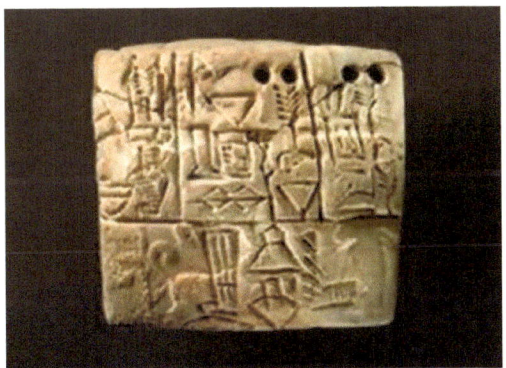

Photo 1.6   Cuneiform Tablet from Ancient Sumaria.

Systems theory goes back to the ancient Sumerians, who believed that systems like these are found in nature. In time, the idea influenced modern science and economics. Examples of systems include the solar system, the life cycle of cells in the body, a family, the economy, and the healthcare system.

A more recent systems theory was developed by Urie Bronfenbrenner (1979) to provide a contextual approach for understanding how children develop. It is a developmental systems theory that displays how each individual's growth and change is nested within various systems that all have the potential to influence the person and be influenced by them. The systems differ and involve social, cultural, economic, political, and global factors, not just psychological ones. Bronfenbrenner envisioned that the systems that influence each person are the microsystem, the mesosystem, the exosystem, the macrosystem, and the chronosystem. The figure below shows examples of the things that are in each system. We will talk more about the ecological systems theory and keep it in mind when we are thinking about how systems interact to influence our health perceptions and experiences (**Photo 1.7**).

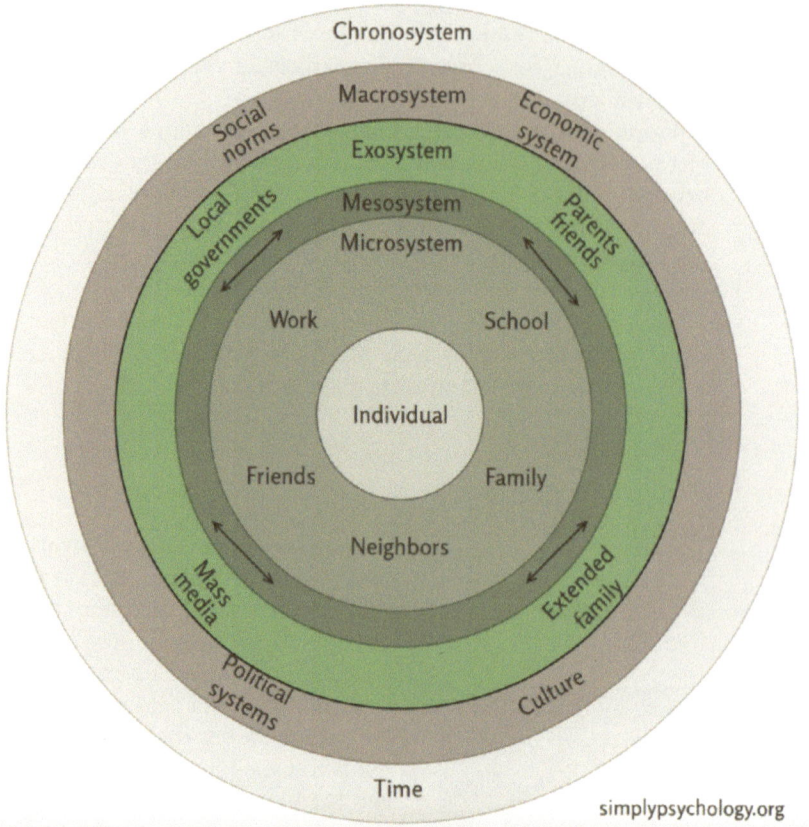

Photo 1.7   Bronfenbrenner's ecological systems theory model—created by Simply Psychology.

The biopsychosocial model teaches us to look at the entirety of human health. Although the individual is still at the center of health, a small change can ripple out to the most distant part of the system [**Photo 1.8**(a–c)] (Kazak, Bosch, & Klonoff, 2012).

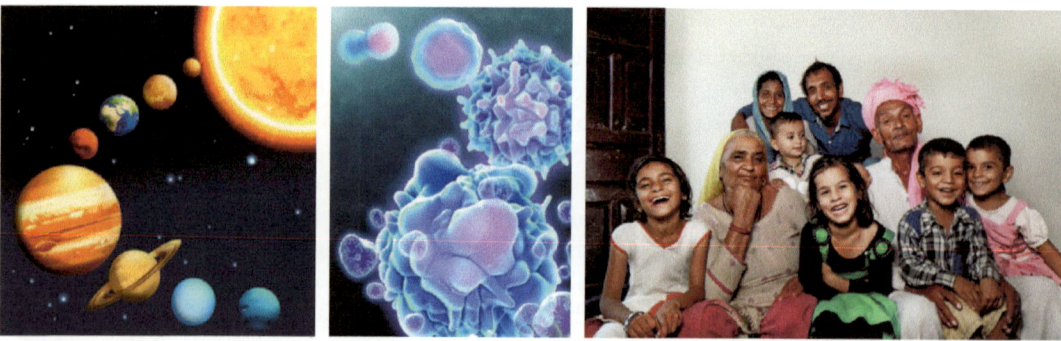

Photo 1.8 (a–c)   Life is made up of many different types of systems. The solar system, cell life cycle, and families are just a few examples.

Subjective and Objective Health

The biopsychosocial model makes clear that health is both an objective state of being and a subjective experience. **Objective health** is the assessment of health from observable measures—such as infection, pain, heart rate, blood pressure, cholesterol, reflexes, and reaction time. Depending on your symptoms, a doctor may ask you to jog on a treadmill to see how that affects your blood pressure and degree of exertion. Physiology and genetics may both influence objective health.

Subjective health is how individuals evaluate their own health status. Think of when your physician asks, "How are you feeling today?" Your answer represents your subjective evaluation of your health. Someone who is feeling energetic, rested, relaxed, and free of pain is more likely to report feeling well. In fact, people with objective signs of illness may report that their health is quite good. Subjective measures of health are often not directly tied to one's actual health status and yet are very predictive of health outcomes and mortality (Idler & Benyamini, 1997). Conversely, some people with no medical ailments perceive their health as poor. For example, people who have illness anxiety disorder, as we see in Chapter 4, have an exaggerated concern for their health, as well as heightened sensitivity to bodily sensations and changes and intense anxiety about the possibility of undiagnosed conditions. College students who scored high on a measure of health anxiety made many more visits to the college health clinic and often turned to prescription drugs for non-medical purposes, mainly as a way to alleviate their health anxiety (Jeffers et al., 2015). This is potentially problematic since the misuse of prescription drugs can be dangerous.

Which measure of health is more important? We need to pay attention to both subjective and objective health. Recently, I asked my students about what they do to stay physically and emotionally healthy. One student, a 20-year-old man, said that he had to be extra vigilant in taking care of his health. Although he had been athletic all his life, he has high blood pressure and high cholesterol levels, and he has a family history of premature death from cardiovascular disease. Outwardly, he is the epitome of health and physical fitness. He is lean, muscular, and young. High blood pressure and high cholesterol levels, two signs of cardiovascular disease, usually emerge in midlife in men who are overweight and sedentary. His subjective experience of his health is now balanced by his knowledge of the objective risks, and, as a result, he can make better decisions to foster a long and healthy life.

At the same time, objective assessments of health are limited. We know that physical, emotional, and social aspects combine to create a sense of well-being, and subjective health is a better index of their interrelationship. One thing to remember is that there are always differences in the experience and evaluation of health. **Interindividual differences**, or differences between people, may include both subjective and objective factors. My athletic 20-year-old student feels strong, has a high quality of life, and is optimistic about the future. Therefore, in a very real sense, he is healthy.

Health Around the World

The biopsychosocial model encourages a global approach to health. Social, cultural, economic, political, and religious factors all influence how people think about their health, and these factors differ dramatically around the world. Health outcomes may differ greatly as well, both globally and within the United States (Kazak et al., 2012). We shall return often to the differences among individuals, communities, nations, and cultures.

Thinking About Health

- ■ Can you identify biopsychosocial factors in your own life that interact to influence your health?

- ■ How could systems theory help explain Sade's situation? Which systems are involved?

- ■ How do objective measures of health conflict with subjective measures? Which measures are more reliable for measuring health?

A Global Approach to Health

Our world has become increasingly interconnected. **Globalization** is the sharing of ideas, values, goods, and services, thanks to travel, the media, trade, and the Internet (Koplan et al., 2009). Yet just as people, information, and currency travel around the globe, so do viruses, health beliefs and behaviors, medical knowledge, and health care. To understand these influences on health and wellness, we need to develop global awareness and think as global citizens (**Photo 1.9**).

Equitable access and outcomes	**Healthcare systems transformation**	**Technology and innovation**	**Environmental sustainability**
Ensuring equal representation, access and outcomes for all	Structuring resilient healthcare systems to provide high-quality care	Cultivating an environment to support innovation in science and medicine	Reducing impact on the environment, preparing for, addressing climate change

Equity as the foundational goal for all change

Photo 1.9   The benefits of health equity.

Source: L.E.K. Consulting; World Economic Forum

	Global health	**International health**	**Public health**
Physical scope	Concentration is on health concerns that affect health in a direct or indirect manner and go beyond one nation	Concentration is on other countries' health concerns, particularly in underserved or poor populations	Concentration is on health concerns of a specific community, city, or nation
Cooperation	Global cooperation and resolutions occur at a global level	Binational cooperation	Cooperation is local, not global
Group care or Individual care	Targets prevention issues in broader population and also individuals	Targets prevention issues on individuals and broader population	Targets primarily prevention plans for broader populations
Health care accessibility	Aims for equal health access among nations and for everyone	Aims to assist those in other countries	Aims for equal health access within a country, city, or community

Source: Information from Koplan et al. (2009).

Table 1.1 Comparison of global health, international health, and public health

The concept of global health is similar to that of public health or international health, but with important differences. As we see in **Table 1.1**, it seeks to improve health and achieve more equal outcomes for all people (Koplan et al., 2009). It also stresses global differences in the experience of health. Understanding health globally is important because there is a high correlation between health and well-being. Although there are many factors that influence the health of people living in a specific country, in general, the better the health of the people who live there the higher their quality of life and feelings of happiness (**Figure 1.4**) (World Population Review, 2023).

The United States, for example, is one of the most diverse and multicultural nations on the planet, yet people in the United States are still likely to agree that health is a personal and collective achievement. It is something we can control. Contrast that with Somalia, on the horn of Africa, where health is a matter of basic survival. Ever since its government collapsed in 1991, the country has been torn apart by war, poverty, natural disasters, and disease (UNICEF, 2018). People live in crowded displacement camps with a lack of access to safe food and water (WHO, 2023b). Infant, child, and maternal mortality are among the highest in the world. Diarrheal disease, respiratory infections, and malaria account for more than half of all child deaths (WHO, 2023b). Cholera outbreaks occur each year from December to June (Emch, Feldacker, Islam, & Ali, 2008). And the incidence of tuberculosis is the highest in the world.

A global approach allows us to look critically at different beliefs, behaviors, societies, and public health policies. People tend to be *ethnocentric*, to not look beyond local beliefs and customs, even in science. Explanations are likely to fail when they do not take into account the context in which we apply them. For example, either a suburban American or a rural Indian

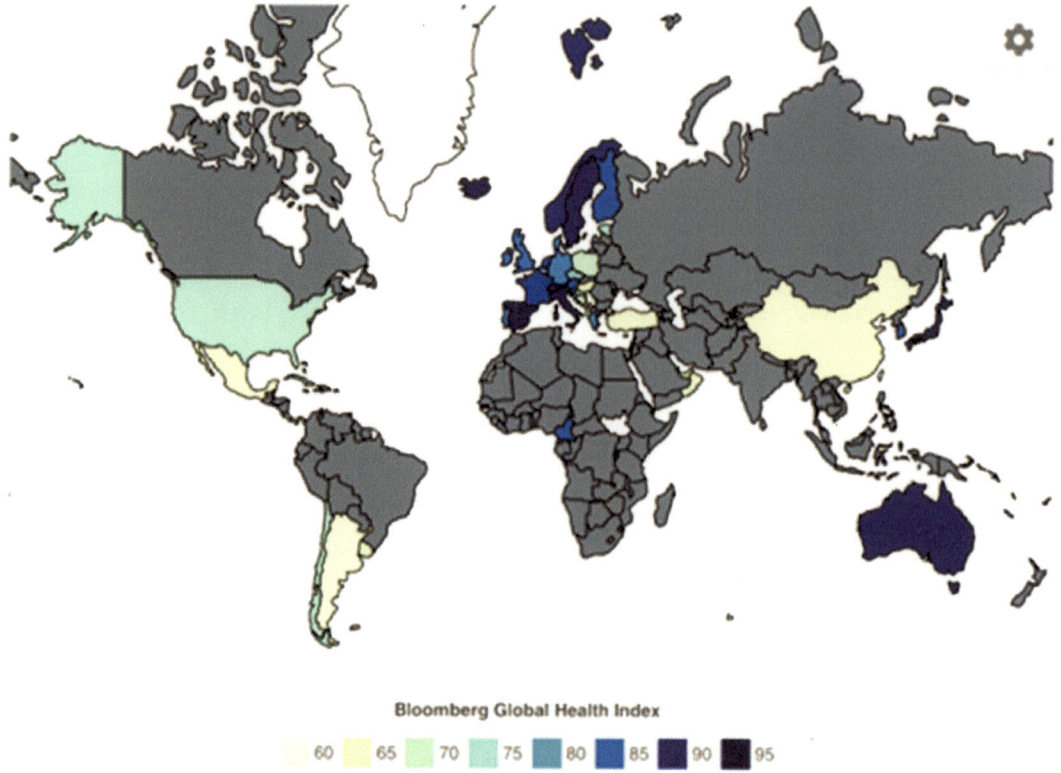

Bloomberg Global Health Index

60 65 70 75 80 85 90 95

Figure 1.4   Healthiest countries 2023.

mother might choose, wrongly, not to have her infant vaccinated against polio, but for very different reasons. In the United States, the risk of exposure to the polio virus is extremely low, a mother might reason, so why to put the child through the pain? Meanwhile, the Indian mother might believe that human health is in the gods' hands and that vaccines are unholy. Both mothers are putting their children and others at risk, but to change their behaviors, we need to understand their beliefs.

Finally, a global perspective highlights areas most in need of help—like Somalia. As the world becomes increasingly open, local health crises can quickly become global health crises. Their problems become our problems, biologically and morally. As health psychologists and global citizens, we have an obligation to share our knowledge and to improve the lives of our neighbors.

Global Health Disparities

Health disparities are differences in overall health, access to quality health care, and health outcomes. These differences may reflect how often a disease affects a group, how many people within the group get sick, and how often the disease

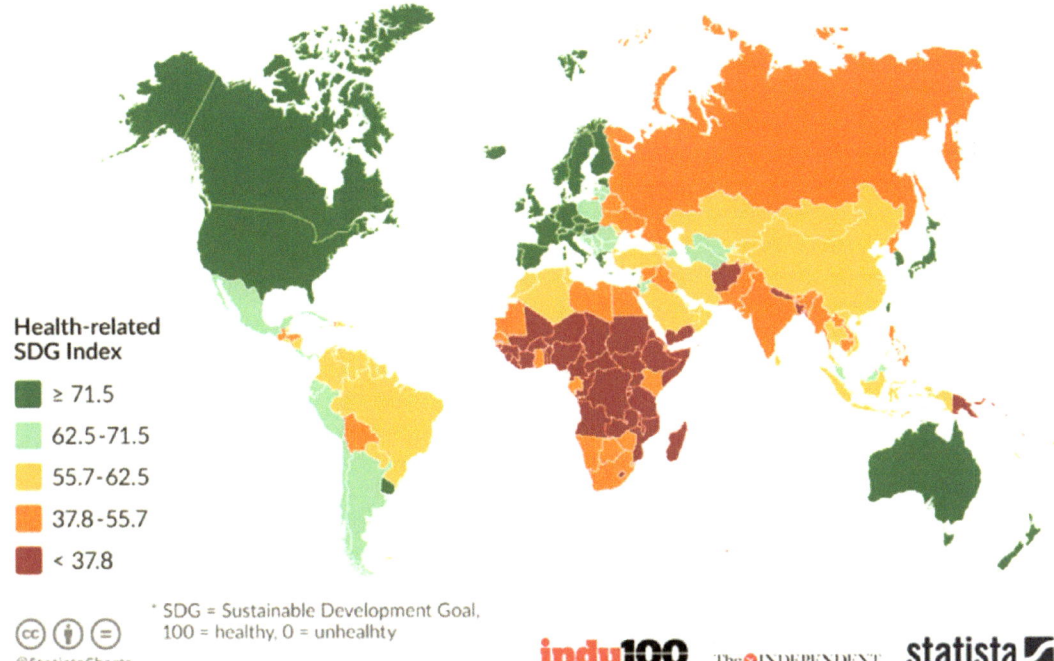

The globe's healthiest & unhealthiest countries visualised

Health-related SGD index scores worldwide in 2015·

Health-related SDG Index

- ≥ 71.5
- 62.5–71.5
- 55.7–62.5
- 37.8–55.7
- < 37.8

· SDG = Sustainable Development Goal, 100 = healthy, 0 = unhealhty

@StatistaCharts

indy100   The INDEPENDENT   **statista**

Figure 1.5   World map representing human development index categories (based on 2021 data, published in 2022). Very high; high; medium; low; no data.

Source: Hunter (2022) The Lancet/Statista

results in death. And the differences are most striking between developed and developing nations (**Figure 1.5**).

Developed nations or nations with developing economies are those with a high average standard of living. Most have fully industrialized economies. As Kofi Annan, the former Secretary General of the United Nations, said, "A developed country is one that allows all its citizens to enjoy a free and healthy life in a safe environment" (Annan, 2000). Japan, Canada, the United States, Australia, New Zealand, Western Europe, and Israel are generally considered developed regions (**Figure 1.6**).

Less Developed Nations or nations with economies that are still developing, have a low level of material well-being. They often have less secure political structures, less stable economies, and less equitable economies. They may suffer from civil war, poverty, famine, and lack of quality medical services. For many who live there, good health may be out of reach.

In economically unstable countries, people are still dying of the kinds of acute infectious diseases that Americans died of during the 1700s. Children are

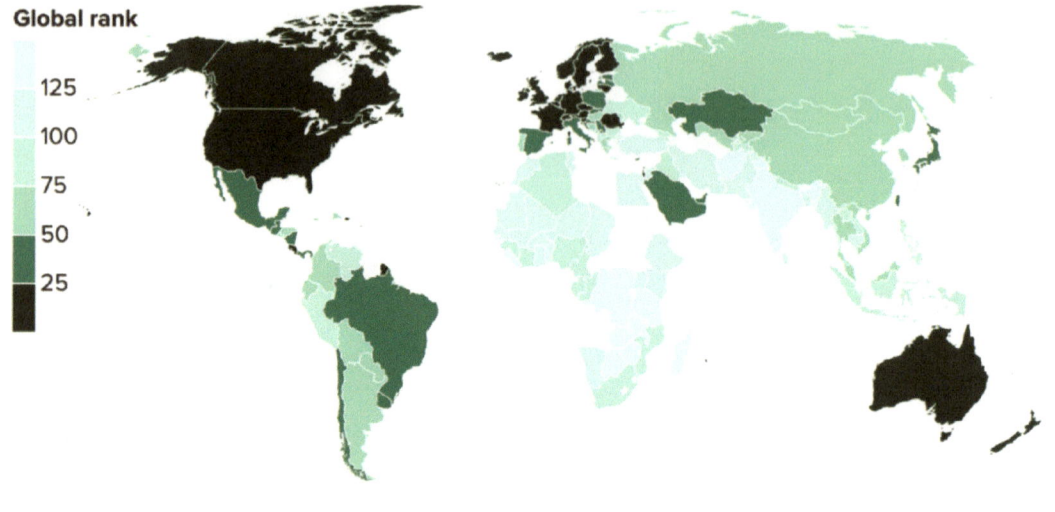

Figure 1.6   Happiest countries in 2023.

Source: The World Happiness Report

dying of malaria and influenza because they do not have access to vaccines and good medical treatment. In these countries, too, HIV is still spreading, and people are still dying of AIDS.

Thinking About Health

■ Why is it important to consider global health issues?

■ How might thinking globally about health influence how you think about your own health?

■ How do health disparities around the world influence our own health care at home?

Health Care in the United States

Note that the countries with the very best health care are not necessarily the wealthiest. **Table 1.2** lists the countries with the strongest economies in the world and the best health care systems, as ranked by the International Monetary Fund and the WHO. Why do they differ? Different countries have different healthcare systems. It is noteworthy that the United States ranks last among

Rank	IMF world strongest economies	WHO world best healthcare systems
1	United States	United Kingdom
2	China	Australia
3	Japan	Netherlands
4	Germany	Norway
5	United Kingdom	New Zealand
6	India	Sweden
7	France	Switzerland
8	Brazil	Germany
9	Italy	Canada
10	Canada	France

Source: Data from Schneider, Sarnak, Squires, Shah, and Doty (2017).

Table 1.2 World's strongest economies and healthcare systems

the seven countries with the strongest economies in the quality and efficiency of health care, access to care, equity of care, and the ability to lead long healthy lives (Thomson, Osborn, Squires, & Reed, 2011). Of those seven countries, only one does not provide health care for all its citizens, and that country is the United States. A lack of universal health care also helps to explain health disparities within the nation.

Health and the Affordable Care Act

Although highly controversial, the Affordable Care Act, which took full effect in 2014, was credited with a significant decline in instances of U.S. citizens without health insurance. Between 2014 and 2016, the number of Americans without health care fell from 18% to 12.7% of the population. However, the marked gains in coverage after the law came into effect are beginning to reverse (Collins, Gunja, Doty, & Bhupal, 2018). Since 2016, an estimated four million people have lost their health insurance, and the uninsured rates have been spiking among lower-income families (Collins et al., 2018). These changes are alarming because too many individuals do not have access to preventive medicine. Nor can they see a doctor when they are ill unless they can pay for care themselves. At the time of writing this book, many Americans in need of medical treatment are unable to afford it.

A lack of health insurance affects treatment-seeking behavior. In recent years, one in every three people in the United States did not seek care because of the expense (Auter, 2017). These people may have been in poor general health or had a serious chronic illness, injury, or disability. These patients may not have visited the doctor when ill, may not have filled prescriptions, may have skipped medications, and may not have followed through with prescribed treatments because of the costs (Auter, 2017). These decisions could have further compromised their health.

Infant mortality is a key indicator of a country's state of health and quality of health care, and the United States is not doing well (Vanderbilt & Wright, 2013). Despite having the biggest economy in the world, the most modern medical services, and the best-trained doctors, the United States has one of the highest infant mortality rates (5.12 per 1000 births) among industrialized nations (CIA, 2018).

Health Disparities Within the United States

Where you live influences your health and wellness—right down to your ZIP (postal) code. What does ZIP code have to do with it? Even today in the United States, there is racial and ethnic segregation in where people live. And health disparities vary as a function of geographic area. For example, Black and Hispanic women who live in segregated urban areas have higher incidences of breast cancer (Pruitt et al., 2015). In addition, Black men have a 14% lower probability of survival and Black women have a 9% lower probability of survival than their White counterparts (Popescu, Duffy, Mendelsohn, & Escarce, 2018). In fact, race and ethnicity are crucial determinants of health because of their enduring links with differences in social and economic resources (Mehta, Lee, & Ylitalo, 2013).

Social determinants of health lead to health disparities. Socioeconomic status (such as income and level of education), unemployment, racial discrimination, neighborhood, social networks, and social support are social factors that impact the incidence of breast cancer, stage of diagnosis, and survival (Coughlin, 2019a, 2019b). Other examples of social determinants that influence health are immigration status, distrust of medical establishments, inadequate housing, food insecurity, and geographic factors such as where you live (Coughlin, 2019a, 2019b).

What may become clear as you think about this is that often times, several of these factors go together. There is **intersectionality** among social factors. For example, Black women often have the greatest socioeconomic challenges and this influences their risk of breast cancer (Mohseny et al., 2016). Here gender intersects with a racial identity which intersects with the level of education which relates to socioeconomic status which impacts health risks (Coughlin, 2019a, 2019b). To understand intersectionality we must appreciate that while each of these social factors by themselves may elevate risk, when they come together or intersect their influence may be magnified. There is an intersection, then, between race and residential segregation that hinges on socioeconomic status, or income. If the socioeconomic status of Blacks were comparable to those of Whites, the White-Black survival gap would disappear **(Photo 1.10)** (Popescue et al., 2018).

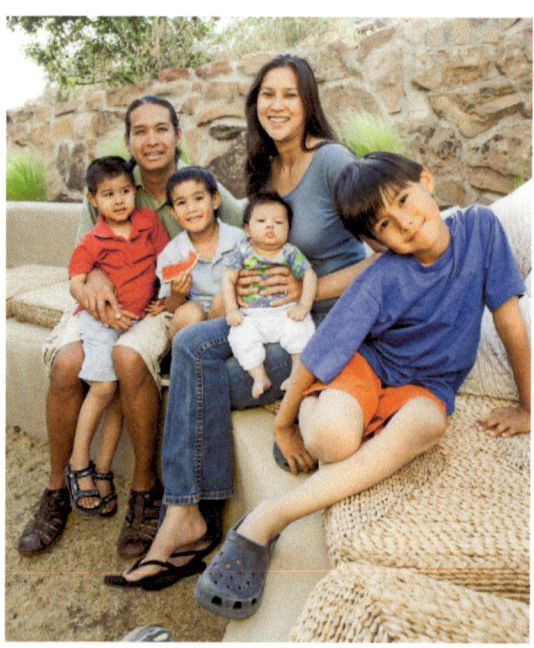

Photo 1.10   What health disparities might this Native American family from New Mexico face that a family from urban New York would not?

Health disparities are striking in communities with low-income, unstable housing, unsafe neighborhoods, limited access to healthy foods and outdoor recreation, and substandard schools (CDC, 2018c). Many organizations, from the American Psychological Association to the Centers for Disease Control and Prevention, are now focused on examining the social determinants of health (**Figure 1.7**).

Social determinants of health are the conditions or environments in which we live, learn, work, play, worship, and grow old, and they influence our mental, cognitive, and physical functioning, our quality of life, and our health risks and outcomes. They also greatly contribute to health disparities.

Other factors, such as gender, sexual orientation, physical or mental disability, education, and income level, relate to health disparities as well. From a developmental perspective, the inequities in health are greatest in infancy and later life (Mehta et al., 2013).

Although national health initiatives emphasize the importance of eliminating health disparities among historically disadvantaged populations, research has only recently begun to examine health outcomes among lesbian, gay, bisexual, and transgender (LGBTQ) people (Fredriksen-Goldsen et al., 2014). But it is clear that LGBTQ individuals face health disparities that are related to societal stigma, discrimination, and denial of their civil rights (McLaughlin, Hatzenbuehler, & Keyes, 2010).

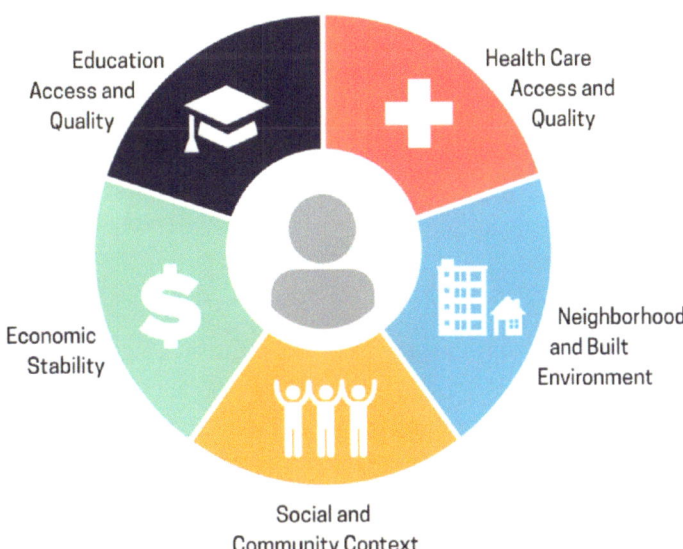

Figure 1.7   The social determinants of health, Healthy People 2023.

There are also health disparities among immigrants to the United States and other countries, who represent a substantial and growing portion of the population (Patterson & Gong, 2009). According to the WHO, globally there are over one billion people worldwide who are immigrants, refugees, or migrants to a new country (WHO, 2022). That is one out of every seven people around the world. Refugee, immigrant, or migrant (RIM) communities are made up of people with diverse backgrounds and experiences and they often face health disparities in their new homes (CDC, 2023c). Some of the factors that lead to these disparities are things like a lack of health insurance, barriers to access to health care, education, and income/wage gaps. Around the world promoting health equity for RIM groups has become a priority.

One study showed that recent migrants in Europe and North America had higher levels of stress that related to a higher risk of metabolic syndrome and cardiovascular disease (Rosenthal, Touyz, & Oparil, 2022). And the stress effects play forward into the future. First-generation adult immigrants and adolescent immigrants develop cardiovascular risk factors later in life (Rosenthal et al., 2022). **Figure 1.8** shows some of the factors that can come together or intersect to influence health in RIM groups.

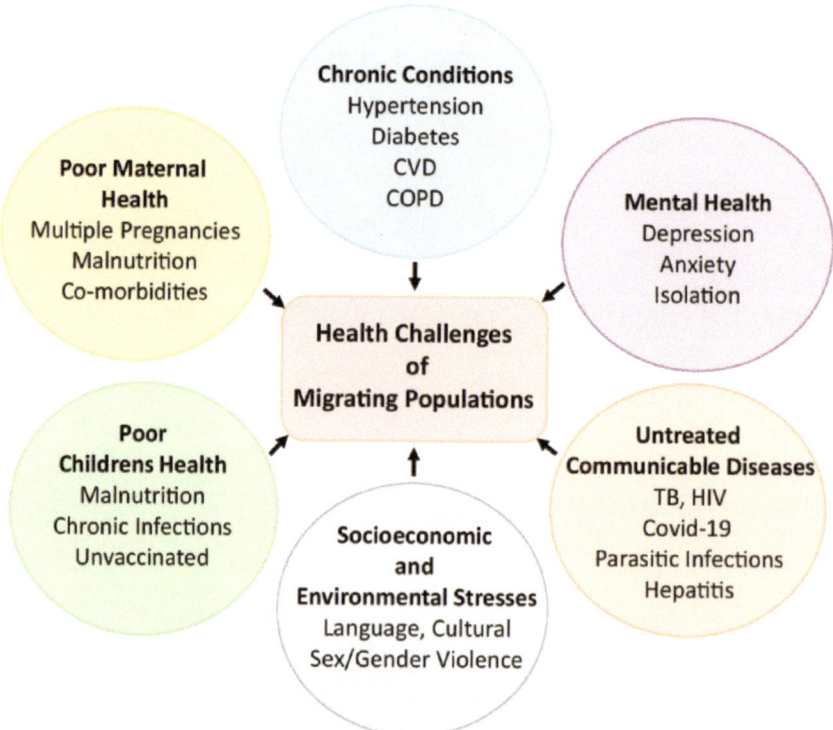

Schematic demonstrating multiple modifiable and non-modifiable factors that contribute to health challenges of migrating populations. CVD, cardiovascular disease; COPD, chronic obstructive pulmonary disease

Figure 1.8   Migrating populations and health: Risk factors for cardiovascular disease and metabolic syndrome.

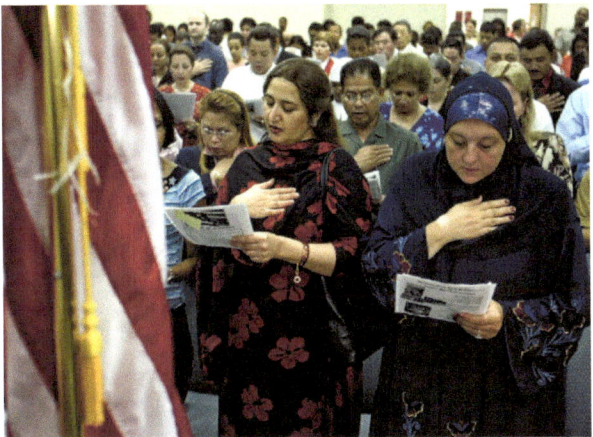

Photo 1.11 These immigrants being sworn in as U.S. citizens may have left developing countries to improve their health and well-being.

Cultural, language, and socioeconomic barriers may all stand in the way of obtaining health care. Immigrants may also lose the health advantages that they had in their home country. For example, obesity rates skyrocket in those who begin to eat a standard American diet (**Photo 1.11**).

Health disparities in the United States are both a public health priority and a civil rights challenge (Bauer & Plescia, 2014), and policymakers, healthcare organizations, and health service providers need to address them. Healthy People 2030, an initiative developed by the U.S. Office of Disease Prevention and Health Promotion, examines and addresses the leading social determinants of health and aims to develop public policy to mitigate them. Perhaps the Healthy People 2030 initiative will be one of many successful U.S. health initiatives to come.

Is Health a Fundamental Human Right?

Could basic health be a fundamental human right? At the very least, it is a fundamental human concern. No matter your age, gender, sexual orientation, socioeconomic status, race, ethnicity, or religion, if you are like most people, you care about your health and the health of those you love. From the moment you wake to the moment you go to sleep; you make decisions that will affect your health and the chances that you become sick. Perhaps today you brushed your teeth, ate balanced meals, wore a seatbelt, exercised, socialized with friends, and listened to relaxing music. Each of these decisions was impactful for your health (**Photo 1.12**). (We will look at what drives good and bad health behaviors in Chapters 3 and 4.)

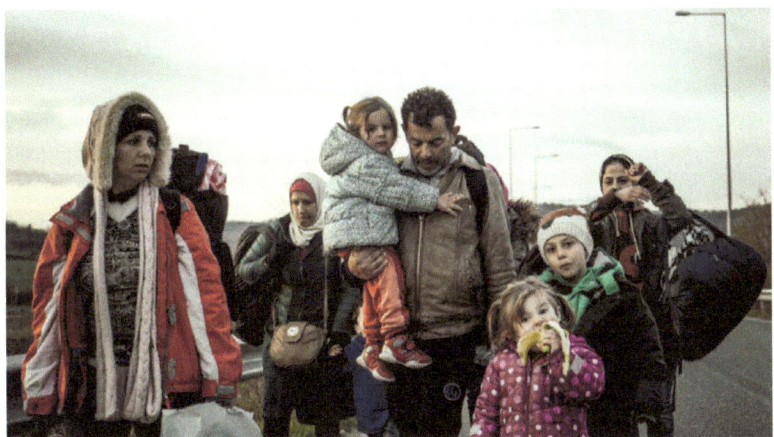

Photo 1.12 Health is a basic fundamental human right, and every person—regardless of citizenship, immigration status, or background—deserves humane treatment.

When we are ill, our health is an even greater concern. Poor health can affect our mood and prevent us from going to work or school. It may interfere with family responsibilities and an active social life. And yet many people lack access to quality health care. Access to care is also highly politicized. Within the United States, the two major political parties diverge sharply on whether to expand or repeal the Affordable Care Act.

The WHO has stated that every human being should have the ability to enjoy good health: "The enjoyment of the highest attainable standard of health is one of the fundamental rights of every human being" (WHO, 1946).

What does this mean? First, nations must provide the bare necessities so that people can achieve and maintain good health. Second, these rights should be enjoyed by all, regardless of age, race, ethnicity, or gender (WHO, 2017b). Adequate food and water, education, proper housing, and freedom from discrimination all contribute to our well-being. Freedom to control one's body (e.g., in the context of sexual and reproductive rights) and to obtain health protections are also fundamental to enjoying the best possible health (WHO, 2017b). From a truly global perspective, health is a basic human right.

Thinking About Health

- Why do factors such as where you live influence health outcomes? How might these factors affect you?
- What roles can individuals and communities play in eliminating health disparities? How can local and federal governments bring about greater equity in health care?
- How can science contribute to the elimination of health disparities?

Historical Views of Health

We have seen how people around the world experience health and disease. How we think about health and health care today is heavily influenced by the history of medicine and psychology. It is these discoveries and developments that have led to our current biopsychosocial approach to health.

Ancient Times

Since the beginning of historical time, human beings have been contemplating health, wellness, illness, and death. The physician who served the Egyptian king in 2600 B.C.E. was considered so important that, after his death, he was worshipped as a god of healing. Of course, it was a very different kind of healing than we recognize today. Documents from between 1900 B.C.E. and 1550 B.C.E., such as the

Rubric No. 197 (Column 39, Line 7):

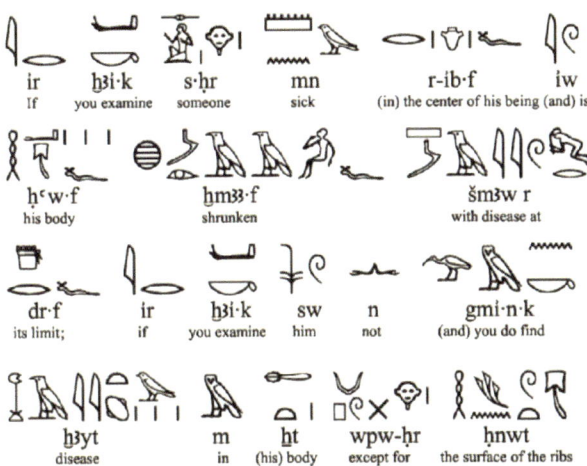

ir	ḥȝi·k	s·ḥr	mn	r-ib·f	iw
If	you examine	someone	sick	(in) the center of his being (and) is	

ḥʿw·f	ḥmȝȝ·f	šmȝw r
his body	shrunken	with disease at

dr·f	ir	ḥȝi·k	sw	n	gmi·n·k
its limit;	if	you examine	him	not	(and) you do find

ḥȝyt	m	ḥt	wpw-ḥr	ḥnwt
disease	in	(his) body	except for	the surface of the ribs

Photo 1.13   The Ebers Papyrus. This ancient Egyptian medical document, containing herbal knowledge, expressed the belief that illness was caused by supernatural forces.

Ebers Papyrus shown in **Photo 1.13**, attribute illness to spiritual beings and supernatural causes. Treatments were in the form of spells and potions to frighten spirits away. Still, the Egyptians were already naming organs of the body. Says one ancient papyrus, "The heart speaks out every limb" (Carpenter et al., 1998). Another contains a detailed description of the brain (Allen, 2005; Breasted, 1930/1991; Ritner, 2001). Could it be that magical thinking prevailed only after other treatments had failed?

In 700 B.C.E., the Greek poet Homer wrote in the *Iliad* that the god Apollo was the "bringer and reliever" of plagues. Although this text still speaks of the power of gods, Greek science and philosophy began just 100 years later. Hippocrates, born in 460 B.C.E., is considered the "father of Western medicine." He argued that disease is not a punishment from the gods, but rather the result of environmental factors, diet, and lifestyle. This idea marked the birth of **dualism**, the belief in the separation of the mind and body. While this was an advance at the time, health psychology today is concerned with the connection between the mind and the body.

Despite his forward-thinking, Hippocrates had a poor understanding of anatomy and physiology. He believed in the **humoral theory of illness**. According to this theory, four bodily fluids (black bile, yellow bile, blood, and phlegm) govern temperament and health. For example, if you had an excess of blood, you were thought to be *sanguine*—courageous, hopeful, and amorous. Although the humoral theory has been invalidated, the legacy of Hippocrates' positive contributions to medicine lives on in the **Hippocratic oath**, a code of ethical conduct that influences current medical practice. One familiar tenet is to "do no harm." The oath is recited by medical students at the White Coat Ceremony when they begin clinical training [**Photo 1.14**(a and b)].

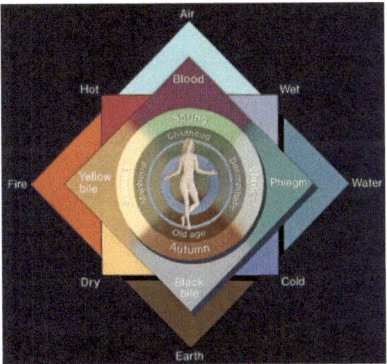
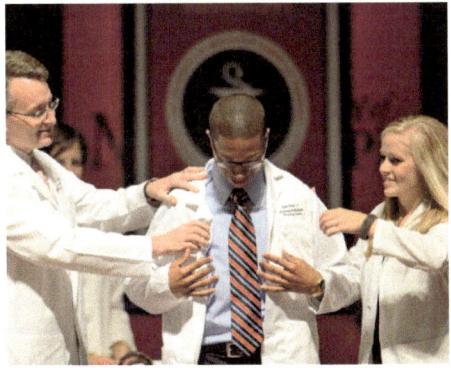

Photo 1.14 (a and b)   Hippocrates expressed the once-popular belief that health was made up of the four humors. However, his importance to the medical field led to the Hippocratic oath, which all medical students must take.

In 180 B.C.E., also in Greece, Galen made the connection between damage to the spinal cord and paralysis. *Pharmacology*, or the science of drugs, took root soon after, including in *De Materia Medica*, a five-volume treatise on herbal medicine. Traditional Chinese medicine also dates to this time, written in the *Huangdi Neijing*, or *The Inner Canon*.

The Middle Ages

The Middle Ages, from roughly the 5th century C.E. to the 15th century C.E., saw extreme health challenges. Despite rapid development in Europe, there were dreadful sanitation practices and no clean running water. Beliefs about health again focused on superstition. Illness was said to result from sins of the soul, and sufferers sought relief through meditation, prayer, herbal remedies, and spiritual healers. None of these were a match for the disease (**Photo 1.15**).

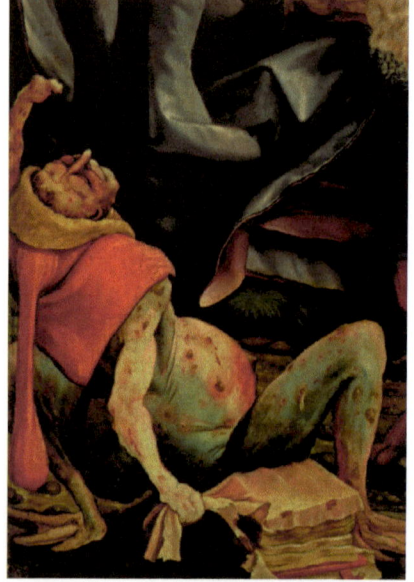

Photo 1.15 This painting shows the effects of bubonic plague, one of history's worst pandemics.

Previously one of the most devastating pandemics in all of history, the **Black Death**, a form of bubonic plague, killed as many as 200 million people, starting with its first outbreak in China in 1328 C.E. In England alone, the Black Death killed between 30% and 60% of the population in just three years (Cohn, 2008). The plague traveled via trade routes such as the Silk Road, transmitted by fleas living on rats that accompanied the traders. The symptoms were awful. A patient's blood turned foul-smelling and almost black. Large, painful, and swollen blisters (or *buboes*) would appear in the armpits, legs, neck, and groin, accompanied by a high fever, delirium, vomiting, muscular pain, and blood in the lungs. An intense desire for sleep only hastened death. Most victims died within four days. You can imagine the devastation the plague wrought, even beyond death and disease. No one knew what caused it or how to treat it.

Now the history and health psychology books include a new pandemic. The COVID-19 (or coronavirus) pandemic is a global pandemic created by severe acute respiratory syndrome coronavirus 2 (SARS-CoV-2). This virus first emerged in China at the end of 2019. It spread from there throughout the world and on January 30, 2020, the World Health Organization declared it a public health emergency of international concern. By the end of May 2023, there were 766,440, 032 diagnosed cases and nearly 7 million confirmed deaths—making COVID-19 one of the deadliest viruses in history. The impacts of this pandemic are not yet over and we will not know the long-term and indirect effects that it has on people's lives and their health for many years to come. We will, however, be thinking a lot about how this global crisis has affected our health and well-being throughout this book.

The Renaissance

The Renaissance began in Italy in the 14th century, bringing with it a rebirth of interest in medical science. Physicians began to study human anatomy, medical treatment, and pharmacology, and surgical procedures were modernized. For

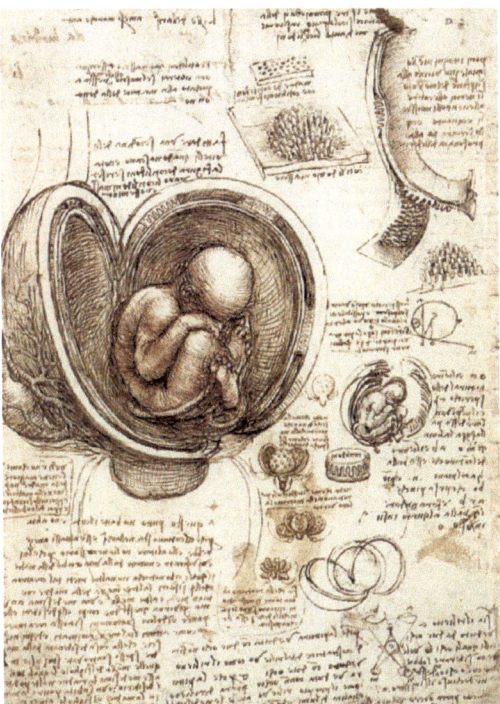

Photo 1.16 Leonardo da Vinci completed a number of anatomical studies, which contributed greatly to the medical field.

example, laudanum (a strong narcotic) was developed to reduce pain. Ambroise Paré, the surgeon to French kings, used a solution of egg yolks, rose oil, and turpentine to bind and heal war wounds. He also tied arteries during surgery to prevent bleeding.

Leonardo da Vinci practiced not just art, architecture, and music; he was also an exceptional scientist who gathered information by dissecting corpses. He diagrammed the functions of the skeleton, illustrated the vascular system, and drew the human fetus into its mother's womb. William Harvey in England advanced the understanding of the role of the heart. He calculated that it pumped 600 pounds of blood each day. Andreas Vesalius, a Flemish anatomist, made major contributions as well (**Photo 1.16**).

Just as important from the point of view of health psychology, beliefs changed. The **germ theory of disease** attributed the disease to microorganisms, the tiny cells we now know as bacteria and fungi. With the development of microscopes, Antoni van Leeuwenhoek could even see them, along with blood and sperm cells. These advances placed medicine in the hands of physicians. This movement—toward science and away from superstition—emphasized the role of the body, rather than the mind, in disease.

The Enlightenment and Industrial Revolution

In the 17th century, René Descartes firmly set apart the mind and the body. He believed that the body functions like a machine, while the mind (or soul) is nonmaterial, although it controls the body. He allowed that when people act "out of passion," the body may influence the mind. For the most part, however, the field of medicine came to see the mind and the body as operating separately.

Later developments included the discovery of **antibiotics**, and drugs to treat infections caused by bacteria. Alexander Fleming discovered penicillin, the first antibiotic, in 1928. If not for him, thousands of soldiers would have died from wound infections and gangrene in World War II. Antibiotics revolutionized health care and gave birth to the pharmaceutical industry.

Another revolutionary advance was the polio vaccine from Jonas Salk. Vaccines work in healthy people by harnessing the body's immune system to fight infection. Since the first vaccine in 1955, and due to the tremendous success of the global polio eradication effort, polio cases decreased by more than 99% in 1988. There was a drop from 350,000 cases to just 118 in 2017, only two countries (Pakistan and Afghanistan) showed cases in 2019 (Rana et al., 2022; Waheed, 2018). However, when COVID-19 happened polio cases began again to increase especially in those two countries. Medical researchers attribute this rise to the disruption that COVID-19 caused in the immunization efforts for polio (Rana et al., 2022). These researchers caution that since the long-term trajectory of the pandemic is unknown it may relate to a resurgence of other epidemic-like diseases like polio. So, although the effort to eradicate polio had been highly successful, the global health impact of the COVID-19 pandemic may impact that.

Thinking About Health

■ What did you find most interesting or surprising about the historical views of health? What can medicine today learn from past mistakes and past discoveries?

■ How have social and cultural facts in the past promoted or stood in the way of proper health care? What parallels do you see between health practices of the past and health care today?

Psychology in the History of Medicine

The dualism of mind and body created a division in healing. Physicians treated problems with the body, while philosophers, priests, and shamans treated problems involving the mind. It wasn't until Sigmund Freud in the late 19th century that the mind and the body were unified once again—a belief known as **holism**.

Psychoanalysis and Health Psychology

Freud, who was trained as a physician, noticed that some patients had symptoms but no physical disorder. The symptoms could be numbness, paralysis, hallucinations, or loss of consciousness. In talking with these patients, Freud came to realize that their symptoms were related to emotional conflict. He believed conflict "converted" into symptoms. He also discovered the powerful therapeutic influence of talk or **psychoanalysis**. As patients discussed their dreams, thoughts, and deep-seated emotions, they often unearthed devastating emotional conflicts, and the mysterious physical symptoms would often disappear. Over time, Freud's theories have become less influential. Nevertheless, he demonstrated that the mind can have a pronounced effect on the body, health, and illness. In a very real sense, health psychology was born.

Psychosomatic medicine examines the relationships between mind and body in health and disease. (In Latin, *psycho* means mind and *soma* means body.) The American Psychosomatic Society, founded in 1930, includes medical professionals, psychoanalysts, and psychiatrists. Its declared mission is to "promote and advance the scientific understanding of the interrelationships among biological, psychological, social, and behavioral factors in human health and disease" (American Psychosomatic Society, 2001). The biopsychosocial model had entered the mainstream.

Still others extended Freud's work, such as Franz Alexander and Flanders Dunbar in the 1930s. They argued that anxiety interacts with the **autonomic nervous system**—the part of the nervous system that controls heart rate, blood pressure, respiration, digestion, perspiration, salivation, body temperature, and more. In this way, stress can lead to hypertension, ulcers, colitis, and rheumatoid arthritis. (We look further at stress-related disorders in Chapters 6 and 7.) Taken together, these developments have led to a very holistic approach to health.

The Lessons of History

As we have seen, the field of health psychology has a lineage that closely follows the history of medicine. Both fields are grounded in science. When we ask why some breast cancer patients benefit from social support (as Sade did) while patients do not, we use the scientific method to find the answers. Just as van Leeuwenhoek advanced medicine by observing blood cells under a microscope, researchers have found through carefully controlled studies that social isolation has a negative effect on the course of cancer (Kroenke, Kubzansky, Schernhammer, Holmes, & Kawachi, 2006). We look more closely at how health psychologists gather information on health and illness in Chapter 2.

We have also seen that health psychology is based on the belief that the mind and body are linked. This is not to say that all illnesses have a psychological cause. Rather, regardless of the cause of disease, each individual will respond to that disease differently because of psychological and social factors that interact with biology. Again, the biopsychosocial model best explains health.

Finally, history demonstrates that beliefs can be understood only within the context of a time and place. Take the Middle Ages. Deadly illnesses were spreading, and people were terrified. In their ignorance, they explained disease with the only belief system available: It was a punishment from God. Today, some groups fear modern medicine because they do not have a clear understanding of how it works. For example, people in northeastern villages in Nigeria are fearful and skeptical when white Western physicians come bearing coolers containing vials of liquids that, a translator tells them, will prevent their children from becoming ill. As we have seen, a mother in a village like that might choose not to vaccinate her children against polio, with deadly consequences. Our job is to look for ways to apply our knowledge to understand the world around us. And when our knowledge does not assist us in helping others, we need to look again at their experience of health. We may yet convince that mother.

Thinking About Health

- What examples can you find of the mind-body relationship in your life?
- How have changes in the patterns of illness over time shaped health psychology and the biopsychosocial approach?

A Lifespan Developmental Perspective

Health psychology is changing, along with the pattern of our lives. We are now living longer, and the leading causes of death have changed. More adults, like Sade at the start of this chapter, are living with chronic illness. A **developmental perspective** considers how the factors that influence health and illness vary across the human lifespan, including both historical and individual changes over time. Although the developmental perspective is based on the biopsychosocial model, it opens up exciting new ways to study health and disease. This long-term view is important to health because the biopsychosocial factors that influence personal choices or how we cope can change over the course of a lifetime. Scientific advances also make it possible to apply human genetics to the diagnosis and treatment of disease.

Living Longer

People around the world are living longer than ever before. Globally, the life expectancy at birth for a child born in 2023 is 73.16 years, compared with just 47.3 years in 1900 (National Center for Health Statistics, 2017). According to the World Population Review (2023d) Monaco, one of the smallest countries in the world, has the highest life expectancy. People born there today have an expected life span of 85.17 years old if they are male, and even longer—88.99 years old if they are female. Most people then did not live through middle age. Many women died in childbirth, and diseases like the Black Death and influenza caused many untimely deaths.

As you can see in **Table 1.3**, the leading causes of death in 1900 were pneumonia, tuberculosis, and intestinal illnesses. These are **infectious diseases**, caused by viruses or bacteria, and are often contagious. They are also acute diseases, rather than chronic illnesses.

When you look at the United States today, you see a very different picture. As Americans are living longer, they instead face chronic illnesses, such

	1900	2018
1	Pneumonia	Heart (cardiovascular) disease
2	Tuberculosis	Cancer
3	Diarrhea/Enteritis	Accidents (unintentional injury)
4	Heart disease	Chronic lower respiratory disease
5	Stroke	Stroke (cerebrovascular disease)
6	Liver disease	Alzheimer's disease
7	Injury	Diabetes
8	Cancer	Influenza and pneumonia
9	Senility	Kidney disease
10	Diphtheria	Suicide (intentional self-harm)

Source: Data from Heron (2018) and Xu, Murphy, Kochanek, and Arias (2016).

Table 1.3 Leading causes of death in 1900 and 2018

as hypertension, diabetes, Alzheimer's disease, and Parkinson's disease, which emerge in later life. There is often no cure for these conditions, and patients will live with them for many years. The goal is to *manage* them so that the progression of disease is slow and the quality of life is preserved.

Take Alzheimer's disease, for example. This is a chronic, progressive neurological disorder most common in people older than 65. Over time, neurofibers (fibers in the brain) get tangled, and plaques build up in the neural pathways. Inflammation occurs, and brain cells die, leading to loss of memory, disordered thinking, language impairments, and personality changes. Eventually, patients can no longer care for themselves or even recognize themselves or others. Although there are genetic markers for Alzheimer's disease, environmental and behavioral factors help determine whether or not it develops. Alzheimer's disease is best understood from a developmental perspective as a late-life disorder, but lifestyle choices such as being physically active earlier in life can offset its development later on. Again, our job is to help people with Alzheimer's disease manage the disorder, provide the care and social support they need, and prevent a more deadly illness. We look further at proper care for people with Alzheimer's disease and other chronic diseases in Chapter 11.

Riskier Lifestyles

Why have the causes of death changed? A lifespan development perspective asks how the many different factors have combined to improve health and well-being. Infectious disease has declined significantly thanks to advances in personal hygiene, better nutrition, and innovative public health measures. Communities introduced water purification and sewage treatment. Landfills and garbage dumps were moved outside the villages. Advances in medical treatments, such as antibiotics and vaccines, were also important (**Photo 1.17**).

Our behavioral choices also affect our lifespan—and not entirely for the better. Several of the leading causes of death relate to lifestyle, such as high-calorie and high-fat diets, lack of exercise, and stress. Obesity is an important risk factor (Centers for Disease Control & Prevention, 2011c).

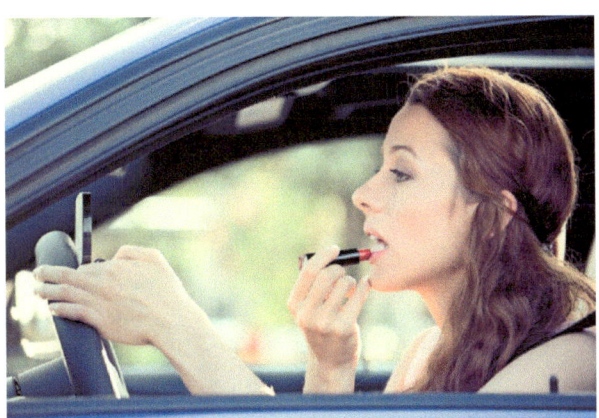

Photo 1.17   Over time, new health risks emerge: Distracted driving is deadly.

Obesity refers to a weight greater than what is considered healthy. More technically, it is defined as a body mass index (BMI) of greater than 30. More than one-third of U.S. adults (39.8%) and 18.5% of children and adolescents have obese. Nearly 50% of college students at Wesley College in Delaware reported they were overweight or obese (D'Souza, Bautista, & Wentzien, 2015). Alabama has the highest rate of obesity, Colorado the lowest, but not a single state in the union has an obesity rate of less than 20%. The main cause of excess weight is an energy imbalance, as we explain in Chapter 5. It occurs when people take in more calories than they burn.

Why is this relevant? Higher BMIs mean greater body fat and greater weight, and the higher these are, the greater the risk of health problems. Heart disease, stroke, and several forms of cancer all relate to diet and weight. So does type 2 diabetes (previously known as adult-onset diabetes), which is a change in the body's ability to regulate blood sugar. If left untreated, it can lead to blindness, gangrene, heart disease, and stroke. Although type 2 diabetes has long been most common in people older than 65, rates are rising in children and adolescents as well. The American Diabetes Association calls this rise an epidemic.

High-fat, high-calorie diets and lack of exercise are not the only health concerns. Other damaging lifestyle choices include smoking, excessive alcohol consumption, not wearing seatbelts, and not practicing safe sex. Tobacco use is still the single largest preventable cause of death and disease in the United States and around the world (CDC, 2023). In the Western Pacific, where smoking rates are highest, 3000 people a day die from tobacco use (**Photo 1.18**).

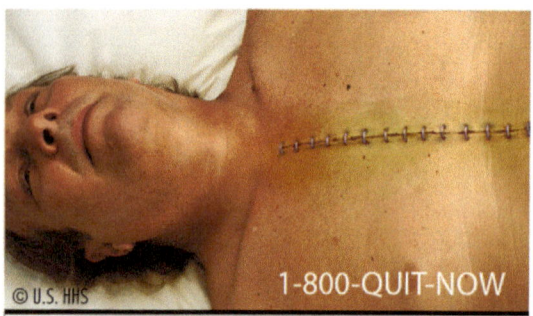

Photo 1.18   The FDA requires cautionary cigarette labels such as this one, which warn the public of health risks.

Health psychologists try to understand why people make the choices they do with regard to their health. For example, although warning labels appear on cigarette packs, public health campaigns, and early education, people still smoke cigarettes. They smoke despite knowing that smoking is bad for their health. And today tobacco use is increasing, especially among adolescents, who have grown up knowing smoking leads to lung cancer. While cigarette smoking declined between 2011 and 2022, the use of e-cigarettes, hookahs, and smokeless tobacco all increased, especially in middle and high school students (CDC, 2023; Park-Lee et al., 2022). Among high school students, nearly 20% use tobacco, with e-cigarettes being the most commonly used tobacco product: Their use increased from 4.5% in 2013 to 85.5% in high school students and 81.5% in middle school students in 2022 (Park-Lee et al., 2022), surpassing the use of all other forms of tobacco in the United States today (Park-Lee et al., 2022). Even more troubling, the availability of flavored tobacco products may be driving increased tobacco use among young people. Why do teenagers gravitate toward these products? What is the impact of this behavior on their development? The answers are more complex than they seem.

We look more at health-compromising behaviors in Chapter 5. Many of the resulting deaths are preventable. Health psychology and understanding the developmental factors that may influence health and health choices can unlock a healthier future.

The Genes for Disease

A lifespan developmental approach opens up new ways to study health psychology. Once we start asking how diseases develop, we can look for answers in our genes, and new technologies are making that possible.

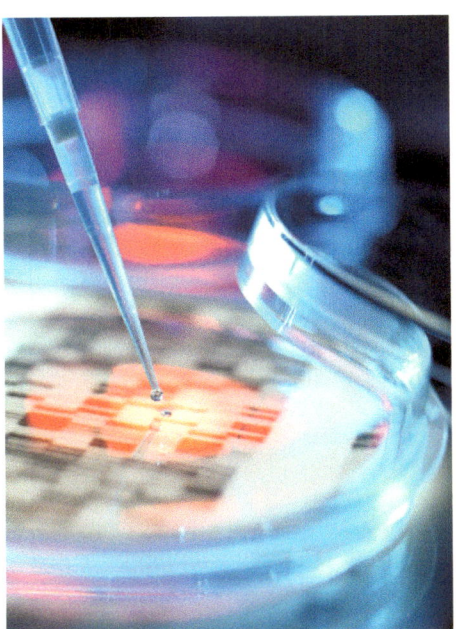

Photo 1.19 Genetic studies help scientists discover what causes certain diseases.

Genes are our biological inheritance from our parents, and two kinds of genes help determine whether we will develop a disease: risk genes and deterministic genes. **Risk genes** may increase the likelihood that we will develop the disease, but they do not directly cause the disease or guarantee that it will happen. In Alzheimer's disease, for example, the most important risk gene is APOE-e4, implicated in up to 40–65% of Alzheimer's cases (Alzheimer's Association, 2023). Each of us inherits a copy of some form of APOE from each parent. If we inherit a single copy of APOE-e4, however, we have an increased risk of developing Alzheimer's disease, and symptoms may appear at a younger age. If we inherit two copies, the risk is even higher. Still, the gene does not guarantee that we will develop the disease (**Photo 1.19**).

Deterministic genes actually cause a disease to develop. Deterministic genes for Alzheimer's disease are found in only a few hundred extended families throughout the world—or less than 1% of all cases. These genes cause *familial early-onset Alzheimer's disease*, in which symptoms usually develop in a person's early 40s or mid-50s. Although these genes are rare, their discovery has expanded our understanding of the disease (Mosconi et al., 2004). Currently, health professionals do not recommend routine genetic testing for Alzheimer's disease. Rather, genetic testing is used primarily in scientific studies of the disease.

What does the future hold? Recent reports present a medical mystery (Kolata, 2016). Patterns of illness may be changing again. Research shows that the incidence of some major diseases like heart disease, some cancers, and dementia is actually declining in wealthy countries (Jones & Greene, 2016). This is good news, but the reasons are still not fully known. The changes are likely due to improved screening, diagnosis, and treatment, or perhaps because people in wealthy countries are making healthier lifestyle choices. Solving this medical mystery is an exciting new challenge for health psychologists.

The Future of Health

Artificial Intelligence and Eating Disorders

Eating disorders are rising at alarming rates worldwide. They are no longer a S.W.A.G disorder—S.W.A.G stands for "skinny" "white" "affluent" "girls"—now eating disorders affect people regardless of their age, gender, racial/ethnic background, socioeconomic status, or where they live in the world. It is important to understand why this potentially life-threatening mental disorder is rising around the globe especially because it can be successfully treated. The escalating rates have been attributed to several recent phenomena: the COVID-19 pandemic, social media, and the use of artificial intelligence in online platforms.

Geoffrey Fowler wrote in the Washington Post (8/10/2023) that the combination of disturbing and triggering fake images as well as harmful and dangerous advice generated by chatbots could be fueling the rise in eating disorders. In his opinion piece, he shares the "guidance" he received from ChatGPT and Google Bard AI on how to induce vomiting, "chewing and spitting" and a weight-loss meal plan with dangerously low calories designed to lose weight quickly—one that no doctor would ever endorse. Fowler also reports that when he typed in "thinspo," a social media catchphrase meaning thin inspiration, he was given disturbing images of women's bodies that were emaciated, skeletal with bones protruding, and alarmingly unhealthy looking. Why is this a problem? Well, research shows that 98% of adolescents and young adults use social media regularly and increasingly seek out health information from sites like TikTok rather than traditional sources such as healthcare providers (Hausmann et al., 2017; Klein et al., 2023; Vogels, Gelles-Watnick, & Massarat, 2022). Although not a scientific study, a large population-based survey conducted by Ireland (2023) showed that across the United States, China, the United Kingdom, Germany, and Japan, 25% of "millennials" reported using social media to discuss health and illness. It is even more concerning that this study showed that 62% of patients with health conditions did not see their doctors as "regular sources of information" and more often turned to online influences and social media for information (who often have no credentials to provide any guidance on medical conditions). But what can we do about the dangerous use of AI and social media for eating disorders?

In his article, Fowler argues that what AI knows about eating disorders is learned from scouring the unhealthy content about eating and body image that is already out there on the internet. Pro-anorexia image generators and chatbots represent the dangers of AI and the internet that Fowler says we are not "talking – and doing – nearly enough about." This situation should anger parents, doctors, mental health providers, and people who have a loved one with an eating disorder. Girls and young women are not the only ones being targeted. Other research by The Center for Countering Digital Hate (2023) shows boys and men are often exposed to toxic ideas of masculinity leading to disordered eating and muscle dysmorphia. For example, viewed over 587 million times in the United States alone, TikTok videos glorify potentially life-threatening bodybuilding images and promote steroid-like drugs to teens further perpetuating dangerous body image disturbances.

There is evidence that AI is unpredictable, inconsistent, using uncredible sources, and presenting made-up facts. As Fowler comments "the problem isn't just AI making things up. AI is perpetuating sick stereotypes we've hardly confronted in our culture. It's disseminating misleading health information. And it's fueling mental illness by pretending to be an authority or even a friend." Social media, and AI in particular, are big business driven by investors, viewers, and advertising dollars. Removing the harmful content about eating and body image from AI and social media is not technically easy. Despite the fact that some of these sites forbid eating disorder content in their usage policies, they do not actively enforce it, and bypassing the filters is easy. Moreover, these companies are not intrinsically motivated nor do they have an economic incentive to care about harmful eating disorder content. So it looks like this problem is one that will continue for the future of our health.

Chapter Summary

Health is not just the absence of disease, but a state of optimal well-being along the illness–wellness continuum. Health psychology examines the psychological influences on health, how and why we become ill, and how we cope with illness. The field is based on the biopsychosocial model, which looks at the many different factors that interact to promote health or illness. We can see enormous health disparities between developed and developing nations, as well as within nations, including the United States. Nonetheless, health, according to the World Health Organization, is a fundamental human right. From a global perspective, we can also see differences in beliefs about health. Historically, advances in understanding and fighting disease came hand in hand with dualism, the separation of mind and body. Psychoanalysis and health psychology, however, have restored the connections. Now that people are living well into old age, the leading causes of death and disability have changed to chronic illnesses and illnesses with a strong behavioral component. These changing patterns demand a lifespan developmental perspective.

Thinking About Health

- How has your own development influenced how you think about your health and how you cope with illness?
- What are the risk factors in your life? Are there any behaviors that you should change for better health? Are you willing to make those changes?
- Thinking about your family history of medical conditions, are there any potential risk factors for your health?

KEY TERMS ▶ health p. 3; illness–wellness continuum p. 3; health psychology p. 4; preventive medicine p. 4; chronic disorders p. 5; acute disorders p. 5; etiology p. 5; epidemiology p. 5; biopsychosocial model p. 9; systems theory p. 11; objective health p. 13; subjective health p. 13; interindividual differences p. 13; globalization p. 14; health disparities p. 16; developed nations p. 17; less developed nations p. 17; dualism p. 25; humoral theory of illness p. 25; Hippocratic oath p. 25; Black Death p. 26; germ theory of disease p. 27; antibiotics p. 27; holism p. 28; psychoanalysis p. 28; psychosomatic medicine p. 28; autonomic nervous system p. 29; developmental perspective p. 30; infectious diseases p. 30; obesity p. 31; risk genes p. 33; deterministic genes p. 33.

CHAPTER 2

Gathering Information on Health and Illness

Learning Outcomes

After reading this chapter, you should be able to:

- **Define** evidence-based practice.
- **Outline** independent (IVs) and dependent variables (DVs)
- **Describe** the field of epidemiology and what epidemiologists do.
- **Explain** the roles of institutional review boards (IRBs) and open science in psychology.
- **Compare** and contrast mortality, morbidity, prevalence, and incidence.
- **Explain** the methodologies used in health psychology.
- **Identify** some cutting-edge areas of research.

"Did you know that 600 new species of bacteria are identified each year? Wow! Over the course of a single infection, bacteria can change their very DNA to survive. They morph just enough to render older antibiotics powerless."

Darius is explaining why he plans to pursue a career as an epidemiologist—a germ chaser. A doctoral student in microbiology, Darius hopes one day to work with the Centers for Disease (**Photo 2.1**).

Control and Prevention (CDC) to help stop life-threatening infections caused by these pesky bacteria. At age 11, he read The Germ Hunter, the biography of Louis Pasteur. Gifted with extraordinary curiosity and imagination, Pasteur was horrified by the effects of rabies and tuberculosis. In the 1830s, he began a lifelong quest to understand and eradicate these and other terrible diseases. To this day, we commemorate his discoveries whenever we drink pasteurized milk. Darius fondly remembers explaining Pasteur's role in milk pasteurization to his mother and sisters over breakfast.

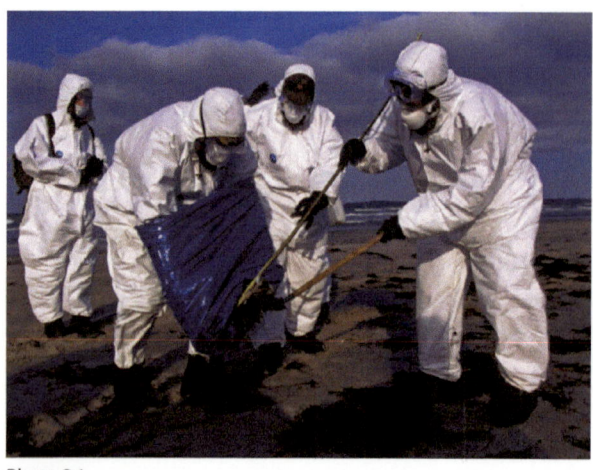

Photo 2.1

DOI: 10.4324/9781032643090-2

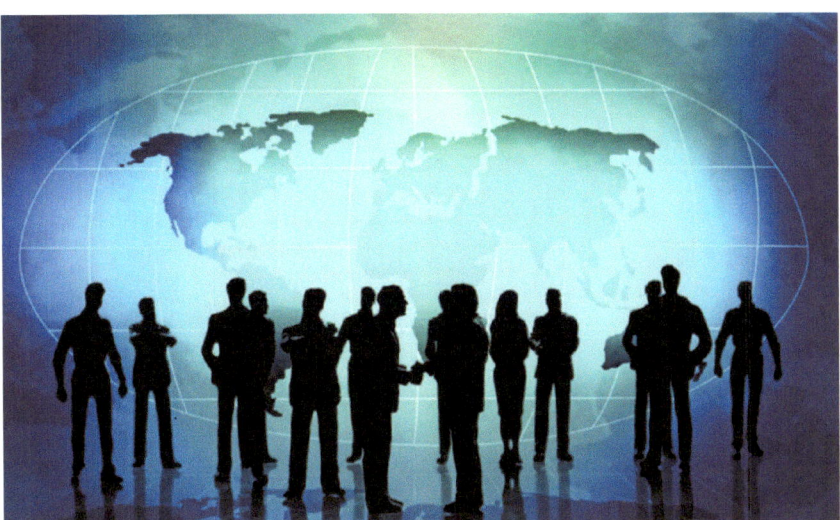

Photo 2.2 Epidemiologists study patterns of illness in populations.

Darius has already had an internship with the CDC's Viral Special Pathogens Branch, studying Ebola in the Democratic Republic of the Congo and Marburg hemorrhagic fever in Uganda. His fieldwork has taken him from corporate offices to war zones, jungles, and deserts. He has collected samples of infections and interviewed people sickened by disease. Darius thinks of himself as a detective. He searches for clues and ways to put them together, and he loves it. He wants to know what causes an outbreak of disease, and how it can infect so many people. Most important of all, what can stop it? What can eradicate disease and prevent future outbreaks? "It's like solving a mystery," he says, and the solution can save lives.

Do you know other people on the front lines in the war against germs? Will you be one of those people someday?

Many scientists from many fields are interested in gaining a greater understanding of health. However, our broadest understanding of world health stems from the work of epidemiologists, like Darius. This chapter asks how researchers gather the information they need to address health problems here and around the world.

We explore how we measure health, illness, disability, and dysfunction. We examine how epidemiologists study the spread of disease and how sound research methods provide health psychologists with solid empirical evidence. We also discuss the ethical issues in science, as well as the challenges facing scientists who work on global health. Finally, we look at some innovative approaches. What we learn will help us become better consumers of health information. We will be better able to evaluate programs designed to prevent and treat illness (**Photo 2.2**).

Evidence-Based Science

Since March 2020, almost every major newspaper has featured articles on the COVID-19 Pandemic. Especially in the early days of this global health crisis, it was hard to make sense of the sometimes conflicting, rapidly changing

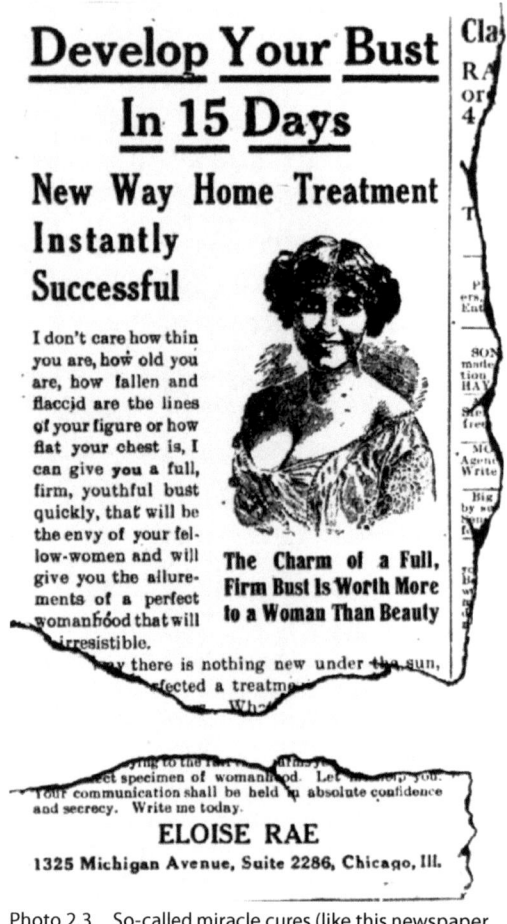

Develop Your Bust
In 15 Days

New Way Home Treatment
Instantly
Successful

I don't care how thin you are, how old you are, how fallen and flaccid are the lines of your figure or how flat your chest is, I can give you a full, firm, youthful bust quickly, that will be the envy of your fellow-women and will give you the allurements of a perfect womanhood that will irresistible.

The Charm of a Full, Firm Bust Is Worth More to a Woman Than Beauty

there is nothing new under the sun, fected a treatme Wh

specimen of womanhood. Let your communication shall be held in absolute confidence and secrecy. Write me today.

ELOISE RAE
1325 Michigan Avenue, Suite 2286, Chicago, Ill.

Photo 2.3   So-called miracle cures (like this newspaper ad promising to "Develop Your Bust") are rarely backed by scientific evidence.

information. This was a perfect example of how our lives are touched by health information. Every day, we are exposed to claims about health. Family and friends suggest home remedies. News stories and product ads promise everything from weight loss to sexual stamina to cures for cancer. Blogs address every condition imaginable. A product may say that it is "proven" to reduce wrinkles, even when no proper scientific evidence supports that claim. Even well-intentioned sources may pass along dubious claims. Not to mention the ongoing debates about vaccines, masking, and the origins of the COVID-19 virus (**Photo 2.3**).

How do we make sense of health information, and how can we identify healthy habits and proper treatment? What will the future look like when technology and health intersect? Dr. Daniel Schiff, co-director of the Governance and Responsible AI Lab at Purdue University was surveyed by the Pew Research Institute and said that advancing technologies like artificial intelligence (AI) have the potential to predict the structure of proteins, identify candidates for vaccine development and diagnose disease based on imaging data and that its impact on the infrastructure of health is "profound." This is more important today than ever before since research shows that, in the USA, up to 79% of Internet users search online for health information (Anderson & Rainie, 2023). Others have called digital access to health information a "super determinant" of health (Turcios, 2023) even more impactful than the social determinants we learned about in Chapter 1 (such as education, employment, and socioeconomic status).

Would you trust AI with your health questions? Recent research on AI chatbots like "ChatGPT" showed that the AI-generated responses to health questions were hard to distinguish from those of actual healthcare providers (Nov et al., 2023). In this study, researchers created hypothetical but realistic patient medical questions and presented them human healthcare providers (e.g., doctors, nurses) and ChatGPT and asked them to respond. They then provided these responses to nearly 400 adults and asked them to identify the source (i.e., medical professional/AI chatbot) and rate how much they trusted the response. Results showed that on average, participants had a hard time telling apart the responses from human medical professionals from the chatbot. Participants also trusted the chatbot's responses. Other research shows that 78% of adults would use ChatGPT for self-diagnosing their medical conditions (Shahsavar & Choudhury, 2023).

To be a skilled consumer of health information, you need a working knowledge of how scientific information is gathered and how to interpret it. You need to know what it means for claims to be based on scientific evidence. You need an understanding of health psychology as evidence-based science.

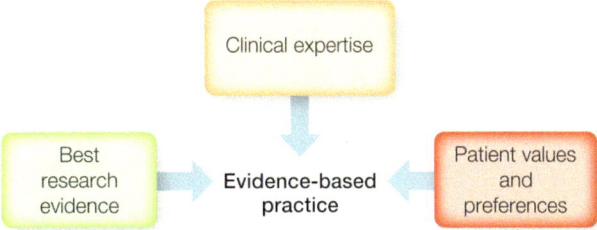

Figure 2.1   Factors in evidence-based practice.

Evidence-based practice, as seen in **Figure 2.1**, is the conscientious application of current scientific evidence to health-related decision-making (Sackett, Rosenberg, Gray, Haynes, & Richardson, 1996). It is based on the best methods of scientific research available, combined with clinical expertise and an understanding of an individual patient's health behaviors, beliefs, and values. Putting prevention and treatment programs to the test allows for greater confidence in their success (Chambless & Hollon, 1998).

Physicians and healthcare providers are trained to evaluate scientific evidence. They know how to provide their patients with health information and medical care that is consistent with the evidence (Davidson, Trudeau, & Smith, 2006). Yet evidence-based practice has gained prominence in psychology in just the last 20 years.

Thinking About Health

■ What factors cause you to question the health information that you encounter?

■ How do you evaluate claims about health and illness?

Measuring Health

Most of what we know today about health, wellness, disease, disability, and death has been generated by scientific research. Scientific research is usually driven by a desire to solve practical problems and to test theories. A **theory** is a set of ideas that explain the world in which we live. In health psychology, theories explain some elements of human behavior. Theories generate statements, or hypotheses, that we can test to determine whether our theory is supported. A **hypothesis** is a proposed explanation for a phenomenon that a scientist seeks to test in a research study.

What Is Epidemiology?

Epidemiology is concerned with measuring health. As we saw in Chapter 1, it is the field concerned with gathering data on health-related issues. We know, for example, that nearly 5.4 million people are bitten by poisonous snakes each year and nearly 138,000 die annually from those bites (WHO, 2021); we know

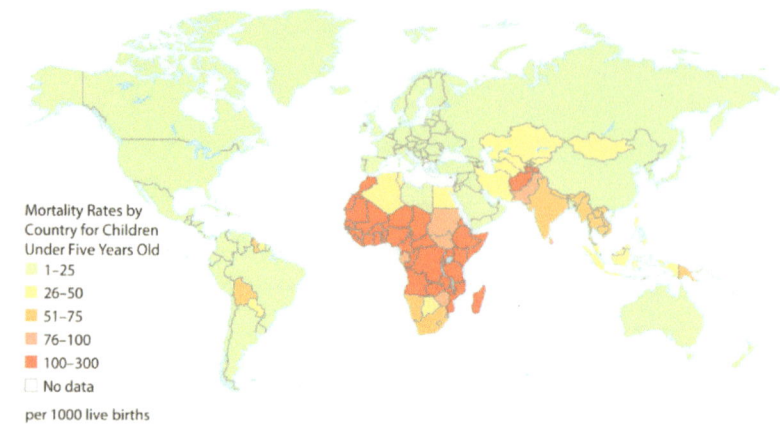

Mortality Rates by Country for Children Under Five Years Old
■ 1–25
■ 26–50
■ 51–75
■ 76–100
■ 100–300
□ No data
per 1000 live births

Photo 2.4   Mortality rates of children worldwide, based on epidemiological data.

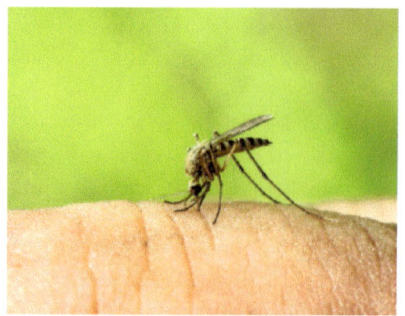

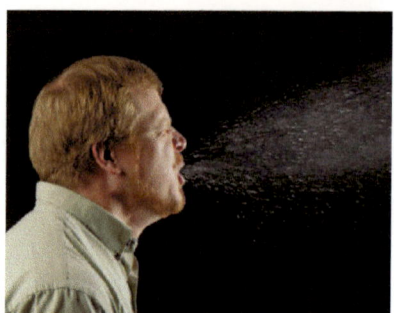

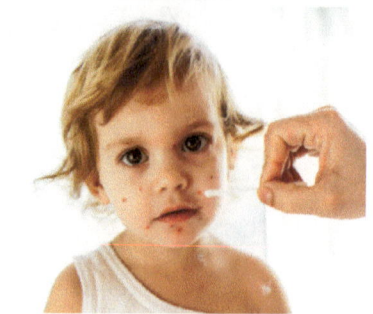

Photo 2.5 (a–c)   Examples of modes of transmission of different conditions (bacterial, respiratory, contagious viral infection).

that because epidemiologists totaled up the causes of death around the world. This number is the **mortality rate** or the number of deaths due to a specific cause. Unfortunately, the mortality rate for snake bites is probably an underestimate because many bites and deaths go unreported.

Epidemiology was first developed to discover the causes of smallpox, typhoid fever, and polio. These are **contagious diseases** that spread through the transmission—of an infectious agent, sometimes by physical contact between people. The field has now expanded to include other diseases, chronic conditions like cancer, and poisonings from the environment.

Epidemiologists gather information from health care providers, medical records, hospitals, and other institutions to track patterns of illness. They also often do field research and interview studies. They look for the risk factors associated with a disease and try to find what may protect us against it. They seek a picture of what is ailing people, and they apply this information to keep health problems under control (**Photos** 2.4 and 2.5).

Epidemiology is also concerned with **morbidity**, the number or frequency of cases of an illness in a specific group at a specific time. In everyday speech, we may think of a morbid person as gloomy and pessimistic, but in epidemiology, the term refers simply to poor health.

Prevalence and Incidence

"Vaping Surges." A recent U.S. news headline shared the alarming increase in adolescent vaping—the largest yearly increase in nicotine use recorded in the past 43 years (University of Michigan Institute for Social Research, 2018). You can read more about this concerning health problem in the In the News feature. How do we know about this increase? Epidemiologists work with numbers and give meaning to data.

Imagine that you read this headline in the newspaper: "New cases of diabetes declined by 20% in the last five years." And yet, a few paragraphs into the article, you read, "The number of people with diabetes is at an all-time high, with 9.4% of the population suffering from this disease." How can something be declining and rising at the same time? The answer requires distinguishing two measures of the frequency of disease: incidence and prevalence. Circling back to snake bites, the prevalence of snake bites is probably an underestimate since so many bites and deaths go unreported. This is because they often occur in rural areas of the world where factors such as the distance to medical care, and the resources of the medical systems to treat and track medical conditions are not ideal.

Incidence is the number of new cases at a given time, while **prevalence** is the total number of cases at that time. The number of new cases may be declining, but each and every new case still adds to the total. In our example, the incidence of diabetes is falling, but the prevalence is not. Incidence is important because it tells us the risk of contracting a disease, whereas prevalence indicates how widespread the disease is and its burden on society. Again, in our example of venomous snake bites, the prevalence of snake bites is expected to increase in the future due to climate change. Researchers at Emory University showed that the likelihood of someone being bitten by a snake increases for each degree increase in temperature (in Celsius). So as temperatures rise globally, the prevalence of snakebites will increase as well. **Lifetime prevalence** refers to the proportion of a population that has, at some point in their lives, had the condition.

The techniques that epidemiologists use to gather data vary, depending on the health problem at stake. **Surveillance** gathers detailed information about health by assessing the magnitude of a problem, or the impact of a disease, by studying cases, or by doing door-to-door interviews. **Descriptive studies** gather information about health status, attitudes, behaviors, or characteristics of a disease. **Analytic studies** apply statistical analysis to study the causes of disease. They are usually undertaken to test a hypothesis, and they look for links between possible causes and the frequency of disease. Together, these methods help identify risk groups to create a profile of a disease. As we see next, health psychologists use some of the same methods.

In the News

A Dangerous New Addiction for Teens

In 2018, the U.S. Food and Drug Administration announced a major crackdown on vaping—specifically, the use of trendy Juul devices (U.S. Food & Drug Administration, 2018). The FDA initiated an undercover sting operation to bust lawbreaking gas stations, convenience stores, and online retailers that sold vaping devices to underage people. Moreover, the FDA demanded that Juul Labs turn over company documents related to the research and marketing of its products, out of suspicion that, despite its alarming toxicology and addictive properties, Juul intentionally marketed to adolescents.

Although the vaping industry argues against claims that flash-drive-like e-cigarettes, candy-flavored vapor, and aggressive social media campaigns are designed to appeal to youth, the FDA is taking a firm stance. "The nicotine in these products can rewire an adolescent's brain, leading to years of addiction," said FDA commissioner Dr. Scott Gottlieb. Although the nicotine content of one Juul pod is equivalent to the amount found in one pack of cigarettes, medical research shows that Juul is more addictive for children than traditional or other e-cigarettes because it delivers the nicotine in a more concentrated manner, leading adolescents to microdose all day long (**Photo 2.6**).

In addition to the FDA's efforts, medical and public health advocacy groups such as the Campaign for Tobacco-Free Kids are working to educate the public on the dangers of vaping. Will they be successful before a new generation of people are addicted to nicotine, the leading preventable cause of death today?

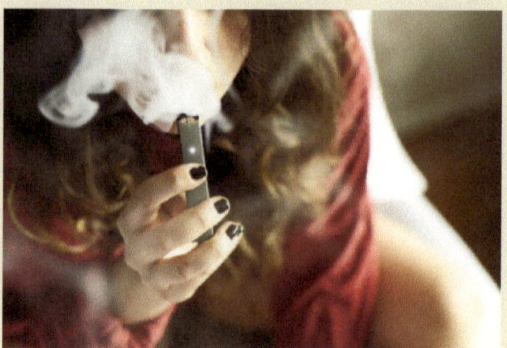

Photo 2.6   A person vaping.

Question: The founders of Juul state that their device is intended to provide a "satisfying alternative to cigarettes" for adult smokers. How would you recommend that Juul accomplish this goal while preventing sales to adolescents?

Thinking About Health

■ How does evidence-based science help health practitioners and health consumers?

■ Think about a news story that involved epidemiologists. What impact did the story have on a health problem?

■ How would you explain the different approaches to gathering information about health and health psychology to a friend?

■ Why are different research methods needed to provide evidence-based knowledge?

Research Methodology

Health psychology draws on data from epidemiology and uses many of the same research designs. However, health psychology also borrows from medical science and the basic research methodologies from psychology. To understand the different research methods, first consider the kinds of evidence they highlight and the variables they put to the test.

Quantitative and Qualitative Methods

Quantitative data are gathered through carefully designed examination, with all the possible factors affecting health determined ahead of time. **Qualitative data** are more open-ended. They are gathered through field observations and open-ended questions, usually with little manipulation of the factors or context. Health psychology is based primarily on quantitative evidence.

Compare two approaches to studying Parkinson's disease, a chronic disorder that makes it difficult for patients to control their movements. In one study, researchers attended weekly meetings of a Parkinson's disease support group. They asked patients to share their experiences of living with the disease, with only a few prompts from the researcher. Each conversation was videotaped. Afterward, researchers watched and listened to the videotapes to see what themes emerged. What similarities and differences could they discern among the interviews? What is it like to live with the disease, in the patients' own words? In the published results, the researchers tried to preserve the flavor of subjective experience and qualitative evidence.

A second study produced quantitative data. Here, too, researchers spoke with patients one-on-one at meetings of the support group, and here, too, they were interested in how older patients cope with the stress of disease. However, in this study, the interviewers asked questions like these:

- On a scale of 1 to 10, with 1 being not-at-all stressful and 10 being extremely stressful, how stressful are the symptoms of your illness?

- Please listen to the following common symptoms of Parkinson's disease. For each symptom, please state the level of pain you experience, on a scale where 1 indicates no pain, 2 indicates some pain, 3 indicates a great deal of pain, and 4 indicates excruciating pain (**Photo 2.7**).

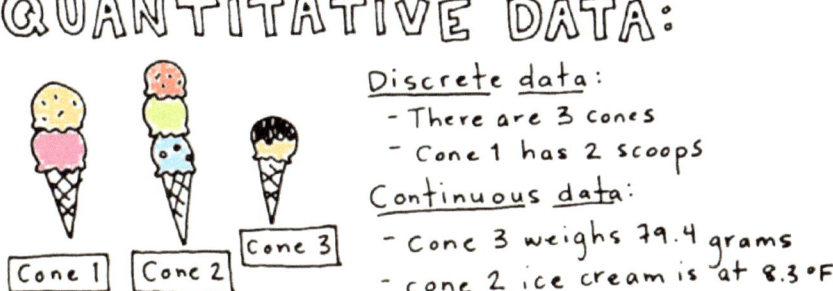

Photo 2.7　Some examples of quantitative data.

Source: Courtesy Allison Horst, Bren, School of Environmental Science & Management at the University of California, Santa Barbara.

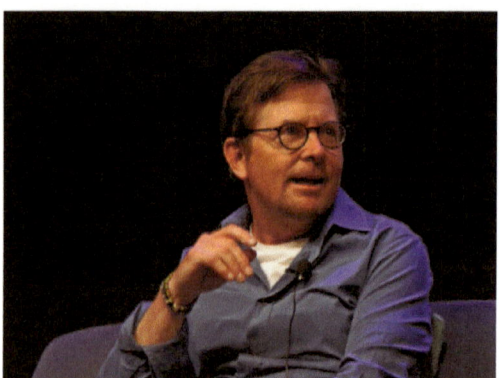

Photo 2.8   An example of a qualitative perspective: "Acceptance doesn't mean resignation; it means understanding that something is what it is and that there's got to be a way through it," says *Back to the Future* star Michael J. Fox, who has lived with Parkinson's disease since 1991.

Afterward, based on respondents' answers, researchers categorized the patients into either a low-stress group or a high-stress group. They could then use statistical analyses to determine whether the high-stress group experienced greater levels of pain than the low-stress group (**Photo 2.8**).

As in this example, qualitative studies aim to explore and describe the quality of experience, while quantitative studies aim to quantify or measure that experience. The first seeks to record the particulars of experience, while the second looks for generalizations from the data. Quantitative research is almost always hypothesis-driven: Researchers know ahead of time what ideas they are testing. A hypothesis is a proposed explanation for a phenomenon that a scientist seeks to test in a research study. In the case of this Parkinson's disease study, the researchers were interested in the impact of stress on the severity of pain. Their hypothesis might have been that Parkinson's patients who have high-stress experience more pain than those with low stress.

Variables

In health psychology, researchers are interested in the causes of illness and wellness. In other words, they are interested in how some factors, or variables, affect others. **Independent variables** (IVs) are the factors that researchers manipulate across different groups or conditions within the experiment. IVs are sometimes called predictor variables; both are used to examine changes in the DV. The main difference between independent and predictor variables is that IVs are manipulated by the experimenter and predictor variables are not. Predictor variables may just be measurements of a psychological construct and are used in nonexperimental designs. In our study of Parkinson's disease, the stress associated with symptoms is the predictor variable. Suppose instead that we subjected some patients to greater stress by, say, asking them to solve a tough problem, while asking other patients to relax. Stress would then be an IV.

Dependent variables (DVs) are the observed or expected outcomes that we record or measure. DVs are also called outcome variables. We are looking to see whether the IVs have influenced the DVs. In our example, we want to determine whether those who experience more stress also experience more pain as an outcome, and so pain is the DV. In empirical studies, researchers aim to determine the effects of the IV on the DV.

Correlation and Causation

Correlational research aims to find links between variables. In our example, researchers examined the links between the amount of stress associated with symptoms of Parkinson's disease and the degree of pain the patient experienced.

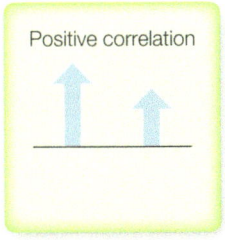

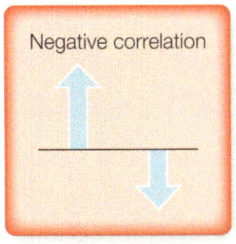

As one variable rises or falls, so does the other.

One variable changes in the opposite direction of the other.

Figure 2.2   Directions of influence in positive and negative correlations.

We might expect that the more stress a patient reports, the more painful his or her symptoms are. This is an example of a **positive correlation** between two variables: As one rises or falls, so does the other. More stress, more pain. In a **negative correlation**, two variables influence each other in the opposite direction: As one rises, the other falls; see **Figures** 2.2 and **2.3**. We might find, for example, that patients with more severe symptoms report less stress because they focus instead on the pain.

We can quantify a correlation using a **correlation coefficient**. The stronger the correlation, the larger the absolute value of the correlation coefficient. Correlation coefficients range from -1.00 (a perfect negative correlation) to 1.00 (a perfect positive correlation). The closer the coefficient is to 0.00 (no relationship between variables), the weaker the correlation is. We say that a correlation is significant if it meets a predetermined **level of significance**, which is reported as a p-value (or probability level). These p values represent the likelihood that you would find a correlation at least as large as the one you found, if there were really no relationship between the variables. So, when we say that the correlation had a p-value below a certain level, we mean that the value reached the threshold at which we are confident that it would be very unlikely if there were truly no relationship. Thus, the two variables are thought to influence each other. Correlational measures are invaluable to both disease detectives (like Darius) and health psychologists.

As useful as these tools are, keep in mind something important: Correlation does not mean causation. In our example, we cannot say that Parkinson's disease causes stress or that stress causes pain. Why not? Because maybe it works

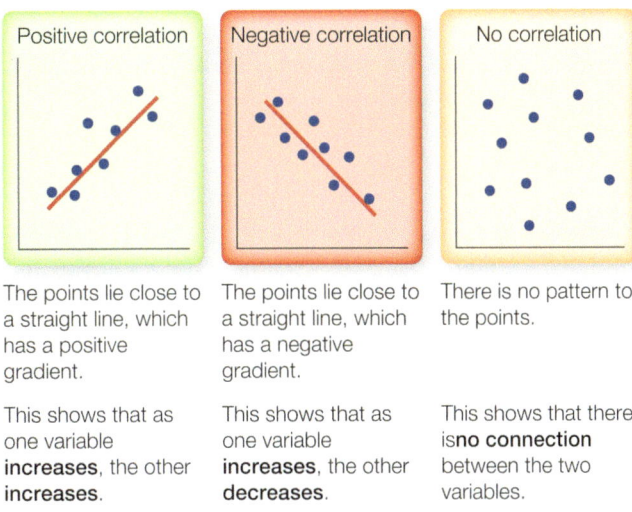

Figure 2.3   Different types of correlations.

the other way around and stress makes people more vulnerable to disease. Or perhaps a third factor has caused both stress and disease. Perhaps the support group is unusual, and a different sample would show a different outcome. Only a strictly designed experiment can provide causality, and only when three conditions have been met:

1. There is covariation, or the IV and the DV are related;
2. there is temporal precedence, or the IV (cause) precedes the DV (outcome) in time; and
3. there is a nonspurious relationship, or no plausible alternative explanation. In other words, the influence of the IV on the DV cannot be explained by some other, unstudied variable.

All we can say for sure, at least for now, is that in our study group, the more severe the disease, the greater the stress and pain.

Thinking About Health

■ Think about a health problem that you have experienced. Can you develop a hypothesis about what caused the problem?

■ What would the IV be? What about the DV?

■ How would you decide whether your hypothesis is right using a quantitative approach? A qualitative approach?

Experimental Studies

Experimental studies take place in carefully controlled laboratory settings. These settings are particularly important in clinical trials that test whether a drug works.

Experimental and Quasi-Experimental Research

Experimental research involves direct manipulation of the variable or variables within a carefully controlled experimental condition; see **Figure 2.4**. **Quasi-experimental research** resembles experimental studies but does not involve random assignment, nor IVs that can be controlled by the researcher. Because there is no random assignment of participants in quasi-experimental designs, we cannot rule out the influence of some unexamined variable, and thus cannot make claims of causality. In our example of Parkinson's disease, the study of quantitative evidence relied on quasi-experimental methods. When researchers recruit participants for studies involving self-report questionnaires, they are most often collecting quasi-experimental data.

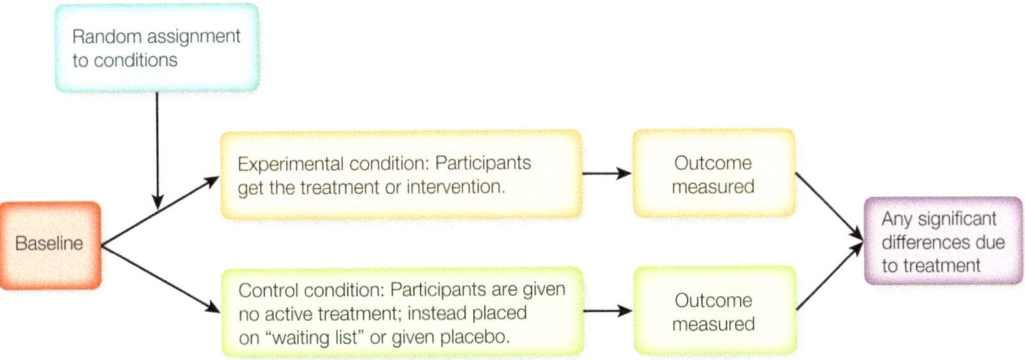

Figure 2.4   Elements of experimental design.

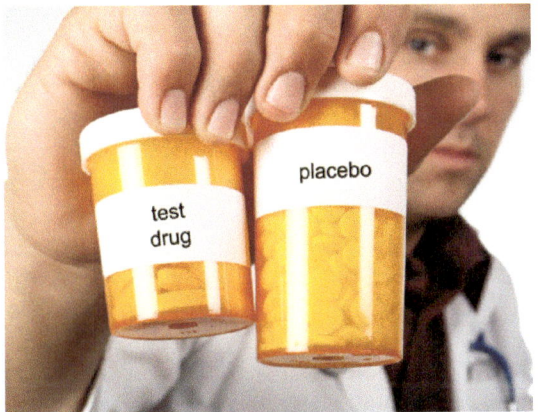

Photo 2.9   In clinical trials, there are often two groups: One receiving the experimental treatment and one receiving a placebo.

In both methods, researchers have defined ahead of time the variables that they wish to examine and the hypotheses that they wish to test. Additionally, researchers define the characteristics of the population under study and recruit participants based on whether they meet those criteria. Yet, in quasi-experimental research, there is still room for the complex, subjective nature of experience (**Photo 2.9**).

Experimental studies randomly assign participants to different conditions. These studies also make use of **a control group**, or a group that is not subjected to the condition we are testing. (We looked at an example of a control group in Chapter 1 Around the World feature when we compared neighborhoods that had been given soap and education about hand washing with those that hadn't.) Say, for example, that we are testing a treatment for Parkinson's disease. We would be sure to include a control group of people not receiving treatment.

Quasi-experimental studies are excellent for establishing differences between groups or links between variables. They can provide support for hypotheses—or prove them wrong.

Yet we still need experimental research to establish a cause. If you read a journal article that states, "This caused that," go back and carefully read the methods section. Were participants randomly assigned? Was there experimental manipulation of the variables? If so, you can have confidence in what the authors are reporting.

Clinical Trials

Consider a new drug for treating pain in Parkinson's patients. Is it effective? Does it have dangerous side effects? Before the drug manufacturer can market and sell the drug, it must gain approval from the U.S. Food and Drug

Administration—and to get that approval, the manufacturer must conduct extensive clinical trials, and carefully controlled studies to see whether the drug works.

Let's imagine a study in which patients with Parkinson's disease are randomly assigned to either an experimental group that receives the new drug or a control group that instead receives a **placebo**, usually an inert substance in the same form as the treatment (placebos are not always pills). Using a placebo is important because simply being treated can affect our minds and symptoms (we explore the placebo effect in greater detail in Chapter 12). In some studies, the control group receives a current treatment, the experimental group receives a new treatment, and the results are compared. In experimental clinical trials, patients are not told to which group they've been assigned. These are called **blind experiments**, because patients are unaware of, or blind to, the treatment they are receiving. In our imagined study, if there is a statistically significant difference between the pain reports of the experimental and control groups, then we can say that the drug had an effect on pain.

It is important to safeguard experimental testing to ensure scientific rigor—especially in testing new drugs. Even if the placebos all look, taste, and smell the same, something else may compromise the study: the researchers. Maybe the doctor acts more excited when handing out drugs that might help or seems more anxious for them to succeed. For this reason, a proper clinical trial is **a double-blind experiment**: No one involved, whether participant or researcher, is aware of the assigned experimental conditions (as seen in **Figure 2.5**).

A slightly different design is used when the treatment is not a drug, so we cannot offer a placebo. Suppose we have developed a program to help patients with Parkinson's disease manage the stress of their symptoms through deep breathing and relaxation, and we want to determine if this program works. The detailed plan of our study, which specifies our experimental, data collection, and sampling methods, is called the **experimental protocol**. Again, we randomly assign patients to the experimental group. This time, however, the control group is assigned to a "waiting list." Patients in the **wait list control group** are told that they are "on call" in case a spot opens up for the new treatment. (Typically, participants in waitlist control groups do not receive treatment until after the completion of the study. So, the wait list group is sort of like the placebo group in a clinical protocol.) We then compare the results of each group, and, if our treatment is effective, we expect to see lower rates of stress in the group receiving treatment. Experimental studies like these provide the evidence-based knowledge that allows practitioners to provide the best care.

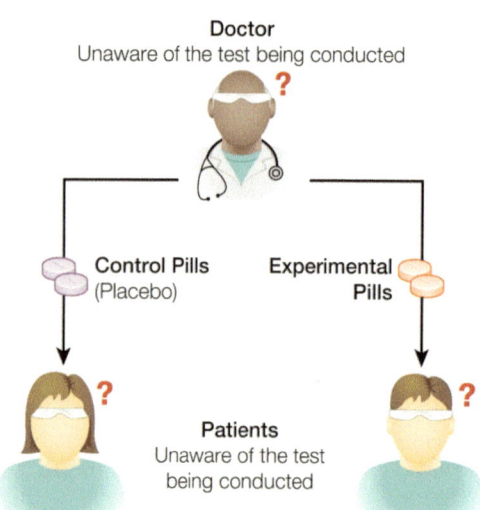

Figure 2.5   The double-blind experiment procedure.

Thinking About Health

- What are the main differences between quasi-experimental and experimental designs?
- Why is it important to know whether a research study is based on quasi-experimental or experimental designs?
- Why is it important to run double-blind experiments?

Cross-Sectional and Longitudinal Designs

In research, we often seek to answer two types of questions: One, how do people compare to one another? And two, how do people change over time? There are two common research designs that allow us to address these questions.

Cross-Sectional Studies

Cross-sectional studies generally collect data from a group (or groups) of people at a specific point in time, taking a "snapshot" of behavior. For example, a cross-sectional study might compare how different age groups care for their health or respond to a treatment. In contrast, **longitudinal studies** follow individuals through their lifespan, determining how they change and grow over time. Longitudinal studies help determine how genetics, environment, and lifestyle influence the risk and development of disease. As Alan Castel (2019) says, "Watching our children grow up or our parents grow old" illustrates how people change over time, and is a way to think about longitudinal research. "Comparing ourselves to our children" illustrates how times change and people differ and is a way to think about cross-sectional research.

Cross-cultural studies: A cross-cultural study, a type of cross-sectional study, can help us understand how cultural differences affect our health. What we learn about disparities in health is often the result of cross-cultural research. For example, one study sought to determine the best way to motivate mothers to have their children vaccinated against human papillomavirus (HPV), a sexually transmitted infection (Lechuga, Swain, & Weinhardt, 2011). The researchers compared three groups of women: Hispanics, whites, and African Americans. Each group was presented with the following two health messages:

- "If you vaccinate your daughter, you can protect her from cervical cancer."
- "If you don't vaccinate your daughter, you miss the opportunity of protecting her from cervical cancer."

The first message was framed as a gain, the second as a loss. The two messages worked equally well to motivate white mothers. However, the "loss" frame worked better for Hispanic mothers and for African American mothers (Lechuga et al., 2011). By examining different groups, the study was able to uncover important cultural differences that affect healthcare decisions and, potentially, health. Other cross-sectional studies may be stratified by age or gender instead of by culture.

Developmental Studies

Developmental studies are concerned with how age or developmental stage relates to some outcome. Both cross-sectional and longitudinal methods can be used in developmental studies. Say we are interested in whether young adults (between the ages of 18 and 25) or older adults (older than 65) are more likely to practice healthful behaviors. To find out, we take two "snapshots," or "cross sections," of the population.

This is a developmental study because we are interested in differences between the two age groups. Recall from Chapter 1 how health psychology takes a developmental perspective, as we shall do often in this book. Here we take age as our IV. We recruit and interview 100 young adults and 100 older adults about their daily health practices. How likely, we ask, are you to do each of the following? We then present choices, such as eating a nutritious breakfast, not smoking, and wearing seatbelts.

Suppose we find that older adults practice more healthful behaviors. We might conclude that, as one gets older, one is more likely to adopt a healthy lifestyle. After all, older adults might be more concerned with living longer. Remember, however, that correlation is not causation. Perhaps today's older adults are always more health-conscious. For example, baby boomers, the generation born between 1946 and 1964, enjoyed America's postwar prosperity. They may have been influenced by the health food craze in America or by nutritional labels that began appearing on food packaging in 1990. Perhaps they are less likely to sit around texting and more likely to complete crossword puzzles or get exercise. Any of these could make them healthier. We speak of groups with a shared experience or lifestyle as cohorts, and we call factors like these **cohort effects**.

How then might age influence health outcomes? To decide, we turn now to longitudinal studies (**Photo 2.10**).

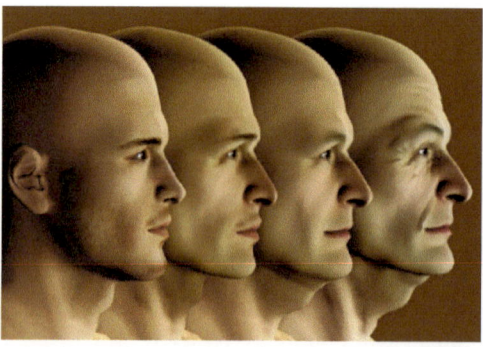 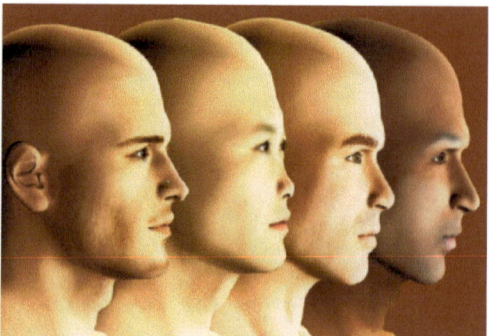

Photo 2.10 (a and b)   Two types of studies are illustrated here: Longitudinal studies (left) follow one person over time (one man at age 20, 40, 60, and 80); cross-sectional studies (right) compare groups of people at the same point in time (men age 20 from different racial/ethnic groups).

Longitudinal Studies

As we now know, a cross-sectional study compares groups of participants at a particular point in time. A longitudinal study, however, follows participants over time, to determine how their behaviors change with age, personal growth, or development. Rather than providing a snapshot, it is more like a movie; see **Table 2.1**. From a lifespan developmental perspective, this is the ideal way to learn about how personal growth influences health.

In our example, as we grow older, do we, in fact, become more conscientious about health? To find out, we would survey a group of young adults and then survey these same participants periodically until they reach old age. We could then see whether their health behavior changed over time.

When we recruit teenagers into a study and follow them over time to see what health issues develop in adulthood, we can see how early experiences shape later behaviors. One longitudinal study surveyed New Zealanders about their use of marijuana between the ages of 18 to 38 and found that, after controlling for tobacco use, those who had smoked pot had poorer dental health, but pot smoking was unrelated to any other health problems in midlife (Meier et al., 2012). Tobacco use, on the other hand, was associated with poorer health outcomes in middle age. By tracking people's health for 20 years, the researchers were able to determine how early risk behaviors play out later in life. This is an example of a developmental longitudinal study.

Prospective and retrospective studies: Some longitudinal studies are also called **prospective studies** because they follow individuals forward through time,

Cohort year of birth	Age							
2000	15	16	17	18	19	20	21	22
2001	14	15	16	17	18	19	20	21
2002	13	14	15	16	17	18	19	10
2003	12	13	14	15	16	17	18	19
2004	11	12	13	14	15	16	17	18
2005	10	11	12	13	14	15	16	17
2006	9	10	11	12	13	14	15	16
2007	8	9	10	11	12	13	14	15
2008	7	8	9	10	11	12	13	14
2009	6	7	8	9	10	11	12	13
2010	5	6	7	8	9	10	11	12

Time of measurement

Indicates a cross-sectional comparison of ages

Indicates a longitudinal comparison of ages

Table 2.1 Comparisons made in cross-sectional versus longitudinal designs

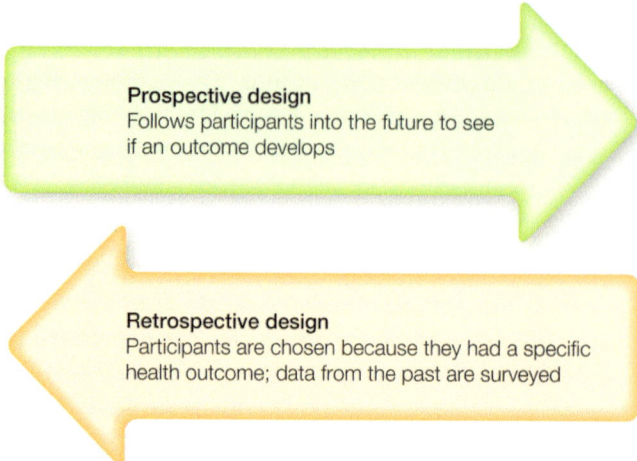

Figure 2.6   Prospective and retrospective designs.

as shown in **Figure 2.6**. How dangerous, for example, is HPV? To answer this question, a study recruited a random sample of 11,088 Danish women between the ages of 20 and 29 (Kjaer et al., 2002). These women were then given annual cervical exams for five years. Nearly half showed no sign of HPV at the start of the study, and they served as the control group. Of the women who did have HPV at enrollment, 80% went on to develop precancerous lesions or cervical cancer. These results highlight the importance of early detection and regular gynecological exams. These health outcomes were discovered by following the development of disease over time.

Retrospective studies look back in time instead, starting with current health status, to discover how past exposure or experience may lead to a present condition; see **Figure 2.6**. This research is called chart review, as it often involves the examination of existing records, much like a doctor in a hospital going over a patient's chart. Let's say a large number of adults are given a diagnosis of tooth decay this year: We might go back and look at their sugar consumption, frequency of dental cleanings, and the amount of fluoride in the water during their childhood years. Our examination might allow us to determine which of those factors led to the development of dental decay in adulthood. Although not as empirically strong as other methods, a retrospective study can help determine what factors influence health. Reliance on existing records is also important for epidemiologists like Darius at the start of this chapter, who could gather important data by examining the causes of death listed on death certificates.

E ach research method can provide valuable information about people and their health.

Evidence-based science helps health psychology reach the goals that we identified in Chapter 1. It allows us to identify the causes of health and illness, to promote and maintain good health, to prevent and treat illness, and, ultimately, to improve health care policy. Just how, though, is research translated into patient care? **Figure 2.7** tracks the steps from testing a new drug to shaping health care.

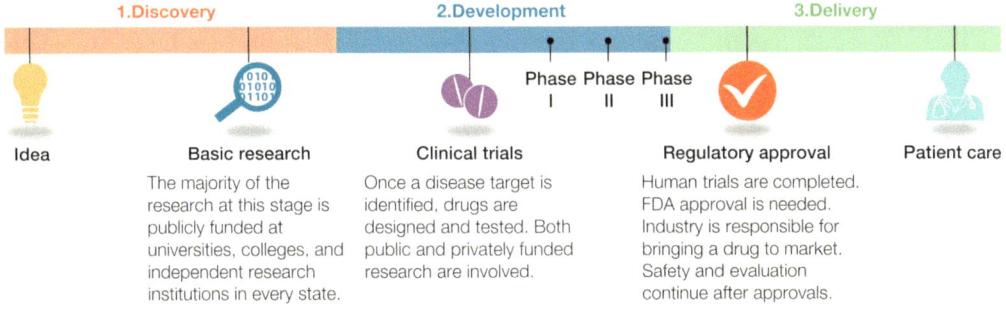

1.Discovery		2.Development		3.Delivery	
Idea	Basic research	Clinical trials		Regulatory approval	Patient care
	The majority of the research at this stage is publicly funded at universities, colleges, and independent research institutions in every state.	Once a disease target is identified, drugs are designed and tested. Both public and privately funded research are involved.		Human trials are completed. FDA approval is needed. Industry is responsible for bringing a drug to market. Safety and evaluation continue after approvals.	

Figure 2.7 Stages in the research process.

Thinking About Health

- How do cross-sectional and longitudinal studies differ?
- Why is a developmental approach so important in health psychology?
- What problems might arise in retrospective and prospective studies and influence the interpretation of the results?

The Ethics of Experiments

Today, any institution in the United States that receives federal funding must protect research participants from harm. Whether they are colleges, universities, pharmaceutical firms, or biotechnology companies, institutions all work within guidelines established for ethical research on humans and animals.

Researchers must gain consent from human participants, and there must be no unnecessary invasive medical procedures. Any scientist planning a study must first gain approval from an **Institutional Review Board (IRB)**. The IRB consists of members of the research institution, the institution's legal counsel, and an additional person, usually someone with medical or legal expertise.

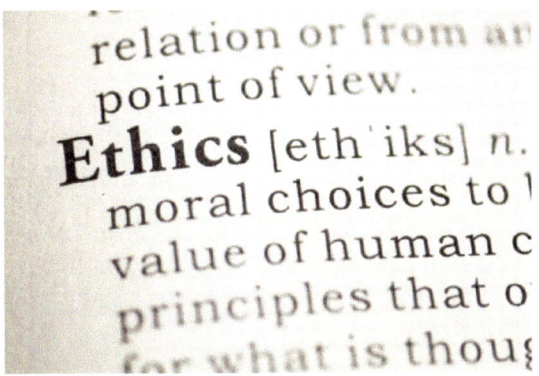

Photo 2.11 Ethics are important in science.

The Tuskegee Experiment

Approval is necessary because research has a tainted past. In the name of science, studies have been conducted that seriously endangered and harmed participants. Some participants were forced to take part or unknowingly took part in studies. One of the most devastating and scandalous medical experiments was also one of the darkest moments in American history (**Photo 2.11**).

The Tuskegee experiment began in Alabama in 1932 and ran for 40 years. Six hundred poor, rural African American sharecroppers (all men) were asked to participate in a study of "bad blood," a local term for illness. In exchange, they were given free medical care and meals. Only later, if at all, did they learn the experiment's real purpose—to examine the effects of untreated syphilis on the body. At the start of the study, 399 of the men had the disease but were never told. A treatment finally became available in 1947, but they were denied it (Danner, Darnell, & McGuire, 2011). They were also subjected to painful spinal taps in order to draw fluids for analysis. And they had to agree to an autopsy to receive free burial insurance. In 1972, when the study ended, only 74 participants were still alive. By then, 28 had died of the disease, and 100 had died from disease-related complications. Forty of their wives were unknowingly infected, and 19 of their children were born with a disabling and often life-threatening form of the disease (Kampmeier, 1974). The U.S. Department of Health, Education, and Welfare shut down the study in 1972, but only after it had become a political embarrassment **(Photo 2.12)**.

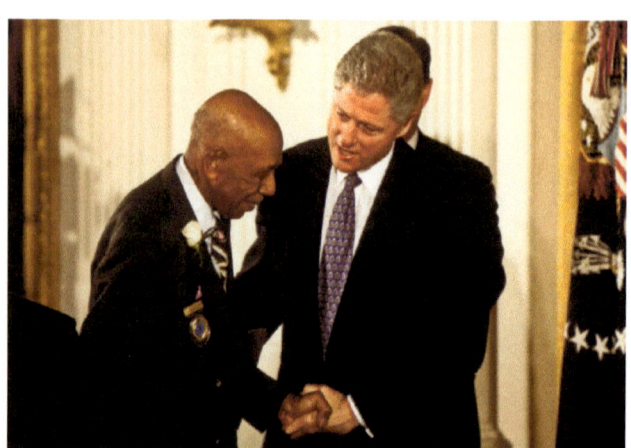

Photo 2.12 President Clinton apologized in 1997 to the survivors of the Tuskegee experiments.

In May 1997, President Bill Clinton apologized in person to the eight remaining survivors. He is quoted as saying,

The eight men who are survivors of the syphilis study at Tuskegee are a living link to a time not so very long ago that many Americans would prefer not to remember, but we dare not forget. It was a time when our nation failed to live up to its ideals, when our nation broke the trust with our people that is the very foundation of our democracy. It is not only in remembering that shameful past that we can make amends and repair our nation, but it is in remembering that past that we can build a better present and a better future.

Codes of Ethics

Another stimulus to ethical reform came after World War II. German physicians had conducted painful and often deadly medical experiments on concentration camp prisoners without their consent (Annas & Grodin, 1992). These atrocities led to the conviction of camp physicians and administrators for crimes of war and crimes against humanity. It also led to the creation of the Nuremberg Code, a 10-point directive for the ethical treatment of human study participants. However, although it was a step in the right direction, the code lacked the force of law and served only as a guideline.

The U.S. National Research Act took the next step forward in 1974. It created a commission to develop and oversee ethical principles for research involving humans. These principles, laid out in the Belmont Report of 1978, became law three years later. Additional protections were signed into law in 1991. Unfortunately, these measures arrived too late to be applied to many classic psychology experiments. The Stanford Prison Experiment (1970s), the Milgram obedience experiment (1960s), and Harlow's studies on dependency in monkeys (1950s), for instance, would not be considered ethical today.

Until recently, the United States was the only country that continued to use chimpanzees in medical research. Chimps were intentionally infected with diseases, such as hepatitis or HIV, and subject to surgical procedures. In November 2015, the National Institutes of Health announced that it would no longer support any invasive research on chimps and that the 300 or so chimps remaining in research facilities would move to a federally approved sanctuary. The Endangered Species Act was modified in 2015, listing chimps as an endangered species, thus making it even more difficult for biomedical science to use chimps in experiments (Echavez, 2015).

Science in the Twenty-First Century

Within the last decade, science, and particularly psychological science, has come under fire in both the popular press and within scientific communities. At issue is whether or not we can trust scientific findings that cannot be replicated. Advocates of the replicability crisis suggest that there are many historically significant findings within the field that are taken as fact, but that cannot be reproduced scientifically today; thus, these findings may no longer explain behavior and should not be used to shape theory and practice in the field. The replicability crisis involves the culmination of three factors: unscrupulous researchers who committed scientific fraud and falsified data, the publication of articles that criticized the research practices of historic studies, and, finally, the failure to replicate these historic studies by a group of researchers affiliated with the Open Science Collaboration (osf.io).

As we have seen in this chapter, health psychology generates knowledge by relying on hypothesis testing and sound empirical methods. However, if a finding from one research study cannot be replicated in another laboratory with a different sample of participants, should the findings be reported and trusted? For example, imagine you are searching for scientific evidence of the most effective natural sleep aid, and you come across a study that touts the many advantages of reading poetry for 30 minutes before bedtime. Before you buy a new poetry book, you would want to evaluate the study's methods and check if other researchers have tested this hypothesis and found the same results. Replication in science is an important issue, and many researchers are now conducting their scientific investigations in ways that allow their empirical methods, hypotheses, data analyses, and findings to be easily tested by others.

Some researchers now provide the data that they have collected from their studies online, free for other scientists to test themselves. This practice, called **open science**, is an important advancement in addressing the replicability crisis (Shrout & Rodgers, 2018). Open science involves full disclosure of all the factors that may have influenced researchers' analyses and findings, including those findings that were not statistically significant. Now, many researchers believe that the "replicability crisis" has led to better science—specifically, to new and important insights and practices that can improve psychological science in the twenty-first century and beyond (Shrout & Rodgers, 2018).

> ## Thinking About Health
>
> ■ How concerned are you about ethics in science?
> ■ What are your views on human or animal participation in medical research?
> ■ How does open science positively affect psychological research?

The Cutting Edge of Science: Advancing Our Understanding of Health

So far, we have looked at research involving people and their experience of health and disease. More and more, however, we can investigate the interplay between genes, the environment, and psychology directly. However, when doing so, we must also take into account global differences in health and beliefs.

Social Genomics and Epigenetics

Social genomics (or social neuroscience) aims to understand genetic, chemical, hormonal, and neural mechanisms using complex technologies and methodologies to examine the reciprocal interactions between biological, cognitive, and social levels of analysis (Slavich & Cole, 2013). It studies how genes and the environment interact to influence health and behavior in ways never seen before.

One approach looks at how emotions can influence genes. Yes, we inherit our genes from our parents, and possessing particular genes leads to such familiar characteristics as eye color and even temperament. However, in one study that examined how emotions influence genes, lonelier people had genes that overexpressed for inflammatory responses to bacterial infections but had a weakened response to viruses. They suffered from greater inflammation but also a higher risk of viral infection (Cole, Hawkley, Arevalo, & Cacioppo, 2011; Cole, Hawkley, Arevalo, Sung, & Cacioppo, 2007). In fact, peer victimization during adolescence, a highly potent source of social stress, can lead to enduring risk for poor mental and physical health by increasing inflammatory responses (**Photo 2.13**) (Giletta et al., 2018).

Childhood adversity, too, may make us more prone to inflammatory responses (Miller et al., 2009). People who grew up in troubled, impoverished, and emotionally challenging conditions compared with those who grew up in high-income and low-challenge environments had greater proinflammatory genes, which put them at greater risk for cardiovascular disease and cancer later

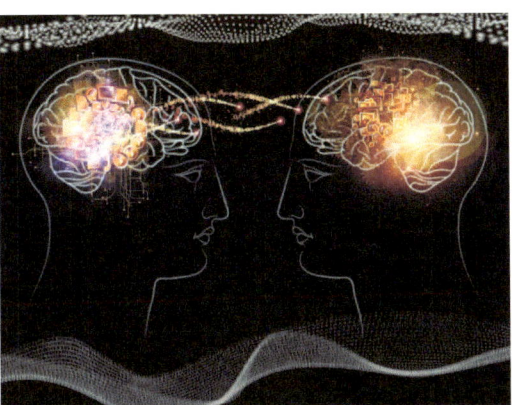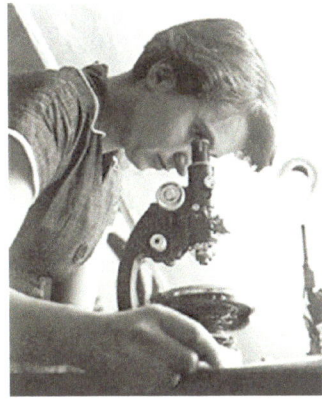

Photo 2.13 (a and b)   Social genomics studies how genes and environment influence health and behavior. This discipline could not exist without Dr. Rosalind Franklin, right, whose experimental data led to the discovery of the structure of DNA.

in life, even if their family incomes improved over time. More generally, our early environment may put us at greater risk of heart disease and cancer by influencing the genetic impact on immune functioning.

Today's advances in genetics officially began in February 1953, when Dr. James Watson and Dr. Francis Crick, guided by the experimental data of Dr. Rosalind Franklin, discovered the structure of DNA, the double helix. DNA is the molecule that carries genetic information from one generation to the next, in the form of chromosomes. Each cell in your body has 46 chromosomes in 23 pairs, half from each parent. Together they make up our genetic inheritance, the **human genome**. These discoveries earned Watson and Crick the Nobel Prize in 1962 (**Photo 2.14**).

In 1991, the United States began the Human Genome Project, with the goal of identifying the nearly 25,000 genes in the body. The project was completed in 2003 (Collins, Morgan, & Patrinos, 2003). These advances gave way to the field of epigenetics, the study of gene expression. **Epigenetics** is the scientific exploration of what factors cause genes to turn on or turn off, thereby influencing what is genetically expressed. Factors such as diet, stressors, or environmental pollutants can trigger a marker on a gene to express or be inhibited from expression.

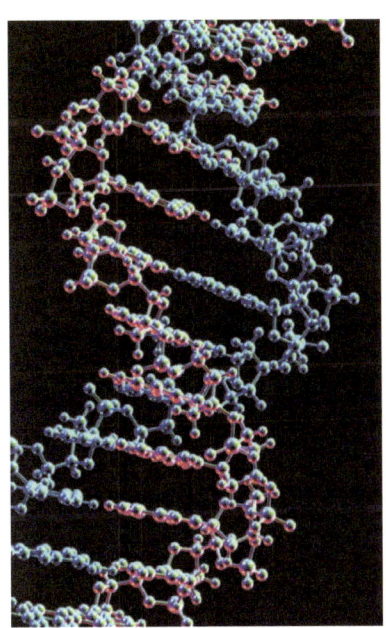

Photo 2.14   The double helix.

In the health field, epigenetics is a popular research area because understanding these markers could provide a different way to treat disease. For instance, removing a bad marker or adding a good marker to change disease outcomes is a real treatment possibility. As we learn the genetic markers for disease, health psychologists can better target treatment and prevention efforts. Thanks to social genomics, we can expect to learn how experience affects our genes as well.

Understanding the Microbiome

In recent years, the gut has been found to play a pivotal role in the complex ecosystem of the human body. The gastrointestinal track, or gut, is the interface between your body and the outside world, serving as the front line of the immune system through constant exposure to molecules and microbes in food and drink. We now know that there are important connections among the gut, the central nervous system, the brain, and our emotional and physical health. Within the gut live bacterial microbes or microorganisms, some that make us sick and some that are critical for health. These microbes contain genetic information referred to as the **microbiome**.

Each of us has a unique microbiome, and the microbiota within it is constantly in flux. We now know that the microbiota-gut-brain axis is critical for health. Stress, for example, can change the internal environment of the gut to make it less hospitable for "good" bacteria while increasing the growth of "bad" bacteria. These changes can influence our brain chemistry and signaling and can alter our moods, pain sensitivity, immune functioning, cognitive functioning, and risk for disease (Johnson & Acabchuk, 2018; Tang et al., 2017). Due to the importance of maintaining a healthy environment for the gut biome, many people have turned to special diets to maintain their health and well-being.

Many factors impact the microbiome, and the gut of each individual is unique. However, the global challenges we face—such as increasing obesity rates, reliance upon processed foods, and widespread use of antibiotics—are impacting the health and diversity of microbiomes.

Improving Science

As you can see from this chapter, the research methods we use are critical for advancing our scientific understanding of the psychological influences on health, health decision-making, behavioral change, and well-being. In the field of psychology more broadly, many of the most famous studies have come under fire because their findings could not be replicated, and this has led scientists to question the credibility and accuracy of some of the research findings we rely on to guide our understanding of psychological phenomena.

The Replication Crisis in psychology became an important topic in the field in the 2010s, when some scientists became skeptical of the way that data was collected, analyzed, and reported in research journals. These questionable research practices led to a series of replication projects where some of the major research studies in the field were conducted again and findings were not replicated. When researchers were only able to reproduce the results in less than half of the studies, the conclusion was that the original research findings were "false positives." This led to scrutiny of how our research practices can lead to false positives, or in rare cases, the fabrication of research findings. Pressure on scientists to "publish or perish" has incentivized them to publish quickly and often and that may have led to less stringent methods. At the same time, the journals that scientists publish in are incentivized to publish surprising and interesting results and that has led to a publication bias toward publishing positive findings rather than reporting when there are no effects. Some have argued that the field is also limited because historically it has only supported, funded, and published research from a small and select group of scholars.

The field of psychology is not alone in this replicability crisis, other fields like economics and medicine have struggled with reproducibility as well.

How can we be sure that the science we consume is valid and reliable? Scientists have pushed for greater transparency in how studies are planned and conducted as well as what the data looks like and how it is analyzed. Several strategies are now being used to achieve this. First, researchers aim to increase the size of their sample and conduct replications within their own studies. Second, we can publicly preregister our hypotheses and study plans ahead of time within some journals and then come back and publish our results. When this is done in the form of a "registered report" the journal will publish the results even if they didn't end up supporting the hypotheses. Finally, we can make our data publicly available for others to use to replicate our findings. These efforts have led to what is known as Open Science, or the movement dedicated to the core beliefs that science should be transparent, credible, reproducible, and accessible.

Global Challenges

In advancing our knowledge of health, global differences raise both practical and ethical challenges. Scientists need to recruit volunteers who are fully aware of what they will be going through, as ethical standards require. Researchers also need funding to cover materials, remuneration for participants, the training of research assistants, and new technology.

The challenges are greater still for researchers who wish to study populations in other countries. They must request approvals from different governments, find collaborators and translators, and convert to foreign technologies. However, perhaps the greatest obstacle has to do with different beliefs about health. People in extremely rural and impoverished areas may view an urban scientist with suspicion, making it harder to obtain experimental and control groups. Perspectives on the urgency of climate change (see the Around the World feature) may vary by geographic region. People may assess their health in ways that make evidence-based research more difficult still. Think of applying the narrowly defined questions of experimental studies to other cultures. Epidemiologists like Darius at the start of this chapter might face concern for their own safety—or for the safety of study participants.

Never has it been more important to develop open lines of communication. Scientists, epidemiologists, and public health workers must find ways to forge working relationships with people around the world (**Photo 2.15**).

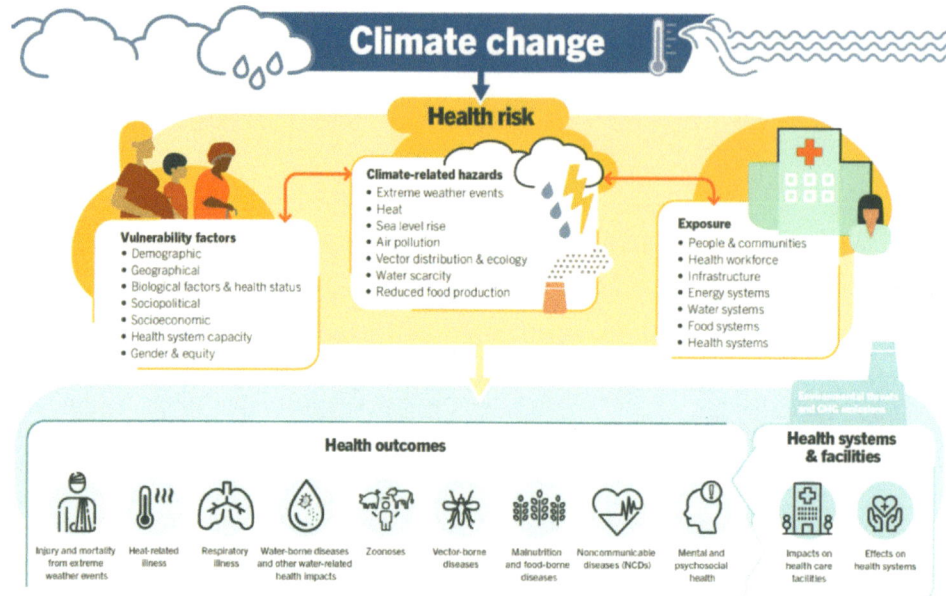

Photo 2.15   How climate change can impact human health.

Thinking About Health

■ If you had a gene that put you at risk for a life-threatening disease, would you rather know or not know about it? Why or why not?

■ Can you see any potential dangers in grouping people based on genetic explanations of health problems?

■ What is the microbiome, and why is it so important for health?

■ What are some of the global challenges that make health research difficult, and how can we overcome them?

Around *the* World

Every day it seems there are news headlines, "Deadly New Year's Day Earthquake Devastates Japan's west coast," "Where did the snow go?" "'Significant damage' reported as storm moves through Britain," and "Germany hit by floods after rainfall hits record highs," that point to the negative effects of climate change. Increasingly those news stories point to the detrimental impact that climate change and the natural disasters it causes have on the health of humans, wildlife, and the planet itself. Over 99% of the worldwide scientific community agrees that human behavior is causing current climate change

through unmitigated greenhouse gas emissions (Lynas et al., 2021). According to the World Health Organization (2024) heatwaves, wildfires, floods, hurricanes and tropical storms, and drought are directly caused by climate change. Moreover, they forecast that between 2030 and 2050 close to 250,000 additional deaths per year will be caused by undernutrition, malaria, diarrhea, and heat stress resulting from climate change and climate disasters. In addition, non-life-threatening conditions related to the environment are also increasing like asthma, Lyme disease, cardiovascular disease, bacterial intestinal diseases, and many others. Climate change impacts our health by disrupting food systems, increasing food, water, and vector-borne diseases, impacting our mental health, the economy, and equality and access to health care and social support systems. People most at risk are those who are most vulnerable and disadvantaged such as women, children, older people, ethnic minorities, disabled people and people with underlying health conditions, migrants or displaced individuals, and those from poor communities.

Each of us can do more to educate ourselves about how our behaviors contribute to global warming and climate change, our own health, and global health. But many people may not be aware of how their behaviors impact the environment. How would you design a research experiment to find out what people know about how their behaviors influence climate change or how climate change influences their health? Who would your participants be? How would you gather information on their knowledge and behaviors? What are your hypotheses? Who would benefit from the results of your study? How could you make an impact on people's knowledge and behavior with this study?

Chapter Summary

Health psychology is an evidence-based science. Epidemiology is concerned with measuring the risks and course of disease through such factors as mortality rate, morbidity, incidence, and prevalence. Research methods used by health psychologists and epidemiologists sometimes differ in the evidence they use and the variables they test. A quasi-experimental design allows for more open-ended answers, while an experimental design is necessary in clinical trials to prove the safety and efficacy of treatment. Cross-sectional studies include cross-cultural research and developmental research. But developmental research can also be longitudinal. Prospective and retrospective research is also longitudinal in that time is a main factor in the gathering of data. Research proposals must gain approval from IRBs to ensure the ethical treatment of human and animal participants. The Human Genome Project and other cutting-edge advances are expanding the range of research methods available. More recent research studies of the microbiome have revealed that the gut is the first line of defense in the human immune system. As scientists continue to apply these methods, we can address global health problems from snakebites to global warming.

KEY TERMS ▶   evidence-based practice p. 39; theory p. 39; hypothesis p. 39; mortality rate p. 40; contagious diseases p. 40; morbidity p. 40; incidence p. 41; prevalence p. 41; lifetime prevalence p. 41; surveillance p. 41; descriptive studies p. 41; analytic studies p. 41; quantitative data p. 43; qualitative data p. 43; IVs (or *predictor variables*) p. 44; DVs (or *outcome variables*) p. 44; correlational research p. 44; positive correlation p. 45; negative correlation p. 45; correlation coefficient p. 45; level of significance p. 45; experimental research p. 46; quasi-experimental research p. 46; control group p. 47; clinical trials p. 47; placebo p. 48; blind experiments p. 48; double-blind experiment p. 48; experimental protocol p. 48; wait list control group p. 48; cross-sectional studies p. 49; longitudinal studies p. 49; cross-cultural study p. 49; developmental study p. 50; cohort effects p. 50; prospective studies p. 51; retrospective studies p. 52; Institutional Review Board (IRB) p. 53; Tuskegee experiment p. 54; open science p. 55; social genomics (or *social neuroscience*) p. 56; human genome p. 57; epigenetics p. 57; microbiome p. 58.

CHAPTER 3

Health Beliefs and Behaviors

Learning Outcomes

After reading this chapter, you should be able to:

- Describe why health promotion and disease prevention are important.
- Compare and contrast the different models of behavior change.
- Define health behaviors, health habits, health goals, and health values.
- Identify potential factors that influence lasting change versus relapse.
- Explain the Alameda County Study: what it found and why it is important.
- Describe the role that health disparities play in health behaviors.
- Outline the factors that promote and. create barriers to good health behaviors.

Elena's New Year's resolution is to lose that "freshman 15," the weight that she gained in her first semester of college. She misses her healthy, athletic self, and she is excited to have received a wearable fitness tracker for the holidays. Each day, it records her steps, the total distance she walks, her heart rate, the calories she burns, and even her sleep—and then shares the data with an online community of fitness buffs like her. She has joined the "quantified self movement," which means knowing yourself through your numbers and encourages people to use electronic devices (such as sensors and wearables) to improve their understanding of health and to gain insights into ways to positively change their health and their lives (Didžiokaite et al., 2018; Feng et al., 2021; Ruckenstein & Pantzar, 2017). One in five people in the United States own a fitness tracker or smartwatch (Vogels, 2020). Sales of Smartwaches are still growing and reached $110 billion dollar revenue in 2023 (Pangarkar, 2024) (**Photo 3.1**).

Fast-forward six months to June. Elena is finishing her second semester in better shape than ever. She walks 10,000 steps every day, works out regularly, and eats healthy meals. She enjoys seeing her progress each day and sharing her fitness goals with her family, friends, and online community.

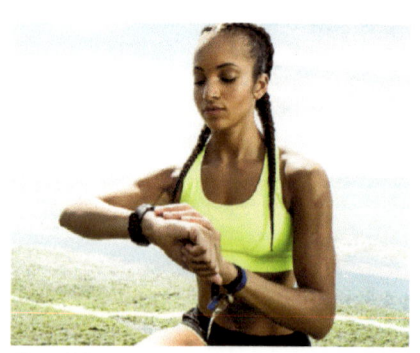

Photo 3.1

Source: Igor Emmerich/Getty Images

DOI: 10.4324/9781032643090-3

They, too, are impressed. All those years as the star of the varsity soccer team are nothing compared to what she has achieved with daily self-monitoring. Technology truly can promote positive changes in behavior. But does it really help people achieve better health?

Like Elena, perhaps you own a self-monitoring device. How does it influence your thoughts and behaviors, from eating to exercise? What does your data say about you? Health and fitness apps are creating an enormous mine of information that researchers are eager to analyze. Self-monitoring devices are everywhere, and research is showing that they help most people make long-term, lasting changes (Mishra et al., 2023). Some people find these devices fun and motivating; for example, Elena loves that she can tell whether she has reached her ideal fat-burning zone in each workout. For other people, self-monitoring can become a source of additional stress (Pogue, 2015).

In this chapter, we ask what influences health beliefs and behaviors. We look at how people make decisions regarding their health and well-being, from daily habits to setting health goals to adhering to treatments for chronic illness. We examine the difficulties in changing behavior and maintaining changes, even after the novelty of devices like Elena's has worn off. As you explore the different theories, ask yourself if they can explain Elena's experiences. As always, health psychologists take a bio-psychosocial approach, considering individual, global, and cultural differences.

Health Promotion and Disease Prevention

Currently, the leading cause of death worldwide is cardiovascular disease (Caceres et al., 2018; WHO, 2023c). Heart disease is preventable. Both men and women can lower their risk by as much as 90% by living a healthy lifestyle (Caceres et al., 2018). In fact, more than half of all deaths and many illnesses could be prevented if people were to change their behaviors in just three areas: tobacco use, obesity, and lack of physical activity (Oddone et al., 2018). The United States has a high prevalence of these three risk factors and the greatest number of preventable deaths of all industrialized nations. In the United States, the COVID-19 pandemic is the fourth leading cause and is also related to elevations in the top three causes of death (Shiels et al., 2022). The United States is not alone in the high incidence of these risk factors (**Photo 3.2**).

How do we tackle these issues? **Health promotion** refers to activities that promote or maintain good health, such as eating right and staying physically active. **Disease prevention** refers to

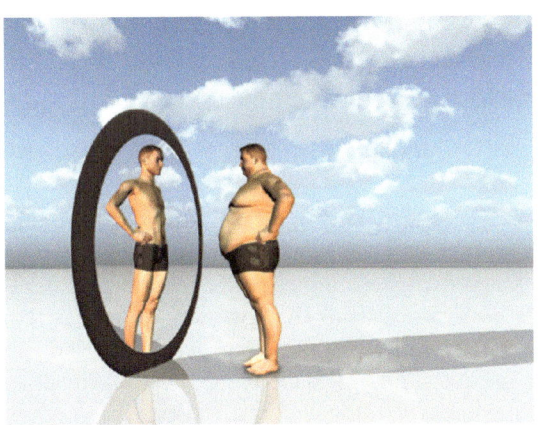

Photo 3.2   Making healthy choices increases life satisfaction in the present. Visualizing our "possible selves" can help us live healthier lives in the future.

actions that reduce the risk of negative health outcomes, such as getting regular checkups and not smoking. In this section, we look at the behaviors and habits that contribute to both promotion and prevention. Achieving the goals of health psychology—health promotion and disease prevention—means developing healthy habits that reduce the risk of negative health outcomes.

Many people strive to be healthy. Although habits ebb and flow across the lifespan, good health and the absence of disease or disability are strongly related to satisfaction with life (Strine et al., 2009). As Eleanor Roosevelt said, "Happiness is not a goal…. It's a by-product of a life well lived." But what leads to a healthy lifestyle? For Elena, it was a fitness self-monitoring 2009). As Eleanor Roosevelt said, "Happiness is not a goal…. It's a by-product of a life well lived." But what leads to a healthy lifestyle? For Elena, it was a fitness self-monitoring device. What about for the rest of us? As we will see next, all it takes is time and setting the right goals.

Health Goals and Health Values

Part of developing good health habits is taking the time to set the right goals. Health goals define the way we envision our future selves, and they play a big part in motivating behaviors. Health-related goals (whether "to be fit," "to run a half marathon," or "to avoid lung cancer") motivate us to engage in healthy behaviors on a day-to-day basis (Frazier & Hooker, 2006). The more important the health-related goal, the more actively we pursue it through healthful decisions and behaviors.

For example, researchers asked adults to imagine or visualize their goals for the future, or for their "possible selves." Participants were then asked how important this future self-representation was, what specific activities they engaged in to make their goals a reality, and if they believed that they would reach their goals in the future. Findings show that the more important the health-related goal, the more daily health behaviors people engaged in, and the more capable they felt of achieving the goal in the future (Dark-Freudeman & West, 2016; Frazier & Hooker, 2006; Hooker & Kaus, 1992). Our health-related possible selves drive health behaviors across the lifespan (Frazier & Hooker, 2006). They influence how we feel about growing older, especially in later life (Turner & Hooker, 2022), they impact our desire to achieve **health goals** and our hope to avoid negative health outcomes, including death (Dark-Freudeman & Bensadon, 2022).

When faced with the need to change behavior (e.g., the need to become more physically active), evoking possible selves is linked to self-efficacy and desired outcomes (Strachan, Marcotte, Giller, Brunet, & Schellenberg, 2017). Future-oriented health images motivate health behaviors even in college students (Hooker, 1992; Ouellette, Hessling, Gibbons, Reis-Bergan, & Gerrard, 2005). In a recent systematic review of adolescents' health risks and health-promoting behaviors simply having a possible self and feeling like you can achieve it was most important for achieving good health outcomes and avoiding negative ones (Corte et al., 2022). Furthermore, when individuals share their possible selves with others, the possibility of changing behaviors in response to health risks increases. For example, when spouses share each other's goals for health, the likelihood that the goals will be attained increases. This can be especially important when facing health stressors such as cancer (Wilson, Barrineau, Butner, & Berg, 2014).

The more central we make a goal, the more actively we pursue it, and the more capable we feel of reaching it (Frazier & Hooker, 2006; Hooker & Kaus, 1992). Some people do it the old-fashioned way—tracking goals with paper and pencil. Others use spreadsheets, apps, and self-monitoring devices. You might find **Figure 3.1** to be a helpful starting point for good health at any age. It is up to you to decide what will work for you, and then to stick to it.

Valuing health and being able to visualize and pursue health-related goals all strongly influence the health behaviors we practice. A **health value** is the intrinsic importance we place on health or health behavior. The more we value good health and think of it as a priority, the more likely we are to practice health-enhancing behaviors and decision-making (Mrus et al., 2006; Rosengard et al., 2001). A health value is the belief that "good health is important."

Health values serve a protective function for health, affecting the health-related behaviors we engage in, and, consequently, our health outcomes (Rosengard et al., 2001). In fact, health values may be imbued with culture. Culture is a broad term that refers to the norms, beliefs, laws, customs, social behavior, and individual knowledge associated with the larger groups that one identifies with (Triandis, 2001). Culture stems from your identities such as gender, race/ethnicity, the country you live in, your religion, or other groups you belong to. There are cultures within many kinds of groups from sexual identity groups to political groups to sports groups. Evidence suggests that when

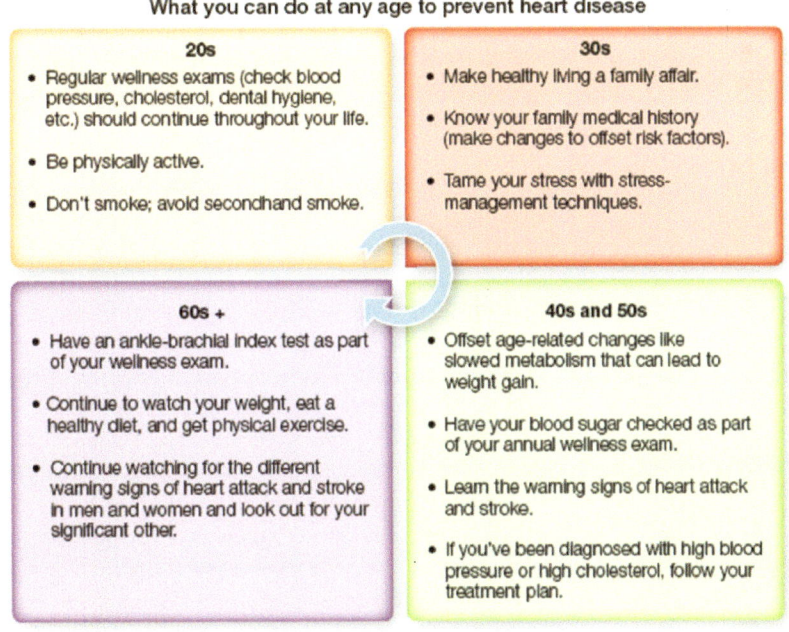

Figure 3.1 Preventing heart disease across the lifespan.

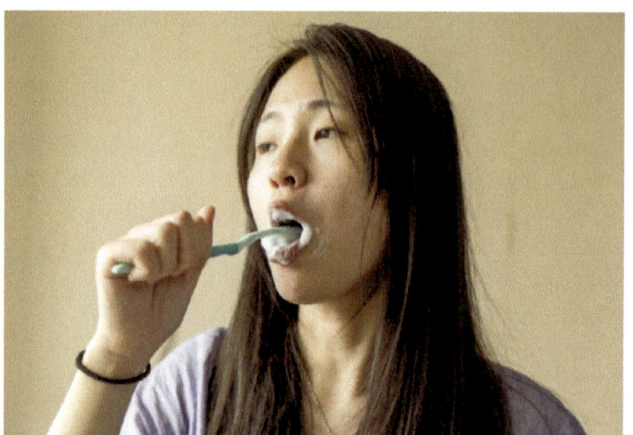

Photo 3.3   Do you value eating fruit? More broadly, what value do you place upon health, and how do your health values influence your health behaviors?

health appeals are framed to be consistent with cultural values of health, more people are motivated to engage in health-promoting behaviors (Spina, Arndt, Landau, & Cameron, 2018). This is one important way to reduce ethnic health disparities. Overall, if you value being healthy, think about your specific health goals, and imagine yourself achieving them (**Photo 3.3**).

Health Behaviors and Health Habits

Health behaviors are actions that promote and maintain good health or stand in the way of good health. Positive health behaviors that increase the chance of good outcomes include wearing seatbelts, using sun protection, eating balanced and nutritious meals, exercising regularly, and managing stress well. Negative health behaviors, in contrast, increase the risk of poor outcomes. Examples include smoking, having unprotected sex, abusing drugs and alcohol, eating foods high in fat and cholesterol, and maintaining a sedentary lifestyle.

The Alameda County Study

Study after study shows that healthful behaviors lead to longer life and higher life satisfaction (Boehm & Kubzansky, 2012; Kao, Lai, Lin, Lee, & Wen, 2005; Uchino et al., 2018). A healthy diet can help prevent diabetes, heart disease, and cancer. Exercise can prevent diabetes and cardiovascular disease, reduce depression and anxiety, and increase muscle strength and quality of life (van Achterberg et al., 2011). And avoiding smoking means avoiding the leading cause of preventable death in the United States today (WHO, 2021, 2023d).

As early as 1965, a classic study made the case for healthful behaviors. The Alameda County Study surveyed nearly 7000 people living in California (Belloc & Breslow, 1972). Residents were asked if they slept between 7 and 8 hours per night, controlled their weight, got physical exercise, limited alcohol to fewer than five drinks per day, did not smoke, ate breakfast every day, and limited snacking between meals (Schoenborn, 1986). People who engaged in most of these healthful behaviors were healthier than those who practiced fewer. Both 9 and 12 years later, the links were clearer still. Men who practiced all these health behaviors had a mortality rate that was 28% lower than men who practiced three or fewer. Women who practiced all seven behaviors had a 43% lower mortality than others (Breslow & Enstrom, 1980). Skipping breakfast and snacking between meals showed the weakest relationships to better health, but the other five behaviors were all very important (Wingard, Berkman, & Brand, 1982).

Research in Alameda County has since linked positive health practices to better mental health, and shown that life satisfaction also predicts mortality

(Berkman & Breslow, 1983; Kaplan & Camacho, 1983; Xu & Roberts, 2010). The Alameda County Study was among the first to examine health habits and health outcomes, and many more studies have continued these inquiries. The Behavioral Risk Factor Surveillance System (BRFSS), for example, is an ongoing U.S. study that collects data on health behaviors, chronic illness, access to health care, and health prevention activities related to the leading causes of death and disability. When five of the original **Alameda County Study** health behaviors (sufficient sleep, nonsmoking, nondrinking/moderate drinking, appropriate body weight, and regular physical activity) were studied, 30% of U.S. adults were found to practice four out of five of these behaviors (Matthews et al., 2017). Although these results are mostly positive, rates of sufficient sleep were consistently low, revealing an important obstacle to reducing chronic disease, disability, and death.

Much has changed since the 1960s. Think of the giant serving sizes in chain restaurants. Think also of the abundance of health information and new technology, like Elena's, that is available today. What are the differences between past versus present health and health behaviors?

Developing Good Habits

Most adults do not meet the basic recommendations to maintain health and avoid chronic illness (Phillips & Mullan, 2023). Even when doctors suggest lifestyle changes to promote health and offset illness, 80% of adults do not change their behavior (Katsaridis et al., 2020; Lennon et al., 2021). This may be because it is often really hard to form a new health habit (**Photo 3.4**).

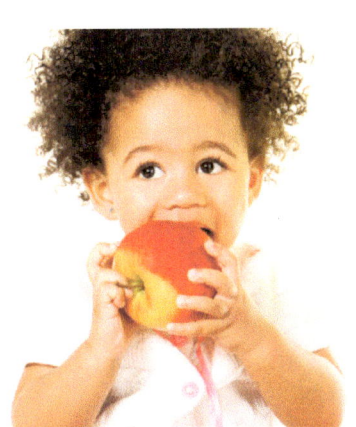

A h**ealth habit** is a health behavior that has become part of daily life, like brushing your teeth. They are learned context-response associations (Fleetwood, 2021; Gardner et al., 2021). Often, environmental cues trigger health habits automatically with little conscious thought or attention. When you wash your hands after using the toilet, using the toilet provides the cue, and washing your hands is the habit. You might not need to give much thought to it; you just do it. While hand washing might be a habit for most people, we often see reminders, as in restaurant restrooms, for those who haven't adopted the habit yet. Habits influence our health behaviors including regular physical activity, a healthy diet, and taking medications (Phillips & Mullan, 2023).

Photo 3.4   Brushing teeth daily is one example of a positive health habit.

Many of our health habits are deeply ingrained and develop early in our lifespan. Like brushing teeth, most habits form in childhood and stabilize around the age of 11 or 12 (Cohen, Brownell, & Felix, 1990). What starts as a response to parental pressure becomes routine. Good parenting includes teaching good health habits. Other health behaviors require mental and physical effort. We need to plan a time each day to go for a run or bike to the gym. Perseverance is the key.

You may have heard that a habit takes 21 days to form (Maltz, 1960). In reality, the time varies from person to person and from habit to habit. The secret is to keep at it; do whatever it is over and over again.

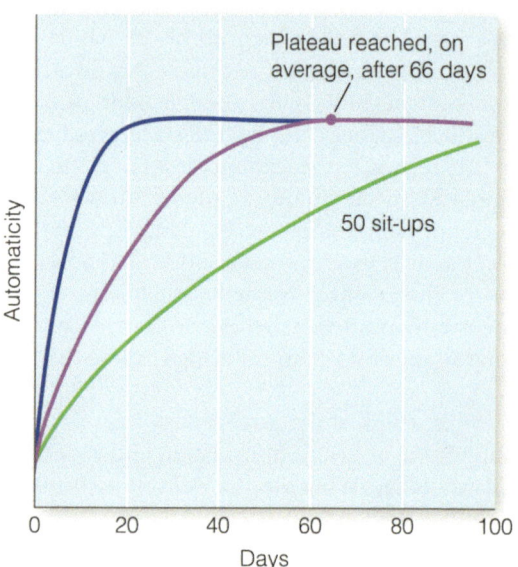

Figure 3.2   Average time it takes to develop a habit.

Source: Data from Lally et al. (2010).

One study asked participants to choose a behavior that they would like to integrate into their lives. It could be flossing, having fruit with meals, or getting 15 minutes of exercise a day (Lally, van Jaarsveld, Potts, & Wardle, 2010). The time it took to become habit ranged from 18 to 264 days, with an average of 66 days of performing it routinely. Habits took hold more quickly for simple actions such as drinking more water than for more elaborate or difficult habits such as doing 50 sit-ups a day, as shown in **Figure 3.2**. The good news is that missing an occasion was not a setback. People got right back on track. Habit researchers now know that the three key things for a new habit to develop our motivation, being capable of making the change, and having the opportunity to repeat the behavior until it "sticks": (Gardner et al., 2021). The basic tenets of developing a health habit, then, are "do it" and "over and over again." Developing healthy habits takes time, but the effort pays off. Once a behavior becomes habitual, it can feel strange to miss a day (Lally, Wardle, & Gardner, 2011).

Healthy behaviors reduce the risk of illness and mortality (Lin et al., 2004; Zyriax & Windler, 2023). Even something as simple as not brushing teeth regularly or flossing can lead to gum disease, and bacteria in the mouth correlate with higher rates of heart disease (Beck, Garcia, Heiss, Vokonas, & Offenbacher, 1996; Sanz et al., 2020), diabetes (Sanz et al., 2018), and respiratory diseases (Herrera et al., 2023), and premature death from all causes (Herrera et al., 2023; Linden, Lyons, & Scannapieco, 2012). As C. Everett Koop, former Surgeon General of the United States, said, "You're not healthy without good oral health" (U.S. Department of Health & Human Services, 2000b). These findings are important for anyone pondering more healthful behaviors, such as consuming fewer calories or less sugar when eating out (see the In the News feature). They are also important for anyone who designs behavioral interventions, such as weight-loss programs. We look more closely at healthful behaviors in Chapter 4.

Thinking About Health

- How do health promotion and disease prevention work together?
- How do health goals translate into action? What health-related "possible selves" do you hope for and fear?
- Do you consider the results of the Alameda County Study relevant today?
- What factors influence the development of health habits?

What Predicts Healthful Behaviors?

In determining who practices different health behaviors, demographics are important (Gottlieb & Green, 1987), but so are individuals' sense of control over their well-being. Together, these differences between individuals can create powerful incentives for, or barriers to, healthful behaviors.

Health Disparities

Globally, disparities in health behaviors extend to gender, race, ethnicity, socioeconomic status, and sexual orientation (Curry et al., 2020; Gorman, Denney, Dowdy, & Medeiros, 2015; Institute of Medicine, 2011; Poulter et al., 2023; Trammell et al., 2023; Vereen et al., 2023). For example, women generally live longer and enjoy better health later in life than men—in part because they make better lifestyle choices (Courtenay, 2000; Lehavot, Hoerster, Nelson, Jakupcak, & Simpson, 2012). Women typically report smoking cigarettes, drinking alcohol, taking drugs, and eating red meat less often than men. Women are also more likely than men to visit their doctors for regular checkups. On the other hand, men tend to exercise more than women do (Verbrugge, 1985). In a large study of Australian older adults (between the ages of 55 and 65) the group labeled as "healthy" (because they engaged in more health behaviors) was 72% women and 53% men (**Photo 3.5**) (Södergren et al., 2014).

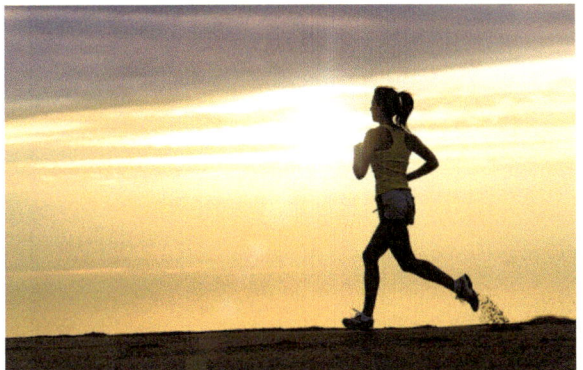

Photo 3.5   What factors predict positive health behaviors such as exercising?

In the News

"Take two grapefruits a day and call me in the morning"

Mounting evidence shows that when doctors prescribe daily expectations for fruit and vegetable intake for their patients, those patients increase their consumption, lose weight and their health improves. It is clearly established that a poor diet (one that is low in fruits, vegetables, and whole grains and high in sodium, sugar, and refined carbohydrates) is related to a higher risk for many chronic health problems including obesity, cardiovascular disease, cancer, and higher mortality from those health problems (Little et al., 2022). Although most people know that a healthy diet is better for them, there are many factors that create barriers to eating more healthful foods. Some factors that create barriers are education and knowledge about health, prices and the affordability of foods, having easy access, and social support. In terms of providing knowledge and stressing the importance of healthy dietary choices for reducing negative health risks, healthcare practitioners have an important role to play. Not only can they provide knowledge but by prescribing increased fruit and vegetable intake they can motivate and support their patients to make better choices. Healthcare provided food prescription programs have been helpful for the pre-natal health of the mother and the fetus (Trapl et al., 2017), to reduce obesity and improve dietary behaviors in childhood (Jones et al., 2020; Ridberg et al., 2019; Saxe-Custack, LaChance, & Kerver, 2024), and for those with hypertension (Trapl et al., 2018) and type 2 diabetes (Bryce et al., 2017; Xie et al., 2021). The recent "Food is Medicine" approaches are growing in popularity and success in the United States, the United Kingdom, Canada, and elsewhere around the globe. It is also a plus that often when health care practitioners provide food prescriptions better quality foods can be obtained through food relief programs. Health care provided food prescriptions have also been used to reduce food insecurity in those who live in poverty. These programs need further study but the early evidence shows promise for helping people overcome obstacles and engage in healthier dietary behaviors.

Question: How would it influence your thoughts, choices, and behaviors if your doctor or health care provider gave you a prescription for fruits and vegetables?

Age, too, is a factor. Children are more likely to practice healthful behaviors, perhaps because of parental pressure. So are older adults faced with the reality of age-related disease (Kasl & Cobb, 1966; Leventhal, Prochaska, & Hirschman, 1985; Martin-Maria et al., 2023), while adolescents and young adults may take greater risks. Although much is known about the risky behaviors of teens, less is known about their health-promoting behaviors. Boys between ninth and twelfth grades are more physically active than girls, but girls practice more safety behaviors, such as wearing seatbelts, and tend to be better at managing stress than boys (Rew, Arheart, Horner, Thompson, & Johnson, 2015). However, all health-promoting behaviors decline in both boys and girls between ninth and twelfth grades (**Photo 3.6**).

Socioeconomic status, a measure of income level and social class, can influence health directly, affecting access to quality health care, a healthy diet, and active leisure activities. Individuals with more economic resources and with higher income typically enjoy better health, lower mortality, less disease, and less disability status (Adler et al., 1994; Antonovsky, 1967;

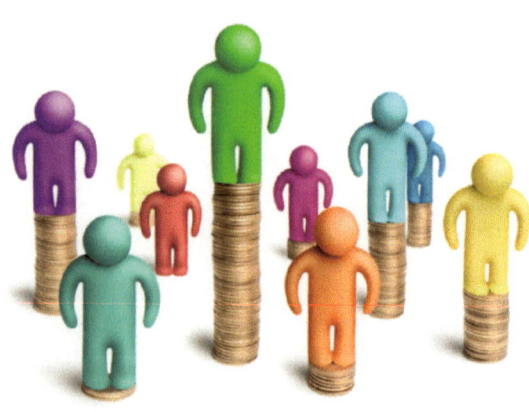

Photo 3.6   Socioeconomic status can create powerful predispositions, or barriers, to healthful behaviors.

Illsley & Baker, 1991). Socioeconomic status is also intertwined with other factors that relate to health outcomes, such as race and education (Adler et al., 1994; King-Meadows & Agarwal, 2024). As we have seen in other chapters, there are interactions among social factors. When there is a confluence of social factors such as gender, education, economic status, migration status, social exclusion, housing insecurity, and inadequate access to quality health care the ability to practice health protective behaviors may be compromised leading to a higher risk for negative health outcomes (Anyiwe et al., 2024).

In general, people with more education are more likely to practice healthful behaviors. They may have learned about the importance of good health and participated in physical education in school. More educated adults also have higher earning potential, and thus more income to invest in their health. Higher levels of education are also related to the development of critical thinking and problem-solving skills that can lead to being a better consumer of health information, making better lifestyle choices, and seeking health care when needed.

Sociocultural factors such as religion and social networking influence health behaviors as well (Almeida, Charles, & Neupert, 2008). Mormons, for example, live 6.6 years longer than the average American (Enstrom & Breslow, 2008; Mason, Toney, & Cho, 2011). The religion's Doctrine and Covenants and Word of Wisdom instruct followers to refrain from tobacco, alcohol, coffee, tea, and illegal drugs. They also stress family life, education, and good health practices, such as moderation in eating (Enstrom & Breslow, 2008; Mason, Toney, & Cho, 2011). In fact, the absence of tobacco accounts on average for only 1.4 of those 6.6 extra years of life (**Photo 3.7**) (Merrill, 2004).

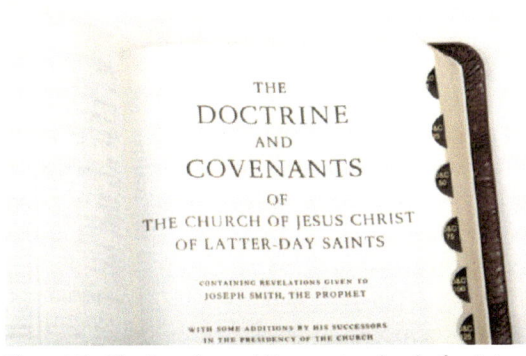

Photo 3.7   The Doctrine and Covenants, a book of scripture, forbids many risky health behaviors for Mormons.

Only recently, unique health needs and health disparities among LGBTQ groups have gained attention. These disparities may exist due to issues of exclusion and disparities related to LGBTQ individuals' use or nonuse of health care, perhaps linked to the fact that primary health care operates predominantly within a heteronormative framework (Hudson & Mehrotra, 2022; Gahagan & Subirana-Malaret, 2018). Consequently, LGBTQ patients may face stereotypes, stigma, and discrimination. For example, lesbian women of childbearing age may feel anxiety about having to explain their sexual orientation when asked, "Are you on birth control?" Cultural competence is important to minimize the health disparities that the LGBTQ community may experience.

Due to avoidance of routine health care, LGBTQ individuals may be at higher risk for and have higher rates of breast and gynecologic cancers, obesity, asthma, diabetes, heart disease, and other chronic conditions (Barefoot, Warren, & Smalley, 2017). Furthermore, when 28 different health-risk behaviors (e.g., diet, exercise, smoking and substance use, risky sexual behavior, driving risks, medical risk-taking, and violence) were tracked across a range of sexual orientation and gender identity groups, findings showed elevated health risks for transgender women (poorer diet and a more sedentary lifestyle); bisexual individuals (substance use); and transgender or pansexual men (higher rates of self-harm; Smalley, Warren, & Barefoot, 2016).

These findings are important because they demonstrate that there are important differences between LGBTQ subgroups, and understanding those differences is key to understanding health disparities. Just as men and women in the larger population face different health risks, so do sexual minorities (lesbian, gay, bisexual, queer, pansexual or omnisexual, asexual) and gender minorities (transgender, genderqueer, nonbinary).

Locus of Control

In addition to the social determinants that influence health, our health behaviors and choices are shaped by our personality—specifically, our sense of control. If you feel that your health is largely out of your hands, you are less likely to practice healthful behaviors. **Health locus of control** is a useful measure of our beliefs about our habits and our health (Rotter, 1966; Wallston, Wallston, & DeVellis, 1978).

People with a high internal health locus of control believe that their decisions make good health likely (**Figure 3.3**). They are less likely to smoke, and they report better health (Turiano, Chapman, Agrigoroaei, Infurna, & Lachman, 2014). Other people may attribute control over their health to external sources instead (see **Figure 3.3**). They are likely to believe that health is a matter of fate, chance, or powerful others. If they become ill, they attribute it to parents, doctors, the environment, or God. Or they were just "in the wrong place at the wrong time."

Which Is Your Locus of Control?

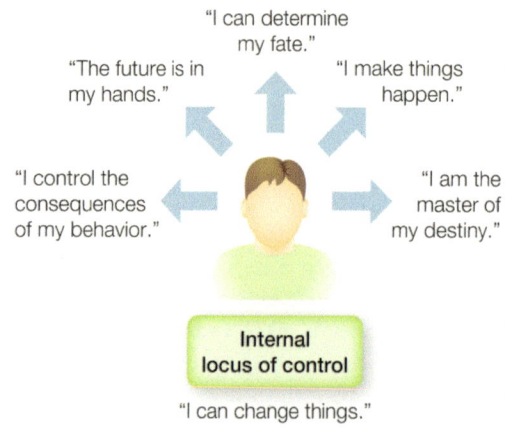
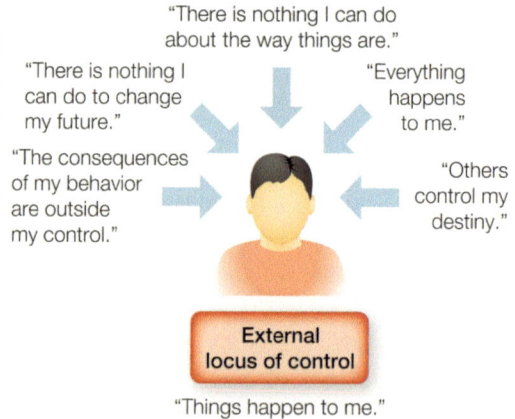

Figure 3.3   Internal versus external locus of control.

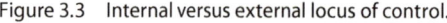

Source: Information from Brandow (2015).

Feeling in control has a protective effect on health. Personal control over one's illness leads to more positive psychological adaptation. In patients with cancer, personal control is related to increased self-esteem, quality of life, and positive mood (Roddenberry & Renk, 2010; Shapiro, Schwartz, & Astin, 1996). Conversely, college students with a high external locus of control report greater levels of stress and illness. They are also less likely to seek treatment for health problems (Roddenberry & Renk, 2010).

You can imagine how living through the COVID-19 pandemic may have influenced people's sense of control over their lives and their health. In one study that compared locus of control before the pandemic (2017) and in the early phases of COVID-19 (i.e., early 2020), both men and women experienced significantly lower internal locus of control during the pandemic than they did in 2017, even though in general their health was the same over time (Würtzen et al., 2022).

Barriers to Healthful Behaviors

Everyday barriers may make positive health behaviors more difficult as well. Some negative health behaviors are just plain appealing. Which would you rather eat right now—a chocolate brownie sundae with whipped cream or a bowl of berries? Even aside from satisfying the physiological addiction, there are positive reinforcements from behaviors such as smoking (Gonzalez, Hogan, McLeish, & Zvolensky, 2010). Some smokers report that smoking relaxes them. To make matters worse, we are bombarded with temptations in the media. That is why the United States and other nations have banned tobacco ads.

Although most Americans value good health and know what choices lead to good health, many still engage in compromising behaviors. Even though smoking prevalence has decreased since 1990, still globally more than 1.14 billion people smoke and over 7.7 million died from smoking-related deaths in 2019 (Jai, Sheng, Han, Li, & Wang, 2024; Reitsma et al., 2021; Sharma & Rakshit, 2022).

According to one report, "nearly the entire U.S. population consumes a diet that is not on par with recommendations" (Institute of Medicine, 2011). At least 75% of Americans consume less than the recommended amount of whole fruits (National Center for Health Statistics, 2010), 88% fail to eat enough vegetables, and 96% fall short of the recommendations for beans and whole grains. With the exception of young children and adolescent boys, up to 98% of Americans do not get enough milk. Moreover, the obesity epidemic is growing worldwide. In the United States, for example, the prevalence of childhood obesity has more than tripled (from 5% in 1978 to nearly 20% in 2020 (CDC, 2022). Worldwide over one in every five children is overweight or obese (Parearroyo, Laja, & Varela-Moreiras, 2019; Taghizadeh et al., 2024). Obesity in childhood is important because once a child becomes overweight or obese weight loss becomes harder and overweight and obesity in childhood are predictive of lifelong overweight and obesity (Leung et al., 2024).

Health behaviors, whether positive or negative, have a direct impact on health outcomes. Longer life and higher life satisfaction are linked to healthful behaviors (Kao et al., 2005). Disease, disability, and premature death are linked

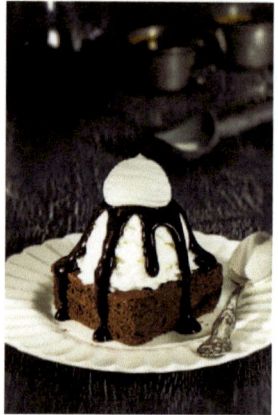 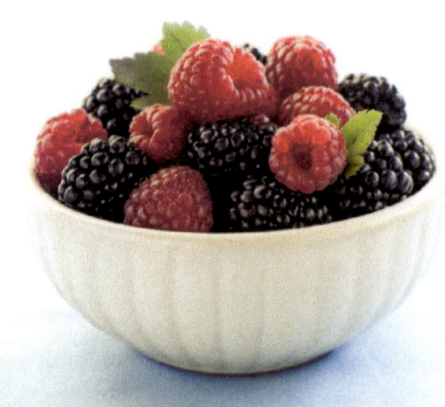

Photo 3.8 (a and b)   Some negative health behaviors—such as eating extremely sugary foods—offer immediate positive (tasty) reinforcement. Which dish would you choose?

to negative behaviors. Adopting a healthy lifestyle, a goal of most people, can nevertheless be a challenge. Certainly, with motivation (and sometimes with help from fitness technology like Elena's) the challenges can be overcome. Some beneficial health practices, such as abstaining from junk food, are hard to maintain, while some negative health behaviors, such as doing drugs, may be maintained because they are immediately pleasurable (**Photo 3.8**).

Thinking About Health

■ What health behaviors and resulting health disparities do you observe in the people around you? On the flip side, what health disparities and resulting health behaviors do you observe?

■ How do personality factors such as locus of control influence your own health?

■ What barriers to changing health behaviors exist in your life?

Why People Practice Health-Promoting Behaviors

We have seen that some people do indeed practice health-promoting behaviors, but why? As we see next, different theories focus on our perceptions of health and illness, the costs and benefits of taking action, our intentions, our readiness to change, and the likelihood of relapse. These different models have been used to explain what motivates, maintains, and derails behavioral change.

The Common-Sense Model of Illness

The common-sense model of illness sees our health behaviors as based on how we perceive our health (Leventhal, Meyer, & Nerenz, 1980; Leventhal, Nerenz, & Steele, 1984). It suggests that we form cognitive representations, mental pictures, of health and illness (Leventhal, Leventhal, & Contrada, 1998).

Say you wake up with intense pain near your belly button. You dismiss it as indigestion, but it persists even after you take an antacid and use the bathroom. Over time, the pain shifts to your right side, and now it hurts when you move or cough. By noon, you are feverish and sick to your stomach. Maybe it was not indigestion after all, but food poisoning or the flu. In other words, when one cognitive representation does not explain your pain, you look for another, based on the best information available.

Where do we look for information? One source is our own experience, such as past bouts with the flu. A second source is people we trust, such as a parent or a doctor, and our cultural beliefs. The third source is how we feel now. What do we do with this information? First, we look for the causes of illness (Hagger & Orbell, 2003; Heijmans, 1998; Moss-Morris, Petrie, & Weinman, 1996). These might be biological, such as a virus, or emotional, such as stress. Causes can also be environmental, such as exposure to chemicals. Second, we consider the consequences of illness on our well-being and ability to function. For example, you may decide at last to seek treatment for abdominal pain when you are not able to perform your daily tasks (**Photo 3.9**).

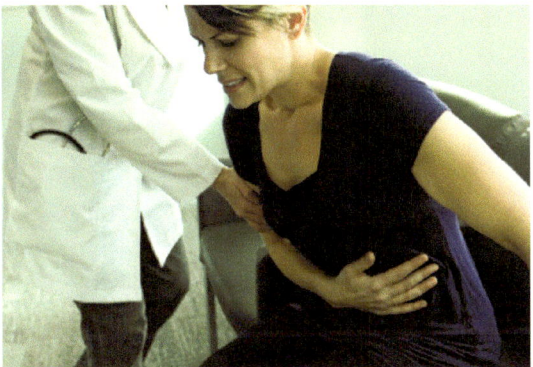

Photo 3.9 How we perceive our health can cause us to react differently to the same symptoms. One person with stomach pain might go to the doctor right away; another might try to push through the pain.

The common-sense model of illness is a parallel processing model: Everything takes place at once. We process the cognitive representations of illness along with the emotional representations of our health. In any given experience, we are thus attending to making sense of the symptoms and managing our emotions. This simultaneous processing of the cognitive and emotional elements of health allows us to cope better (**Figure 3.4**).

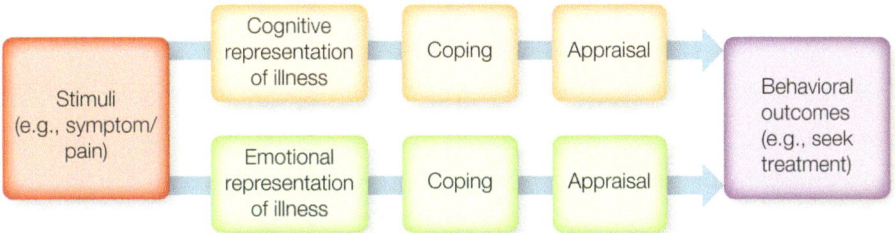

Figure 3.4 The common-sense model of illness.

Bear in mind, though, that the common-sense model focuses on representations, and these are not always so cut and dry. The representations include the labels we are taught to assign to our symptoms, such as food poisoning, and our emotions, such as the distress that unexpected or painful symptoms may cause. They also include our beliefs about illness (Lau & Hartman, 1983), and they influence how we cope with and what we do in response to health threats. Maybe you tell yourself, "If I rest and take aspirin, the pain will go away." Someone else might think differently: "If I see the doctor, I will find out what is causing this pain." These different decisions are likely to be the outcome of different representations, and ultimately they can make a big difference in our health and well-being. If it turns out that your pain was from appendicitis, for example, you'd have had a better outcome if you'd seen a doctor right away.

The Health Beliefs Model

The health beliefs model explains health behaviors as actions aimed at getting results (Becker, 1979; Becker & Rosenstock, 1984; Janz & Becker, 1984; Rosenstock, 1966). It argues that we set goals for ourselves and ask ourselves what it will take to achieve those goals. We then weigh the perceived benefits of acting against the barriers that stand in the way.

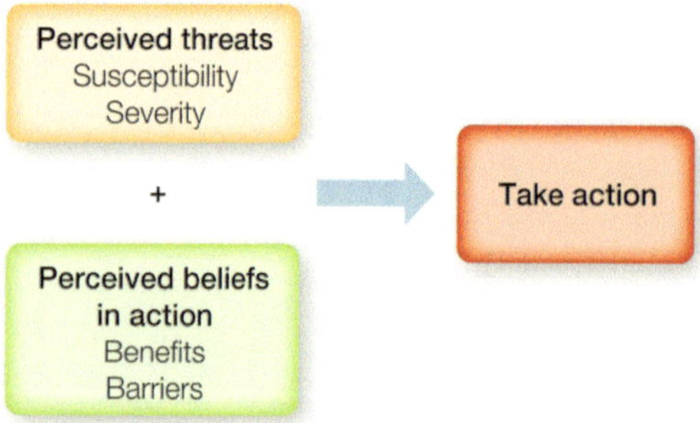

Figure 3.5   The health beliefs model.

According to the health beliefs model, whether a person practices a specific health behavior depends on a cognitive assessment of two factors: the perceived threat of a health problem and the belief that taking action will reduce the perceived threat. As you can see in **Figure 3.5**, the perceived threat of a potential health problem is based on two additional assessments. First is perceived susceptibility, how one sees one's risk associated with the perceived threat. The greater the perception of risk, the greater the likelihood of engaging in behavior to reduce that risk. The second is perceived severity, the perception that there will have serious consequences if the risk becomes a reality.

Our taking action also depends on its perceived benefits and the perceived barriers. This kind of cost–benefit analysis helps us decide whether taking action will indeed reduce the threat. If taking action is expensive, difficult, time-consuming, or disruptive to our lives or plans, then the costs will seem to us to outweigh the benefits, and we may not act.

Say we wish to avoid sexually transmitted infections (STIs) and unplanned pregnancy. We might decide that wearing a condom is an effective way to do just that. It sounds straightforward enough, but we are in fact weighing several factors (Maiman & Becker, 1974). We have assigned a value to our goal and weighed the threat of illness. That includes how vulnerable we think we are to STIs and the severity of the illness. We also have to believe that our actions will reduce the threat at a cost that we can afford. If we think that condoms are ineffective, expensive, difficult to use, or disruptive to our lives, then the costs may seem to outweigh the benefits. We may then look for another solution—or not act at all.

One last factor may tip the scale toward positive health behavior—a strong cue to action. Cues to action can be as simple as receiving a postcard to remind you that it is time to make your dental appointment, or as significant as a major, health threat. Suppose that after an unprotected sexual encounter, a friend begins to experience scary symptoms. A doctor might confirm that this friend does not have an STI (whew!), but using protection against STIs next time will feel much more urgent (**Photo 3.10**).

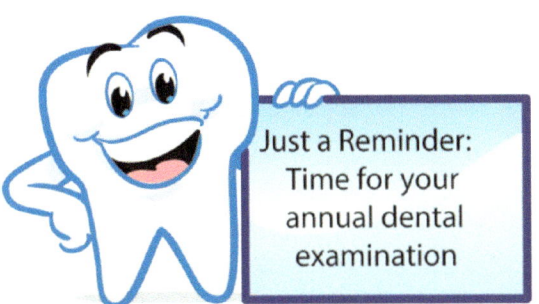

Just a Reminder: Time for your annual dental examination

Photo 3.10 Dental reminder cards can be a cue to action encouraging health.

The health beliefs model suggests that health professionals will get better results if they do more to explain the benefits of proper care and to reduce the hassles. Consider **colonoscopy**, one of the most widely used screening tests for colon cancer. This test requires several days of preparation, including a strict diet of clear liquids to cleanse the colon, accompanied by a liquid or a pill to stimulate bowel movements. The procedure, which is done under general anesthesia, involves the insertion of a long, flexible instrument about ½-inch wide with a camera on the end. The instrument is inserted into the rectum and up through the length of the colon. If necessary, small amounts of tissue are taken for analysis. Women who see the benefit of early detection are more likely to get a colonoscopy (Frank, Swedmark, & Grubbs, 2004). Thus, in weighing the hassles and discomfort associated with this procedure against the benefits of early detection of colon cancer, many choose the benefits over the costs.

The health beliefs model has been effective at predicting who will engage in healthful behaviors and why. It also points to the many individual differences standing in the way. Age, gender, ethnicity, social class, personality traits, and medical knowledge all influence our perceptions of costs and benefits. People with fewer economic resources may be less likely to seek treatment because of the expense, while people with the experience of a given health threat may be more likely to seek treatment, regardless of the cost. It all depends on our lives and beliefs about health.

The Theory of Planned Behavior

The theory of planned behavior sees health behaviors as the result of our intentions (Ajzen & Madden, 1986; Fishbein & Ajzen, 1975). Like the health beliefs model, it takes into account our values and our hopes of success. However, it gives greater weight to our intentions to succeed.

The theory has its roots in the idea that we will act in a way that best helps us accomplish our goals (Fishbein & Ajzen, 1975). Say that, like Elena at the start of this chapter, you want to lose weight. Unlike her, you might decide that

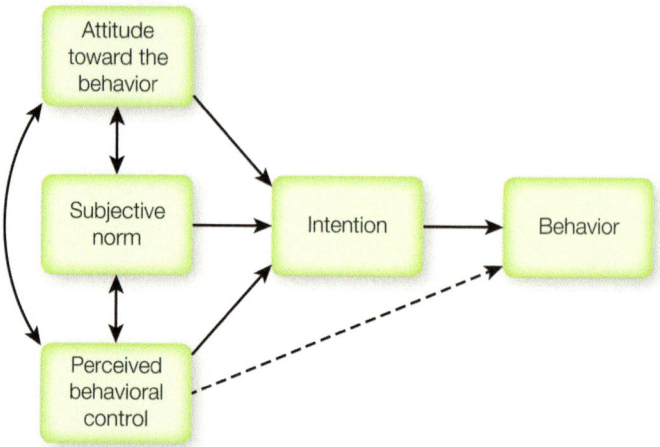

Figure 3.6   The theory of planned behavior.

it is easier to reach your goal by eating less since exercise requires more time and hard work, so you make that your goal. However, even the best of intentions do not always work out. Perhaps your goal is derailed by the temptation of Halloween candy or Valentine's Day chocolate, or by the easy availability of enormous portions at your favorite restaurant.

To make sense of the conflicts, the theory of planned behavior also takes into account what shapes our intentions (**Figure 3.6**). That includes our feelings about the behavior, what other people think of our behavior, and our sense of control (Ajzen & Fishbein, 1980; Fishbein & Ajzen, 1975). Recall that Elena made a firm resolution, and she found support for it in the online community. Her new fitness monitor also gave her confidence that she could achieve her goals.

Let's work through another example. Jennifer smokes, and lately, her friends have been making her life miserable. They ask her to go outside by herself to smoke because none of them like the smell, telling her that it is "gross." Jennifer wants to quit, but she also knows that she is dependent on nicotine. Will she quit?

To answer, we look first at her attitude regarding the behavior. Jennifer believes that if she quits, she will be happier and healthier. Second, we look at subjective norms, and the influence of others from her point of view. Jennifer feels social pressure, and she knows that her friends would be happy and supportive if she quit. Third, we look at her perceived behavioral control (Bandura, 1991; Murphy, Stein, Schlenger, & Mailbach, 2001). For Jennifer, this is the weakest link because she feels dependent on nicotine; still, she knows that she can quit if she tries. So she makes a decision, sets a start date, and consciously intends to quit. Jennifer throws out her remaining cigarettes and declares to her friends that she is quitting. The first few days are hard, but each day is one more day of successful behavioral change.

The theory of planned behavior successfully predicts condom use among college students (Sutton, McVey, & Glanz, 1999), heterosexual men and women (Gredig, Nideröst, & Parpan-Blaser, 2007; Muñoz-Silva, Sánchez-García, Nunes, & Martins, 2007), rural Ethiopians (Molla, Åstrøm, & Berhane, 2007), and female drug users and sex workers in China (Gu et al., 2009). The theory has also been applied to the use of oral contraceptives to prevent pregnancy (Doll & Orth, 1993; Peyman & Oakley, 2009), mammograms to screen for breast cancer in women (Tolma, Reininger, Evans, & Ureda, 2006), prostate and colorectal cancer screening in men (Sieverding, Matterne, & Ciccarello, 2010), sunscreen to reduce risk of skin cancer (Pertl et al., 2010; Potente, Coppa, Williams, & Engels, 2011), and preventive dental care (Lavin & Groarke, 2005). It applies, too, to weight-loss programs (McConnon et al., 2012; Nejad, Wertheim, & Greenwood, 2004) and habits of regular exercise (de Bruijn, 2011).

There are also developmental shifts in behavioral change. Willingness to change is predictive of change in substance use in early adolescence (around age 13), whereas it is the intention to change that helps older teens (around age 16). As a result, older teens with greater experience show more reasoned behavioral change (Pomery, Gibbons, Reis-Bergan, & Gerrard, 2009).

The Transtheoretical Model

The **transtheoretical model of illness** (or stages of change model) sees a change in health behavior not as an event but as a process (Prochaska, 1994; Prochaska, DiClemente, & Norcross, 1992).

For actor Robert Downey, Jr., this means a lifelong process. Describing his experience with drug addiction, Downey once said, "It's like I have a loaded gun in my mouth and I like the taste of metal" (Fleming, 2010). The actor, known on-screen as Iron Man and Sherlock Holmes, has cycled from stardom to the depths of addiction many times. He claims that his father introduced him to drugs at age 8, leading him to have problems with addiction ever since. Downey has been arrested several times on drug-related charges, spent time in prison, and left rehabilitation programs only to return to using drugs and alcohol later on.

Downey finally kicked his addictions in 2003. He attributes his success to yoga, kung fu, and the support of his wife, Susan Levin. Remembering his past also helps him live for the future. "I don't pretend it didn't happen," he said (Fleming, 2010). He has conquered his addictions and is committed to a substance-free life. Still, he knows that he faces a long battle: "I'm a veteran of a war that is difficult to discuss with people who haven't been there" (Fleming, 2010).

It takes time to build up the incentive to change—and even then, when one is ready, it takes preparation and commitment. Yet behavioral change is possible. The transtheoretical model breaks the process down into five stages, each

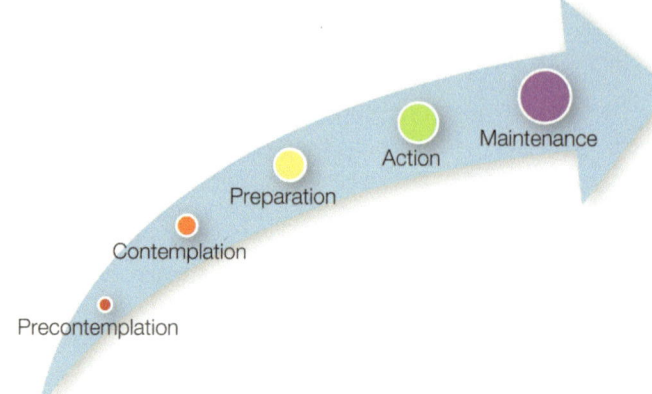

Figure 3.7   The transtheoretical model of change.

a distinct stage of readiness to change (**Figure 3.7**): (1) precontemplation, (2) contemplation, (3) preparation, (4) action, and (5) maintenance (Prochaska et al., 1994). Unlike our earlier models, the transtheoretical model of change focuses on the individual rather than on outside influences. If a person tries to change a behavior when he or she is not yet ready for change, the attempt will fail. If health practitioners try to deliver information on improving an unhealthy lifestyle to someone who is not ready to hear it, it will fall on deaf ears (**Photo 3.11**).

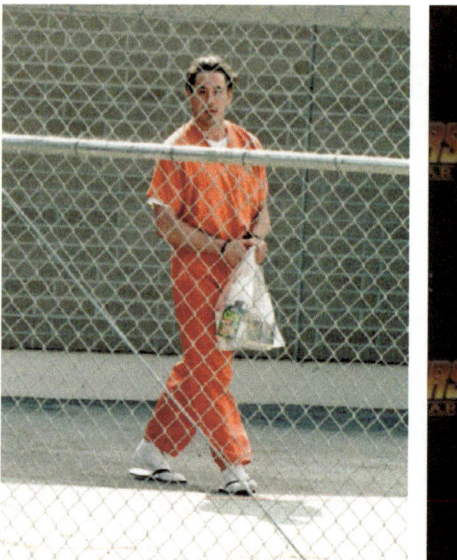
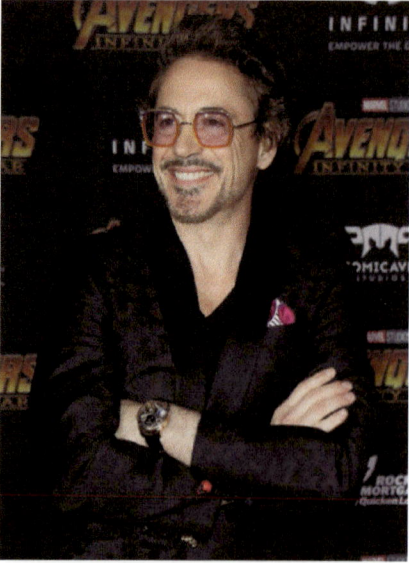

Photo 3.11 (a and b)   Actor Robert Downey, Jr., has struggled with addiction in the past but is committed to the long process of recovery. The transtheoretical model of illness exemplifies this process.

In the first stage, precontemplation, there is no intention to change. Significant others, friends, and employers may be aware of a problem, but the individual is not. As far as that person is concerned, "I have my faults, but there is nothing that I need to change" (DiClemente & Huges, 1990). In fact, recognizing a problem behavior is the first step toward changing it.

In the second stage, contemplation, the individual recognizes that the behavior is unhealthy, but is still not ready to commit to change. People can stall in this stage for years. They may know the direction that they need to take but are not ready to take it. Or they may be weighing the pros and cons of taking action.

People in the third stage, preparation, have moved to the point of wanting to work on a problem. They might set a date to quit smoking or research fitness centers. However, they have not yet quit smoking or started exercising. They are not quite ready to take action.

In the fourth stage, action, they take the leap. "I spent some time thinking and talking about change, but now I am doing something about it" (DiClemente & Huges, 1990). This stage requires a significant commitment of time and energy. It also requires setting specific criteria for change, such as the number of visits to the gym each week.

The final stage, maintenance, involves an ongoing effort to make the change last. People have reached this stage if they have continued their new behavior for six months or longer. Especially in the case of addiction, this stage is still a fragile period. It requires effort, commitment, and support.

Perhaps because the model has received so much attention, it has encountered extensive criticism (Armitage, 2009; Armitage & Arden, 2012; Herzog, 2008; Lamb & Joshi, 1996).

Some critics point out that diet, exercise, and other habits are too complex to be addressed at the level of the individual alone. Nevertheless, the transtheoretical model has helped thousands of people, and it can be useful in therapeutic settings as well. It has been applied to alcohol and substance abuse, stress, anxiety and panic disorders, depression, domestic violence, delinquency, HIV and AIDS, eating disorders and obesity, lack of exercise, refusal to undergo mammography screening, not taking prescribed medicine, unplanned pregnancy, and sun exposure (Prochaska, Johnson, & Lee, 2009). Consistently, behavioral change is most successful when the individual is ready for change.

The Relapse Prevention Model

Behavioral change is always a challenge, but even harder is maintaining the change (Dubbert, Rappaport, & Martin, 1987). **Adherence** to a health goal or medical recommendation refers to whether the person's behavior is consistent with medical or health advice, stated goals, or a behavioral change. Essentially, adherence is whether someone sticks with a change.

Every December 31, 35–50% of all Americans make a New Year's resolution. Most common are resolutions to quit smoking, lose weight, or begin an exercise routine (Curry & Marlatt, 1985; Marlatt & Kaplan, 1972; Norcross, Ratzin, & Payne, 1989; Poll, 2018). But only 20% (or one out of every five people) keep and adhere to their New Year's resolutions until the following June (Ballard, 2018).

Many people who try to break old habits make several unsuccessful attempts before they succeed (Brownell, Marlatt, Lichtenstein, & Wilson, 1986). **Relapse** is returning to a substance or behavior after a period of abstinence (Hendershot, Stoner, Pantalone, & Simoni, 2009), and relapse rates for unhealthy eating and addictive disorders are between 50% and 90% (Marlatt & Gordon, 1985; National Institute on Drug Abuse, 2012). However, the U.S. National Institute on Drug Abuse (NIDA) wants people to know that relapse does not mean that treatment has failed. Due to the chronic nature of drug addiction, "relapse is a normal part of recovery" (NIDA, 2018b). However, for some, drug relapse can be very dangerous and even life-threatening.

In one **meta-analysis**, a study that compiles the results of many previous studies, around 75% of patients adhered to their treatment programs (Bosworth, Oddone, & Weinberger, 2006). Adherence rates were highest for treatments for arthritis, gastrointestinal disorders, HIV, and cancer (Bosworth et al., 2006). Adherence was lower for treatments for pulmonary diseases, diabetes, and sleep disorders. Why the difference? It may be because treatments for pulmonary diseases, diabetes, and sleep disorders have a behavioral component. Adherence is usually lowest for changes in lifestyle, such as exercising more, eating more healthfully, and not smoking. And that does not count the many people who try to change on their own, without treatment.

Who Relapses and Why? The models that we have explored thus far are helpful in predicting the process of behavioral change and when a person will begin to change; see **Table 3.1**. They are less able to predict how long that change will last. The relapse prevention model (see **Figure 3.8**) provides a framework for understanding relapse and preventing it (Marlatt & Gordon, 1980).

Who is most likely to stick with a plan? Many factors can inhibit or promote change (DiMatteo, Haskard, & Williams, 2007; Shumaker, Ockene, & Riekert, 2008). Marital problems, loneliness, family conflict, mental health problems, and substance abuse can all stand in the way of adherence; so can financial strains or lack of access to medical services. Long, intensive treatment is harder

Theory	Premises
Common-sense model of illness	Representations of health and illness are based on cognitive and emotional responses to cues.
Health beliefs model	Goals are based on the perceived threat of illness (susceptibility and severity) and the benefits of action.
Theory of planned behavior	Intentions are based on attitude toward the behavior, subjective norms, and perceived behavioral control.
Transtheoretical model	Change will be most successful when it occurs at the right stage of readiness.
Relapse prevention model	Relapse occurs when covert antecedents build up and immediate precipitants create a high-risk situation.

Table 3.1   Models of behavior change

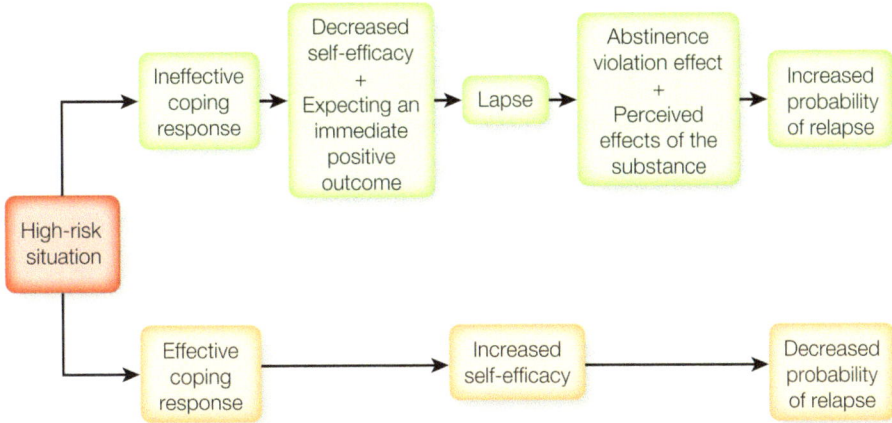

Figure 3.8   A Cognitive-behavioral model of the relapse process.

Source: Information from Parks, Anderson, and Marlatt (2003).

to follow, especially for long-standing problems or conditions with no obvious symptoms (Bosworth et al., 2006; Polivy & Herman, 2002). In turn, the more serious the illness seems to the patient, the greater the adherence (DiMatteo et al., 2007).

The relapse prevention model identifies certain high-risk situations that commonly lead to relapse. These situations can be high risk because of the **immediate determinants**, the precipitating factors that pose the most danger and highest risk of relapse. They could be physiological, such as the pain of drug withdrawal, or emotional, such as the feeling of being vulnerable and alone. They could be environmental, such as renewed exposure to a drug, or interpersonal, such as loss of family support. The factors depend on the individual (Witkiewitz & Marlatt, 2007), but negative emotions are almost always a risk for drug addicts (Baker, Piper, McCarthy, Majeskie, & Fiore, 2004).

Less obvious factors, such as losing one's equilibrium because of stress, are **covert antecedents**. These are the day-to-day activities, demands, and desires that put someone at risk of relapse (Marlatt & Gordon, 1985). They can be as simple as memories of the pleasurable experiences of a drug. When demands like these outweigh the pain associated with the drug and the desire to change, they can lead to cravings. Covert antecedents work by slowly wearing down resolve and the ability to cope (Larimer, Palmer, & Marlatt, 1999).

When faced with a high-risk situation, it is a person's coping response that will determine whether or not they relapse (Lox, Martin Ginis, & Petruzzello, 2010). When coping efforts are closely tied to the goal and self-efficacy is high, the person will feel that they are in control and less susceptible to relapse. On the other hand, if they are not coping well, have lower self-efficacy, and feel the pull, desire, or reinforcement of engaging in the behavior they are trying to abstain from, they will lapse. Their lapse may lead to guilt and helplessness, and that, in turn, may lead to letting go of the goal. This is the **abstinence violation effect**; each lapse can make the next lapse more likely (Larimer et al., 1999). In the end, whether a situation results in relapse depends on one thing—the individual's ability to cope (Hendershot et al., 2009).

We have already seen the importance of self-efficacy, a feeling of competence. For some former alcoholics, "falling off the wagon" makes them redouble their resolve to quit. Others, however, feel only that they have failed and are unable to succeed. Self-efficacy goes hand-in-hand with coping efficacy. Developing effective coping strategies for dealing with behavioral change in the face of life's challenges is crucial to treatment (see Chapter 7).

Global Perspectives

Our different models of behavioral change have at least one thing in common: They show that beliefs about health help determine success. As we have seen again and again, cultures and society mold those beliefs. They shape personal experiences, how health information is conveyed and interpreted, and how diseases are treated (Farr & Marková, 1995; Furnham, Akande, & Baguma, 1999). (See the Around the World feature to learn more about which cultures and societies live the longest, healthiest lives as a result of their common health behaviors.)

In economically stable countries, people are more likely to trust natural-world explanations of ill health (Helman, 2001). Supernatural explanations are more common in nonindustrial nations, such as Laos and Uganda (Furnham et al., 1999). Immigrants to developed nations do not easily give up their beliefs (Jobanputra & Furnham, 2005). Gujarati Indian immigrants to England are still more likely than native British to believe in the influence of the "evil eye." Younger immigrants hold much the same beliefs as older immigrants. As the overall population changes in developed nations, healthcare practices may need to change to accommodate differing perspectives on health.

Thinking About Health

■ How can you apply each behavioral model to your own health choices?

■ If you wanted to change a specific health behavior, which model would be your best guide and why?

■ Have you ever experienced the abstinence violation effect? What were some of the factors that influenced the violation?

Around *the* World

Who are the healthiest people in the world, where do they live, and what do they have in common?

Blue Zones, for one thing. Blue Zones are places where people live long, healthy, happy lives. The term was coined by *National Geographic* author Dan Buettner, who, with a grant from the National Institute on Aging, began researching hot spots of longevity. He published his findings in the November 2005 National Geographic magazine story "The Secrets of Long Life." Over the next few years, he uncovered more regions where people live very long lives, and he identified the commonalities among them in his 2015 book, The Blue Zones Solution: Eating and Living. The book quickly became a New York Times Best Seller.

So, where are the Blue Zones? There are five areas—in Europe, Latin America, Asia, and the United States—that have the largest number of centenarians in the world. Buettner and his team of medical scientists, epidemiologists, anthropologists, and demographers found that people who live in Blue Zones share common health behaviors. They eat well (usually a plant-based diet), drink wine in moderation, sleep well (according to their body's needs), and exercise regularly. They also spend time relaxing to reduce stress, cultivate good social support networks, engage in their communities (including faith-based ones), and have family and friends who support their healthy lifestyles. Buettner found that people in these Blue Zones had less incidence of heart disease, diabetes, obesity, and cancers, and lower rates of cognitive dysfunction. Many lived to see their one-hundredth birthday! This age is significant because the average life expectancy for a baby born in the United States today is 78 years.

Results from many studies, including the Danish Twin Study (Herskind et al., 1996), show that only about 20% of our lifespan is attributable to genetics. The Blue Zones support the notion of environmental and behavioral factors that contribute to longevity. Interestingly, many of the health behaviors shared by centenarians are the same health behaviors investigated in the Alameda County Study of the 1960s.

Question:
What lifestyle changes would you or your family and friends need to make in order to live "blue" lives?

Helping with Behavioral Change

What programs work best to promote positive health behaviors? Almost all the theories we have discussed have been used to design and test potential interventions. Once we identify the influences on change, we can apply what we have learned to encourage, guide, and support change.

M any people are able to make a behavioral change by themselves, without assistance from other people. Most ex-smokers have quit on their own, often by using a nicotine replacement program (gums, patches, sprays, lozenges, or tablets) available at the pharmacy. For others, however, a more structured approach can help. Many of those who are involved with behavioral interventions either at the individual level (as with psychotherapy) or at the group level (as with work or school interventions) develop their interventions with the models we have discussed in mind. All of these people or places can provide tools to help change behavior and maintain changes for positive health outcomes.

Psychotherapy

Many people seek help with behavioral change from psychologists, psychiatric social workers, and other therapists. The therapist gets to know the individual and can tailor suggestions to the client's needs.

Suppose, for example, that a morbidly obese woman in her thirties is seeking treatment for weight loss. The therapist might explore emotional issues associated with food, interpersonal issues that create distress and prompt eating, and problems with self-esteem and body image. The therapist may apply any of the models we have discussed to help guide the patient toward changing her behavior. The therapist can then help the woman become aware of the emotional and environmental cues to eating and teach her effective emotional responses. However, one-to-one therapy like this is expensive and may be out of reach for the people who most need help.

Primary Health Care

Many people first learn of the need to change their health behaviors from their primary care physician or other health care professionals. Consider a 60-year-old man who recently had a heart attack. It was totally unexpected, and he had immediate surgery to open his arteries and repair the damage. When he returned to work, he was asked how he was doing. "I'm doing fine," he said, "except that my doctor told me to quit smoking." Of course, that would be a good chance to help ensure a long and healthy life. "But," he said, "it's hard because smoking is how I relieve stress."

A health crisis can be the "wake-up call" to better habits. A physician has the credibility to influence patients in a positive way. A patient might be told, for example, that he or she is "a heart attack waiting to happen unless you lose weight." Physicians can also provide information to help the patient make changes or can suggest specialists, such as a nutritionist, who will help. Many physicians offer leaflets on diet and nutrition provided by the American Diabetes Association and the American Heart Association.

Managed care facilities often have programs at minimal cost to those with health insurance. Because many of these programs are offered to groups, patients also receive valuable social support.

The Workplace and Schools

Many large organizations offer wellness programs that focus on weight loss, exercise, smoking cessation, alcohol abuse, and stress management. These programs devise incentives, create motivation, and cultivate social norms associated with healthful behaviors. They provide valuable support for changes in behavior.

Your own university may offer fitness programs for students, faculty, and staff, promoting weight loss, health, and wellness. Your university or organization may also provide other services, such as nutrition counseling. Unfortunately, workplace interventions sometimes have low enrollment rates, and their efficacy is still unclear (Goldgruber & Ahrens, 2010).

Primary and secondary schools have the potential to reach many more people (Katz, 2009; Maes & Boersma, 2004). Schools already have programs to help with nutrition, exercise, alcohol and drug abuse, tobacco use, and sexual activity. Most children learn early on that smoking is bad for them, and schools around the United States celebrate "Red Ribbon Week," a week dedicated to teaching students about the dangers of drug use and encouraging them to be drug-free. Many schools are also adding more nutritious options at meal times and removing unhealthy choices from vending machines (**Photo 3.12**).

Schools also influence how much physical activity children get. Most students have physical education each day, while younger students have "recess," a period for free play. Many middle and high schools encourage students to become involved in fund-raising for cancer, heart disease, and other illnesses by participating in walks, bake sales, or other events such as Relay for Life and Jump Rope for Heart.

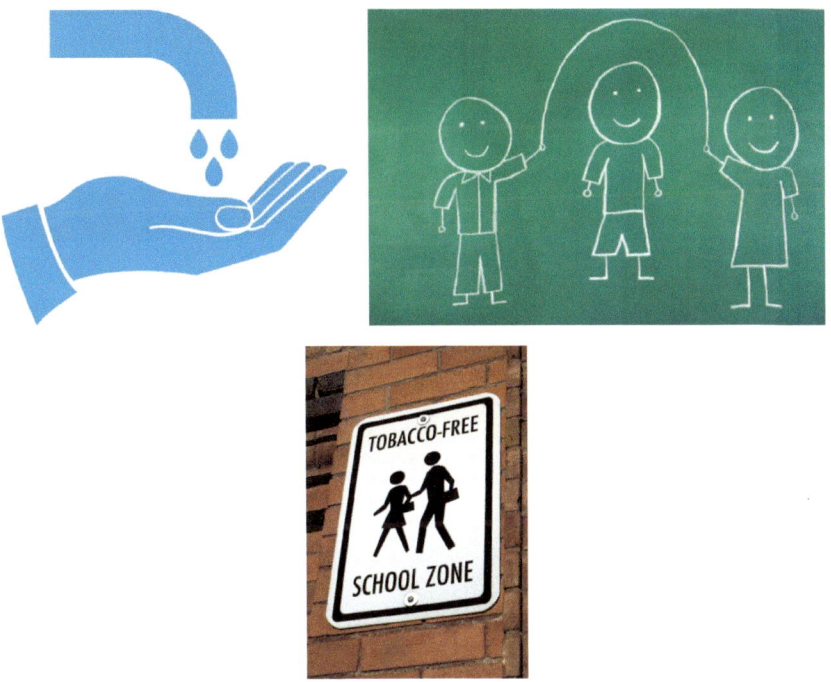

Photo 3.12 (a–c)   Behavior change messages are everywhere. Primary and secondary schools, in particular, have the potential to affect the daily behavior of children, whether by encouraging hand washing, exercise, or a tobacco-free lifestyle.

The Community

Social engineering uses the environment to shape behavior. Think of the fluoride in our water to prevent tooth decay, airbags in cars, designated smoking areas in public places, and taxes on tobacco, plastic bags, and soda. Most workplaces and universities now prohibit smoking anywhere on campus, making it inconvenient to continue the habit, while offering water bottle refilling stations in every building, creating more opportunities to stay hydrated. Situations like these can change behavior without individual engagement. Some find social engineering liberating; others consider it a dangerous form of social control. What do you think?

Generally, community-based interventions can promote good health (Estabrooks, Bradshaw, Dzewaltoski, & Smith-Ray, 2008; Thompson, Coronado, Snipes, & Puschel, 2003). They can affect large numbers of people, educating and engaging them. They can make use of the media, social organizations, door-to-door campaigns, and other grassroots efforts. For example, people in each county in the state of Kansas were encouraged to participate in Walk Kansas, a team-based program that helps people lead a healthier life (Estabrooks et al., 2008). Five years later, participants in 97 counties had maintained their new activity levels, and the number of counties participating increased over the period.

Can the idea of community extend to the Internet? Elena, from our chapter opening story, thinks so, but what do you think? Regardless, people who want to adopt positive health behaviors should know that they are not alone.

Thinking About Health

■ How might each model of behavior change be applied within the context of workplace and school interventions?

■ How can social engineering be used to positively shape health behaviors?

Chapter Summary

Behavioral change is always a challenge, but the benefits of behaviors that promote health and prevent disease are worth the effort. Positive influences on health habits include the goal of a long and healthy life and a sense of personal control. Barriers to practicing these positive health habits include lower socioeconomic status and a sense that our health is largely out of our control. Different models of why people adopt health behaviors focus on perceptions of health, the costs of adopting new behaviors, intentions, readiness to change, the temptation to relapse, and cultural differences. Every day, more workplaces, schools, medical professionals, and communities are encouraging people to practice healthful behaviors.

KEY TERMS ▶ health promotion p. 63; disease prevention p. 63; health goals p. 64; health value p. 65; health behaviors p. 66; Alameda County Study p. 67; health habit p. 67; health locus of control p. 72; common-sense model of illness p. 75; health beliefs model p. 76; colonoscopy p. 77; theory of planned behavior p. 77; transtheoretical model of illness p. 79; adherence p. 81; relapse p. 82; meta-analysis p. 82; relapse prevention model p. 83; immediate determinants p. 83; covert antecedents p. 83; abstinence violation effect p. 84; social engineering p. 88.

CHAPTER 4

Health-Enhancing Behaviors

Learning Outcomes

After reading this chapter, you should be able to:

- **Define** health-enhancing behaviors and explain why they are important for good health.
- **Describe** the psychological constructs related to practicing health-promoting behaviors.
- **Describe** the basic guidelines for a health healthy diet and exercise plan.
- **Explain** the health disparities that affect health-enhancing behaviors.
- **Outline** the biopsychosocial factors that promote and create barriers to healthy diets and exercise.
- **Identify** potential developmental influences on positive health behaviors.

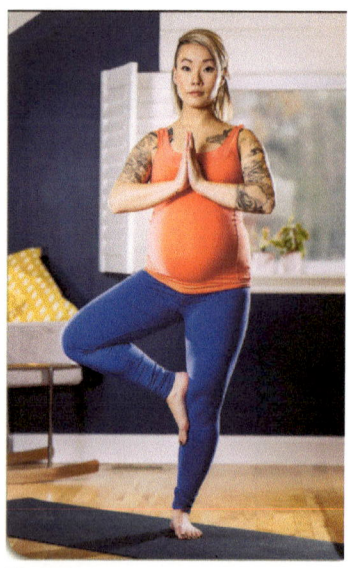

Photo 4.1

Source: Sisoje/Getty Images

Sydney was a healthy 130 pounds when she became pregnant at the age of 32. Excited to give her baby the best-possible start in life, she did everything she could to have a healthy pregnancy: she watched what she ate, enrolled in yoga classes for pregnant moms, and avoided alcohol, secondhand smoke, and other unhealthy situations. The only problem was her cravings. Popcorn, cheese, potato chips, and peanut butter cups, which she had always enjoyed, suddenly seemed irresistible!

Given that she was being so healthful in other areas, Sydney considered her increasing indulgence in these "treats" to be okay. Her doctor had told her that gaining up to 30 pounds during the pregnancy would actually be helpful in supporting the baby. But by the time her daughter was born, Sydney was nearly 50 pounds heavier than her prepregnancy weight. What had initially been sporadic cravings for unhealthy foods had developed into daily unhealthy habits (**Photo 4.1**).

Once she had recovered from the birth, Sydney resolved that it was time to return to her former, healthy weight. Applying the same enthusiasm and resourcefulness that had helped her have a healthy pregnancy, she cleaned her home of the salty, fatty foods she had craved. She made sure her refrigerator and her diet once again

DOI: 10.4324/9781032643090-4

included plenty of fruits, vegetables, whole grains, and protein. Within months, the improvements to her diet resulted in weight loss—but not nearly enough to return her to her prepregnancy weight. Was she truly living as healthfully as possible?

One day, in line at the coffee shop, Sydney overheard two new moms talking about how much fun they had had at a spinning class that morning. Perhaps high-intensity physical fitness was exactly what Sydney had been looking for. With her usual determination, she began to research fitness programs to see what might work for her. At local gyms, she tried spinning, Pilates, and barre classes but quickly realized that she loved the CrossFit program the most. Although it was intimidating at first, Sydney realized that she loved challenging herself and working with her team and her trainer.

After two months of CrossFit, Sydney had not only lost the last of her pregnancy weight—she also was stronger and fitter than she had ever been before. She had more energy, was proud of herself, and loved the way her body felt. Most importantly, she felt that the good health and positive energy that being strong and fit provided made her a better parent. She was happy to promote the value of exercise and fitness to her child—and to be the best version of herself that she could possibly be.

Sydney improved her life by turning to **health-enhancing behaviors**, the things we do that maintain and promote good health, well-being, and longevity. Through this process, she learned a lesson about the importance of self-efficacy—or, how to stop focusing on what you can't do, and to focus instead on what you can do.

From the Alameda County Study in Chapter 3, we know the basic behaviors that lead to good health: maintain a healthy weight; eat nutritious, balanced meals; do not skip breakfast; avoid snacking; do not smoke; drink in moderation; exercise regularly; and sleep seven to eight hours a night. All of these behaviors are important for many reasons, but most of all because they make poor health and disease less likely later on. A healthy diet and regular exercise, for example, can significantly lower the risk of obesity, heart disease, diabetes, and cancer. There is no true Fountain of Youth, but we can take steps to ensure good health and longer lives.

Now that we have an understanding of what it takes to achieve good health, we will look more closely at health-enhancing behaviors. What are they, and what predicts who will practice them? In this chapter, we will explore the behaviors that can lead to better health and offset chronic illness. In Chapter 5, we will examine the biopsychosocial factors that present health risks that can lead to either positive or negative health outcomes. In both chapters, you will see that these factors include genetics and lifestyle, personality and behavior, social support, and cultural identity.

Healthy Diet

Perhaps the most crucial step toward good health is maintaining a healthy weight through diet and lifestyle (see **Table 4.1**). What, however, is a healthy diet? Ask your friends, and you may hear things like "eat three square meals a day" or "don't eat sugary foods." But the complete answer is much more complex. A healthy diet is one that maintains or improves your health, protects

1. Try to burn as much energy as you eat, and try to eat as much energy as you burn, as healthy weight is a balance between these two.
2. Increase consumption of plant foods, particularly fruits, vegetables, legumes, whole grains, and nuts.
3. Limit intake of fats and oils, and avoid saturated fats (those that become solid at room temperature, such as coconut oil and most animal fats, including those found in red meat, dairy, and eggs). Prefer unsaturated fats (which remain liquid at room temperature and include most plant-based oils and foods). Eliminate trans fats.
4. Limit intake of granulated sugar.
5. Limit salt and sodium consumption from all sources and ensure that any salt consumed is iodized.

Source: Information from World Health Organization (2015a).

Table 4.1 Who dietary recommendations

against malnutrition, and lowers the risk of chronic diseases (World Health Organization [WHO], 2024c). Eating a healthy diet is also good for the environment. A healthy diet now is a mostly plant-based diet, which relates to lower greenhouse gasses, less use of fresh water, and a reduction in overuse of land.

The Food and Agriculture Organization of the United Nations has established food-based dietary guidelines to create a basis for worldwide nutrition and health. These science-based guidelines provide advice on the foods and food groups that lead to the consumption of good levels for required nutrients, to promote overall health and prevent chronic disease (Food and Agriculture Organization of the United Nations, 2024). Over 100 different countries have established the recommendations to their own specifications considering the state of general nutrition, food availability, cultural culinary factors, and eating habits of their people. This link (https://www.fao.org/nutrition/education/food-dietary-guidelines/home/en/) allows you to search by country.

Within the United States, the U.S. Department of Agriculture (USDA) is tasked with setting nutritional guidelines, with the aim of combating the rising rates of obesity and such chronic illness as diabetes. **Table 4.2** shows the prevalence rates of different nutrition-related conditions in the U.S. today. As you can see, nearly 75% of adults in the United States are overweight or have obesity, and this is most common in midlife (between the ages of 40–59). The USDA revises and publishes these guidelines every five years so that all Americans can be aware of what they should consume each day to be healthy and offset disease. The guidelines are also useful for institutions such as public schools, government cafeterias, hospitals, and nursing homes.

The U.S. Dietary Guidelines Advisory Committee met in January 2025. Their goal is to provide independent, scientific recommendations that are health equity-based and inform the current USDA guidelines. Those guidelines were consistent with the United Nation's advocate for a plant-based diet with an abundance of colorful fruits and vegetables, whole grains, seeds and nuts, low-fat or nonfat dairy, seafood, and beans. The guidelines emphasize the importance of limiting dairy, consuming only healthy oils, and avoiding saturated

Health conditions	Statistics
Overweight and obesity	■ Over 74% of adults are overweight or have obesity ■ Adults ages 40–59 have the highest rates of obesity (43%) of any age group with adults 60 years and older having a 1% rate of obesity ■ About 40% of children and adolescents are overweight or have obesity; the rate of obesity increases throughout the childhood and teenage years
Cardiovascular disease (CVD) and risk factors	■ Heart disease is the leading cause of death ■ Over 18 million adults have coronary artery disease, the most common type of heart disease ■ Stroke is the fifth leading cause of death ■ Hypertension, high LDL cholesterol, and high total cholesterol are major risk factor in heart disease and stroke ■ Rates of hypertension and high total cholesterol are higher in adults with obesity than those who are a healthy weight ■ About 45% of adults have hypertension (defined as a systolic blood pressure > 130mm Hg and/or a diastolic blood pressure > 90 mm Hg) ■ More Black adults (54%) than White adults (46%) have hypertension ■ Nearly 4% of adolescents have hypertension ■ More than 11% of adults have high total cholesterol ≥ 240 mg/dL ■ 7% of children and adolescents have high total cholesterol ≥ 200 mg/dL
Diabetes	■ Almost 35% of adults have prediabetes, and it is highest in those over age 65 (48%) compared to other age groups ■ Almost 90% of adults with diabetes are overweight or have obesity ■ About 210,000 children and adolescents have diabetes, including 187,000 with type 1 diabetes ■ From 6% to 9% of pregnant women develop gestational diabetes
Cancer	■ Colorectal cancer in men and breast cancer in women are among the most common types of cancer ■ About 250, 520 women will be diagnosed with breast cancer this year ■ Close to 5% of men and women will be diagnosed with colorectal cancer at some point in their lifetime ■ More than 1.3 million people are living with colorectal cancer ■ The incidence and mortality rates are highest among those age 65 and older for every type of cancer
Bone health and muscle strength	■ More women (17%) than men (5%) have osteoporosis ■ 20% of older adults have reduced muscle strength ■ Adults over 80 years, non-Hispanic Asians, and women are at the highest risk for reduced bone mass and muscle strength

Source: U.S. Department of Agriculture and U.S. Department of Health and Human Services. Dietary Guidelines for Americans, 2020–2025. 9th Edition. December 2020. Available at DietaryGuidelines.gov.

Table 4.2   Prevalence of diet-related health conditions in the United States

and trans fats. One recommendation that many Americans may not like is the cap on sugar consumption. The Dietary Guidelines for Americans 2020–2025 set added sugar intake at no more than 10% of daily calories or fewer than 12 teaspoons per day. The American Heart Association has even stricter limits and suggests that we should not consume more than 100 calories per day in added sugar (that is six teaspoons or 24 grams). An average 12-ounce can of cola alone has more than 10 teaspoons of sugar. That means that drinking just one can of soda can put us in danger of exceeding the daily limit! Right now, our average daily intake of sugar is 17 teaspoons every day (CDC, 2024a), and includes all forms of sugar, including high-fructose corn syrup. For optimal health, we should all try to avoid as much added sugar as possible.

The typical American diet has a long way to go to be healthy.

The Impact of Fast Foods

With each update to the USDA guidelines, we can expect to see changes in school lunches and nutrition labels. We can also expect public health and educational campaigns to create awareness and bring about positive health behaviors (**Photos 4.2 and 4.3**).

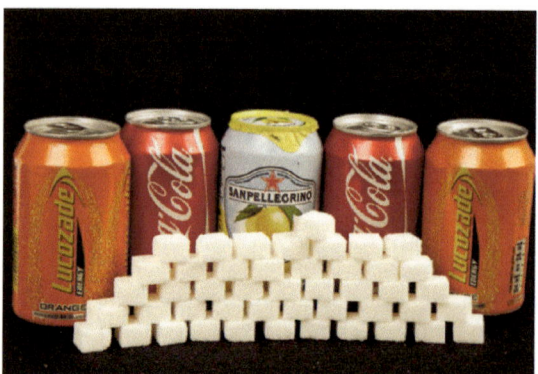

Photo 4.2   A single soft drink may contain more sugar than the USDA recommends consuming in an entire day.

Source: Geoff Abbott/Alamy

One reason that the American diet is currently so unhealthful is our reliance on high-calorie fast foods. These foods are quick, easy, and inexpensive to eat, but they significantly increase the risks of obesity, high cholesterol, hypertension, cardiovascular disease, metabolic syndrome, diabetes, and cancer (Steele et al., 2023). One recent study from Norway also showed for children's exposure to the high-calorie food of fast food restaurants had negative effects on cognition and higher body mass (Abrahamsson et al., 2023). Fast food meals often contain extremely high levels of sugar and sodium, and they are often fried in saturated fats as well. The average meal from a fast-food restaurant can contain more than 800 calories.

Fast foods are made mostly from low-quality ingredients to cut costs. They are loaded with preservatives for shelf life, color additives to look appealing,

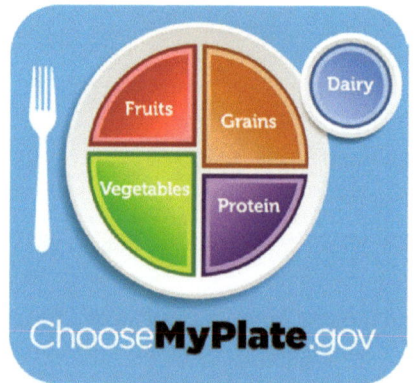
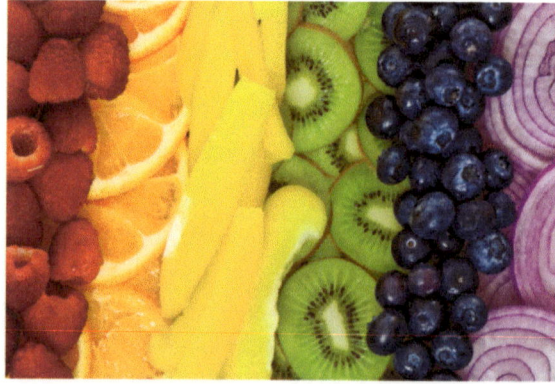

Photo 4.3   The USDA created this diagram (left) to represent an ideal healthy diet, including many fruits and vegetables (right).

Source: James McQuillan/Getty Images

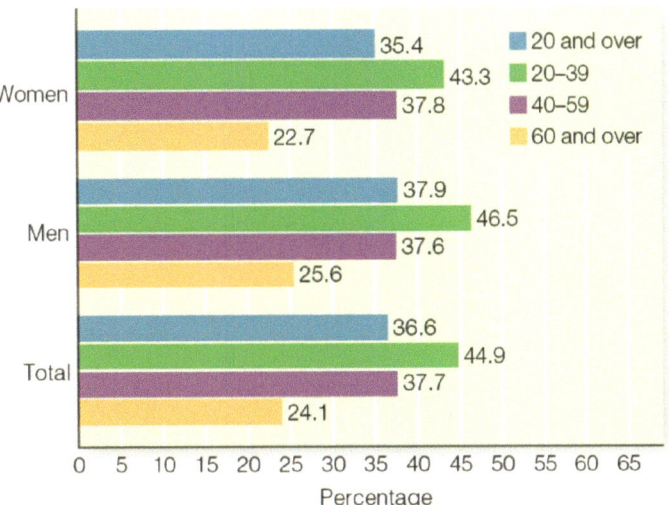

Figure 4.1   Daily fast-food consumption by sex and age in the United States.

Source: Data from Fryar et al. (2018)

stabilizers and texturizers to maintain consistency, emulsifiers to thicken, bleach to disinfect and deodorize, and softeners to give what the industry calls "mouth appeal." (See the In the News feature for an example of a controversial measure that the food industry has taken to cut costs.) Processed foods also contain artificial sweeteners, which are sweeter and more cost-effective than sugar.

Nevertheless, the results are clear: We love our fast food! Getting a meal from a fast food restaurant is often seen as a special treat for children (Sajjad, et al., 2023; Seo et al., 2011) and this can lead to rising rates of obesity and food-related diseases (Sajjad et al., 2023). In one study, 91% of parents reported buying lunch or dinner for their children from fast-food chains like McDonald's, Burger King, Subway, or Wendy's, usually more than twice per week (Harris et al., 2017). In college-aged adults, there are increased risks for nutritional problems due to changes in lifestyle, time constraints, and social factors and that is why close to 40% of students in a recent study said they consumed fast food at least one time in the last 15 days (Arslan et al., 2023). Some studies show that university students eat fast food almost every day! (Arslan et al., 2023). And on any given day, nearly 37% of Americans consume fast food (Fryar, Hughes, Herrick, & Ahluwalia, 2018; see **Figure 4.1**).

The Typical American Diet

The typical American diet is high in calories and low in nutrition. Most Americans barely eat the suggested amount of fruits and vegetables, much less a colorful selection of them.

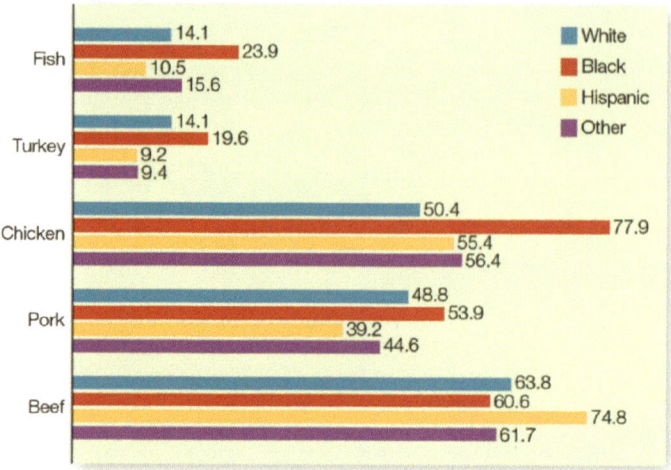

Figure 4.2   Meat consumption by race or ethnicity in the United States. Data shown are in retail weight per person per year.

Source: Data from USDA, Economic Research Service (2013)

Given the sociocultural diversity in the United States today, the typical American diet is changing. For example, while overall more chicken is consumed than beef or pork (as **Figure 4.2** shows), Hispanic Americans consume more beef. Gender and age differences appear in consumption as well. Men consume more calories per day than women, but also more meat (as shown in **Figure 4.3**). Adolescence is a period of increasing autonomy, especially in food choices, and developmental change can affect healthy eating (Shearer et al., 2015).

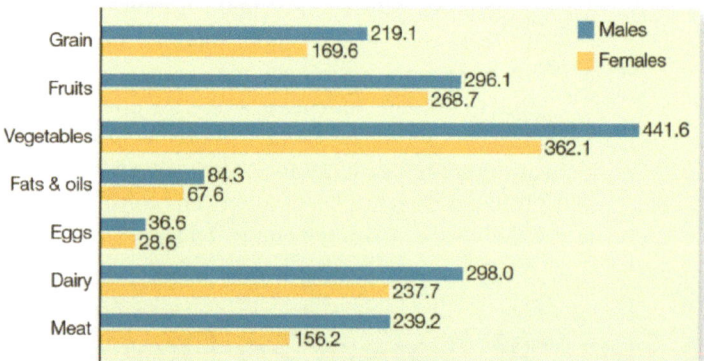

Figure 4.3   Food consumption by gender in the United States. Data shown are in retail weight per person per year.

Source: Data from USDA, Economic Research Service (2013)

Health disparities also influence food consumption. Higher levels of education and greater interest in nutrition (a health value; see Chapter 3) are related to consuming fewer calories, sugar, and carbohydrates (Ma, Ailawadi, & Grewal, 2013).

In the News

If you care about what you eat, surely you will want to know what it is that you are eating. However, that may not be as easy as you think (**Photo 4.4**).

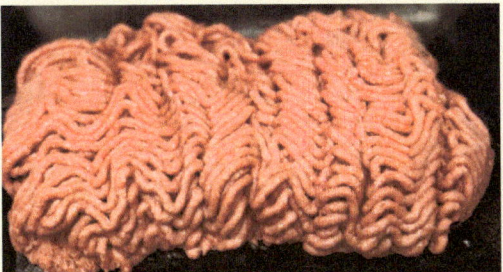

Photo 4.4 "Pink Slime": What's in Your Hamburger?

Source: REUTERS/Alamy

There is red meat—and then there is "pink slime." The term refers to beef trimmings, once used only in dog food and now added as filler to most ground beef. According to Gerald Zirnstein, it is found in 70% of the ground beef at the supermarket. As a scientist at the U.S. Department of Agriculture, Zirnstein coined the term. Now, as a whistleblower, he won't buy it.

"It's economic fraud," he told ABC News. "It's not fresh ground beef…. It's a cheap substitute being added in." Excess fat is spun out, and the remainder is sprayed with ammonia to make it safe to eat. You probably did not plan on consuming ammonia with your hamburger, but there it is. In 2012, ABC News broadcast a news series exposing the use of "pink slime" and was sued for $1.2 billion by the largest U.S. beef producer, Beef Products Inc., for making false claims.

Concerns over the safety of meat are not new. In his 1906 book The Jungle, Upton Sinclair described the workplace in the meatpacking industry in the United States. His novel created an uproar that led to important industry regulations, including the Pure Food and Drug Act that same year. Yet, in 2013, Europe was rocked by the addition of horse meat to common food. Starbucks, the coffee chain, was found to use a red dye from crushed beetles in some of its bakery and drink products. Chicken nuggets were found to contain less actual chicken meat and more of whatever is left over from meat processing. Although many of these products may not be harmful, we have a right to know what we are eating.

Debate continues over the effects of readily available nutritional information on consumer behavior. "Pink slime," however, does not have to appear on the label. Over the objections of their own scientists, USDA officials consider it meat. If you want to try to avoid it, look out for labels such as "finely texturized beef" or "boneless lean beef trimmings"—these refer to "pink slime." Unfortunately, unless you grind your own beef, it will be difficult to avoid "pink slime" entirely. As beef prices rise, more meat-processing plants are using it (Russell, 2014).

Question: If you eat red meat, does knowing about "pink slime" make you want to change your eating habits? How can you protect yourself from food fraud?

Developmentally, adolescents, especially African and Hispanic American teens, are disproportionally at risk for obesity and metabolic disease (Taveras, Gillman, Kleinman, Rich-Edwards, & Rifas-Shiman, 2013; see **Figure** 4.4). Twenty-two percent of African American teens and 25.8% of Hispanic teens are obese compared with 14% of white teens in the United States today. And boys are more likely to be obese than girls (NHANES, 2018). Two modifiable dietary

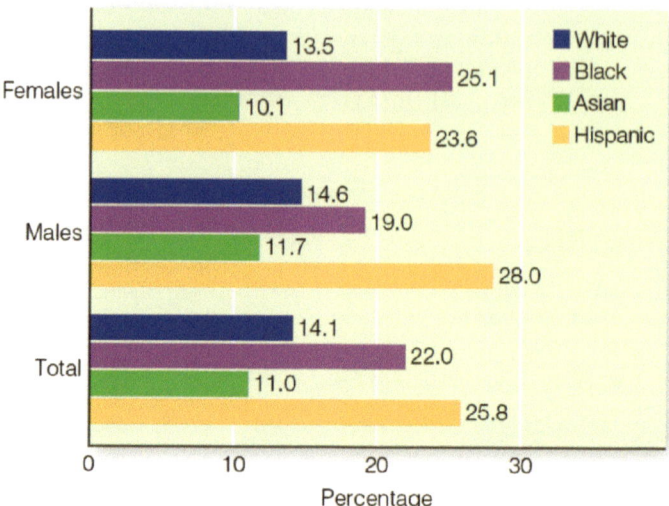

Figure 4.4   Prevalence of obesity in youth by gender and race or ethnicity in the United States.

Source: Data from Fryar et al. (2018)

factors that influence obesity in these groups are a high intake of added sugars and a low intake of dietary fiber.

For instance, African American and Hispanic-American teens consume more calories from sugar-sweetened beverages than white teens (Shearer et al., 2015; Wang, Bleich, & Gortmaker, 2008).

Thinking About Health

■ How does your diet compare to the UN or USDA guidelines?

■ Are you more concerned about how the food you eat is made, or about how it tastes?

■ What aspects of your diet are you willing to change to enhance your health?

Diet Around the World

Geography, culture, climate, and economics all influence a population's diet and, ultimately, its health. How do we go about comparing healthy diets around the globe? One benchmark is **life expectancy**, or how long, on average, people live (**Photo 4.5**).

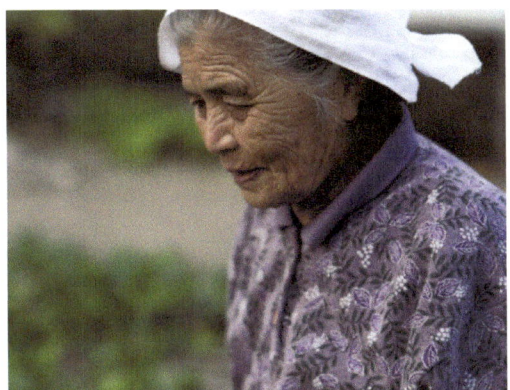

Photo 4.5   This woman is one of many Okinawan centenarians. Okinawans tend to live longer, healthier lives than the rest of the world because of their healthy diets.

Source: Chris Willson/Alamy

The highest number of centenarians (people aged 100 years old or older) reside in several key areas: Loma Linda, California; Nicoya, Costa Rica; Sardinia, Italy; Ikaria, Greece; and Okinawa, Japan. While each of these Blue Zones (regions whose residents live much longer than those who live elsewhere; see Chapter 3) has unique community attributes that help people maintain good health, such as an association with the Seventh-day Adventist Church (Loma Linda) or an agricultural lifestyle (Okinawa), there are commonalities across the lifestyles—and particularly within the diets—of the people who live the longest (Buettner, 2005). Not smoking, eating a plant-based diet (especially one that includes legumes), moderate physical activity, social engagement, and investment in a family are the important commonalities that lead to long lives.

Food Scarcity

One in 10 people currently alive is undernourished (that is 811 million people worldwide; FAO, IFAD, UNICEF, WFP, & WHO, 2023). In some countries, people are starving, and a healthy diet is nearly impossible to attain. Malnutrition is the cause of over one-third of childhood deaths in developing countries where essential foods are simply unavailable (Bill & Melinda Gates Foundation, 2024). Famine, a widespread shortage of food, can be caused by poverty, crop failure, and environmental pressures, political upheaval, or policy decisions. It has been suggested by the United Nations that the COVID-19 pandemic has exacerbated world food scarcity and famine (United Nations, 2023). In sub-Saharan Africa, for example, famine is devastating. Even within the United States, there is food scarcity. **Food scarcity** (or food insecurity) refers to having uncertain or limited access to nutritionally adequate and safe foods.

Although food scarcity correlates with poverty, not everyone who experiences food insecurity is poor (Palar et al., 2018). Worldwide, 811 million people went hungry in 2023—that is one out of every ten people (United Nations, 2023). Food scarcity and malnutrition have the most devastating effects on children and the elderly.

Despite the fact that the United States has one of the largest economies in the world, many of its residents are starving; see **Figure 4.5**. In 2023, 28 million American households reported food insecurity in the previous month: They did not know where the next meal would come from (United States Census Bureau, 2024). Over five million Americans reported very low food security that significantly disrupted their eating patterns. Of these people, 99% said that they were worried that their food supplies would run out before they had money to buy more; 95% said that they could not afford to eat balanced, nutritious

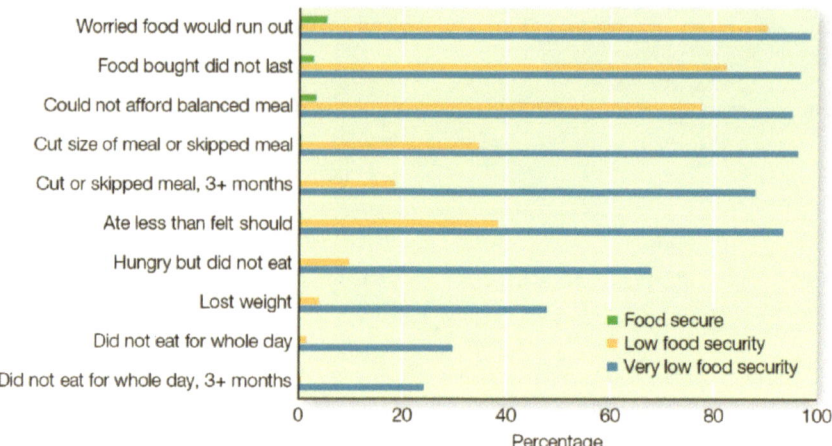

Figure 4.5   Percentage of U.S. households reporting indicators of food insecurity by food security status.

Source: Data from Coleman-Jensen et al. (2018)

meals; 96% said that they'd had to cut the size of meals or skipped meals altogether to save food; and 68% reported being hungry, but unable to afford to eat (Coleman-Jensen et al., 2018). Most often, food insecurity is found in households with incomes near or below the poverty line, in single-parent households, in households headed by women living alone, in black- or Hispanic-headed households, and in rural households (Coleman-Jensen et al., 2018).

There is some good news, though. Overall, from 2014 to 2017, the number of Americans with food insecurity went down from 14% to 11.8% of households (or from approximately 17.4 to 15 million households; Coleman-Jensen et al., 2018). This is a significant improvement. However, many Americans who are taking advantage of federal food and nutrition assistance programs are still going hungry. The global and national problem of food scarcity is yet to be fully addressed.

Thinking About Health

■ Which regions of the world live the longest and have the healthiest diets?

■ What recommendations would you make to alleviate food scarcity, both in the United States and worldwide?

Who Eats a Healthy Diet and Why

When it comes to nutrition, education is critical, but knowledge alone is only a part of the story. A large majority of American adults (95%) already believe that balance, moderation, and variety are essential to healthy eating (van den Bree, Przybeck, & Cloninger, 2006). Research shows that most people (83%) are aware

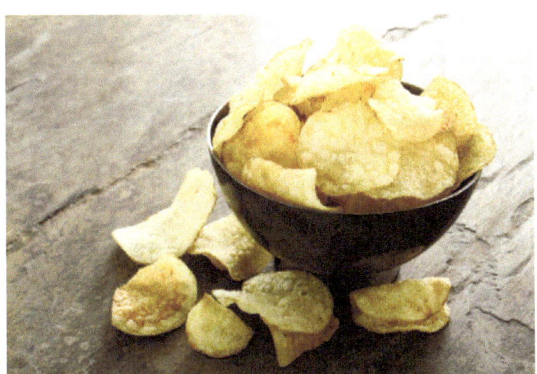

Photo 4.6 Did you know? Potato chips were invented in 1853 by native American/African American George Crum in Saratoga Springs, New York. While working as a Chef at A Local Resort, he was annoyed when a customer kept sending his french fries back because they were too thick. So, Crum cut the potatoes as thin as possible.

Source: Neil Iangan/Shutterstock.com

that what they eat affects their health (Lachance, 1992). Too often, however, this knowledge does not translate into behavior (Kant, Block, Schatzkin, & Nestle, 1992; Subar et al., 1995). Some studies show that only 3% of the U.S. population regularly eats the recommended amounts in each food group (**Photo 4.6**) (Kant et al., 1992; van den Bree et al., 2006).

How do food preferences form? Biological, psychological, and social factors all help to explain why people do not make healthier choices. We generally eat what we like, what we are familiar with, and what is easily available to us. For many of us, eating is associated with family, friends, and celebration. Let's look at both genetic and environmental factors. One important caveat at the outset is that current scholars in biology and psychology firmly and strongly believe that genetic and environmental factors cannot be separated (Lickliter & Witherington, 2017). There is no such thing as "biological inheritance" (Lickliter & Moore, 2023), and in order to fully understand any health-related concept, we must consider both and understand that they work together to produce outcomes.

The Biology of Eating

Did you know that your (and Sydney's) weakness for doughnuts and potato chips may be innate? What you like to eat, when and how much you eat, and how quickly you convert food calories to energy are all dictated in part by genetics. Our predisposition toward sweet and salty foods, like our dislike of bitter and sour tastes, is in our genes. Parents even pass their own unique food likes and dislikes on to their children through their genes (Kral & Rauh, 2010). In fact, in adolescence, genes have been found to influence preferences for vegetables, fruit, starchy foods, meat or fish, dairy products, and snacks (Smith et al., 2016). Recent research shows that vegetarianism (not eating meat, fish, shellfish) is 77% heritable (Wesseldijk, Tybur, Boomsma, Willemsen, & Vink, 2023).

Our genetic predispositions are shaped by learning and experience too. Eating habits and dietary preferences acquired in childhood last well into adulthood (Kelder, Perry, Klepp, & Lytle, 1994; Scaglioni, Salvioni, & Galimberti, 2008). Still, we are not slaves to our genes. From birth, our parents cultivate environments that may give rise to healthy eating or obesity. Your own lifestyle choices also play a large role.

How can we assess the interplay of genes and learning when it comes to diet? Twin studies have helped show how genetics influence our eating (Carnell,

Haworth, Plomin, & Wardle, 2008; Smith et al., 2016). They confirm that preferences for desserts, vegetables, and fruits are highly heritable, as are preferences for high-protein foods, such as meats and fish, and sensitivity to bitterness (Breen, Plomin, & Wardle, 2006; Kral & Rauh, 2010; Russell & Worsley, 2008; Smith et al., 2016). Strangely enough, **neophobia**, a fear of trying new things, is heritable, too (Faith, Heo, Keller, & Pietrobelli, 2013).

For our prehistoric ancestors, an aversion to strange tastes helped them avoid eating toxic things (Cassells, Magarey, Daniels, & Mallan, 2014). Today, however, neophobia can be unhealthy. It can lead to a poor diet because it reduces the variety of foods eaten (Cooke, Haworth, & Wardle, 2007; Knaapila et al., 2007). Neophobia shows an interesting developmental pattern. It in children is most prevalent between the ages of two and six (Dovey et al., 2008) but it emerges again in late adulthood (Soucier et al., 2019; van den Heuvel, Newbury, & Appleton, 2019). In a study of six hundred 2- to 6-year-olds, those with greater neophobia ate fewer fruits, vegetables, and meat, but neophobia was not correlated with the consumption of dairy foods, cakes, or cookies (Cooke, 2004). Not surprisingly, young children are more open to trying new cakes or cookies than new fruits and vegetables (Cooke, 2004). In older adults, neophobia was related to a more limited diet, luckily it had no impact on overall health (Costa, Carrión, Puig-Pey, Juárez, & Clavé, 2019).

Biologically speaking, the brain—specifically, the hypothalamus—controls appetite, energy use, and body weight. It adjusts our food intake in relation to our level of physical activity. That is why if you have had a particularly physically active day and burned a lot of calories, you may feel hungrier than normal. Hunger is a signal from your hypothalamus that you need to eat to replenish energy stores. Disruptions in the functioning of the hypothalamus can result in overeating.

Our genes, in large part, dictate not just our food preferences, but also our appetite, so that we meet our daily needs. Those needs, in turn, vary from person to person, depending on our **basal metabolic rate (BMR)**, the calories that the body needs to carry out such basic functions as breathing, heart pumping, converting food to energy, and sleeping.

Diet and the Environment

So, is diet driven by genes or behavior? The answer is both. For some people, maintaining a healthy weight is harder than for others, but not just because of their genetically determined appetite (Carnell et al., 2008). We all share an environment of easily accessible, super-sized foods, and yet each of us has our own history of learning.

Food preferences begin to develop in the womb. Flavor compounds are transmitted from the mother's diet to the fetus through the amniotic fluid (Beauchamp & Mennella, 2009). Still other flavors are transmitted in nursing, through breast milk or infant formula (Mennella, Kennedy, & Beauchamp, 2006). Later, parents influence not only the types and amounts of foods served but also the social context of eating (Kral & Rauh, 2010) (**Photo 4.7**).

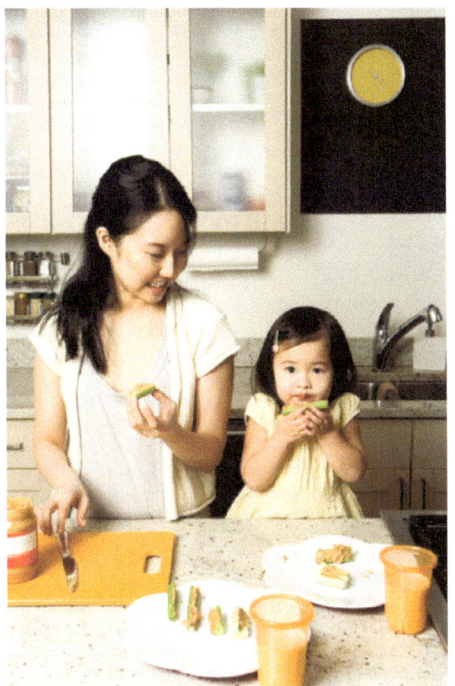

Photo 4.7   This mother is encouraging healthy habits by introducing nutritious snacks at an early age.

Source: Getty Images

Look again at neophobia. Kids can easily pick up their parents' aversion to trying things. Some parents may not make healthy foods available or may not encourage their kids to try new foods (Tan & Holub, 2012). On the other hand, pressuring kids to lose weight, to eat only healthy foods, or to eat only what the parent dictates may backfire. All may cause a child to associate eating well with stress, leading him or her to avoid it. In turn, super-picky eaters may create overprotective parents who cater to their kids (Cardona Cano et al., 2015; Johnson, Goodell, Williams, Power, & Hughes, 2015). Because these parents become anxious when their kids don't eat, they tend to serve mostly the foods that they know the child will eat (Cardona Cano et al., 2015).

Parents are important role models in children's food choices and should always encourage kids to try new things. They can allow children to make their own food choices while monitoring what they eat to make sure that they are healthy (Tan & Holub, 2012). When children observe mothers eating a new food or food that they may previously have disliked, they are more likely to try it again (Kral & Rauh, 2010). When parents eat healthy foods or make healthy foods readily available, children are more likely to eat them too (Cullen et al., 2003; Miller, Moore, & Kral, 2011).

The Importance of Family Dinners

Something as simple as the timing of dinner can have an impact on food consumption. Eating after 8:00 p.m. is linked to consuming more calories, greater reliance on fast food, and obesity (Baron, Reid, Kern, & Zee, 2011; Bo et al., 2014; Jones 2018). Late eaters lose weight more slowly and are at greater risk of diabetes as well (Lopez-Minguez, Saxena, Bandín, Scheer, & Garaulet, 2018; Scheer, Morris, & Shea, 2013). They also consume fewer calories at other meals and often skip breakfast (de Castro, 2009).

Three family routines can lead to healthier eating: Regularly eating dinner together, limited time spent watching TV and playing computer and video games, and adequate nighttime sleep are all associated with a lower prevalence of obesity (Anderson & Whitaker, 2010; Taveras et al., 2012). Unfortunately, although most 12-year-olds have family meals nearly seven nights a week, only 25% of 17-year-olds eat meals with family. In families that eat fewer than three meals together a week, 45% leave the TV on while eating, and 33% say that conversation is minimal. Families that don't often eat meals together usually have less pleasant dining experiences when they do. There is also more tension within the family, and children are much less likely to think their parents are proud of them (Taveras et al., 2012). A large-scale systematic review of family mealtimes show its protective factors on children. Specifically, the greater frequency of family meals together is related to a better overall diet, lower rates of obesity, lower risky behaviors, better academic performance, and better mental health and well-being (Snuggs & Harvey, 2023).

Family time around meals matters—and not just because it instills good eating habits. It is an important foundation for a child's development as well. Interesting research findings show that the COVID-19 pandemic had a positive effect on family dinner. At the height of the shutdown, participants reported a greater frequency of family meals and that these meals contributed to feelings of closeness mitigating the stress of the pandemic (Marks et al., 2023).

Thinking About Health

- What biopsychosocial factors influence your diet?
- What dietary choices and preferences may run in your family?

A Healthy Weight

Before we consider weight and what is considered healthy for long-term wellness, it is important to address the psychological consequences of how weight and a "healthy" weight are defined. There is a lot of social stigma and weight-shaming in our culture and it has led to many negative outcomes for people who struggle with their weight. In fact, the internal struggles that people have with their weight are, in part, a function of the pressures that societies, cultures, and the social media place upon them. Human beings are highly sensitive and attuned to the attitudes of others (Latané & Wolf, 1981) and are influenced by the implicit and explicit cultural and social norms about what is "good, right, proper, valued, and beautiful" (Ravary, Baldwin, & Bartz, 2019). These implicit and explicit anti-"fat" and "fat shaming" attitudes are incredibly detrimental to the mental and physical health of people whose weights are not deemed as socially "acceptable" or "normal." The "thin ideal" in American culture is responsible, in part, for the poorer mental health of overweight/obese people and the detrimental body image issues associated with people with eating disorders. Body dissatisfaction is highly associated with depression, lower self-esteem, risky health behaviors, eating disorders, and lower overall quality of life (Pellizzer & Wade, 2023). In an effort to combat body shaming, the "body positivity" movement arose largely through social media with hashtag #bodypositive, for example. This movement focused on countering the "thin ideal," promoting acceptance of all body shapes, and encouraging people to love the body they have (Cohen, Newton-John, & Slater, 2021). Although this movement is a step in a positive direction, it too has had a profound effect on the emotions and self-esteem of people who struggle with weight (Davies et al., 2020). Recently, a focus on more truly appreciating

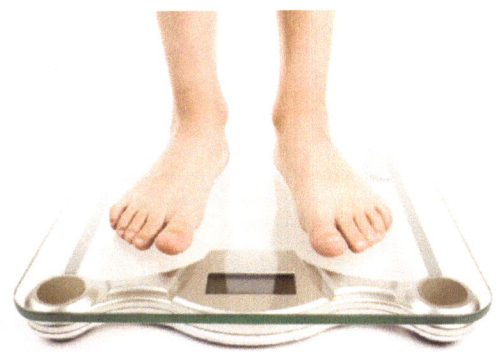

Photo 4.8   The number on the scale is not the sole indicator of healthy weight. Medical professionals evaluate several other factors, such as BMI, waist-to-hip ratio, and lifestyle.

Source: Sychugina/Shutterstock

one's body just as it is, appreciating the unique and individual differences in bodies more generally, and focusing on the functions and strengths of our unique bodies can lead to more neutral and less negative self-talk and body appreciation (Pellizzer & Wade, 2023). This approach captures body neutrality or the recognition that bodies change as do our emotions about them, therefore it is ideal to observe our bodies without judgment while focusing on what they can do for us. This is a diversity-affirming approach that has the potential to destigmatize cultural expectations about "ideal" bodies and provide a more psychologically and physically healthy approach to discussions of weight and body shape. Therefore, in this section, we talk objectively and without judgment about the science that looks at how body weight correlates with health outcomes (**Photo 4.8**).

If you are curious about whether or not you may have implicit biases regrading weight and body shape you can take this self-test to find out…. https://implicit.harvard.edu/implicit/Study?tid=-1

The best way to maintain a healthy weight is through regular exercise and well-balanced, nutritious meals. First, though, we need to define healthy weight—it is not just a number that you see when you step on the scale.

Body Mass Index

Medical professionals rely on several factors to determine a healthy weight. The first is **body mass index** (BMI), a measure of your body fat based on your height and weight. You calculate BMI by multiplying your weight in pounds by 703 and then dividing by your height in inches squared:

$$BMI = \frac{weight}{height}\ ()*703 \frac{lb}{2}\ (in2)$$

For example, if you weigh 150 pounds and your height is 5'5" (65"), your BMI is [150 × 703 ÷ (65)2] = 24.96. There are many online BMI calculators that can help do the math.

Once you know your BMI, you can determine whether you are within a healthy range; see **Table 4.3** and **Figure 4.6**. (Special BMI tables apply to children, because, developmentally, their bodies need a different proportion of fat to lean tissue to mature normally.) BMI is used both in scientific studies of weight (Burkhauser & Cawley, 2008) and by healthcare professionals.

Nevertheless, the BMI system can misclassify people (Holt et al., 2023). BMI for adults may not always predict body fat accurately, because different people have different body shapes and proportions. BMI categories, as depicted in **Figure 4.6**,

	BMI (kg/m²)	
Classification	**Principal cutoff points**	**Additional cutoff points**
Underweight	<18.50	<18.50
Severe thinness	<16.00	<16.00
Moderate thinness	16.00–16.99	16.00–16.99
Mild thinness	17.00–18.49	17.00–18.49
Normal range	18.50–24.99	18.50–22.99
		23.00–24.99
Overweight	≥25.00	≥25.00
Preobese	25.00–29.99	25.00–27.49
		27.50–29.99
Obese	≥30.00	≥30.00
Obese class I	30.00–34.99	30.00–32.49
		32.50–34.99
Obese class II	35.00–39.99	35.00–37.49
		37.50–39.99
Obese class III	≥40.00	≥40.00

Source: Data from World Health Organization (2016a). Note: Although this table is based on the calculation of BMI in meters and kilograms, it displays exactly the same cut-off points as BMI calculated with height and weight in pounds and inches.

Table 4.3   The international classification of underweight, overweight, and obese adults according to BMI

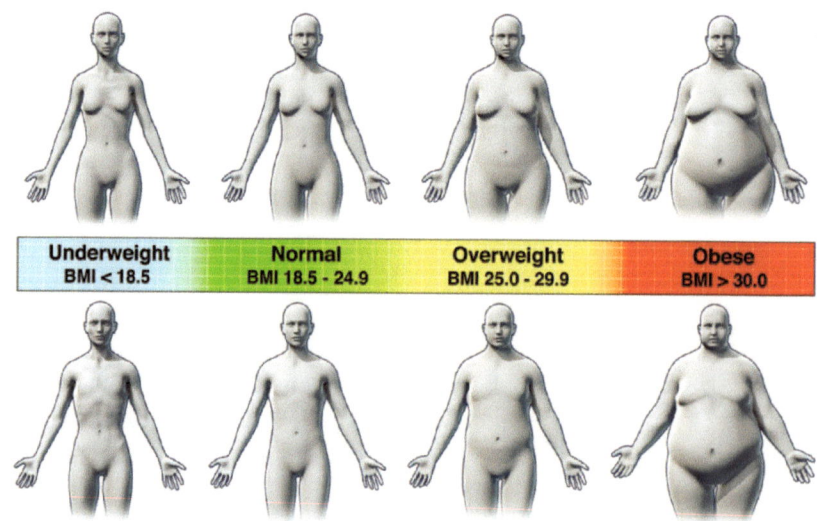

Figure 4.6   Pictoral BMI classifications.

Source: EVAN OTO/Science Source

were constructed on "average" males and females, but BMI can overestimate the amount of body fat in athletes and people with a muscular build. Conversely, in older people or people with less muscle tone, BMI may underestimate body fat. This is because people who have a good deal of muscle weigh more. Also, BMI does not distinguish among different types of fat or where it is distributed, which may be more indicative of health. Moreover, since BMI is calculated based on age and height, it becomes less accurate as a person grows older. This is because as we age we lose height. We shrink! Men lose an average of 5 centimeters and women lose an average of 6 centimeters by age 80 years old (Holt et al., 2023; Sorkin et al., 1999).

BMI also differs across populations. BMI is less accurate at classifying men than women, and it may exaggerate the differences in obesity between white men and African American men (Burkhauser & Cawley, 2008). At the same time, it may minimize the differences between white non-Hispanic women and African American women (Burkhauser & Cawley, 2008). Many Asian people have relatively low BMIs but are still at high risk of type 2 diabetes and cardiovascular disease (Expert Consultation, WHO, 2004).

Do we need better measures of body fat altogether? As it turns out, we already have some. We can use calipers to take measurements from around the body. We can also use dual-energy X-ray absorptiometry. This technique for measuring body composition can distinguish between the amount of body fat and lean muscle mass by sending a harmless electrical signal through the body to record the impedance or resistance to the electric current. Finally, the underwater hydrostatic weighing technique uses Archimedes' principle of displacement: The more water that is displaced when a person gets into a measuring tub, the greater the body fat. We may not need to complicate our lives with measures like these, but, at the very least, BMI should be interpreted through the lens of lifestyle, age, and ethnicity.

Body Fat and BMI

BMI also cannot take into account the shape of your body or where body fat is distributed on the body.

The **waist-to-hip ratio**, based on the circumference of your waist and hips, can point to where fat is stored. The risk of poor health increases with a waist greater than 35 inches for women and 40 inches for men.

Fat around your middle (called central obesity) is more dangerous than fat around other parts of the body, like your hips, thighs, and buttocks. Belly fat indicates fat deposits around the internal organs (see **Figure 4.7**). Abdominal fat puts you at higher risk for cardiovascular disease, hypertension, diabetes, cancer, and a decline in cognitive functions (Kim, Kim, & Park, 2016; Lee, Pedley, Hoffmann, Massaro, & Fox, 2016; Sato & von Haehling, 2023; Sato et al., 2018; Sponholtz et al., 2016). One study followed 359,387 participants from nine European countries over nearly ten years (Pischon et al., 2008). The results were striking. When BMI was held constant, those who died had significantly higher waist-to-hip ratios than those who did not, and the larger their waistlines were, the more likely they were to die.

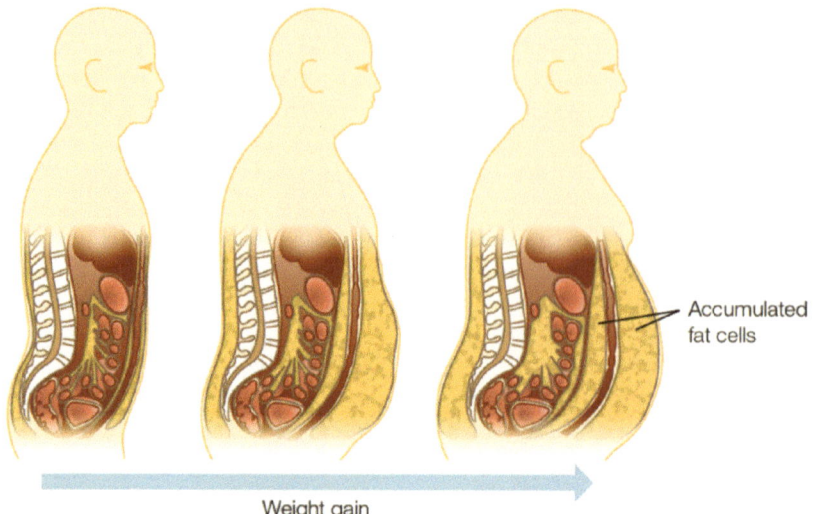

Figure 4.7   How fat accumulates in the abdomen.

Fat around the waist has also been shown to set you up for forgetfulness, confusion, and dementia in later life (Whitmer et al., 2008). Those with the largest waistlines had double the risk of dementia over those with the thinnest waistlines. The greatest risk was for those who were obese with greater belly fat. Middle-aged obese people with excess belly fat had 3.6 times greater risk of dementia than did people of normal weight with low belly fat. Being overweight or obese at midlife independently increases the risk of dementia, Alzheimer's disease, and vascular dementia later in life (Xu, Atti, Gatz, & Fratiglioni, 2011). The larger the waistline, the greater the risk.

Stress and Weight

How, then, does the presence of belly fat lead to so many negative health outcomes? One explanation is that abdominal fat increases in response to stress (Rebuffé-Scrive, Walsh, McEwen, & Rodin, 1992). Stress is a topic we will take a deep dive into in Chapter 6. For now, stress is defined as any negative emotional state accompanied by biochemical, physiological, cognitive, and behavioral changes aimed at removing, altering, or adjusting to its effects (Baum, 1990). Stress has been linked to many negative mental and physical health outcomes such as depression, anxiety, hypertension, ulcers, atherosclerosis, osteoporosis, obesity, and mortality (Heshmati, Luzi, Greenway, & Rebello, 2023).

But How Does Stress Lead to Weight Gain?

Weight gain in response to stress can be due to a change in eating habits, less physical activity, lower cortisol levels, or poor sleep (Geiker et al., 2018; Heshmati et al., 2023). Belly fat that develops as a result of stress is called stress-related weight gain.

People who tend to put on weight in the middle also tend to react badly to stress (Davis, Twamley, Hamilton, & Swan, 1999; Epel et al., 2000). The reason is that fat tissue is a strong producer of **cytokines**, the cell-signaling protein molecules that help regulate the immune system. Some cytokines (anti-inflammatory cytokines) reduce inflammation and promote healing, while others (proinflammatory cytokines) produce fever, increase inflammation, destroy tissue, and make diseases worse (Dinarello, 2000). When abdominal fat triggers a greater production of the second type of cytokines, it can lead to cardiovascular disease, diabetes, stroke, and dementia.

The Evolutionary Foundations of Fat

All fat is not created equal. Why? The puzzle is still being teased apart but the answer most likely relates to hormones. Just above we considered the role of abdominal or central obesity. When adipose tissue accumulates in the abdominal area, it is related to higher risks for diseases such as hypertension, diabetes, heart disease, and some cancers and this is true for both men and women (Power & Schulkin, 2008). However, men and women differ in the patterns of where adipose tissue is most often stored in the body and how it is metabolized and used as energy. These differences relate to sex and reproductive hormones.

Female hormones like estrogen cause women to store fat in the hips, thighs, legs, and buttocks for more successful pregnancy, birthing, and breast-feeding (Singh, 1993). Gluteofemoral fat, the fat on the butt and hips, is actually a sign of strong fertility and metabolic health. In contrast, men are more likely to accumulate fat in the abdomen and upper body (Singh, 1993). These sex differences may have biological roots; however, their psychological impact cannot go unmentioned. A recent study showed that women who stored fat in their abdomen were more likely targets of fat shame and stigma than women who stored fat in the hips, thighs, and buttocks (Krems & Bock, 2023). These findings show that weight stigma can be shape-sensitive. Nevertheless, in both sexes, early humans evolved and adapted to store fat more easily, a problem for today's sedentary lifestyles and high-calorie diets.

Weight Across the Lifespan

What about today? What makes you underweight, overweight, or a healthy weight? Your weight is based primarily on the number and size of your fat cells. Both the number and the size of the fat cells are significantly larger in severely obese people than in nonobese people (Brownell, 1982). Moderately obese individuals have about the same number of fat cells as nonobese individuals, but the size of the fat cells is larger.

What determines the number, size, and distribution of our fat cells? As we mentioned at the beginning of the chapter biology and environment always interact to produce outcomes. Nevertheless, your physique is shaped first by genetics, specifically how tall you are, and your body shape is encoded in your genes. However, early feeding patterns, including a lack of proper nutrition during infancy, can also influence your weight. Poor eating habits, especially in the adolescent years, but even in adulthood, can also increase the size of the fat cells. This means that childhood and adolescence are windows of vulnerability, making it especially important for parents (such as Sydney) to promote healthy food choices, balanced nutrition, and exercise.

Age-related changes affect weight gain as well. As the body changes in midlife, the metabolism slows down. Middle-aged people may consume the same number of calories per day as they did when they were younger, but those calories will not be burned at the same rate. Unless middle-aged people reduce the number of calories they consume or get more exercise to burn the extra calories, they will slowly and steadily gain weight.

Other changes that come with age also affect body shape. Many older adults eat less than they did before, and this has risks of its own. You will recall that middle-aged adults with excess belly fat may be at risk for dementia later in life. Yet weight loss, too, may be a marker of impending Alzheimer's disease (Johnson, Wilkins, & Morris, 2006). Patients with Alzheimer's tend to be thinner than other older adults, though the reasons have long been elusive. Some men begin losing weight at least six years prior to receiving the diagnosis of Alzheimer's disease (Stewart et al., 2005). Recent studies show that higher body mass may serve a protective function against the development and progression of this disease (Sun et al., 2020). Why might weight loss relate to the development of Alzheimer's disease? First, the disorder may cause older adults to forget when to eat. Second, it may cause apathy, anxiety, irritability, or depression, all of which can reduce appetite and the ability to prepare food (Feldman & Woodward, 2005; Grundman et al., 2004). Third, the disease may cause atrophy in areas of the brain that regulate appetite, energy expenditure, and a stable body weight (Grundman, et al., 2004). It may also be that with higher body mass there is higher brain weight which buffers the brain atrophy and neuropathological changes that occur in Alzheimer's disease (Sun et al., 2023). The linkages among weight in later life and the onset and progression of Alzheimer's disease are still under study.

Regardless of your age, maintaining a healthy weight is crucial for offsetting disease and disability. A healthy, nutritious, balanced diet is the key.

Thinking About Health

■ How might your genetic predisposition storing adipose tissue and your environment contribute to your weight? Are you at risk of certain health outcomes as a result of your weight?

■ What dietary changes might you make to offset any potential risks you might have?

■ What are some of the negative health outcomes associated with being overweight or obese?

Who Maintains a Healthy Weight and Why

So far we have considered how genes, family, stress, and age influence what we eat, our body fat, our metabolism, and the shape of our bodies. However, there is a lot of evidence of the powerful influences of personality on health behaviors. Our sense of control, self-efficacy, emotional intelligence, and personality also influence whether we are able to maintain a healthy weight.

Self-Control and Self-Efficacy

Many of us think of gaining weight as a matter of poor self-control (Wills, Isasi, Mendoza, & Ainette, 2007). **Self-control** is the ability to control desires, emotions, and behaviors (Carver, 2004). It involves overriding our habitual or automatic responses and our strong impulses (Gailliot & Baumeister, 2018). It takes self-control not to pick up that candy bar at the grocery store, just as it took self-control for Sydney to expunge her home of unhealthy foods after her pregnancy. Self-control is one form of conscious self-regulation, and, from a biological standpoint, can be traced to brain functioning—specifically, the anterior cingulate cortex in the prefrontal cortex (Banfield, Wyland, Macrae, Münte, & Heatherton, 2005). Although self-control was previously thought to be a personality trait (Tangney, Baumeister, & Boone, 2004), more recently, it has been considered a limited resource. Each act that requires self-control can decrease that resource, making it harder to maintain willpower (Gailliot & Baumeister, 2018).

Faced with sweets and other tempting foods, those with less self-control end up eating more or failing to stick to a diet. They often make unhealthy choices and have greater difficulty losing weight (Crescioni et al., 2011). People who are higher in self-control are more likely, for example, to report eating breakfast regularly (Junger & Van Kampen, 2010). And those who have higher self-control also tend to have lower BMIs (Junger & Van Kampen, 2010; Konttinen, Haukkala, Sarlio-Lähteenkorva, Silventoinen, & Jousilahti, 2009). Self-control is predictive of a healthy diet and weight control (de Ridder, Geenen, Kuijer, & van Middendorp, 2008). In longitudinal studies, children with less self-control were more likely to become obese as they got older (Duckworth, Tsukayama, & Geier, 2010; Francis & Susman, 2009). Higher levels of self-control also bolster those who want to lose weight, helping them stick to their diets (Crescioni et al., 2011).

One of the most intriguing questions about human nature that has fascinated scholars for millennia is how we successfully regulate our desires in the pursuit of longer-term goals (Werner & Ford, 2023). When you think about eating a healthful diet, when one is tempted by things that are less healthful but motivated to lose weight, have more energy or because the doctor has told us eating healthy is the way to reduce our risk of disease, we are faced with conflict.

Self-control is important to resolving the conflict among conflicting goals (Inzlicht et al., 2021). Anyone who has had this struggle knows what it feels like to eat ice cream despite the doctor's orders to avoid high-fat, sugar-laden foods. Most research on self-control has focused on what happens when we fail at self-control and the importance of having willpower (Baumeister, 2018). It has been argued that willpower is a limited resource; however, this is a counterproductive way of thinking. But learning how to say "no" is not the answer and some researchers now believe that "willpower is overrated" (Werner & Ford, 2023).

There have been several theories of self-control that are usefully applied to health behaviors such as pursuing a healthy diet and maintaining a healthy weight. One is the dual-process model of self-control (Metcalfe & Mischel, 1999) which posits that there is a conflict between "hot" emotional states (e.g., impulsivity and "cravings") and a "cold" rational cognitive state (e.g., restraint, inhibition). To exert self-control in health decision-making, one must overcome the "hot" impulse and drive with the "cold." In the value-based choice model, our choices have subjective value for us. For one person, in the moment the value of choosing a brownie sundae might be much stronger than the value of choosing a fruit bowl. The conflict is among taste value and health value. When the weight of the value of one choice exceeds the other that is what we choose. To exert more self-control, one must reevaluate the value of the choices. Cosme and colleagues tested these two models using neurobiological data (i.e., activation in the brain during dietary decision-making) and found that the value-based choice model outperformed the dual process model for dietary decisions (Cosme, Ludwig, & Berkman, 2019).

One interesting way to think about how one's self-control relates to a health behavior like eating a healthy diet comes from Integrative Self-Control Theory (Hofmann, Dohle, & Diel, 2020; Kotabe & Hofmann, 2015). According to Hofmann and colleagues (2020; see also Kotabe & Hofmann, 2015), there are seven psychological "hubs" of self-control:

Desire: an emotional process that motivates behavior
self-control goal: a mental representation of the desired end state
self-control conflict: the competition between temptation now and end states later
self-control motivation: the extent to which one seeks to control the temptation
self-control capacity: the mental resources one has to override temptation to achieve long-term goals
self-control effort: the actual amount of self-control capacity that is called upon to avoid temptation in service of long-term goals
enactment constraints: unexpected things in the environment that interfere with either desire or self-control.

Let's run through an example. Miguel is a college athlete on the wrestling team. He must keep his weight within his weight class in order to be able to compete. On the weekends he hangs out with friends who coax him into drinking games like beer pong, "drunk jenga," or quarters, and there is always pizza, lots and lots of pizza. Putting aside whether you think this is a healthy lifestyle or not, Miguel is always torn because he has a strong desire to maintain a healthy weight so that he can run track that is in conflict with his desire to be with friends and have fun—these are both desires. When he envisions himself winning a wrestling match this is his self-control goal. The self-control conflict is the emotional state he is in at the moment when his friends are prodding and teasing him to "have fun" (his immediate temptation) and his vision of winning his next match (his long-term goal that requires self-control at the moment). The stronger his feelings about meeting his weight requirements and competing the more self-control motivation he has. Given that he's a pretty smart guy, Miguel can usually recall or think of things that help him to stick to his goal and exert his self-control (self-control capacity), and most of the time he finds a way to avoid actually playing the beer games and will indulge in only one piece of pizza (self-control effort) so he can go home feeling good about having reconciled his desires so that he can stick to his goals. There was a time though when he had lost a hard-fought match and was feeling really down, that night at the party, he was not really thinking too much about his next match and just wanted to feel good in the moment, so he surprised his friends and won beer pong! That night the enactment constraints (losing the match, feeling bad, and his momentary desire to feel good) overrode his long-term goals.

Self-control is an important psychological resource that explains why it may be so hard to stick to a healthy diet and maintain a healthy weight in the face of so many choices that are not consistent with those goals. You might want to think about your own thoughts when you are faced with two competing choices, one that is immediately more desirable and satisfying and one that you know is ultimately better for your long-term health. How do you choose? Engaging in more mindful dietary decision-making may help your long-term health.

Self-efficacy is a belief in one's ability to succeed or reach a goal (Bandura, 1995), and it can help greatly with health behaviors (Zhang et al., 2019) and weight loss and maintenance (Clark, Abrams, Niaura, Eaton, & Rossi, 1991; DePue, Clark, Ruggiero, Medeiros, & Pera, 1995; Elfhag & Rössner, 2005; Rodin, Elias, Silberstein, & Wagner, 1988; Stich, Knauper, & Tint, 2009). Self-efficacy is based upon our past successes and failures in reaching goals in spite of obstacles and challenges, and it is a potent motivator of behavior (Bandura, 1998). We can have self-efficacy in one situation but not in others. One student may have very high self-efficacy for doing well on her exam in Health Psychology but have very low self-efficacy for choosing not to have a large popcorn at the movie theatre. Because it is context-specific, researchers have examined eating self-efficacy (Clark et al., 1991) and its role in long-term weight management (Latner et al., 2013; Oikarinen et al., 2023; Varkevisser et al., 2019). Eating self-efficacy refers to the ability to resist eating when faced with challenges including eating tempting but less healthful foods or eating too much. Compared to people with low eating self-efficacy, those who have high eating self-efficacy typically engage in more healthful choices, they are able to stay at a healthy weight and when they lose weight they are better able to maintain it overtime (Oikarinen et al., 2023). Eating self-efficacy has also been an important factor for those who are successful in obesity treatment (Miller et al., 1999). One recent study showed that people overweight or obesity who had low eating self-efficacy had more difficulties (i.e., low cognitive restraint, high uncontrolled eating, high emotional eating and high binge eating) than those with higher eating self-efficacy and this was true for both genders (Oikarinen et al., 2023). These authors argue that their findings shed light on the challenges that people with obesity or overweight confront and point to an avenue for intervention—eating self-efficacy, like self-efficacy for any domain can be changed especially as one encounters more successes in their goal pursuit. Eating self-efficacy when high may even serve a protective function helping people make better choices and achieve their dietary and weight goals.

It is related to our health goals and to our possible selves (see Chapter 3). Self-control in the face of temptation is enhanced when you are confident that you will not give in. Self-control and self-efficacy go hand in hand in eating and weight management.

Personality and Eating

From a psychological perspective self-control and self-efficacy can be considered a part of who we are, or a resource that we have. Our personalities definitely relate to and drive our choices and behaviors. Personality then plays an important role in both risk and protective health behaviors such as eating a healthy diet and maintaining a healthy weight. Personality has been examined in relation to the development of overweight and obesity (Gerlach et al., 2015).

Is there a personality type related to obesity? Early research found that people with an aggressive personality were more likely to have an unhealthy diet and less likely to stick to positive dietary changes (Milligan et al., 1997). Early studies also found links between obesity and impulsivity, boredom, a pessimistic attitude, and anxiety (Fassino et al., 2002).

Other studies single out five personality traits: neuroticism, extraversion, openness to experience, agreeableness, and conscientiousness (Costa & McCrae, 1984). These traits, often called **the Big 5**, are found to some degree in most adults, and most of us have some blend of all of them. They influence how a person experiences the world and copes with stress, and they can have a major impact on healthy behavior.

Someone high in neuroticism tends to experience negative emotions, such as anxiety, anger, worry, self-consciousness, and guilt. Even psychologically stable people may be high in neuroticism. **Neuroticism** is related to higher BMIs (Terracciano et al., 2009). **Extraversion** is the tendency to be outgoing, warm, and sociable. Although it has not been found consistently to relate to weight, some studies have found that extraverted people have higher BMIs (Kakizaki et al., 2008; Magee & Heaven, 2011). In contrast, more conscientious individuals may have lower rates of obesity and lower BMIs (Brummett et al., 2006). **Conscientiousness** is characterized by feeling more comfortable with rules and expectations, and highly conscientious people may be less likely to indulge or overeat: They choose to do things that are health-enhancing (Goldberg & Strycker, 2002).

A systematic review of a large body of literature showed that Neuroticism, Impulsivity, and sensitivity to reward appear to be risk factors for overweight and obesity, whereas conscientiousness and self-control may have protective functions and reduce the risk of overweight and obesity (Gerlach et al., 2015). After decades of research on the links among personality and overweight and obesity, there are some clear and consistent findings showing linkages among personality and these outcomes. Several studies show that personality interacts with other factors such as socioeconomic status so it is impossible to really account for its role in weight (St-Amour et al., 2023). The bottom line though is that there is no one Big 5 personality trait associated with obesity but a host of biopsychosocial factors that interact to create weight-related challenges for people.

Recently, interest has grown in the personality trait of emotional intelligence. Emotional intelligence refers to our ability to recognize our own emotions both positive and negative, and those of others, and to use this information to guide our thoughts and behaviors (Mayer & Salovey, 1997; Salovey et al., 1995). Emotional intelligence is like being able to "read the room" and respond appropriately so that we feel good and others do too. Emotional intelligence in general helps us to understand ourselves and to adapt to environmental demands. In that way is serves a self-regulatory function helping us cope. It has been found to be instrumental in living a healthy life (Dai et al., 2021). A recent systematic review showed that across 26 different studies, both cross-sectional and longitudinal, there is a consistent finding that higher emotional intelligence relates to lower overeating leading to being overweight (Favieri et al., 2021).

Emotional intelligence is also related to body image dissatisfaction. Body image is a representation that we have of our own bodies and it can be associated with both positive and negative emotions. Emotional intelligence interacts with body image to influence weight, weight maintenance and weight loss, and eating disorders (emotional intelligence then is a key factor in the regulation of a healthy diet and weigh management, and health related-quality of life (Pollatos et al., 2020).

Taken together, these studies suggest links between personality traits and weight, but why? It could be that being obese affects personality, taking its toll on one's emotional state. In this way, a high BMI may lead one to experience greater levels of negative emotions. Alternatively, personality, established early in life, may influence how stress is experienced, eating habits, and other behaviors that may increase the tendency to gain weight. Like many psychological factors, keeping a healthy diet and maintaining weight is likely to be determined by the dynamic interaction of multiple complex factors. Nevertheless, you can think about your personality and the degree of self-control, self-efficacy, specific traits you may have as well as your emotional intelligence, and be on the lookout for how they may shape your choices around food, eating, and weight.

Patterns of Eating

Personality also influences weight through lifestyle choices and eating behaviors (Elfhag & Morey, 2008; van Strien, Frijters, Bergers, & Defares, 1986). Patterns of eating could be considered personal traits or patterns of behavior. **Restrained eaters** consciously restrict their eating to control their caloric intake and body weight (Cavanaugh, Kruja, & Forestell, 2014; Houben, Nederkoorn, & Jansen, 2012). **Emotional eaters** tend to eat in response to negative emotions such as anxiety, anger, depression, disappointment, and loneliness. Finally, **external eaters** eat in response to food cues, such as the sight, smell, and taste of foods.

Emotional and external eating styles are associated with higher body weight (Elfhag & Linné, 2005) and more unhealthy consumption of foods high in calories, fat, and sugar (Elfhag, Tholin, & Rasmussen, 2008; van Strien, 2000). Emotional eaters likely overeat in response to a variety of cues, not limited to negative emotions (Bongers, de Graaff, & Jansen, 2016). In one study, across four different conditions—(1) a negative mood manipulation (listening to sad music), (2) a positive mood manipulation (listening to happy, upbeat music), (3) food exposure (their favorite foods and snacks), and (4) a control condition (time spent solving puzzles)—emotional eaters ate more than nonemotional eaters, especially when they were experiencing negative emotions, regardless of the food cues (Bongers et al., 2016). Some research shows that people who have difficulty regulating their emotions, especially anxiety, are more likely to be emotional eaters, and this is linked to higher rates of disordered eating (Bazo Perez et al., 2023). Does this research confirm the role of negative emotions in eating? The jury is still out. To complicate things further, external eaters are not more likely to be obese (Rodin, 1981), although they may still have weight problems.

Where do different eating styles come from? According to one theory, emotional eating relates to depression and has its roots in early childhood (Elfhag & Morey, 2008). Mood, however, is not the whole story, even for emotional eaters. They also tend to have less self-control, be less conscientious, and be more easily discouraged. You can probably also see the connection between emotional intelligence and emotional eating. Another useful term here is impulsiveness, the inability to resist desires, control urges, and tolerate frustration (Piedmont & Ciarrocchi, 1999). As we saw earlier in this chapter, not allowing children to eat certain things, like sugary cereal or cookies, can backfire. It can increase a child's impulsiveness and lead to weight gain (Rollins, Loken, Savage, & Birch, 2014). Adolescence, a highly emotional period, is a critical period in the development of unhealthy eating behaviors and eating disorders (Zhu, Luo, Cai, Li, & Liu 2014). For emotional eating, the family environment is critical.

External eaters, who are susceptible to food cues (Schachter, Goldman, & Gordon, 1968), also tend to be higher in neuroticism (although not as much as emotional eaters), impulsive, and less self-disciplined. Personality, especially a tendency toward external eating patterns, lies behind the "what-the-hell-effect" (Baumeister & Tierney, 2012), or counterregulatory eating. Suppose that you are watching your weight, but you go out to dinner for your friend's birthday. You've shared appetizers and eaten a huge meal, and then the dessert cart comes. You are stuffed and know that you shouldn't have a dessert, but then you think, "I've already blown my diet, so I might as well." As this example suggests, often people can monitor their eating quite well until the very day they indulge—and then their resolve goes out the window

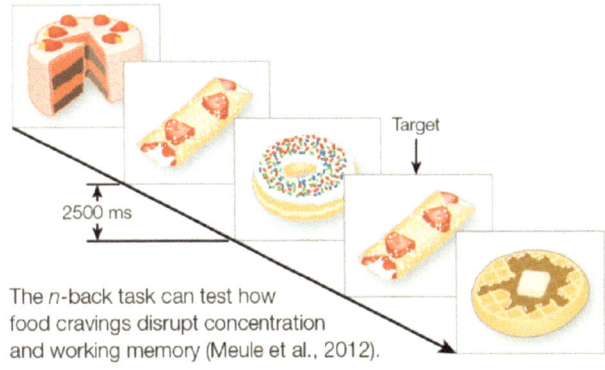

Target

2500 ms

The *n*-back task can test how food cravings disrupt concentration and working memory (Meule et al., 2012).

Photo 4.9   The n-back task can test how food cravings disrupt concentration and working memory.

Source: Research from Meule et al. (2012)

(Baumeister & Tierney, 2012; Gailliot & Baumeister, 2018). This effect is bad for diet, health, and morale, and is psychologically similar to the abstinence violation effect (see Chapter 3).

Food cravings can exhaust our cognitive resources and create cognitive impairments (Meule, Skirde, Freund Vögele, & Kübler, 2012). In other words, food cravings make it difficult to concentrate and interfere with working memory. To test this, scientists have used a technique called the n-back task displayed in **Photo 4.9**. Here, participants are presented with a series of pictures of high-calorie sweet and savory foods and neutral objects and asked to indicate whether each matches a picture that they have seen before. People who have food cravings (especially for chocolate!) show slower reaction times and make more errors when given pictures of unhealthy food than of something less crave-worthy.

If we are all vulnerable to the appeal of food, how do restrained eaters manage not to indulge in overeating? They carefully monitor the types of foods they eat, the number of calories they consume, and their overall weight (Boschi, Iorio, Margiotta, D'Orsi, & Falconi, 2001; Elfhag & Linné, 2005; Lowe, Doshi, Katterman, & Feig, 2013). They may also be more effective at losing weight (Elfhag & Morey, 2008).

But even restrained eating can be bad for health. It may relate to greater neuroticism, especially in children and teenagers (Heaven, Mulligan, Merrilees, Woods, & Fairooz, 2001). Continual restraint may signify body dissatisfaction and struggles with food and eating, and may even put us at risk of eventual overeating and eating disorders (Stunkard & Messick, 1985; Tuschl, 1990). In sum, restraint in the face of temptation is good, but if we are overly strict with what we eat all the time, we may eventually be overwhelmed by temptation.

Do you eat when you feel hungry? Do you eat only until you feel satisfied and full? If so, you are an intuitive eater. **Intuitive eaters** eat when they feel hunger and stop eating when they feel full (Tribole & Resch, 2003; Tylka, 2006; Young, 2010). They are not preoccupied with food and dieting, and they do not restrict their food choices based on whether foods are "good" or "bad." Yet they often end up choosing healthier foods and maintaining a healthy weight. They also have less chronic dieting, binge eating, and other disordered eating behaviors. They eat what their bodies need. Among healthy young adults, men are more trusting of their bodies to tell them when and how much to eat (Denny, Loth, Eisenberg, & Neumark-Sztainer, 2013). A recent large-scale meta-analysis showed that highly intuitive eating was associated with numerous positive outcomes like positive body image, higher self-esteem, and greater well-being, whereas those who are

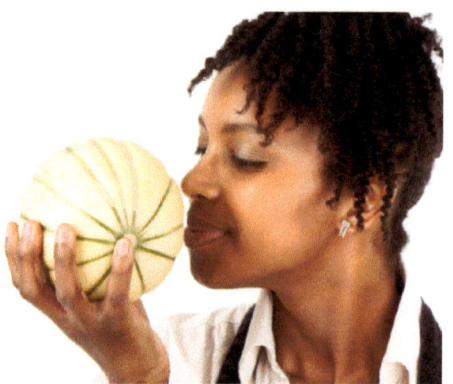

Photo 4.10   Some people actually crave healthy foods: intuitive eaters.

Source: Samuel Borges Photography/Shutterstock

not intuitive eaters were more likely to display pathological eating, disturbances in body image and other forms of psychopathology (Linardon et al., 2021). These findings show how adaptive intuitive eating is for a healthy diet and weight (**Photo 4.10**).

Intuitive eating is generally healthy eating. In contrast, extensive food restriction stands in the way of the body's normal cues. The more people diet, the less they are in tune with hunger and satiety, and that puts them at risk for disordered eating (Costanzo, Reichmann, Friedman, & Musante, 2001; Herman, Polivy, Lank, & Heatherton, 1987).

As we can see, many different attributes, beliefs, and behaviors have been examined to predict positive and negative health outcomes with regard to food and eating (Kerin, Webb, & Zimmer-Gembeck, 2019). Understanding the patterns that emerge when various behaviors come together is important for helping people eat more healthfully and create optimal health outcomes (Kerin et al., 2019).

Thinking About Health

■ What psychosocial, emotional, and personality factors influence eating behaviors?

■ Can you identify the potential problems that arise from restrained, emotional, external, and intuitive eating patterns?

■ If you have tried dieting, has it worked for you? Why or why not?

The Importance of Exercise

If you want to live longer, exercise. If you want to be healthier, exercise. If you want to avoid cardiovascular disease, cancer, diabetes, and many other chronic and debilitating diseases, exercise. If you want to lose weight, exercise. If you want to have less stress and sleep better … you get the point.

The costs of inactivity are high. Worldwide, physical inactivity will cost $300 billion by 2030 in health care and lost productivity unless more countries "scale up" and implement policies to get people moving (WHO, 2022). Globally, nearly 28% of adults and 81% of adolescents do not meet the WHO's recommended levels of physical activity (WHO, 2022). A scientific review of medical records of over 100,000 people spanning a 30-year period shows that those who met the U.S. Department of Health and Human Services' current recommendations for moderate to vigorous weekly exercise had between a 19 and 21% lower risk of death from all causes than those who did not (Lee et al., 2022). Regular physical activity is beneficial for both mental and physical health for people of all ages and abilities and the great news is….it is never too late to begin being active!

How Much Exercise Is Enough?

Physical activity is beneficial in any form and includes walking, cycling, dancing, swimming, weightlifting, playing sports, and even cleaning the house! We define **physical activity** as "anything that gets your body moving." And more specifically any bodily movement that requires energy expenditure.

However, the guidelines now urge two complementary types of physical activity each week (see **Figure 4.8**). **Aerobic exercise** (or cardio) raises your heart rate and strengthens the heart and lungs. Cardio gets your heart pumping and gets you breathing harder. You want to reach an intensity at which you "break a sweat." **Resistance training** (or strength training) builds muscle mass and conditioning. It is as simple as using your own body weight to build muscle mass—think sit-ups, push-ups, squats, and lunges! The minimum recommendation for healthy adults is 150 minutes per week of aerobic exercise at moderate intensity and strength training two or more days per week. That training should include working all major muscle groups—legs, hips, back, chest, abdomen, shoulders, and arms. And for those of us who find it hard to work exercise into our busy schedules, there is great news: You do not need to exercise every day to get the benefits (O'Donovan, Lee, Hamer, & Stamatakis, 2017). Just one or two sessions per week can reduce mortality, heart disease, and cancer. Just move!

Adults Need a Mix of Physical Activity to Stay Healthy

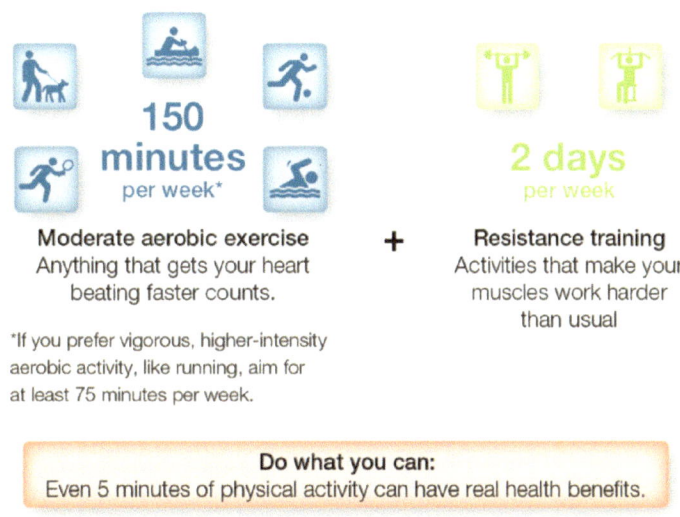

Adults need a mix of physical activity to stay healthy.

150 minutes per week*

Moderate aerobic exercise
Anything that gets your heart beating faster counts.

*If you prefer vigorous, higher-intensity aerobic activity, like running, aim for at least 75 minutes per week.

+

2 days per week

Resistance training
Activities that make your muscles work harder than usual

Do what you can:
Even 5 minutes of physical activity can have real health benefits.

Figure 4.8   Physical activity guidelines for Americans.

Source: Data from U.S. Department of Health and Human Services (2018)

The Overall Benefits of Exercise

Sydney's story at the start of this chapter is an example of the benefits of strength training and conditioning. What she was able to accomplish after her pregnancy was admirable, but not remarkable—anyone can perform and benefit from regular physical activity. Whether walking the dog or running a marathon, exercise provides long-term health benefits for everyone.

The significance of exercise for a healthy lifestyle cannot be understated. At any age, exercise provides many healthful benefits beyond weight control and weight loss. It also prevents or delays such conditions as osteoporosis, high blood pressure, diabetes, and heart disease. Exercise even helps to improve memory and to offset memory problems in older adults. In the brain, it elevates levels of neurochemicals, like serotonin, that increase feelings of well-being, decrease stress, and buffer against anxiety and depression. In fact, research shows that exercise stimulates the growth of new stem cells in the brain (Blackmore, Golmohammadi, Large, Waters, & Rietze, 2009). Active children sleep better, do better in school, and feel better about themselves, not to mention that kids who exercise are on a path to greater health throughout their lives.

The benefits of exercise, then, are physical, cognitive, and mental. So are the costs of a sedentary lifestyle. Let's look at each in more detail.

The Physical Benefits of Exercise

Aerobic exercise increases the efficiency of the **cardiorespiratory system**, which includes the heart and lungs, improving their ability to transport blood and oxygen through the body. Go for a jog and you can feel the effects of exercise on your heart and lungs immediately. Within the cardiovascular system, exercise improves blood flow, reduces resting heart rate, reduces blood pressure, improves cholesterol level (increasing high-density lipoprotein, or "good cholesterol"), and strengthens the heart itself so that it pumps more blood per beat. A strong heart is a healthy heart. Good heart health reduces the risk of heart disease, stroke, diabetes, and hypertension.

In the **respiratory system**, which carries oxygen-rich blood throughout your body, regular exercise increases maximum oxygen consumption and improves lung capacity. Although exercise doesn't change the lungs themselves, it does make them more efficient at using oxygen. Exercise also helps to strengthen your **immune system**, which defends against disease-causing microorganisms (Miles, Huber, Thompson, Davison, & Breier, 2009). When your immune system is weakened, it becomes more vulnerable to invading germs and bacteria. And when your immune system is strong, you enjoy better health. The risk of catching a cold or flu or having a severe bout of either if you do get sick, is lower if you exercise moderately (**Photo 4.11**).

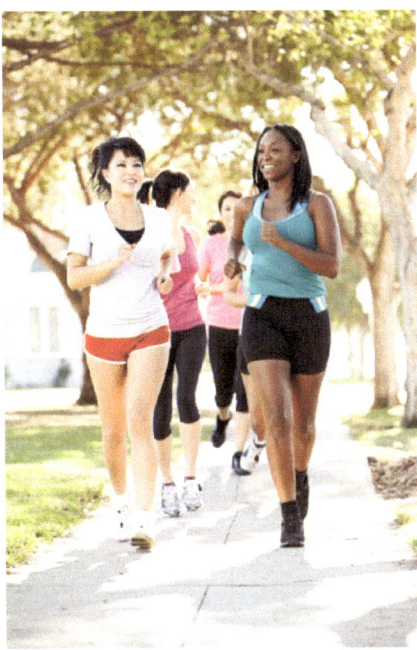

Photo 4.11   Exercise with a friend! You will be more inclined to stick to your exercise routine.

Source: Monkey Business Images/Shutterstock

The Cognitive Benefits of Exercise

Regular exercise positively influences **cognitive functioning**, the processes concerned with knowing, perceiving, attention, and remembering. Moderate-intensity exercise leads to improvements in reaction time, executive functioning, and working and short-term memory functioning. Across the lifespan, research shows the benefits of exercise on cognition (Colzato, Kramer, & Bherer, 2018). For example, aerobic exercise throughout childhood is beneficial for attention and performance (Raine et al., 2018). In adolescence, and especially in the classroom, regular exercise promotes attention, task-related concentration, and achievement of goals (Ludyga, Pühse, Lucchi, Marti, & Gerber, 2019). In older adults, in particular, the evidence is growing that physical activity and physical fitness are associated with better cognitive functioning (Peven, Grove, Jakicic, Alessi, & Erickson, 2018), enhanced brain functioning (ten Brinke, Hsu, Best, Barha, & Liu-Ambrose, 2018; Voss et al., 2010), prevention of brain atrophy (Colcombe et al., 2006), and even growth and regeneration among neurons and greater plasticity in the brain (Greenwood & Parasuraman, 2010). Plasticity, or neuroplasticity, refers to a process in which neural pathways in the brain reorganize, or new pathways develop in response to experience. Given the evidence, some gerontologists argue that exercise can promote brain growth in seniors (Liu-Ambrose, Nagamatsu,

Voss, Khan, & Handy, 2012). Not only does exercise significantly decrease age-related cognitive impairment, but it may also offset and slow the progression of Alzheimer's disease (Weinstein et al., 2012).

At any age, the evidence shows that physical exercise can promote positive changes and offset neurodegeneration in the brain, providing enormous benefits for cognitive functioning and well-being (Mandolesi et al., 2018).

The Mental Health Benefits of Exercise

People who exercise regularly also enjoy better mental health. Exercise is immediately uplifting, and has long-term benefits for emotional well-being. Even a single session of exercise reduces self-reported anxiety and depression and increases positive mood (Anderson & Brice, 2011; Steptoe & Cox, 1988). It can take only 10 minutes of walking to lift yourself out of a funk (Anderson & Brice, 2011; Ekkekakis & Petruzzello, 2000; Hansen, Stevens, & Coast, 2001). And the positive effects of exercise continue to boost mood for up to 24 hours afterward (Sibold & Berg, 2010). After a 10-week exercise program, participants experienced significantly improved self-esteem as well (Desharnais, Jobin, Côté, Lévesque, & Godin, 1993). All else being equal (age, health, income level), people who exercised had one to five fewer days of poor mental health than those who did not exercise (Chekroud et al., 2018). The benefits are strongest when people exercise 30–60 minutes per day for three to five days a week. And not all exercise is equally beneficial—popular team sports and cycling are best! (Chekroud et al., 2018).

People who suffer from mood disorders, such as depression, can benefit from exercise. Those who are physically active are less likely than those who are inactive to become depressed (Otto et al., 2007). In a clinical trial, patients with major depressive disorder were assigned randomly to one of four conditions: supervised exercise, home-based exercise, antidepressant therapy, or a placebo pill (Blumenthal et al., 2007). Remarkably, exercise turned out to work as well as pharmacological treatment. After the first four months of treatment, patients in the exercise groups experienced less depression and greater remission of their symptoms, equivalent to those taking antidepressant medications and greater than those taking placebo. One year later, the people who continued to exercise still had lower rates of depression than their less-active counterparts (Blumenthal et al., 2010). In another study, people who had recently recovered from an episode of major depression, but who were still experiencing bouts of sadness, were prescribed 15 minutes of acute physical exercise daily. Even this little bit of exercise helped protect against life's stressors. As exercise levels increased, so, too, did mood and patients' abilities to cope with difficult life situations (Mata, Hogan, Joormann, Waugh, & Gotlib, 2013).

Exercise is also beneficial for treating and perhaps preventing anxiety. Some people are said to experience anxiety sensitivity: They have a heightened awareness of the physiological cues of anxiety, including increased heart rate, rapid breathing, and perspiration—a "fear of fear" (Reiss, Peterson, Gursky,

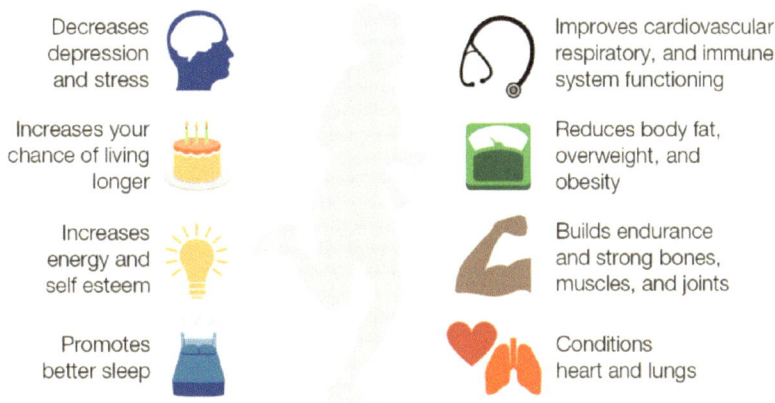

Photo 4.12 The benefits of exercise.

& McNally, 1986). And these people are also at greater risk of panic attacks. Exercise may offset that sensitivity (Smits et al., 2008). In one study, participants learned to associate physiological cues with exercise instead of threat or danger. Other researchers simulated an anxiety attack in participants by exposing them to carbon dioxide, which triggers increased heart rate, breathing, dry mouth, and dizziness. Physically active participants were less likely to panic (Smits, Tart, Rosenfield, & Zvolensky, 2011).

Furthermore, exercise has been found to increase the quality of life for those who suffer from chronic illnesses. Thirty-six studies examined in a meta-analysis showed that, for women undergoing breast cancer treatments, it didn't matter what kind of exercise they did—any exercise improved their quality of life (Zhang, Li, & Liu, 2019). For patients with pulmonary fibrosis (a lung disease), exercise lessened symptoms (Wittman & Swigris, 2019). In patients with multiple sclerosis, aerobic exercise improved cognitive functioning, lifted depression, and reduced fatigue (Sandroff, Pilutti, & Motl, 2019). And for Parkinson's patients, who may have difficulty moving, exercise in many forms can be helpful. From aerobics to yoga to tai chi, the benefits are massive (Raje et al., 2019). These are just a few of the many recent studies showing how exercise, even in the context of disease, can have positive benefits (**Photo 4.12**).

Sitting Too Much Can Be Lethal

Although exercise is important, the amount of time we spend sitting around is also a powerful predictor of health—for the worse. Among middle-aged Scottish men, those who reported spending two or more hours a day sitting at a screen had two times the risk of heart attack and other heart problems (Stamatakis, Hamer, & Dunstan, 2011). More troubling still, those who spent four or more hours watching TV and using computers were 50% more likely to die (of any cause) than those who were less sedentary, even if these men also exercised. Over the course of a week, men who spent more than 23 hours sitting (watching TV or sitting in their cars while commuting) were more likely to die of heart disease than those who spent 11 hours or more a week being more active (Owen, Healy, Matthews, & Dunstan, 2010).

Exercise Snacking

Instead of reaching for the potato chips or the cookies, how about an exercise snack? "Exercise snacks" is a term introduced by Dr Howard Hartley (2007) to refer to brief, sporadic bursts of vigorous-intensity exercise lasting less than one minute. Just think about that. If you haven't been exercising because you don't have the time—maybe you do! All it takes is a minute of running up a flight of stairs, doing a few squats while you sauté your veggies for dinner, or walking the hallway of your dorm at a fast clip. The goal is a short burst of activity that gets your heart rate up for a short time. The more frequently you snack on exercise the better it is for your health. In one study healthy but sedentary college students engaged in exercise snacking by rapidly running up and down three flights of stairs, three times a day (morning, lunchtime, and late afternoon) every day for six weeks (Jenkins et al., 2019). These students were not doing any other form of physical activity. However, after six weeks they had gained aerobic fitness and better oxygen consumption and muscle strength in their legs compared to the non-training control group (Jenkins et al., 2019). Many studies show that we should spend less time sitting because it is bad for our health (Healy et al., 2008; Moore et al., 2022), just getting up every so often and doing jumping jacks for 60 seconds, running up the stairs, or doing a few squats as you watch a commercial can get you in better shape.

Without question, today's work environment has changed everything. Many more people spend time sitting while commuting to work or while working at an office computer. What is striking about the Scottish study is that the sedentary time was leisure time or discretionary time. Those men chose to spend those hours in front of their TVs. Thus, lifestyle choices are key to health.

Thinking About Health

■ Do you think that the U.S. government's guidelines for exercise are an effective framework for maintaining good health?

■ What are some of the many benefits of exercise? How do you benefit from exercise?

Who Exercises and Why

Individuals who were active in sports as children continue to exercise throughout their lives. Some research shows that people who enjoy exercise come from families in which physical activity is valued—exercise is something that family members do together.

Most of the same psychological factors discussed above for maintaining a healthy diet and weight also apply to exercise.

One crucial factor here is self-efficacy: Those who feel capable of exercising do it and benefit from it. Finally, once physical activity on a daily basis becomes a habit, maintaining that lifestyle is easier.

Still, many more do not get enough exercise. An online search shows that in 2017, 38,477 health clubs existed in the United States, and more than 60 million Americans had gym memberships. Yet, on average, 80% of Americans do not get the recommended amount of physical activity (Piercy et al., 2018). And Americans are not alone. Lack of exercise may be a factor in 1 of 10 premature deaths around the world each year—roughly equivalent to the number of deaths caused by smoking.

Barriers to Exercise

Why don't people get enough exercise? In one survey (Sallis & Howell, 1990; Sallis et al., 1992), the 10 most common reasons for not exercising were the following:

1. Lack of time
2. Inconvenience
3. Lack of self-motivation
4. Not enjoying exercise
5. "Exercise is boring"
6. Low confidence in one's ability to be physically active
7. Fear of injury or recovering from injury
8. Inability to set personal goals and monitor progress
9. Lack of encouragement, support, or companionship from family and friends
10. No safe, convenient place to exercise.

Additionally, people report that cost, fatigue, family, work, and other obligations make it hard to prioritize physical activity (Salmon, Owen, Crawford, Bauman, & Sallis, 2003). However, people who report enjoying physical activity are twice as likely to make time for it (Salmon et al., 2003).

How can motivation tip the scales in favor of exercise? Think back again to Sydney—a typical person with a busy life and many demands on her time. Imagine what barriers she had to overcome in order to work out and become strong. Can you think of some of the ways in which exercising helped her, beyond just losing the weight that she gained during pregnancy? Think of the ways in which strength training and the commitment to exercise gave her life new purpose and meaning. Do you find her story motivating?

Cross-Cultural Differences in Exercise

Although the health club trend developed in the United States, people exercise all over the world. In fact, some unique trends are found in other countries.

In China, walking backward is a common way to exercise, as it benefits leg muscles that are not normally used. It also improves balance and posture, and—according to ancient rumors—can reverse your karma and offset senile dementia. In Japan, every morning, Radio Taiso broadcasts a series of warm-up and stretching exercises designed to raise energy levels and unite people in promoting good health. Students, employees, and family members all stop what they are doing and perform these morning exercises together. Capoeira, a Brazilian tradition, combines dance, acrobatics, music, and martial arts in a form of exercise that increases strength and flexibility, while improving balance, coordination, rhythm, and heart health. Capoeira was thought to have been invented by African slaves who were actually practicing martial arts while pretending to dance (**Photo 4.13**).

Another form of dance that is great exercise is belly dancing, often found in the Middle East. It is both a cardiovascular exercise and a great strengthening workout for core abdominal muscles. Yoga, an ancient form of physical and mental discipline, is practiced in India to gain harmony between the body and the mind. There are many different kinds of yoga, but all of them increase flexibility, tone the muscles, and help to achieve peace of mind. In contrast to the calming effects of yoga, today the hottest workout in Delhi is "laughter yoga." Hundreds of people gather to giggle, guffaw, and whoop it up. Maybe laughter really is the best medicine.

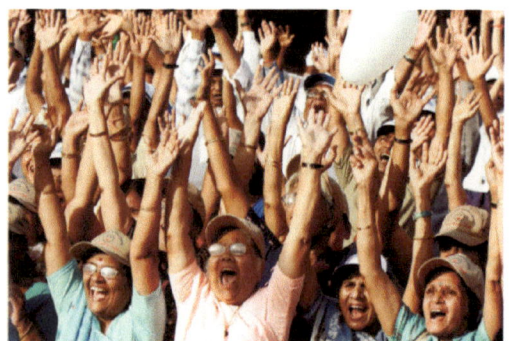 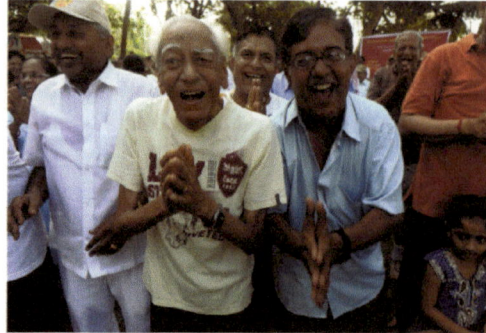

Photo 4.13   "Laughter Yoga" not only exercises the body but can also lift the spirit!

Thinking About Health

■ What are some of the barriers to exercise?

■ How can you eliminate the barriers that make exercise hard for you?

Sleep

In addition to a healthy diet, weight management, and physical activity, sleep is crucial for cognitive, emotional, and physical functioning. As an Irish proverb says, "A good laugh and a long sleep are the best cures in the doctor's book." Yet most people do not get nearly enough sleep to be fully functional during the day.

Sleep's Benefits and Sleep Debt

Although everyone is different, on average, healthy adults need seven to eight hours of sleep each night. Those who sleep only four or five hours each night experience significant negative physical and behavioral consequences. Not sleeping enough or getting a bad night's sleep is related to high blood pressure, weakened immune system functioning, and a higher risk of diabetes, stroke, cancer, and cardiovascular disease. It also negatively impacts mood, sex drive, and weight gain. However, those who sleep more than seven or eight hours per night may have higher mortality rates than those who sleep fewer hours (Knutson, 2010; Youngstedt & Kripke, 2004). An Australian study, by far the largest ever done in the Southern Hemisphere, found that a person who sleeps too much, sits too much, and isn't physically active is more than four times as likely to die early (Ding et al., 2016). As the study's author put it, "When you add the lack of exercise into the mix, you get a 'triple whammy.'"

Feeling alert and well-rested depends on getting those seven to eight hours of sleep night after night. Without that, you may suffer from the cumulative effects of loss of sleep over time, or **sleep debt**. Just a few nights of poor sleep will cause you to go into sleep debt.

Sleep debt may have serious consequences on your daily functioning and your long-term health and well-being. Not getting enough sleep on a regular basis can lead to significant impairments in attention, reaction times, learning, and memory; increased risk of auto accidents, substance abuse, and psychiatric conditions; an increase in BMI; and a greater likelihood of being overweight or obese. One recent study showed that middle-aged adults who got fewer than six hours of sleep a night developed plaques in their arteries (Domínguez et al., 2019), characteristic of the development of atherosclerosis, or heart disease (see Chapter 10) (**Photo 4.14**).

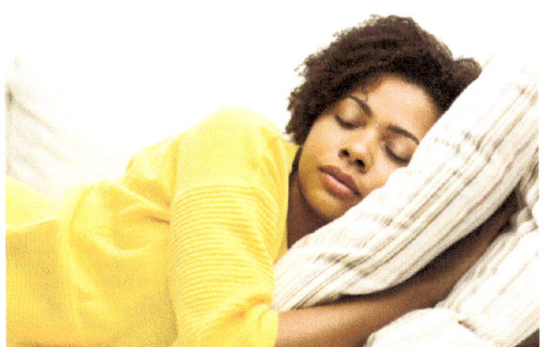

Photo 4.14   Some research shows that women sleep more than men.

Source: Burgard and Ailshire (2013). Syda Productions/ Shutterstock

Age	Sleep needs (hours)
Newborns	12–18
Toddlers	14–15
School-age children	12–14
Infants	11–13
Preschoolers	10–11
Teens	8.5–9.25
Adults	7–9

Source: Data from National Sleep Foundation (2015).

Table 4.4   Average sleep needs for different age groups

Differences in the Need for Sleep

Once again, however, getting too much sleep may not be beneficial, either. Clearly, sleeping too little and sleeping too much are both bad for your health.

There are many individual differences in the amount of sleep needed because each of us has our own unique **circadian rhythm**—the biological cycles that carry us from day to night and night to day. There are also substantial differences in the optimal amount of sleep needed across the lifespan, as **Table 4.4** shows.

Optimal sleep duration is the longest early in life, with newborn infants spending 18 of 24 hours sleeping. This amount of sleep is crucial for early development. However, as children age, their sleep needs change, and adolescents can manage eight-and-a-half to nine-and-a-half hours of sleep. People often find that their sleep becomes lighter and less restful with age, so those older than 65 may need more sleep each day than when they were younger. Many older adults also have chronic medical conditions that may interfere with sleep. As a result, many older folks nap more, which, unfortunately, may make nighttime sleep more elusive. Older adults also spend less time in deep sleep—the stage of sleep with the most benefits.

The Architecture of Sleep

A good night's sleep involves passing through several important stages. In addition, there is a major distinction between two types of sleep, called REM and NREM.

Each stage of the **sleep cycle** is differentiated by the type of brain waves observed and other physiological characteristics. The cycle begins each night when the body signals that it is time to sleep by boosting the circulating levels of adenosine, the neurotransmitter that signals readiness to sleep.

Adenosine effectively powers down the body's waking functions, such as attention, memory, and reactions to physical stimuli. As circulating levels of adenosine increase, our feelings of drowsiness increase, and we begin to enter **NREM (non-rapid eye movement) sleep**. It is during this phase that the first three states of sleep occur. Stage 1 (or N1) sleep is characterized by slow eye movements and slow relaxation of the voluntary muscles (arms, legs, face). Some people experience sudden jerky movements during this stage, known as **hypnic myoclonia (or myoclonic jerks)**. These "sleep starts," which may feel like falling, happen when the motor areas of the brain receive spontaneous activation. Usually, this transitional period is brief, lasting between 5 and 10 minutes. During a full night's sleep, Stage 1 accounts for 5% of our total sleep. People who wake up during this period do not even feel as if they had been sleeping.

Next, we move into Stage 2 (or N2) sleep. During this stage, we become less aware of our surroundings, our body temperature drops and our breathing and heart rates slow. This stage lasts for about 20 minutes each time we cycle through it, accounting for nearly 50% of our time asleep, in total. During Stage 2 sleep, brain waves become more rapid and rhythmic and produce little bursts of activity known as **sleep spindles**. Sleep spindles are linked to neurologic activity, which is thought to help the integration of new information into our knowledge base. It also facilitates memory processing (Saletin, Goldstein, & Walker, 2011; Tamminen, Lambon Ralph, & Lewis, 2013). Recent research has also discovered that changes in N2 sleep can be indicative of later disease. Older adults who show a reduction in N2 sleep and changes in sleep spindles may develop cognitive impairment (Taillard et al., 2019). Sleep studies that examine sleep spindles as biomarkers may help to identify older people at risk for dementia.

Perhaps even more astonishing is the finding that, during Stage 2 sleep, the brain gets a nightly bath! During N2 sleep, channels in the brain open, and cerebrospinal fluid (CSF) flows in and cleanses the brain, washing away the daily accumulation of metabolic waste (Iliff & Nedergaard, 2013; Nedergaard, Iliff, Benveniste, & Deane, 2018). When this waste is not removed, plaque can build up in the brain, leading to Alzheimer's disease, stroke, and other dysfunctions. Poor sleep and a lack of N2 sleep can have long-term negative impacts on health.

When the brain waves become deep and slow (high-amplitude delta waves), we have entered Stage 3 (or N3) sleep. This is the deepest stage of NREM sleep. At this time, we become much less responsive to things around us. Sleepwalking (parasomnias), sleep talking (somniloquy), and night terrors occur during N3 sleep, and it is generally difficult to wake someone from this stage of sleep. But because these stages are the deepest, they are also the most restorative. During Stage 3 sleep, our blood pressure drops, our muscles become more relaxed, our energy is restored, and tissue growth and repair occur. Growth hormones in children and young adults are also released, making this stage essential for development.

REM (rapid eye movement) sleep is a hallmark of the last stage of sleep. This sleep stage is marked by intense activity in different parts of the brain and can appear like wakefulness, even though people are temporarily paralyzed (with

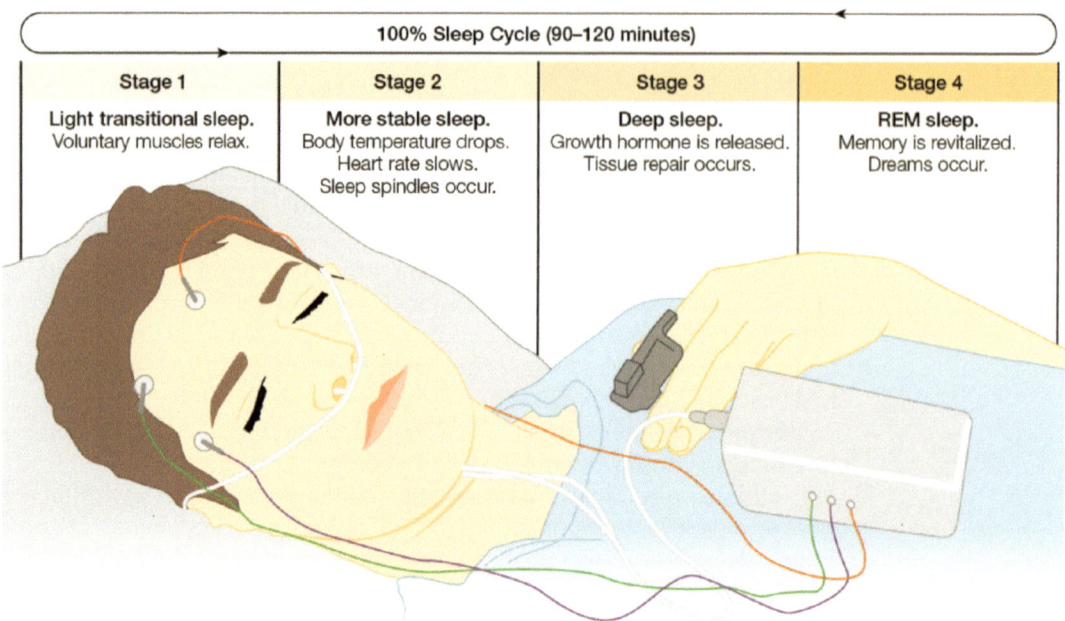

100% Sleep Cycle (90–120 minutes)			
Stage 1	**Stage 2**	**Stage 3**	**Stage 4**
Light transitional sleep. Voluntary muscles relax.	**More stable sleep.** Body temperature drops. Heart rate slows. Sleep spindles occur.	**Deep sleep.** Growth hormone is released. Tissue repair occurs.	**REM sleep.** Memory is revitalized. Dreams occur.

Figure 4.9   The stages of sleep.

no voluntary motor movement). NREM sleep accounts for 75% of the time we spend sleeping at night; REM encompasses the remaining 25% (see **Figure 4.9**). The first REM stage usually begins 90 minutes after we fall asleep, and we enter it again every 90 minutes. Throughout the night, we move in and out of the stages of sleep, usually going from Stage 1 to Stage 2, then to Stage 3, and then back through Stages 3 and 2 again before entering REM sleep. Depending on how long we sleep, we make four or five complete cycles through the stages each night. However, unless we wake up at some point during the night, we do not re-cycle through Stage 1. The sleep cycle includes several brief periods of wakeful-ness intermittently throughout the night as well. With age, people spend more time awake, which can lead to feelings of fatigue during the day.

REM Sleep

As we now know, after about 70–90 minutes of sleep, we enter REM sleep. This stage is characterized by rapid eye movement, increased breathing, and increased brain activity. REM sleep is a paradox because, although brain activity increases significantly, our bodies actually become more relaxed, to the point of mild paralysis of voluntary muscles (like your hands, arms, or legs). The brain activity during REM sleep looks much like brain activity when we are awake, with high alpha and beta wave activity. Our breathing becomes rapid, irregular, and shallow during REM, and our heart rate and blood pressure increase.

It is during this stage that dreaming occurs. The function of dreams is still not fully understood (Schredl, 2018). They may represent neuronal connections being made and unmade, forming the basis for our thoughts, memories, mental functioning, and even emotional processing (Hartmann, 1996). REM sleep helps the nervous system develop in early life, facilitating some kinds of learning throughout the lifespan and playing a crucial role in the repair, reorganization, and formation of new connections in the brain (Hartmann, 2007).

Despite its importance, each REM cycle is rather short. The first REM cycle of the night typically lasts only 10 minutes. During the course of the night, the distribution of time spent within each stage changes so that the periods of REM sleep increase. You thus spend the most time dreaming in the early morning before you wake up, and you get the most restorative deep sleep earlier in the night, shortly after falling asleep.

Across the human lifespan, the amount of time we spend in each sleep stage changes. In later life, less time is spent in deep sleep. As a consequence of this and other age-related changes, older people wake more often during the night. Conversely, during infancy and early childhood, the percentage of time spent in REM sleep is highest. In fact, infants spend as much as 50% of their sleep in REM sleep. The percentage of REM sleep begins to decrease in adolescence and young adulthood when only about 20% of sleep is REM sleep.

Seep Hygiene: How Can You Improve Your Sleep?

How do you sleep? Do you have difficulty powering down after a busy day? Do you wake up during the night and have difficulty falling back asleep? Do you feel rested when you wake up? There are many ways to measure the quality of your sleep—and many ways to improve it (see **Figure 4.10**).

Many fitness-tracking devices—including our phones—now allow us to track our sleep in detail. These apps can tell us how much time we spend in each phase of sleep and can help us make our own connections between how well we've slept and how well

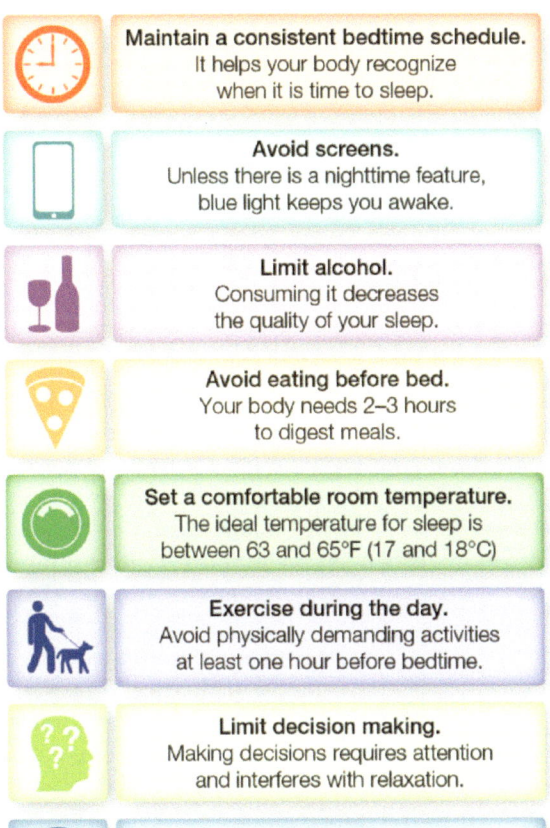

Maintain a consistent bedtime schedule.
It helps your body recognize when it is time to sleep.

Avoid screens.
Unless there is a nighttime feature, blue light keeps you awake.

Limit alcohol.
Consuming it decreases the quality of your sleep.

Avoid eating before bed.
Your body needs 2–3 hours to digest meals.

Set a comfortable room temperature.
The ideal temperature for sleep is between 63 and 65°F (17 and 18°C)

Exercise during the day.
Avoid physically demanding activities at least one hour before bedtime.

Limit decision making.
Making decisions requires attention and interferes with relaxation.

Unwind.
Establish a relaxing, comfortable environment for sleep in your home.

Figure 4.10   Steps to improve sleep.

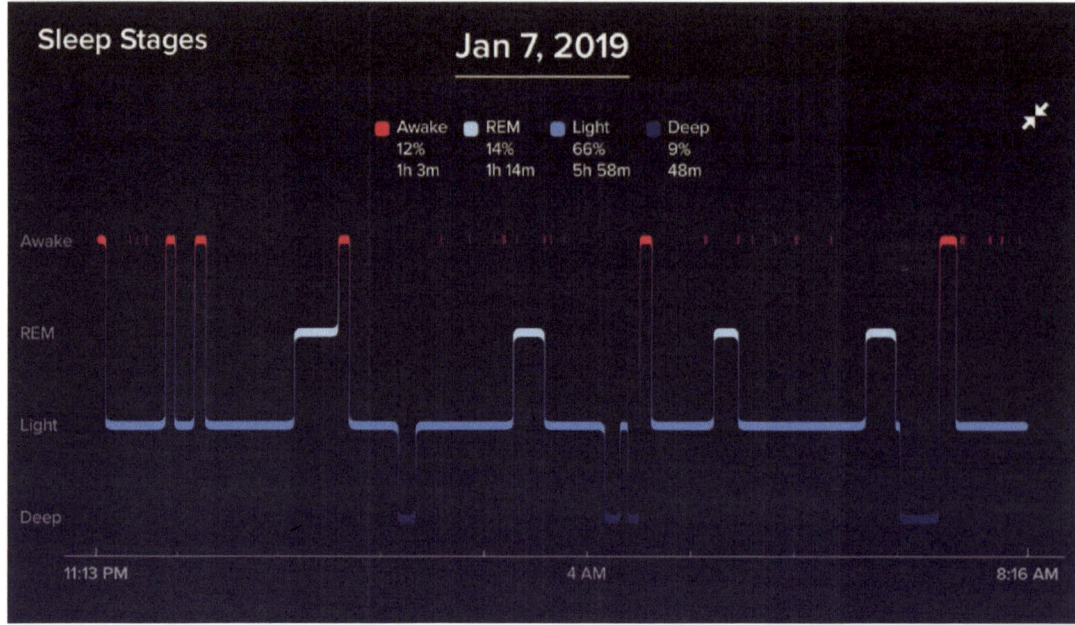

Figure 4.11   Sample night of sleep as tracked by a Fitbit.

we function during the day. **Figure 4.11** shows the results of one night's sleep, as tracked by a Fitbit.

With growing concerns about how our sleep is being compromised, and the negative health outcomes that can result from this, many health practitioners are advocating better **sleep hygiene**—the practices that lead to better sleep. But how do you really know if you've slept well? One good indicator is if you wake up feeling rested and if you have the energy to get through the day. Our perception of our sleep quality is highly subjective. We often consider how deep we think we slept, if we fell asleep easily, slept a good amount of time, didn't wake up too often during the night, and waking easily feeling well rested. For those college students 59% have low sleep quality (Yildirim, Onder, & Avci, 2020). Some factors that reduce sleep hygiene and leave people feeling unrested are caffeine consumption which makes it harder to fall asleep, reduces time asleep, and causes more wakings during the night; consumption of energy drinks and sugar-sweetened beverages, skipping breakfast, eating irregularly, and eating an unhealthy diet also contribute (Shimura et al., 2020). The use of electronics before sleep is also detrimental, making it harder to fall asleep, poorer sleep quality, and difficulty getting up in the morning (Amra et al., 2017). You can also imagine the negative impact of stress and worry on sleep. In a meta-analysis of the sleep experience of COVID-19 patients (people who tested positive for COVID-19) had more sleep problems than those testing negative and health-care workers during the COVID-19 pandemic (Jahrami et al., 2021). However, there are other studies that showed that during COVID-19 lockdown people slept better than pre-pandemic (Staller & Randler, 2021). That led sleep scientist, Michael Scullin and his team (Gao & Scullin, 2020) to wonder whether the stress of the pandemic would cause worse sleep, for sleep to remain unchanged, or for sleep to actually improve. Using longitudinal, cross-sectional, and retrospective data of nearly 700 American adults in the early phases of COVID-19, they found that overall, for most people in the study, sleep was unchanged or even improved. Those for whom sleep worsened (25% of the sample) reported more stress due to caregiving, an adverse impact on their lives due to COVID-19, being a shift worker, and having COVID-19 (Gao & Scullin, 2020). Other studies also showed the negative impact of the COVID-19 pandemic on sleep (Hyun et al., 2021).

In addition to the tips provided in **Figure 4.10**, the Around the World feature describes a unique (and contentious) practice for improving sleep hygiene for infants.

We have seen how a healthy diet, exercise, and sleep can contribute to positive health outcomes. What are some other behaviors that can improve our health? Let's look at some important examples of preventive health care.

Thinking About Health

- Why is adequate sleep a health-enhancing behavior?
- If too much sleep is correlated with higher mortality, could the cause run the other way—with poor mental or physical health leading to too much time in bed? In light of the studies we have examined, which direction seems more likely to you?
- What can you do to improve the quality and quantity of your sleep?

Question: Babies Who Chill

For ages, parents and grandparents in Scandinavia have left their babies out in the cold—literally! In Norway, Sweden, Finland, and Denmark, it is common practice to wrap the little ones up in lots of blankets and place them in strollers outside to sleep, even in the dead of winter. A Swedish colleague reported that, in Stockholm, one often sees prams (strollers) parked outside on the sidewalk while parents socialize and enjoy a convivial lunch inside a restaurant as temperatures dip to 23 degrees F (−5°C). Even some nurseries encourage outdoor naps. In fact, most daycare centers in Sweden have outdoor naptime even when it is snowing. (Of course, if the temperatures drop too low, they cover the prams with blankets.) (See **Photo 4.15**.)

This practice is believed to have taken hold in Finland in the 1920s when infant mortality rates were high (Tourula, Pölkki, & Isola, 2013). Air quality outdoors was thought to be better than indoors, and napping in fresh air was believed to prevent rickets, strengthen the

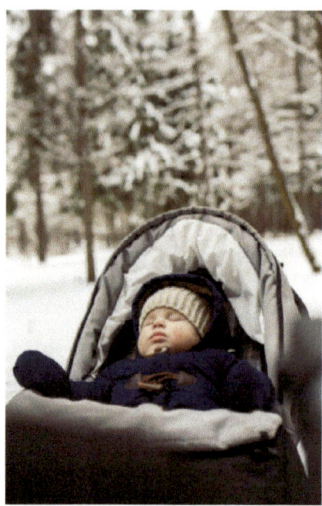

Photo 4.15   Scandinavian babies nap outside even in the winter.

Scandinavian parents report that napping in the cold leads to longer naps, which is beneficial for developing babies (Tourula et al., 2013). Scandinavians also believe that outdoor napping—even in the coldest temperatures—leads to happier, more energetic, and more well-adjusted children who are better able to sleep through the night and sleep under challenging conditions (Tourula, Isola, & Hassi, 2008). Parents who place their kids outdoors for naps also argue that it is healthier for them to be outside in the winter rather than indoors where germs are thriving. Regardless of the reasons why these practices have endured for generations, there is a growing body of research to support the benefits (Tourula et al., 2013; Tourula, Fukazawa, Isola, Hassi, Tochihara, & Rintamäki, 2011). However, while this practice is culturally acceptable in the Nordic countries, Scandinavian parents have been arrested in the United States for leaving their kids outside in the cold.

What are the benefits of napping outdoors? What problems could arise from this practice?

blood, and offset disease. These cultural norms have endured, and now, in Norway (and elsewhere), babies are put outdoors to nap when they are as young as two weeks old.

Other Health-Enhancing Behaviors

Regular preventive health care and dental care are essential to good health. Although children are often required by their schools to have regular physical examinations, some adults, with no such requirements, also get annual medical exams. These adults place value on health and are willing to make efforts to preserve it. People who regularly practice this health-enhancing behavior tend to be older, more highly educated, primarily white, and of higher socioeconomic status.

Despite the fact that the cause is not known, most cancers can be prevented. Cancer is actually not a single disease but a group of diseases that share the common feature of the uncontrolled growth and spread of abnormal cells, when if not treated can lead to death. According to the American

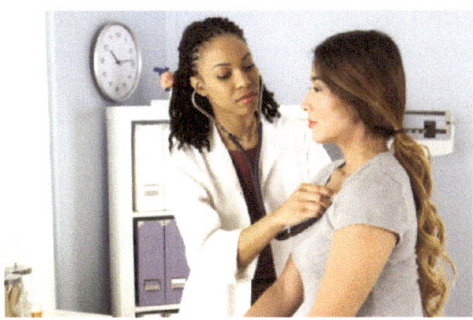

Photo 4.16   Regular doctor visits can help catch health issues before they become dangerous.

Source: Rocketclips, Inc./Shutterstock

Cancer Society, over 2 million new cancer cases and 611,720 cancer deaths were projected for the United States in 2024 (American Cancer Society, 2024). That is roughly 1,680 deaths per day. The good news is that these figures represent a 33% decline in overall death rates due to cancer from its peak in 1991 (American Cancer Society, 2024). Decrease in tobacco use, better screening, early detection and treatment, and preventive health behaviors have all contributed. Death rates due to cancer should continue to decline in the four major cancer sites—the lungs, the colon or rectum, the breasts, and the prostate (**Photo 4.16**) (American Cancer Society, 2024).

Still, individuals can do much more to prevent and offset their risk of developing cancer (see Chapter 11 for more information on cancer). What health-enhancing behaviors are associated with cancer prevention? Furthermore, what behaviors can make everyday life activities—such as driving and sex—safer as well?

Breast Cancer Prevention

About one of every eight American women will get breast cancer during her lifetime, making it the second leading cause of cancer in women (American Cancer Society, 2024). Maintaining a healthy weight, using hormone replacement therapy, drinking alcohol, and not being physically active are some of the lifestyle factors that relate to increased risk of breast cancer. Many women know from their obstetrician or gynecologist about the benefits of routine breast exams. Early detection is the key.

A **mammogram** is a screening and diagnostic tool that involves a low-energy X-ray of breast tissue. Mammography has a proven track record for early detection and treatment of breast cancer. Originally, the U.S. Preventive Services Task Force recommended that women aged 45 or older should have a mammography annually, a recommendation that the American Cancer Society endorsed. In 2009, the task force revised these guidelines to state that mammograms are not needed until age 50 and then only every two years. This reflects the much greater benefits of mammography to women in their sixties, but also the psychological impact of a false-positive result and fear of unnecessary radiation exposure from early treatment. However, this revised recommendation may lead to underdiagnosis. It may cause 20% of breast cancers to go undetected (Arleo et al., 2013). More alarmingly, over 50% of these undiagnosed cancers may be invasive, having spread through the breast tissue.

Both the task force and its critics agree that the decision to conduct annual mammograms before age 50 should be made on an individual basis, in consultation with one's physician. It should take into account any family history of breast cancer. In the meantime, routine manual breast exams should be conducted in annual gynecology visits.

Colorectal Cancer Screening

The third most common type of cancer originates in the colon or rectum. It is also the third leading cause of death in both men and women in the United States today (American Cancer Society, 2024). Colorectal cancers often begin with the growth of a **polyp**, or noncancerous tumor, in the inner lining of the colon or rectum. Some polyps can become malignant forms of cancer. The chance of a polyp turning from benign to malignant depends on the type of polyp and whether it is found and treated early.

According to the U.S. Preventive Services Task Force, regular screenings are advised from age 45 onward. This screening involves high-sensitivity fecal occult blood testing (in which stool samples are examined for the presence of blood), sigmoidoscopy (a test in which a lighted camera is used to examine the lining of the rectum and colon), and a **colonoscopy**. In this last test, a flexible tube called a colonoscope is threaded all the way up the colon to examine the tissue and collect any tissue samples that look problematic. These screening tests have been found to be highly useful for early detection, but many people do not get them.

The main barriers to early detection of colorectal cancers are lack of knowledge or awareness on the part of patients, anxiety about cost or lack of insurance coverage, fear of the procedure itself, and lack of regular or current contact with a physician. Some patients report that their physicians did not inform them of the screening, and some physicians report that patients expressed anxiety and embarrassment about the procedure (Klabunde et al., 2005). Public health officials need to make more efforts to inform the general public of the benefits of screening and alleviate any concerns or barriers.

Sun Protection and Skin Cancer

Another public health concern linked to cancer is the lack of regular sunscreen use. The primary risk factor for all skin cancers is sun exposure—specifically, ultraviolet radiation. In climates with a great deal of sunlight and in latitudes that have more intense sun exposure, the incidence of skin cancers is higher. Those who work or play in the sun without protecting their skin are at highest risk. Using tanning beds and lamps is also very dangerous, and there is a movement to enact strict legislation on tanning salons in the United States.

Sunscreen and sunblock are effective protections against skin cancer, but their use varies tremendously. One international meta-analysis based on 91 journal articles found that the reported use of sunscreen varies from 7% to 90% (Kasparian, McLoone, & Meiser, 2009). The same investigation also showed that only between 8% and 21% of individuals have annual clinical examinations for skin cancer. These findings show that some people are very conscientious about their skin cancer risk, while others are not.

Of all cancers, skin cancer is the most common in the United States—one in five Americans will develop it at some point in their lives (American Academy of Dermatology, 2019; American Cancer Society, 2024). New invasive melanoma diagnoses were projected to be 100, 640 in 2024 (American Cancer Society, 2024). Statistics show that incidence is highest in women before the age of 50 and then the rates rise much faster in men. This gender difference represents historical recreational and occupational exposure in men, and an accelerated exposure to ultraviolet radiation from indoor tanning salons for women, despite public health campaigns to educate people on the dangers of unprotected sun exposure and indoor tanning salons (Kuhrik, Seckman, Kuhrik, Ahearn, & Ercole, 2011; Quintanilla-Dieck & Bichakjian, 2019). But skin cancer does not discriminate—people of all skin colors can develop melanoma. Unfortunately, it can be harder to diagnose those with darker skin tones because of the assumption that they are protected by melanin and because the lesions themselves may be harder to detect (American Academy of Dermatology, 2019).

There are three basic types of skin cancers. **Basal cell carcinomas** appear as raised, pink, waxy bumps that have superficial blood vessels and a slight depression in the center of the bump. They rarely metastasize. **Squamous cell carcinomas** are red, rough, or scaly, and somewhat raised skin lesions. They develop on skin that is exposed to sun, most frequently the head, neck, ears, lips, back of hands, top of feet, and forearms. Squamous cell carcinomas metastasize in 2% of cases.

The most dangerous type of skin cancer, **melanoma**, is a cancer that forms in cells that produce pigment (or melanin). Melanomas appear as black or brown skin lesions with irregular borders and coloration. They are sometimes raised, but can also be flat like freckles. Melanomas can develop on skin that previously appeared normal or within an existing mole. Some 77% of deaths related to skin cancer are due to melanomas. They have a high fatality rate because the cancer cells break apart and spread throughout the body. Yet there is a strong chance of successful treatment if melanomas are caught early on.

The best way to tell if a freckle is cancerous is to consult a dermatologist, who can examine your skin for sun damage or precancerous skin lesions.

Warning signs are a sore that does not heal, new growth or a spread in the pigment (or color) of a spot, redness or swelling of a bump, itching or tenderness, or any change in the surface of a mole (National Council on Skin Cancer Prevention, 2016).

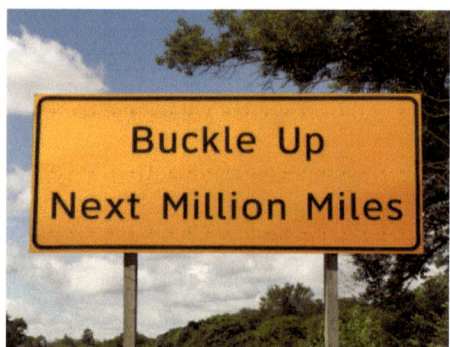

Photo 4.17   The simple habit of buckling your seatbelt can save your life.

Source: trekandshoot/Shutterstock

Seatbelt Use

In 2017 alone, car crashes killed 37,133 people. The good news is that this is a 2% decrease in fatalities from 2015 (National Highway Traffic Safety Administration, 2018b). The cause of these deaths is drivers' behaviors: speeding, drunk driving, running red lights, aggressive driving, fatigue, and distracted driving—that is, talking on the phone or texting while driving (National Highway Traffic Safety Administration, 2018a) (**Photo 4.17**).

One of the easiest health-enhancing behaviors to practice is buckling up. Seatbelt use in the United States has reached an all-time high, with 91.9% of people buckling up (National Highway Traffic Safety Administration, 2024), and vehicular fatalities decreasing. Still, in 2017, more than half (between 53% and 62%) of teens and adults who were killed in car accidents were not wearing their seatbelts (National Highway Traffic Safety Administration, 2018b).

Wearing a seatbelt regularly is one of the most significant behaviors that you can do to prevent death and disability. So why doesn't everyone wear their seatbelts? Here are some of the reasons people give:

- If you have airbags, you don't need to wear a seatbelt.
- Seatbelts can trap you in a fire or underwater.
- If you aren't going far, it doesn't matter.
- Being in a truck makes you safer.
- I'm a good driver, so I don't need to wear one (**Photo 4.18**).

These beliefs are all false. For example, research shows that airbags can be deadly when you do not have your seatbelt on. Routine trips around town and short trips on the highway are often the most dangerous. In fact, most fatal crashes happen within 25- to 40-mile-per-hour zones.

Seatbelt use is important for all of us, whether passengers or drivers. Seatbelts worn in trucks, SUVs, and vans save lives just as in cars, reducing the risk of fatal injury by 60%. Finally, self-confidence in driving ability is a good thing, but one needs to protect oneself from other drivers, too.

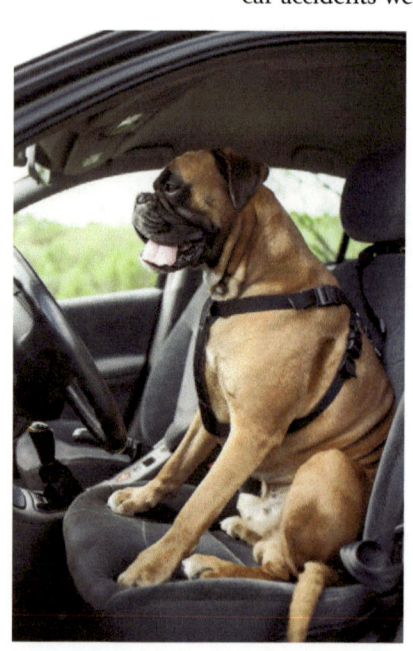

Photo 4.18   Buckle up yourself and your furry friends!

Source: walik/Getty Images

Safer Sex

Both men and women are capable of neglecting another important health-enhancing behavior: safer sex. Is that the same as safe sex? Not exactly.

Safe sex is the practice of using protection to prevent unintended pregnancy and exposure to **sexually transmitted infections (STIs)**. These are viral infections or diseases that are transmitted through sexual contact with an infected partner. The U.S. has the highest rates of STIs. Worldwide. There are more than 25 different STIs but the most common are chlamydia, gonorrhea, hepatitis B virus, herpes, HIV, HPV, syphilis, and trichomoniasis. Globally, more than one million new cases of STIs are acquired every day (WHO). In 2022, the number of new cases of STIs 2as 26 million in the United States, and almost half of these new cases were in people between the ages of 15 and 24 years old (CDC, 2024c). This figure is alarming—it wasn't that long ago that syphilis had nearly been eradicated, and other forms of STIs were at historic lows.

And these rates may be underestimated because many cases go unreported and undiagnosed (CDC, 2024). The U.S. Institute of Medicine has referred to STIs as a "hidden epidemic" with tremendous health and economic consequences (Eng & Butler, 1997). What's more: More than half of Americans will experience an STI at some point in their lifetimes (Koutsky, 1997).

Sex is rarely 100% safe. The only way to guarantee safe sex is to be in a relationship in which both partners are free of any STIs, neither partner has sex with anyone outside the relationship, and contraception is used to prevent unwanted pregnancy. Outside of this framework, it is best to practice safer sex.

Safer sex is sexual engagement that is respectful, pleasurable, and freely consented to by both partners, and that reduces the risk of unintended pregnancy or infections. It does not involve the exchange of any blood, semen, or vaginal fluids from one partner to another. Two crucial factors in safer sex are knowing if either partner is a potential carrier of an STI and maintaining open communication between partners. Communication is often the biggest obstacle to safer sex for young adults. Starting that conversation with a potential partner can be difficult, but it is necessary. Even when using condoms to protect against infection, genital warts and genital herpes can still be transmitted, because the condoms do not always cover the infected area. So, talking about safe sex is key to preventing unwanted exposure.

Chlamydia, gonorrhea, syphilis, and trichomoniasis are all easily treated when diagnosed early, but many of these infections go untreated because they often display no symptoms. They can have significant health consequences beyond themselves. If left untreated, both chlamydia and gonorrhea put women at higher risk for chronic pelvic pain and a life-threatening ectopic pregnancy. They also increase a woman's risk of becoming infertile.

Condoms cannot entirely protect against HPV, the fastest-growing STI, making communication between partners that much more important. HPV is, however, preventable. Although there are no treatments once someone has contracted the virus, young men and women can now get vaccinations before they become sexually active. The CDC and most physicians recommend the vaccine for 11- to 12-year-olds. The vaccine also reduces the risk of cervical cancers that can result from HPV. Safer sex and vaccination are thus important health-enhancing behaviors (**Figure 4.12**).

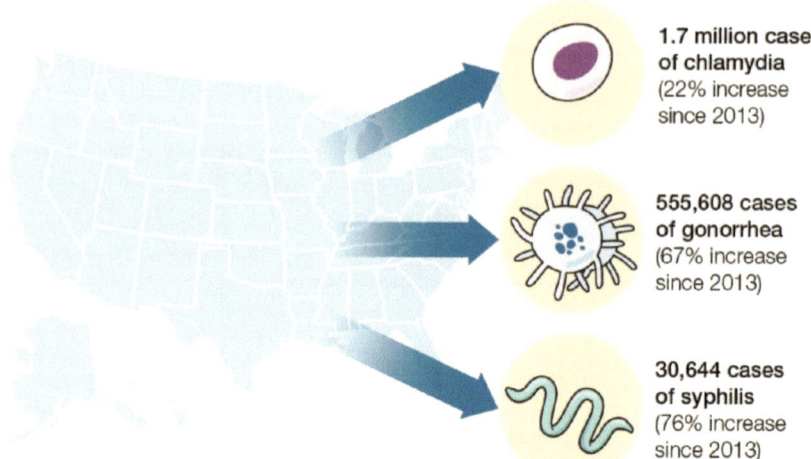

The State of STIs in the United States

1.7 million cases of chlamydia (22% increase since 2013)

555,608 cases of gonorrhea (67% increase since 2013)

30,644 cases of syphilis (76% increase since 2013)

Anyone who is sexually active is at risk.

Some groups are more affected:

· Young people (aged 15–24)
· Gay and bisexual men
· Pregnant women

Without treatment, STIs can cause:

· Increased risk of HIV
· Long-term pelvic or abdominal pain
· Pregnancy complications

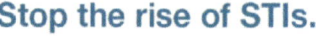

Stop the rise of STIs.
Follow these three steps:

Talk openly about STIs with your partners and health care providers.

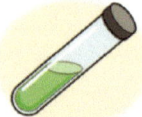

Get tested for STIs regularly.

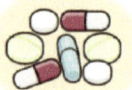

Get treatment if you have an STI.

Figure 4.12   The state of STIs in the United States.

Source: Data from CDC (2018d)

Thinking About Health

■ What preventive measures do you currently take against cancer? How will the measures you take change as you age?

■ How do you react to the rationales that people give for not wearing a seatbelt?

■ What steps do you take to protect yourself against STIs?

Chapter Summary

Health-enhancing behaviors can significantly reduce the risk of disease and disability. Lifestyle factors, such as a healthy diet, a healthy weight, and regular exercise, ensure a higher quality of life and greater well-being for everyone. Getting adequate sleep, practicing preventive medicine, wearing sunscreen, wearing seatbelts, and practicing safer sex are all choices that can lead to a longer, healthier life.

KEY TERMS ▶ health-enhancing behaviors p. 91; life expectancy p. 98; food scarcity (or *food insecurity)* p. 99; neophobia p. 102; basal metabolic rate (BMR) p. 102; body mass index (BMI) p. 105; waist-to-hip ratio p. 107; stress and weight p. 108; cytokines p. 109; self-control p. 111; self-efficacy p. 113; Big 5 p. 114; neuroticism p. 114; extraversion p. 114; conscientiousness p. 114; restrained eaters p. 115; emotional eaters p. 116; external eaters p. 116; intuitive eaters p. 117; physical activity p. 119; aerobic exercise (or *cardio)* p. 119; resistance training (or *strength training)* p. 119; cardiorespiratory system p. 120; respiratory system p. 120; immune system p. 120; cognitive functioning p. 121; sleep debt p. 127; circadian rhythms p. 128; sleep cycle p. 128; NREM (non-rapid eye movement) sleep p. 129; hypnic myoclonia (or *myoclonicjerks)* p. 129; sleep spindles p. 129; REM (rapid eye movement) sleep p. 129; sleep hygiene p. 132; mammogram p. 135; polyp p. 136; colonoscopy p. 136; basal cell carcinomas p. 137; squamous cell carcinomas p. 137; melanoma p. 137; sexually transmitted infections (STIs) p. 139; safer sex p. 139.

CHAPTER 5

Health-Compromising Behaviors

Learning Outcomes

After reading this chapter, you should be able to:

- **Define** what health-compromising behaviors are, why they put our health at risk, and why people engage in them.
- **Describe** theories that explain why people take risks with their health.
- **Explain** the developmental window of vulnerability in adolescence.
- **Describe** the opioid epidemics, and the personal and public health consequences associated with each.
- **Identify** the biopsychosocial factors that influence health-compromising behaviors.
- **Describe** the various interventions used to treat health-compromising behaviors.

Taylor was a typical kid, with a typical childhood. She played softball and the violin, had lots of friends, got good grades, and enjoyed a close relationship with her parents and two older sisters. She and her siblings enjoyed parties, but drugs and alcohol were not a problem, and none drank more than the occasional beer. When Taylor went away to college—on a softball scholarship, at that—her parents were proud, and her future looked ever so bright (**Photo 5.1**).

In a crucial game during her freshman year, Taylor injured her ankle and was prescribed an opioid pain medication: OxyContin. The pain in her ankle was bad, but the stress was worse—suddenly, she was unable to play sports, afraid that she might lose her scholarship, and exhausted from getting around campus on crutches, all while trying to manage her coursework. The pain medication dulled the pain and her anxiety, making her feel blissfully relaxed and happy. She very

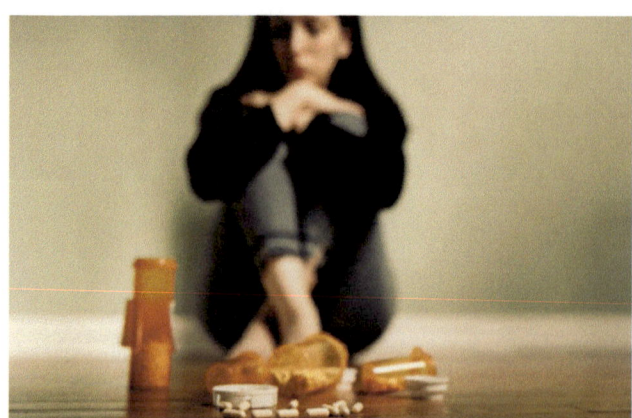

Photo 5.1

DOI: 10.4324/9781032643090-5

quickly found herself addicted to these powerful pills. When she could not convince the campus physician to prescribe more, she turned to another opioid: heroin. Her behavior was not uncommon—80% of heroin users report having misused prescription pain medication first (Severino et al., 2018). Taylor was having the time of her life.

She began lying to everyone. She convinced her parents to send her money for make-believe crises, and she stole valuables from roommates, teammates, and friends. Eventually, she got kicked off the softball team for being high at practice, her grades plummeted, and she lost her scholarship. Her world spiraled further into despair and addiction, until she was sleeping in the local park and begging for money to buy more drugs. Only when she was found unconscious and unresponsive in a public restroom did the police take her in and call her parents.

Several days later, Taylor woke up in a treatment facility. Her parents and sisters brought family photos, trophies from when she was a star softball player, and her violin. Her family members and personal belongings filled the room. Finally, a nurse asked the ultimate question: "Do you want to die?"

Taylor struggled to find an answer. On the one hand, she was aware of the depths that her life had sunk to. On the other hand, she was terrified to confront life without opioids. The question marked the first day of the long, hard road to recovery. There were many dark moments, but Taylor has been sober now for one year. She is one of the lucky ones—she survived and is in recovery. Others are not so fortunate—every day, 130 people die of an opioid overdose in the United States, a number 16 times higher than the number of overdose deaths in 2020. Fortunately, Taylor was not a casualty of the current Opioid Epidemic in America (U.S. Department of Health and Human Services, 2024).

"Only those who will risk going too far," T.S. Eliot wrote, "can possibly find out how far one can go." Do you know someone like Taylor who has experienced substance abuse and addiction? What causes people to lose control of their health and fall into risky lifestyles?

In this chapter, we explore health-compromising behaviors, the kind that may put your health at risk. Many health risks are due to factors outside of the individual, such as poverty, famine, pollution, or unsafe working conditions. Yet many more risks are personal choices, and some can become addictive. All can lead to negative health outcomes—from being overweight, to being diseased, disabled, or dead. For the sake of our well-being, we need to understand the prevalence of these behaviors, the factors that lead to them, the health outcomes associated with them, and treatment options for them. Changing health habits is hard. This chapter also looks at the challenges of reducing health risks.

What Is Health-Compromising Behavior?

A **health-compromising behavior** is an activity with a frequency or intensity that puts an individual's health or well-being at risk. It may lead to poor health, disease, disability, injury, or death (Steptoe & Wardle, 2004). The idea of "risky behavior" may conjure up images of drag racing, skydiving, and high-stakes poker. Yet we all make decisions that involve some degree of risk several times a day: "Should I wear shorts or pants today?" "Eww, do these leftovers smell okay to you?" "We didn't drink that much, so we can still drive, right?" Sometimes, a pattern of behavior can present serious threats to our health.

In Chapter 4, we looked at the excuses people make for skipping health-enhancing behaviors: "I don't need to wear a seatbelt because I'm just going down the road to the convenience store." Yet people who make decisions like these may be engaging in seriously health-compromising behaviors. Health-compromising behaviors can take several forms, whether we avoid what is good for our health, or actively put our health at risk. Some behaviors, such as smoking or unprotected sex, are always risky. Others, such as alcohol consumption, are fine in moderation but can become dangerous very easily. A biopsychosocial approach can help us understand why some behaviors present great risks to our health.

Kinds of Risk

At some point in our lives, most of us engage in activities that put us at risk. Sometimes, however, these behaviors become habits or addictions that are very hard to change. The greater the number of risky behaviors we engage in, the greater our risk of disability and death. Over the past two decades, roughly 50% of deaths each year in the United States have been due to personal behaviors (Alzahrani, Watt, Sheiham, Aresu, & Tsakos, 2014; Mokdad, Marks, Stroup, & Gerberding, 2004). Understanding health risks and why people take them is important because many of these health behaviors can be changed and many negative health consequences are preventable.

Risks to health are both short term and long term. In the short term, unprotected sex may lead to unwanted pregnancy and sexually transmitted diseases. Alcohol abuse, drunk driving, and failure to wear a seatbelt all raise the immediate chances of injury or death. In the long term, poor diet, lack of exercise, smoking, and substance use may contribute to high blood pressure, obesity, heart disease, and diabetes. Substance use in the teen years is often linked to substance abuse and arrests during adulthood.

A combination of risky behaviors increases the risks, and some combinations are more lethal than others. In a longitudinal study of nearly 20,000 middle-aged and older adults, smoking elevated the risk of mortality for everyone, but death rates were especially high when smoking was combined with heavy drinking and physical inactivity (Shaw & Agahi, 2012). In a study of Scottish men (Hart, Morrison, Batty, Mitchell, & Davey Smith, 2010), 25% of those who smoked and drank heavily did not make it to their sixty-fifth birthdays. Conversely, when smokers had healthy diets, their risk of death was high, but not as high as for smokers who had unhealthy diets and did not exercise (Ford, Bergmann, Boeing, Li, & Capewell, 2012). In another study, risky sexual behaviors such as sexting (sharing sexually suggestive or explicit images as text messages) were significantly related to substance use (Benotsch, Snipes, Martin, & Bull, 2013). Presumably, when one is under the influence of a substance, inhibitions are lowered and other risky behaviors are more likely to occur.

A recent systematic review showed that for people who currently or previously smoke tobacco, there is a much higher risk of dying from COVID-19 (Gallus et al., 2023; Patanavanich et al., 2023). In fact, smoking and alcohol use increased exposure, duration, severity, and likelihood of hospitalization of all variants of the COVID-19 virus and exacerbated the problems for those who have "long covid" (or symptoms that last for years after contracting the virus) (Rodriguez-Miguelez et al., 2023). When we think about how these risk factors come together to impact health, we see how complicated understanding risk can be.

Many risky behaviors are preventable. We will see how these behaviors represent personal choices that can be modified and changed. Understanding why people take risks with their health is the cornerstone of preventive medicine. It can help us develop effective public policy and medical and psychological intervention to reduce risk and provide support for those who need it. More broadly, understanding why people take health risks gives us insight into personality, decision-making, and the adaptability of human behavior (Llewellyn, 2008).

Why Take Risks?

Sigmund Freud, "the father of psychoanalysis," argued that people are drawn to risky behaviors because of a "death drive." Thanatos, as he called it, is an unconscious drive propelling us toward death, self-destruction, and the return to an inorganic state as a life-less object (Freud, 1920). He saw this drive in opposition to a drive for life—a life-giving drive toward creativity, survival, and sex (**Photo 5.2a and b**).

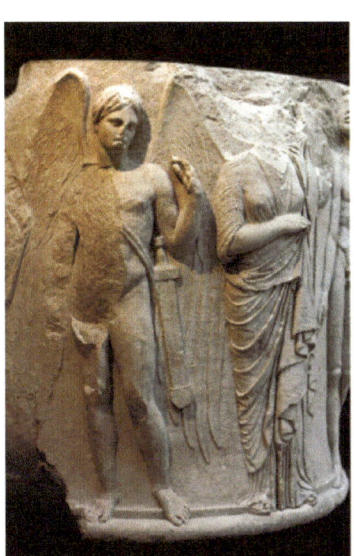 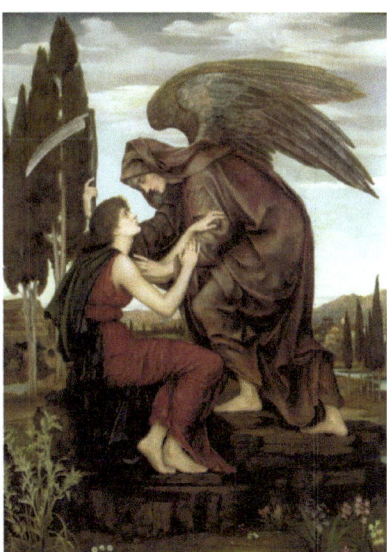

Photo 5.2   Throughout history, death has been personified. Classical Greeks called it Thanatos (left, in an ancient sculpture); for many others, it was the Angel of Death (right, in a painting by Evelyn De Morgan, c. 1881).

Although Freud's theory is intriguing, multiple complex forces lie behind health-compromising behaviors. In reality, health-compromising behaviors are biopsychosocial and must be appreciated at many levels. Some of the forces behind risky behaviors are unconscious and biological in nature. And some are conscious, personal choices aimed at experiencing excitement and pleasure.

From an evolutionary perspective, risk-taking is a necessary part of life, because it is a natural outcome of "survival of the fittest." Those who take risks and survive to reproduce may be passing on genes that lead to stronger and better-adapted offspring. Those who don't survive do not. It was, after all, the risk-takers who climbed the tree to get the ripest fruit or fought off the saber-toothed cat. Are you a risk taker? See **Table 5.1**.

Decisions regarding risk also involve our personalities: Some people are risk takers and some are risk averse. Our emotions—high arousal and anticipation of reward—will increase risk-taking, but so does the day-to-day need to make choices.

Neurobiology also plays a part. fMRI studies show that specific regions of the brain, the nucleus accumbens, and the anterior insula, light up when someone considers a choice involving risk. Developmentally speaking, as we will see, risk-taking is highest during adolescence years. Teens, especially boys, take more risks in every domain of their lives than their adult counterparts (Casey, Kosofsky, & Bhide, 2014).

In short, the causes of risky behavior are many and varied, and each represents just one piece of a complex puzzle (Petraitis, Flay, & Miller, 1995). More than 40 different theories have been put forth to explain the development of substance use alone (Lettieri, Sayers, & Pearson, 1980).

Answer each question on a scale of 1 (not likely at all) to 7 (extremely likely)
How open are you to. . . ?

1. Trying drugs other than alcohol or marijuana
2. Missing class or work
3. Leaving a social event with someone you just met
4. Driving after drinking alcohol
5. Having sex without protection
6. Leaving tasks and assignments until the last minute
7. Making a scene in public
8. Snow skiing or water skiing
9. Betting on a football game
10. Punching or hitting someone with a fist

The closer your score is to 70, the more of a risk-taker you are. The lower your score, the more risk-averse you are.

Source: Information from National Geographic (2011).

Table 5.1   Are you a risk taker?

Theoretical Approaches

Some of the many theories of risky behavior have focused on why people do the things they do. When faced with any decision, we engage in a cost-benefits analysis, weighing the risks against the benefits. A smoker may choose to smoke in social situations to feel less anxious, despite concerns about lung cancer. **Problem-behavior theory** sees risky behaviors, especially in adolescence, not as thrill-seeking or accidental but, rather, as purposeful, goal-directed behavior (Jessor, 1987, 1992; Jessor & Jessor, 1977). Maybe we want to be cool, to fit in, or simply to have fun, and that is more important to us than any potential risks. In the calculus of risk, education, health values, a sense of social control, and positive relationships with adults can help protect us (Jessor, Van Den Bos, Vanderryn, Costa, & Turbin, 1995).

The **theory of triadic influence** brings together the different models of health behavior to map out what leads people to take risks (Flay & Petraitis, 1994). This theory proposes that our behaviors are shaped by several streams of influence—biological and personal factors, social context, and environment influences (see **Figure 5.1**). For example, a smoker may have a biological predisposition to nicotine sensitivity, a sense of social competence when smoking, and a need to reduce anxiety experienced in social contexts. He or she may also spend a great deal of time in an environment in which others smoke.

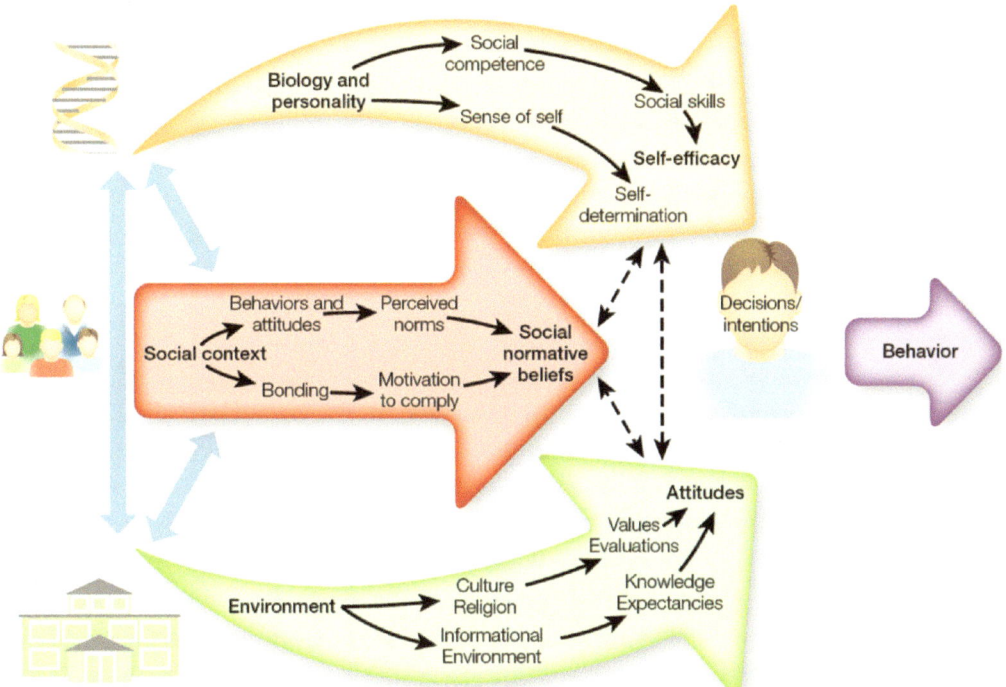

Figure 5.1   Theory of triadic influences.

Source: Information from Flay (2005)

We can also distinguish between **levels of causation** to predict behavior. Some factors have an immediate influence on our behavior; others do not. The more control we have over these influences, the more likely they are to influence our behavior. For example, society-level causes, like our culture, are not under our control. Community-level predictors, such as our relationships with peers, partners, or parents, have a bit more influence on our behavior. And finally, individual-level factors—our specific decisions, intentions, motivations, and experiences—have a very close and direct influence on our behavior. Each of these levels influences our behavior, but the individual level is the most predictive (Snyder & Flay, 2012). For example, if someone suffers from social anxiety, she may drink more to reduce that anxiety. Drinking affects the feeling of anxiety directly by depressing it. Other causes are not so direct. For example, her drinking may be motivated by peer pressure and the larger goal of fitting in.

Here is an example, you are driving and pick up your phone to check an incoming text, as you do your car begins to swerve off the road. You have a near miss with a mail box jerking the car back onto the road and gasping for breath. The danger of the moment causes you to chastise yourself and put your phone away. The danger of the moment, the fear response, and the threat to your safety may cause you to avoid that risky behavior in the future. However, imagine that you got a text while driving and checked while maintaining attention to the road. You are likely to feel like you can "multi-task" while driving quite well and be more likely to check an incoming text next time. **"Risk creep"** refers to when we become more and more comfortable or tolerant of risky behavior (Logg et al., 2022). Risk creep can happen when we experience a "near miss" and come out o.k. or when an event that might have had a negative outcome did not. Risk creep is the spread of risk-taking behavior, and it is influenced by our experiences, trial-and-error, and social learning (Logg et al., 2022). **Social learning theory** can explain risky behavior as well as the phenomenon of risk creep. We adopt risky behaviors through social learning when we observe others and learn which behaviors to engage in or not based on the consequences we observe. When people engage in risky behaviors and do not experience consequences, they will likely engage in them again, engaging in risk creep.

Risk creep was apparent during the COVID-19 pandemic. A 5-month long longitudinal field study followed people when they left their homes after the lockdown in the United States (and before COVID-19 vaccines were available; see Logg et al., 2022). The goal was to track perceptions and behaviors over time and participants reported on how many times they left home to engage in different activities (that ranged in terms of necessity and risk exposure). For example, a non-discretionary necessary day-to-day activity was leaving home to get food whereas a discretionary less necessary, and more risky behavior was attending a social event in a large group. Over the five months, people's nondiscretionary activities didn't change much. But when people saw others engaging in discretionary activities, their own engagement in those riskier activities increases the very next week! People in this study experimented with risky behavior and when there were no adverse consequences they showed a creeping tolerance of the risks. The authors concluded that risk creep was associated with social learning and influenced people's behavior during the COVID-19 pandemic (Logg et al., 2022).

Lastly, and foremost among research on substance use disorder (SUD), is the **brain disease model of addiction**, the idea that addiction is a disease of the brain. This model is consistent with emerging neurobiological and social genomics research that identifies brain regions, neurochemicals, and specific genes that may be linked to risky behaviors and disease outcomes. According to this theory, fundamental biological processes, when disrupted, can lead to profound changes in decision-making abilities, emotional regulation, and behavioral control (Volkow, Koob, & McLellan, 2016). Skeptics claim that insufficient neurological evidence for this model exists, but, in doing so, they overlook the biopsychosocial nature of the brain—that addiction may be caused by complex interactions among brain circuitry, as combined with environmental, psychological, and social factors. As we move through this chapter, we will approach health-compromising behaviors from a biopsychosocial point of view in order to understand how they develop, and how they can be changed.

Why Do Risky Behaviors Cluster Together?

Think about the last time you were at a party. Was there drinking? If so, how many people drinking were also using other substances, smoking, or vaping? In movie or television scenes set in a bar, especially before widespread antismoking campaigns, a person was almost never seen drinking without a cigarette in hand. Someone under the influence of alcohol is also more likely to have unprotected sex or end up in a car with a drunk driver. Risky behaviors seem to compound one another, and some combinations are more lethal than others. But why?

The theory of triadic influence offers one explanation: Some behaviors have similar consequences. For example, alcohol and nicotine abuse are linked because both regulate our emotions, and both can be triggered by the same social cues (like social anxiety). Different behaviors can also contribute to one another because they are part of the same dynamic system—a cluster of behaviors that changes with peoples' experiences (Flay, Snyder, & Petraitis, 2009; Lerner, 2006). It follows that interventions to help people change risky behaviors can be most effective when they address these behaviors together (Lippke, Nigg, & Maddock, 2012) (**Photo 5.3**).

Other explanations for risky behaviors' **comorbidity**, the presence of two conditions at the same time, come from advances in neuropsychology and social genomics and theories such as the brain disease model of addiction. For example, a study of 1.2 million people found that two addictive substances—nicotine and alcohol use—have several things in common (Liu et al., 2019). Aside from being pleasurable, they are both heritable, and may involve similar neurochemical, neurostructural, and behavioral systems. Genetic risk scores for smoking and alcohol also significantly predict later use of cocaine, amphetamines,

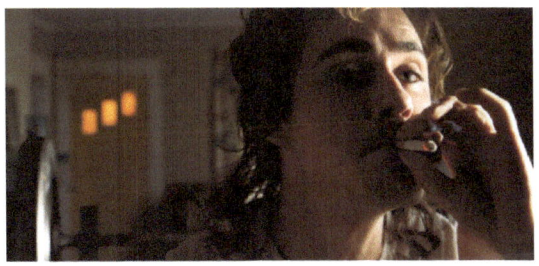

Photo 5.3   Social cues for risky behaviors often emerge on film and television. Recently, streaming services such as Netflix have come under fire for their frequent and glamorized portrayals of smoking. The series Stranger Things has proven to be the worst offender, showing instances of tobacco usage in every episode of its first and second seasons (Truth Initiative, 2019).

Source: Netflix/Kobal/Shutterstock.com

hallucinogens, ecstasy, and cannabis (Chang et al., 2019). We will explore these connections further when we dive into understanding addiction.

The model still leaves some open questions: Why are some patterns of risk more dangerous than others? What portion of the overall increase in risk can be attributed to each individual behavior? How much do health-enhancing behaviors lower the risks? Whatever the answers, the risks change when we consider behaviors together.

Adolescence: A Window of Vulnerability

For teenagers, the balance tips in favor of high emotions and risk-taking (Giedd, 2008). Adolescence is a period of rapid change. During this time, we explore identities with new-found autonomy and self-determination (Erikson, 1968; Galliher & Kerpelman, 2012; Syed & Seiffge-Krenke, 2013). In other words, we are more likely to seek novel experiences and try new things, such as nicotine, alcohol, and other substances. This makes adolescence a window of vulnerability for many risky behaviors.

Health-compromising behaviors are a leading cause of death among those aged 10–24 in the United States, according to the Youth Risk Behavior Surveillance System (Kann et al., 2018). This national longitudinal study, which began in 1990, has collected data from more than 4.4 million high school students on their engagement in health behaviors that contribute to the leading causes of social problems, disability, and death. Six categories of health behaviors are assessed: (1) behaviors leading to unintentional injury and violence; (2) sexual behaviors related to unintended pregnancy and STIs; (3) alcohol and drug use; (4) tobacco use; (5) unhealthy dietary behaviors; and (6) inadequate physical activity. The most recent wave of data collection shows that 74% of deaths in American high school students resulted from four causes: car crashes (22%), other unintentional injuries (20%), suicide (17%), and homicide (15%). One of the most dangerous behaviors that contributed to these deaths was distracted driving—specifically, driving a car or other vehicle while texting or emailing (62.8%). Other risky behaviors that students reported engaging in within the previous month were unprotected sex (46.2%), alcohol use (29.8%), marijuana use (19.8%), taking pain medications without a prescription (14.4%), vaping (13.2%), and smoking cigarettes (8.8%). All of these behaviors directly and negatively impact health and well-being. To illustrate the concept of comorbidity, results show that high school students who reported misusing prescription opioids had a 59.4% likelihood of misusing alcohol and a 44% likelihood of smoking marijuana (Jones et al., 2020).

Nonetheless, not all adolescents are harming themselves. In fact, two distinct profiles have emerged: Some teens engage in very few risky behaviors and practice more health-enhancing ones, while others engage in many risky behaviors and few health-enhancing ones (Hair et al., 2009; Zweig, Lindberg, & McGinley, 2001). But who falls into which category, and why? Standard theories of behavior change (see Chapter 3) are not very good at predicting adolescents' risky behaviors, because their behaviors are not often planned in advance. Rather, they happen impulsively, in the heat of the moment, and often when there is social pressure (Lane, Gibbons, O'Hara, & Gerrard, 2011). Adolescents may not think through the consequences of their behaviors and may end up doing things they might not have done under other circumstances. These actions are simply not planned behaviors. Why is adolescence highlighted by impulsivity and risk-taking?

Research in neuroscience points to developmental changes in the brain as one reason risk-taking and impulsivity increase between childhood and adolescence, peaking in the middle teens (Heitzeg, Hardee, & Beltz, 2018; Steinberg, 2010). Specifically, changes in teens' socio-emotional systems can lead to greater reward-seeking behavior and physiological arousal, especially in the presence of peers (Steinberg, 2008). These changes take place in the brain's **dopaminergic system**. This system originates in the midbrain where the neurotransmitter dopamine is produced, and dopamine is responsible for moderating the hormones that influence arousal, learning, emotional processing, sensitivity to social pressure, social bonding, and self-consciousness. Evidence across different species—from rats to humans—shows that, during adolescence, the brain is "reward-centric"; that is, it has a heightened sensitivity to stimulation and experiences that are pleasurable (Doremus-Fitzwater & Spear, 2016). Thus, adolescents are hard-wired to take more risks in pursuit of greater rewards.

Although the window of vulnerability for risky behaviors is in adolescence, everyone may engage in unhealthful behaviors at some point in life. People who continue behaving unhealthily throughout adulthood are at the greatest risk of disease, disability, and death. We look next at some of the most common risk factors: being overweight or obese, **eating disorders**, **substance use** and abuse, and risky sexual behaviors.

Culture and Risk Behaviors

It has been said that the COVID-19 pandemic was one of the biggest challenges facing mankind in recent history (Liu & Yang, 2023). Containing the spread of the virus depended on changing perceptions of risk and risky behaviors on every level of society from the individual up to world leaders. In the United States, to stem the spread and contain the virus required coordinated efforts from state and local governments to implement stay-at-home orders, canceling major events, increasing testing, and protective behaviors such as mask-wearing and social distancing. However, despite these efforts and the warnings of public health officials, many Americans resisted these ideas (Bogel-Burroughs & Peters, 2020). Many people put their health at risk by violating these protective guidelines and took to demonstrating and protesting in public places (Mervosh et al., 2020). This is in contrast to the even more extreme responses taken in Asian countries such as China, Singapore, and South Korea. In those countries, the public was supportive of these recommendations and the virus was kept under control. Research showed that in countries with more collectivist societies, there were significantly fewer COVID-19 cases and significantly fewer deaths when compared to individualistic cultures like the United States (Rajkumar, 2021). Other research showed that in collectivistic countries like Thailand, South Korea, and the United Arab Emirates more people wore masks and the culture was generally more risk-averse (Kasdan & Campbell, 2020; Lu et al., 2021; Liu & Yang, 2023). Research also shows that people from individualistic cultures had a lower perception of risk for the pandemic than those from collectivistic cultures (Dryhurst et al., 2020). Even within the United States, there are variations that map on to the collectivistic/individualistic distinction. For example, rural Southeastern Alaska Native people relied on traditional and historic knowledge grounded in their cultural beliefs to adapt to and cope with the threat of COVID-19 (van Doren et al., 2023). These community-centered nonindividualistic behaviors gave them resilience in the pandemic, their indigenous cultural beliefs were highly protective against the virus.

> ### Thinking About Health
>
> ■ In your opinion, which theory of risk best explains health-compromising behaviors?
> ■ Why do risky behaviors cluster together?
> ■ What are the biopsychosocial reasons that adolescence is a window of vulnerability?
> ■ What factors explain your own risky behaviors?

Substance Use

Our opening story about Taylor shows how even the most innocuous circumstances can evolve into dangerous lifestyle choices. Health-compromising behaviors are often synonymous with high-risk behaviors, leaving people prone to injury, disease, financial loss, prison, or death (Kelley, Schochet, & Landry, 2004; Llewellyn, 2008; Turner, McClure, & Pirozzo, 2004). Among the most dangerous health-compromising behaviors is substance use—the use of tobacco, alcohol, or illicit drugs.

What Substances Are Abused?

A **psychoactive substance** is any substance that crosses the blood-brain barrier and affects the central nervous system—in particular, brain functioning. The results can be alterations in sensations, perceptions, mood, consciousness, cognitive processes, or behavior. Psychoactive substances are usually used recreationally to alter consciousness. Because these substances act directly on the reward centers in the brain, their use is often psychologically reinforcing. They may promote euphoria or heightened arousal and alertness. This, in turn, can lead to an increased need and desire for the substance, increased tolerance, and withdrawal symptoms. In other words, it can lead to dependency or addiction. When dependency occurs, and the substance is harmful or hazardous, it can create difficulty controlling the use of the substance and it may eventually interfere with daily life.

Some frequently misused drugs are depressants (such as alcohol, barbiturates, and benzodiazepines), stimulants (such as tobacco, amphetamines, cocaine, and MDMA [ecstasy]), hallucinogens (such as LSD), and opioids (such as codeine, heroin, and morphine). Anabolic steroid use to improve athletic performance has become a concern in recent years as well. **Table 5.2** shows each of the major substances, their effects on the body, and their health risks (**Photo 5.4**).

Drug	Examples	Acute effects	Health risks
Tobacco	Cigarettes, cigars, bidis, smokeless tobacco	Increased blood pressure, heart rate	Chronic lung disease; cardiovascular disease; stroke; cancers of the mouth, pharynx, larynx, esophagus, stomach, pancreas, cervix, kidney, and bladder; acute myeloid leukemia; adverse pregnancy outcomes; addiction
Alcohol	Liquor, beer, wine	Low doses: euphoria, mild stimulation, relaxation, lowered inhibition. Higher doses: drowsiness, slurred speech, nausea, emotional volatility, loss of coordination, visual distortions, impaired memory, sexual dysfunction, loss of consciousness	Increased risk of injuries, violence, fetal damage in pregnant women, depression, neurologic deficits, hypertension, liver and heart disease, addiction, fatal overdose
Cannabinoids	Marijuana, hashish	Euphoria, relaxation, slowed reaction time, distorted sensory perception, impaired balance and coordination, increased heart rate and appetite, impaired learning, memory, anxiety, panic attacks, psychosis	Cough, frequent respiratory infection, possible mental health decline, addiction
Opioids	Heroin, opium	Euphoria, drowsiness, impaired coordination, dizziness, confusion, nausea, sedation, feeling of heaviness in the body, slowed or arrested breathing	Constipation, endocarditis, hepatitis, HIV, addiction, fatal overdose
Stimulants	Cocaine, amphetamine, methamphetamine	Increased heart rate, blood pressure, body temperature, metabolism, feelings of exhilaration, energy, mental alertness, tremors, reduced appetite, irritability, anxiety, panic, paranoia, violent behavior, psychosis	Weight loss, insomnia, cardiac or cardiovascular complications, stroke, seizures, addiction
Club drugs	MDMA (ecstasy), Rohypnol (roofies), GHB (liquid ecstasy)	MDMA: mild hallucinogenic effects, increased tactile sensitivity, empathic feelings, lowered inhibition, anxiety, chills, sweating, teeth clenching, muscle cramping. Rohypnol: sedation, muscle relaxation, confusion, memory loss, dizziness, impaired coordination. GHB: drowsiness, nausea, headache, disorientation, loss of coordination, memory loss	MDMA: sleep disturbances, depression, impaired memory, hyperthermia, addiction Rohypnol: addiction GHB: unconsciousness, seizures, coma

Table 5.2   Health risks of substances   (*Continued*)

Drug	Examples	Acute effects	Health risks
Dissociative Drugs	Ketamine (special K or vitamin K), PCP and analogs (angel dust, peace pill), *Salvia divinorum* (salvia, Sally-d), dextromethorphan (DXM; cough and cold medicines)	Feelings of being separate from one's body and environment; impaired motor functioning. Special K: analgesia, impaired memory, delirium, respiratory depression and arrest, death PCP: analgesia, psychosis, aggression, violence, slurred speech, loss of coordination, hallucinations DXM: euphoria, slurred speech, confusion, dizziness, distorted visual perceptions	Anxiety, tremors, numbness, memory loss, nausea, death
Hallucinogens	LSD, mescaline, psilocybin	Altered states of perception and feeling, hallucinations, nausea. LSD and mescaline: increased body temperature, heart rate, blood pressure, loss of appetite, sweating, sleeplessness, numbness, dizziness, weakness, tremors, impulsive behavior, rapid shifts in emotion. Psilocybin: nervousness, paranoia, panic	Flashbacks, hallucinogen persisting perception disorder
Other drugs	Anabolic steroids	No intoxication effects	Hypertension, blood clotting, cholesterol changes, liver cysts, hostility and aggression, acne. In adolescents: premature growth stoppage. In males (of any age): prostate cancer, reduction in sperm production, shrunken testicles, breast enlargement. In females: menstrual irregularities, development of beard and other masculine characteristics

Source: Information from NIDA (2016a, 2016b).

Table 5.2   Health risks of substances (*Continued*)

Regardless of what substance a person is addicted to, **substance use disorder (SUDs)** are not the result of personal failings, a lack of willpower, character, or the ability to control the use of the substance. People do not choose to be addicted to substances. The repeated use of addictive substances powerfully alters the brain's chemistry and how it functions to create a neurobiological disorder. Addictive substances, whether it is nicotine, alcohol, or drugs, lead to drastic changes in brain functioning that reduce the person's ability to control their use. We now recognize that addictions are diseases not dissimilar from heart disease or cancer. Therefore, we no longer use pejorative terms that imply blame, shame, and stigma. Instead, consistent with the Diagnostic and Statistical

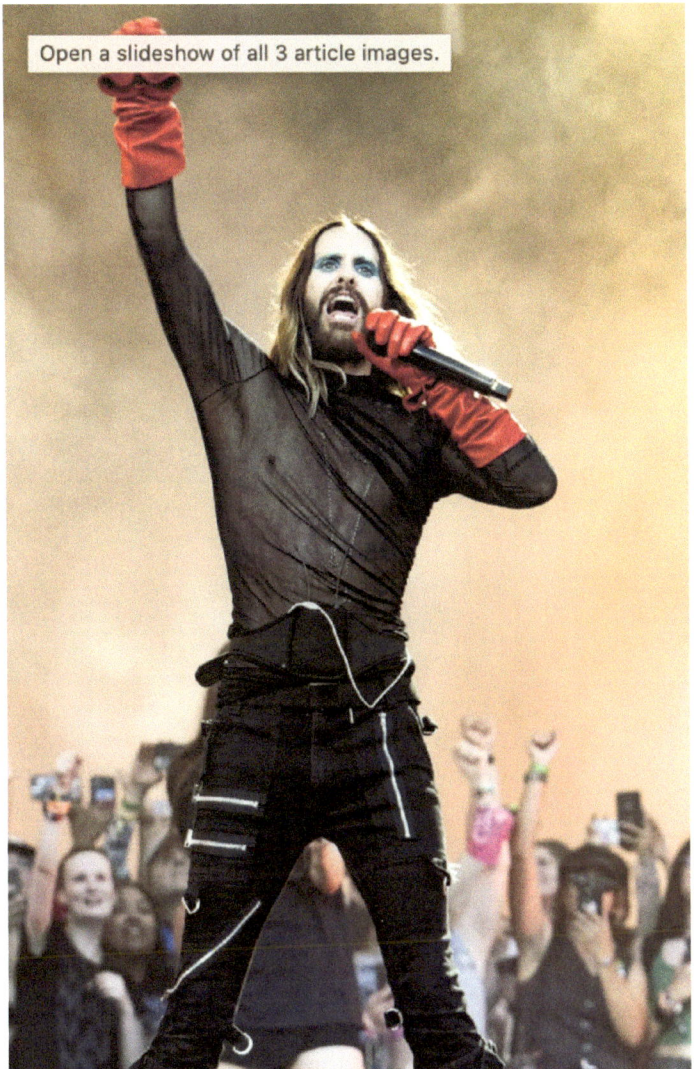

Photo 5.4   Jared Leto in PageSix interview: "I had a moment of clarity,…I had an epiphany. There were two paths that I could take in life. I guess is the only way I can describe it." Fortunately, He Says "I took that path. I've had very close friends that didn't, and they're not here anymore. Many."

Manual of Mental Disorders (DSM-5), most medical and psychological professional associations, and scientific journals, we use "person-first language" to distinguish the person from their diagnosis or their perceived membership in a stigmatized group. To that end, in this chapter, we talk about people with SUDs.

SUD is the cluster of behavioral, cognitive, and physiological problems that develop from substance abuse and dependence. In its most severe form, SUD represents addiction to a substance. SUD is a chronic brain disorder that people can and do recover from. In the most recent revision of the Diagnostic and Statistical Manual of Mental Disorders (DSM-5; American Psychiatric

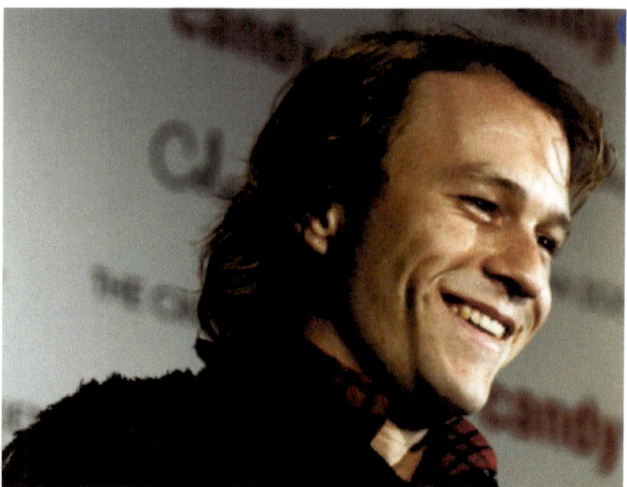

Photo 5.5   Heath ledger, Australian actor who played the joker in The Dark Knight died on January 22, 2008 of an accidental overdose that resulted from prescription drug abuse.

Source: Jemal Countess/Wireimage

Association, 2013), a diagnosis of SUD is given if two or more of the following criteria are present: when drug use interferes with relationships; when it interferes with the ability to fulfill school, work, or family obligations; or when it results in dangerous behaviors or legal difficulties (**Photo 5.5**).

Men typically have higher rates of drug use and SUD than women do but evidence suggests that women are in many ways more vulnerable to this disease (Towers et al., 2023). The "telescoping effect" in sometimes seen in addiction and SUD. It refers to the accelerated course and faster transition from initiation of substance use to meeting the criteria for a diagnosed disorder and seeking treatment. One common example of the telescoping effect is that women more often meet the criteria and seek treatment for SUD sooner than men do (Towers et al., 2023). The telescoping effect was originally observed and replicated may times with alcohol use but has been found for stimulants, nicotine, methamphetamine, opioids, cannabis, and other addictions such as gambling (Towers et al., 2023). With regard to substance use, animal models show that females develop features of addiction such as compulsive use, enhanced motivation, and stronger cravings for the drug, and greater relapse than male animals. This may be due to biologic factors such as the influence of female ovarian hormones on the dopamine reward pathways that serve to reward and reinforce the addictive effects of drugs leading to SUD (see Towers et al., 2023).

Is Substance Use Decreasing?

There is good news and bad news on this front. As we have seen, adolescents are especially vulnerable to risky behavior. Substance use increases during adolescence and peaks in early adulthood (Brown et al., 2008; Narendorf,

Fedoravicius, McMillen, McNelly, & Robinson, 2012). The good news is that, compared to 2022 in 2023 alcohol use remained stable for children in Grades 8 through 12 (Miech et al., 2018). Over 11% of 8th graders report nicotine vaping and this number was stable from 2022 to 2023. Older children (grade 12) reduced their nicotine vaping over that period from over 27% to 23%. Cannabis use and cannabis vaping remained stable across adolescence. Nearly 30% of 12th graders reported smoking cannabis and 20% reporting vaping cannabis over the last year. Measured for the first time in 2023, use of Delta-8-THC (a psychoactive byproduct from the Cannabis sativa plant) was found to be at 11% for 12th graders. This trend in substance use will be tracked going forward. There was also stability in illicit drug use other than marijuana from 2022 to 2023 and the use of narcotics (excluding heroin) decreased to an all-time low of 1.0%. Perhaps most interesting is the stable rate of abstaining from substance use altogether. In 2023 63% of 12th graders reported not using marijuana, alcohol, or nicotine over the past month.

The bad news is that despite the stable rates of most substances in teenagers in the United States, there was an alarming rise in overdose deaths between 2010 and 2022. Overdose deaths were due to illicit fentanyl (a potent counterfeit synthetic drug made to resemble prescription medication). These counterfeit pills are much more dangerous and life-threatening. It is paradoxical then that while drug use is not rising in adolescence and young adulthood, it is becoming more dangerous and more fatal (**Figure 5.2**).

There are interesting differences in substance use between college students and their peers who do not go to college (NIDA, 2018a). College students smoke less marijuana and fewer cigarettes, vape less, use fewer synthetic drugs, and use fewer narcotic pain killers. However, college students tend to drink more alcohol than their noncollege peers. They also mix alcohol with energy drinks (and other stimulants; see the In the News feature) more frequently, a dangerous combination that can lead to overintoxication, increased likelihood of driving under the influence, and alcohol poisoning (Williams, Housman, Woolsey, & Sather, 2018). This mix has also been found to increase other risky behaviors, such as risky sex, sexual victimization, and increased aggression (Ball, Miller, Quigley, Eliseo-Arras, 2018). Can you see how risky behaviors compound one another?

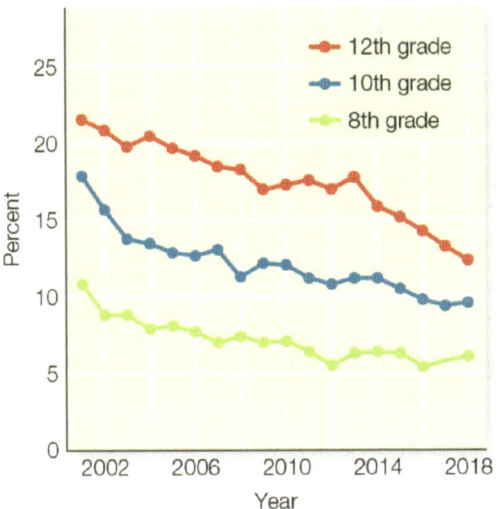

Figure 5.2 Percentage of students who have used any illicit drug other than Marijuana in the past year.

Source: Data from NIDA (2018c)

From what we have learned, we can expect that these health-compromising behaviors have multiple causes, and a biopsychosocial perspective gives us the best understanding of both use and treatment. We look next at each of the major types of substances.

In the News

Social Media and Sexual Risk

Heavy social media use increases the likelihood of sexting, transactional sex, and risky sex (Purba et al., 2023). Teens who are on TikTok, Instagram, Snapchat, and YouTube every day are more likely to engage in risky behaviors. Kids as young as 10 years old are using alcohol, drugs, and tobacco and engaging in anti-social and risky sexual behavior as a result of spending a lot of time on social media. Publa and colleagues (2023) showed that a minimum of two hours per day can double the odds of alcohol consumption when compared to kids who are on social medial less than two hours per day. However, most adolescents report spending between three to five hours a day on social media (Vente, Daley, Killmeyer, & Grubb, 2020).

Social media was shown to be one of the main socializing factors along with peers and family that influence how adolescents think about sex. People of all ages are accessing pornography at a much greater rate today and this has been linked to increased engagement in risky sexual behaviors (Mubasshera, 2024). Excessive and problematic pornography consumption is related to a greater incidence of cyber dating violence in adolescents (Morelli et al., 2024). One out of every eight teens reports having engaged in self-injury and over 25% have shared sexually explicit messages and these rates increase with the number of social media platforms they interact with (Vente et al., 2020).

It's not just health behaviors though. The Publa study also showed that frequent social media consumption increased by 73% the risk of anti-social behaviors including bullying, aggressive behavior, physical assault, delinquent, and criminal behaviors, and it nearly tripled the risk of gambling. The window of vulnerability in the teenage years is magnified when social media is involved.

Question: What are the dangers some other dangers of social media for people of all ages?

Thinking About Health

- What is SUD?
- What substances can be misused, and what are the potential short- and long-term effects on the body and health?
- Why might substance dependence rates be decreasing?
- Is the trend likely to continue? Why or why not?

Smoking and Nicotine

Through tobacco use, nicotine is one of the most heavily used and addictive drugs. The tobacco epidemic is now one of the world's biggest health threats – killing around 8 million people yearly worldwide (WHO, 2021, 2024d). Although tobacco use has decreased over time, it remains the single leading cause of preventable disease, disability, and death in the United States (CDC, 2024c; WHO, 2021, 2024c).

Health Risks

One out of every 10 deaths worldwide is caused by tobacco (WHO, 2024c). Nearly every organ in the human body is harmed by smoking (CDC, 2024c). One-third of all cancers and 90% of all lung cancer cases are due to cigarette smoking. Lung diseases, such as chronic bronchitis and emphysema, are caused by smoking, and tobacco use also significantly increases the risk of heart attack, stroke, aneurysm, heart disease, and vascular disease. It is also linked to leukemia, cataracts, and pneumonia (U.S. Department of Health and Human Services [USHHS], 2014). Worldwide, the World Health Organization has found that approximately 7 million people a year die as a result of tobacco use, and that number is likely to rise to 2.2 billion by 2050 unless the smoking trends can be reversed (Mackay, Eriksen, & Eriksen, 2002).

According to the Centers for Disease Control and Prevention, more than 16 million Americans live with diseases that are caused by smoking (CDC, 2024c). Every day, 1300 people die as a result of cigarette smoking. Smokers die, on average, 10 years earlier than nonsmokers (Jha et al., 2013). And those not killed by smoking are often sickened by it. Think of it this way: For every person who dies from smoking, 30 more suffer from at least one tobacco-related illness (CDC, 2024c).

Smoking affects not just the smokers themselves. Approximately 41,000 nonsmokers die each year from exposure to secondhand smoke. Living with a smoker is nearly as dangerous as smoking oneself. Pregnant women who smoke also increase the risk of learning and behavioral problems in their children. Smoking during pregnancy is associated with increased risks of miscarriage, stillborn or premature births, and low-birth-weight infants. Pregnant women who smoke more than one pack of cigarettes a day are doubling the risk that their child will become addicted to tobacco in the future (**Photos 5.6** and **5.7**).

Photo 5.6   Fowler JS, Logan J, Wang G-J, et al. Low monoamine oxidase B in peripheral organs in smokers. Proceedings of the National Academy of Sciences of the United States of America. 2003;100(20):11600–11605. Copyright (2003). National Academy of Sciences, USA.

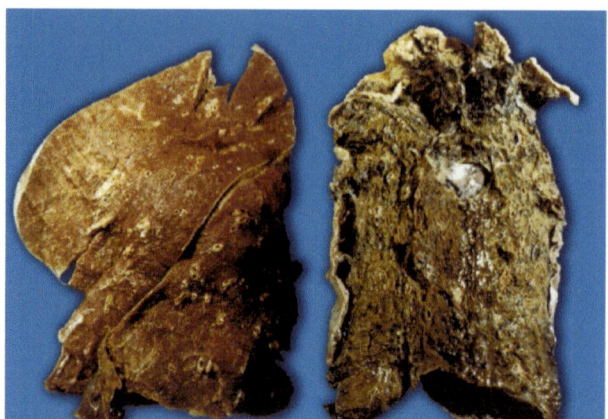

Photo 5.7   (Left) Using neuroimaging, scientists can see the effects of nicotine throughout the body and (right) comparison of a healthy lung (left) and the lung of a smoker (right).

Source: ARTHUR GLAUBERMAN/Science Source

Why People Smoke

Despite an all-time low in smoking rates among adolescents, too many young people still smoke. If smoking rates continue among young people in the United States, one out of every 13 kids age 17 or younger who are alive today will die due to smoking-related illness later on (Jha et al., 2013).

Cigarettes, e-cigarettes, vapes, cigars, pipes, snuff, and chewing tobacco all contain nicotine, which is highly addictive. Nicotine is absorbed into the bloodstream whenever a tobacco product is used. Once it enters the bloodstream, it activates the adrenal glands to release the hormone epinephrine (or adrenaline), which then stimulates the central nervous system, leading to increased blood pressure, respiration, and heart rate. Nicotine works in the brain to increase the levels of dopamine, a neurotransmitter that, we have learned, stimulates the brain centers that signal reward and pleasure. Over time, the drug creates long-term changes in the brain, and users become both physiologically and psychologically addicted. As with any SUD, quitting is not easy. Withdrawal symptoms include irritability, attentional difficulties, increased appetite, sleep disturbances, and powerful cravings for tobacco.

The addictive power of nicotine cannot be underestimated. Nicotine has been shown to be as addictive as alcohol, cocaine, or heroin (CDC, 2016b). Most smokers know that tobacco use is harmful, and many want to quit. Seven of every 10 adult smokers report wanting to quit smoking (CDC, 2011d). Although it is difficult to quit, success is possible. The good news is that there are actually more former smokers today than there are smokers (Center for Behavioral Health Statistics & Quality, 2015).

If so many people want to quit, why are so few able to do so? Understanding addiction to nicotine is still an active area of research. **Pharmacogenomics**

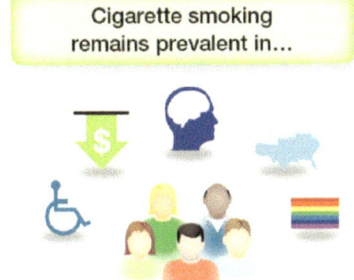

Cigarette smoking is down, but almost 38 million American adults still smoke

Cigarette smoking remains prevalent in…

- Men
- Adults 25–64 years old
- Less educated people
- Americans below the poverty level
- Midwesterners and Southerners
- Uninsured or underinsured people
- Disabled people
- Psychologically distressed people
- Native and multiracial Americans
- LGBTQ people

Strategies to reducing cigarette smoking overall include…

- Implementing smoke-free laws
- Running mass media campaigns
- Raising tobacco prices
- Making access to quitting resources easy

Photo 5.8   Information from CDC (2018e).

studies how genes influence the response to drugs and medications. Studies on twins show that about 40% to 70% of the risk of addiction to nicotine depends on one's genes (Agrawal & Lynskey, 2008). It appears that people who are able to quit have a gene that causes them to metabolize nicotine more slowly. These "slow metabolizers" generally smoke fewer cigarettes a day as well (**Photo 5.8**).

Treatments for Smoking Cessation

Although many smokers quit without help, many people need some form of treatment to help them. Several treatment options exist, including both pharmacological and behavioral approaches. Nicotine replacement therapies, such as a nicotine patch or gum, deliver a small and continuous dose—small enough that patients do not become dependent on them. Over time, the dose is lowered until no nicotine is dispensed. The idea is to reduce the withdrawal symptoms that often drive smokers back to smoking. Social engineering, social support, individualized therapy, and group therapy can significantly enhance the effectiveness of nicotine replacement therapies and lead to long-term success.

Another pharmacological treatment is antidepressant medication. Bupropion, approved by the FDA for the treatment of nicotine addiction in 1997, helps to alleviate cravings and other symptoms of withdrawal. More recently, varenicline tartrate has been used. This medication blocks the brain receptors that respond to nicotine so that quitters who try smoking again will not receive the same neurochemical rewards. Cutting-edge research is also exploring the use of hypertensives as well as the feasibility of a vaccine that stimulates the production of antibodies that block nicotine absorption in the brain.

Recently, many people have turned to e-cigarettes or vapes to help them quit smoking tobacco, believing that these options are less harmful than smoking cigarettes. In fact, e-cigarettes were originally designed for the purpose of helping smokers quit. While e-cigarettes and vapes are significantly safer than traditional cigarettes, there is limited evidence that they are useful for smoking cessation (Hartmann-Boyce, Begh, & Aveyard, 2018). Two large, randomized clinical trials of smokers trying to quit showed that smokers who used e-cigarettes with nicotine were able to refrain from smoking for 6–12 months, compared to those who tried to quit using e-cigarettes without nicotine (Hartmann-Boyce et al., 2016). However, the concern is that using e-cigarettes for smoking cessation causes a transfer of addictions—from a cigarette addiction to a nicotine addiction. For example, one French study showed that over half the people who used e-cigarettes to quit smoking were still using the e-cigarettes 6 months later, and reported that they continued to use them out of fear of returning to smoking (Borup, Mikkelsen, Tønnesen, & Christrup, 2015; Etter & Bullen, 2011; Hartmann-Boyce et al., 2018; Pasquereau, Guignard, Andler, & Nguyen-Thanh, 2017). So, the jury is still out, and more research is needed, in determining whether e-cigarettes or vapes are helpful to those who want to break their addiction to nicotine.

Behavioral treatments are crucial as well in addressing the psychological aspects of nicotine addiction. For smokers, having nicotine at certain times and under certain circumstances becomes a habit. Part of the challenge in quitting is that smoking has become part of the fabric of life. Self-help materials are available, as are cognitive behavioral therapy and counseling. These can teach the smoker to recognize stressful situations that may lead them to smoke. These materials can help with developing alternative coping strategies, relaxation techniques, and problem-solving skills. Social support is instrumental, and many people have turned to nontraditional therapeutic groups such as Nicotine Anonymous and Internet support groups for help. However, in order to be effective, behavioral treatments must be appropriate for the individual.

It takes a long time to break a smoking addiction. Up to 80% of those who try to quit, even with help, will relapse at least once (Borland, Partos, Yong, Cummings, & Hyland, 2012). Perhaps they tried to quit, or felt pressured to quit, before they were fully ready. Think back to the transtheoretical model in Chapter 3: There is no simple road to success, because there is no one factor behind health-compromising behavior. A person has to be emotionally, cognitively, and behaviorally ready to change. And behavioral change will involve lifestyle changes as well. It takes vigilance to maintain behavioral change, and it can take years of maintenance for the change to take hold.

When quitting is successful, the effects are immediate. Quitters begin reversing the negative effects of smoking within 24 hours—blood pressure and the chance of heart attack both decrease. Long-term benefits include a reduction in the risk of stroke, cancers, and coronary heart disease. Recall that smokers die, on average, 10 years sooner than non-smokers—quitting can add years back to the lifespan. A man who quits at age 35 will, on average, add five years to his life expectancy just by quitting. Kicking the habit is a great thing to do, so quitters should not be afraid to seek support.

Thinking About Health

- What effects does smoking have on the body?
- Who smokes, and why?
- What are the most effective treatments for smoking addiction?
- Why is there concern about the effectiveness of e-cigarettes and vapes for smoking cessation?

Drinking and Alcohol

Alcohol is everywhere. It has played a significant role in almost all human cultures. Some say that the very foundation of civilization centered on the cultivation of grains for beer—agriculture was not for bread alone (Fraser & Rimas, 2010; Social Issues Research Centre, 2016). Moreover, the near-universal use of alcohol throughout human evolution has led some to speculate that drinking alcohol must have powerful adaptive benefits. Since its beginning, probably in the Neolithic period (4000 B.C.E.), drinking has been a largely social activity, and it endures as a common feature of traditions, celebrations, holidays, religious observances, and family dinners.

Nevertheless, alcohol is related to at least 230 different types of diseases that negatively impact people's health and that is not considering alcohol use disorder. Worldwide three million people die annually due to alcohol and in the United States, there are 95,000 alcohol-related deaths annually (NCDAS, 2024; WHO, 2024d). To put that into perspective that is around 261 alcohol-related deaths per day in the United States, and as many as 30 people die each day due to drunk driving (NCDAS, 2024). Here is another sobering statistic, of the nearly 7,500 homicides in the United States each year, 40% of the perpetrators who were convicted were under the influence of alcohol when they committed murder.

In the United States, more than half of all adults (older than 18 years) report that they drank in the last month (Substance Abuse and Mental Health Services Administration [SAMHSA], 2021). Worldwide, the recommended low-risk limits on alcohol consumption vary greatly by country; however, based on data from around the world, the lowest risks for death and disability were associated with consumption of 100 grams (or 3.5 ounces) per week or less (Wood et al., 2018). This is significantly less than is standard in the United States.

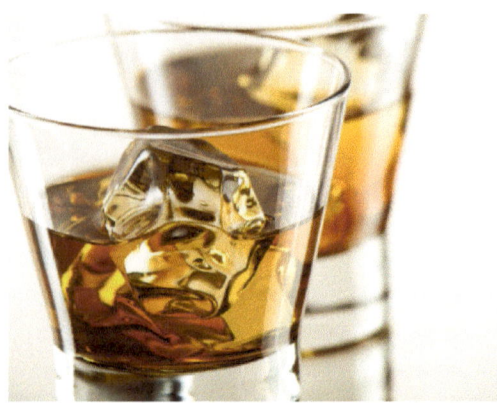

Photo 5.9   Drinking just two whiskies can impair your cognitive functioning.

In the United States, a woman who has one drink per day is a moderate drinker, whereas a man who has two drinks per day is a moderate drinker. Among college students, 53% said they drank in the last month, nearly 33% engaged in binge drinking (five or more drinks on one occasion), and 8% were heavy drinkers (five or more drinks on one occasion more than five times in the last month; SAMHSA, 2021). Most of us are able to drink responsibly. However, for some, alcohol is no longer just a social activity. It has become part of their daily lives, a danger that they cannot do without or control. Overall, alcohol abuse kills 3 million people per year worldwide (**Photo** 5.9) (WHO, 2024d).

How Much Is Too Much?

It's likely that most adults will be inebriated at some point in their lives. Because alcohol is so ever-present, any of us could drink to excess. Drinking in a social context can be pleasurable, and many people like how alcohol affects them. They may feel more social, more confident, less inhibited, funnier, more relaxed, or more excited when they drink. For most people, there is no harm in having a few drinks, as long as they are not driving. No one should ever get behind the wheel of a car if one has had too much to drink.

Stress can also impact alcohol consumption. For example, alcohol consumption increased drastically in response to the COVID-19 pandemic, as did alcohol-related illnesses and deaths. The increase was more than over the last 50 years. The stress associated with the pandemic included severe illness, grief, disrupted schooling and social life, feelings of isolation and loneliness, food insecurity, shortages, and changes in diet and exercise, job loss, and economic hardship made it hard for many to cope. Many people turned to alcohol to help them cope. It is not uncommon for people to turn to alcohol in times of extreme stress (Rodriguez et al., 2020; Schmidt et al., 2021). Research shows that there were similar spikes after the bombings of the World Trade Centers on 9/11 2001 and after Hurricane Katrina in August 2005 in New Orleans (Beaudoin, 2011).

Researchers credit the social isolation for the increase in alcohol consumption during the COVID-19 pandemic. During the pandemic, those with existing alcohol-related illnesses were more likely to have complications and to die from them (White et al., 2022). Figure on alcohol-related deaths during the pandemic.

The Health Consequences of Alcohol Misuse

The term "alcoholic" is a pejorative term that conveys stigma. Historically, substance misuse in general has been portrayed as a moral failing rather than a disease and a serious mental health condition. Rather than labeling individuals a more thoughtful approach is to understand the extent to which a person's drinking is causing problems in their lives.

Unhealthy alcohol use, a technical term developed by the National Institute of Alcohol Abuse and Alcohol use disorder (NIAAA), refers to drinking four standard drinks per occasion. For men, unhealthy alcohol use is 14 drinks per week (4 drinks in a single occasion), and for women, it is seven drinks per week (3 in a single occasion). Unhealthy alcohol use is also called at-risk alcohol use, either of which at higher levels of drinking can create greater problems and become Alcohol Use Disorder.

A person with **alcohol use disorder** may have a hard time controlling their drinking, they have a high tolerance for alcohol, and they experience withdrawal symptoms if they try to wean themselves from alcohol. They have a daily need for alcohol and an inability to cut back. They may also go through periods of binge drinking and experience occasional blackouts or loss of memory for events that occurred while drinking. People with alcohol use disorder often report several failed attempts to regulate or control their drinking, and they continue drinking despite legal or health problems. Some drink early in the morning or throughout the day to maintain elevated blood-alcohol levels and to avoid debilitating withdrawal symptoms.

Alcohol **use** Disorder is diagnosed by the DSM-5 in a range from mild to severe depending on the number of symptoms identified below. Specifically, alcohol use disorder involves a problematic pattern of alcohol use that leads to significant distress or problems functioning. Symptoms of AUD include:

- Drinking more alcohol or over a longer period than originally intended.
- Unsuccessfully trying to cut down or control alcohol use.
- Craving, or a strong desire or urge to use alcohol. (Wanting a drink so much it's difficult to think of anything else.)
- Drinking that interferes with responsibilities at home, at work, or at school.
- Continuing to use alcohol even when it causes problems with family and friends.
- Giving up important social, occupational, or recreational activities because of alcohol use.
- Repeatedly using alcohol in physically hazardous situations.
- Developing a tolerance to alcohol (needing more alcohol to get the same effect).
- Experiencing withdrawal symptoms such as shakiness, restlessness, nausea, or sweating after stopping or reducing drinking.

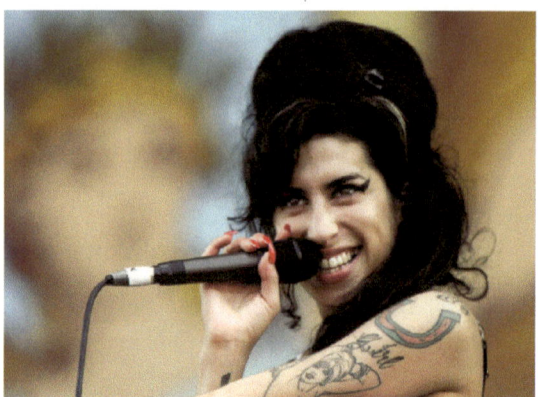

Photo 5.10   Musician Amy Winehouse died of alcohol poisoning in July 2011, at age 27. Her blood alcohol content was 0.42% at the time of her death, five times the minimum to count as intoxicated under the law. According to the Coroner who examined her, "The unintended consequences of such potentially fatal levels was her sudden death" (Hechinger, 2011).

Source: Matt Cardy/Getty Images

Having at least two of these symptoms in the last year is indicative of an alcohol use disorder. Two to three symptoms indicate a mild disorder, four to five symptoms indicate a moderate disorder, and six or more symptoms indicate severe alcohol use disorder.

Drinking, even small amounts daily and occasional intoxication do not by themselves make a diagnosis of alcohol use disorder (**Photo 5.10**).

Overall, the main factor in determining the health consequences of alcohol use is how much alcohol a person drinks—with one fatal exception. It takes just one night of drinking—and only a minimal amount of alcohol in the bloodstream, at that—to impair functioning enough that one could die behind the wheel of a car. In the United States, 37 people are killed every 38 minutes in traffic accidents involving alcohol every day of the year, and this is a 14% increase since 2020 (Stewart, 2023). In 2021, 13,384 people lost their lives the same way. Aside from alcohol-related traffic accidents, however, most of the health consequences of alcohol abuse are cumulative, the result of many years of habitual drinking.

One of the most common health outcomes of alcohol abuse is liver damage, known as **cirrhosis** of the liver. This occurs over time, as scar tissue forms and blocks the flow of blood to the liver, disrupting the processing of nutrients, hormones, and proteins. Symptoms include loss of appetite, weakness, fatigue, jaundice, itching, and easy bruising.

Another possible health consequence is a cumulative impairment in neurological and cognitive functioning. Excessive consumption of alcohol over time can lead to a thiamine (vitamin B1) deficiency caused by malnutrition, which, in turn, can damage or destroy nerve cells in the brain. This is **Korsakoff's syndrome**, named for Sergei Korsakoff, the nineteenth-century Russian neuropsychiatrist who identified it. Its symptoms include amnesia and memory loss, not unlike what is seen in dementia. The brain regions indicated in this disorder are the medial thalamus and the mammillary bodies in the posterior hypothalamus. These parts of the brain's limbic system are responsible for memory and emotion. Korsakoff's patients will often confabulate to fill in the information that they do not remember. Additional symptoms include apathy and disorientation (Harper, 2009; Parsons & Prigatano, 1977). It is only possible to diagnose Korsakoff's after death, through autopsy, but up to 78% of **people with alcohol use disorders** show some amount of brain pathology of this disease (Goldstein & Shelly, 1980; Ridley, Draper, & Withall, 2013).

It has been said that alcohol is both a tonic and a poison. It has also been said that moderate alcohol use, such as a glass of red wine at dinner, can be good for your health. Indeed, some research supports the idea that moderate drinking can offset heart disease (Goldberg, Mosca, Piano, & Fisher, 2001). At the same time, cancer deaths due to alcohol consumption have increased by 60% (Nelson et al., 2013). Just three or more drinks per day increase the risk of death from seven different kinds of cancer, including breast cancer in women and cancers of the mouth and throat in men. Even just one-and-a-half drinks per day have been linked to more than 35% of these deaths from cancer (Nelson et al., 2013). Timothy Naimi, a researcher involved in that study, suggests that when it comes to cancer, "the less you drink, the better."

Another serious health consequence of alcohol use is **fetal alcohol syndrome** (FAS), the leading cause of mental retardation in the Western world (Abel & Sokol, 1986). When a woman drinks during pregnancy, the alcohol crosses the placental barrier, where it can interfere with the development of the growing fetus. During pregnancy, consumption of alcohol causes a variety of mental and physical defects, including stunted fetal growth, low fetal weight and low birth weight, facial deformities, and damage to neurons. Brain damage due to pre-natal drinking may result in poor memory, attention deficits, impulsive behavior, poor reasoning abilities, and a predisposition to drug addiction and other mental health problems. The U.S. Surgeon General recommends that pregnant women abstain completely from alcohol.

Alcohol has other health consequences as well, such as accidental drowning, falls, electrical shocks, homicides, suicides, and other risky behaviors. Drinking alcohol before going on a date increases the chance that the couple will have sexual intercourse—often without any discussion of potential sexually transmitted infections (STIs), pregnancy, or condom use (Griffin, Umstattd, & Usdan, 2010). College students across the United States (specifically, in California) reported drinking alcohol regularly, and 12% of them reported that they were sexually active and had been diagnosed with an STI at least once. The reported rate of drinking and unprotected sex in the Midwest was even higher (25%), and the STI rates were two times higher in females than in males (Cooper, 2002).

In at least half of all rapes and sexual assaults, the male perpetrators reported drinking alcohol (Abbey, Zawacki, Buck, Clinton, & McAuslan, 2004). Of acquaintance rapes, 46% occurred when one or both parties had been drinking (Griffin et al., 2010).

Alcohol Myopia

Have you ever had the experience of waking up after a night of partying with friends and being embarrassed when you remembered something that you did or said? Drinking alcohol lowers inhibitions and interferes with rational thought—but how? **Alcohol myopia theory** suggests that when people are under the influence of alcohol, they become unable to process information deeply (Kaly, Heesacker, & Frost, 2002; Steele & Josephs, 1990). Intoxicated people focus on a much more limited range of environmental stimuli and take longer to understand what is going on around them (Steele & Josephs, 1990). In a sense, they become nearsighted, much like people with ordinary myopia.

Ordinarily, myopia is a visual impairment. Nearsighted people have poor vision for objects at a distance, but perfectly good vision for objects that are nearby. In much the same way, intoxicated people focus on the here and now and miss the bigger picture. They also make impulsive decisions at the moment without thinking about the future consequences. Without the larger context of past experiences and memories, or the foresight to think about the future, they fail to attend to the consequences of their choices. That makes it more difficult for them to inhibit risky or aggressive behaviors. In one study, women watched videos of potential dating partners (Murphy, Monahan, & Miller, 1998). Half the women drank alcohol prior to watching the videos and the other half did not. Intoxicated women rated an attractive but sexually risky man as having better relationship potential than did sober women (Murphy et al., 1998). This study supports the theory of alcohol myopia and demonstrates how alcohol can influence our perceptions and choices.

These are only some of the most common health consequences of alcohol abuse. Although alcohol is a socially accepted part of our lives, it represents a serious threat to health and is a major public health issue when alcohol use gets out of control.

Treatment of Alcohol Abuse

One of the biggest obstacles in treating alcohol use disorder is overcoming the withdrawal symptoms. Almost all people with alcohol use disorders experience some degree of withdrawal when they quit, ranging from mild shakes to delirium tremens, a condition that includes confusion, hallucinations, convulsions, autonomic instability, and even death. They go through detox, or detoxification, as alcohol dissipates from the system, and 5% of them may need medical assistance. Detoxification treatment can take place in a hospital or detox treatment facility. It includes close monitoring of vital signs and, in some cases, the use of benzodiazepines (tranquilizers such as Valium, Librium, or Ativan) to help ease the discomfort of withdrawal. It can take up to seven days for the last traces of alcohol to be eliminated from the system. Once this threshold is reached, and patients are no longer addicted to alcohol, the goal is then to provide the psychosocial tools they will need to cope with life without alcohol and to prevent relapse.

Behavioral conditioning can help break the learned addiction to alcohol. Some treatment programs rely on Antabuse, a chemical that makes patients vomit when it is paired with alcohol. Over time, people with alcohol use disorders come to associate vomiting with alcohol consumption and develop such a negative response to the sight or smell of alcohol that they no longer desire it.

One of the oldest and best-known treatment programs is People with alcohol use disorders Anonymous (or A.A.). This is a social network or fellowship of people who understand alcohol use disorder from personal experience. A.A. is a 12-step program that helps recovering people with alcohol use disorders deal with life without alcohol and stay sober. Many other programs are now based on the same 12 principles (see **Table 5.3**).

These are the original 12 steps as published by People with alcohol use disorders Anonymous:

1. We admitted we were powerless over alcohol—that our lives had become unmanageable.
2. Came to believe that a power greater than ourselves could restore us to sanity.
3. Made a decision to turn our will and our lives over to the care of God, *as we understood Him*.
4. Made a searching and fearless moral inventory of ourselves.
5. Admitted to God, to ourselves, and to another human being the exact nature of our wrongs.
6. Were entirely ready to have God remove all these defects of character.
7. Humbly asked Him to remove our shortcomings.
8. Made a list of all persons we had harmed, and became willing to make amends to them all.
9. Made direct amends to such people wherever possible, except when to do so would injure them or others.
10. Continued to take personal inventory, and when we were wrong, promptly admitted it.
11. Sought through prayer and meditation to improve our conscious contact with God *as we understood Him*, praying only for knowledge of His will for us and the power to carry that out.
12. Having had a spiritual awakening as the result of these steps, we tried to carry this message to people with alcohol use disorders and to practice these principles in all our affairs.

Source: The Twelve Steps are reprinted with permission of People with alcohol use disorders Anonymous World Services, Inc. ("A.A.W.S.") Permission to reprint the Twelve Steps does not mean that A.A.W.S. has reviewed or approved the contents of this publication, or that A.A. necessarily agrees with the views expressed herein. A.A. is a program of recovery from alcohol use disorder only—use of the Twelve Steps in connection with programs and activities which are patterned after A.A., but which address other problems, or in any other non-A.A., does not imply otherwise.

Table 5.3 The twelve steps

One of the program's major precepts is that participants acknowledge that they cannot control alcohol and accept that they can never drink again. This may be one of the most challenging parts of quitting through A.A., because alcohol has become part of their lives, and, as we have noted, alcohol is part of the social fabric of life. Alternative programs to break the addiction to alcohol, therefore, encourage learning to drink responsibly. These programs teach skills for coping with the presence of alcohol in social situations, which may be a more realistic approach.

It is hard to measure the success rate of A.A. and other programs because many people with alcohol use disorders relapse. Yet many people report successfully breaking free of their dependence on alcohol. Regardless of the method through which people with alcohol use disorders break their addiction, the health benefits are many.

Thinking About Health

- Can you point out the differences between social and problem drinking patterns in the people around you?
- What is alcohol use disorder, what is alcohol use disorder, and what is a high-functioning people with alcohol use disorder?
- What are some of the short- and long-term health consequences of alcohol abuse?
- What are the most effective treatments for alcohol addiction?

Marijuana Use and Substance Abuse

The origins of marijuana, a plant with medicinal properties, can be traced back to the ancient world. Although evidence is scant, ashes from archeological sites show that its medicinal use began around 400 C.E. (Zias et al., 1993) and that it was used extensively more than 5000 years ago in what is now Romania (Bennett, 2010). **Marijuana** is what we call the *Cannabis sativa* plant when it is used as a drug. Marijuana has many everyday names, such as *pot* or *weed*, but scientists refer to marijuana as **cannabis**, and the chemical compound derived from the drug is called tetrahydrocannabinol, or **THC**.

Across history, cannabis has been a medicinal staple. It has been mixed into teas and tinctures and smoked to treat pain and other ailments. It became known in the United States for its medicinal properties in the mid-1800s. Although cannabis was widely used in the nineteenth and early twentieth centuries in the United States, federal restrictions began in 1937, and, by 1970, its use was prohibited under federal law. Recently, however, medical and popular opinions on cannabis have been shifting, and it has now been legalized for medicinal use in 23 states (see **Figure** 5.3).

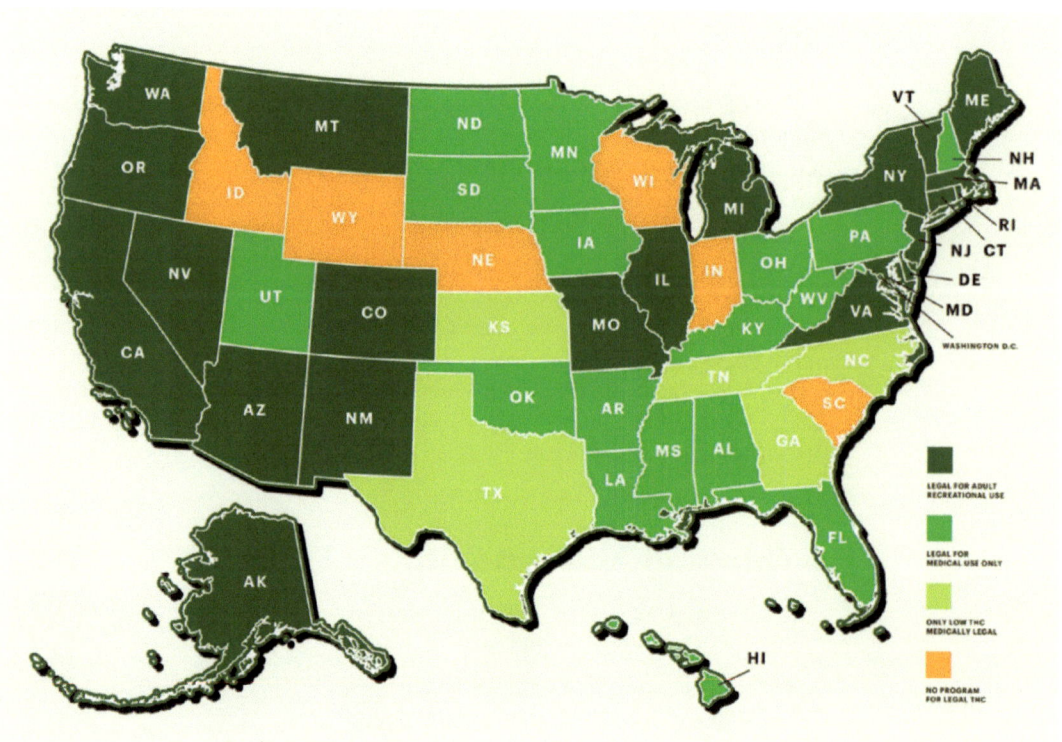

ROLLING STONE
Figure 5.3   As of 2024, a map of marijuana legalization in the United States.

Marijuana and Public Opinion

As of 2019, marijuana was legal in all but 17 states. Medical marijuana was available in 33 states, and recreational smoking was legal only in 10. What **Figure 5.3** shows is that most Americans have voted to legalize and decriminalize marijuana.

Many patients who suffer from painful, debilitating illnesses have benefited from medical marijuana. Legalization of marijuana (both medical and recreational) is spreading globally, and many people see no reason that marijuana should not be legal, especially for medical purposes. However, those who oppose making medical marijuana legal feel very strongly that doing so would increase drug use of all kinds and put an undue burden on law enforcement. Let's look at the evidence.

The majority of Americans are now in favor of legalizing marijuana for the first time in more than four decades of polling (Saad, 2023). In fact, 70% (seven of every ten) Americans now support legalizing marijuana, a figure that represents a new record (Saad, 2023). In one recent survey, 50% of American adults reported having tried marijuana, and 17% of American adults reported using it regularly. Some 55 million Americans reported using it in the last year and that is higher than the number of people who smoke nicotine (approximately 37 million according to the CDC).

Of those who reported smoking it, more than half (53%) cited a medical reason as at least part of the reason, but almost as many (47%) said they used it "just for fun." Fewer and fewer adolescents believe that smoking pot is harmful or dangerous (Meier et al., 2012). More teens are trying it, and trying it at earlier ages, and more are using it daily. Between the ages of 18–29, over 21% of young adults report having used cannabis in the last year (Meier & White, 2018).

Although young adults smoke pot more frequently than other age groups, roughly 3–5% of people over age 50 have also smoked pot in the last year (Choi, DiNitto, & Marti, 2016). This is a 71% jump over previous years (Han et al., 2017). Interestingly, this research shows that most older people who currently use marijuana began using it before the age of 18 (Lloyd & Striley, 2018). Men (54%) are more likely to smoke pot than women (42%), and a majority of both whites and blacks have tried marijuana, compared with only 34% of Hispanics. Clearly, public opinion in the United States is changing. But is the public opinion right? (See **Photo 5.11**.)

"Some of my finest hours have been spent on my back veranda, smoking hemp and observing as far as my eye can see."

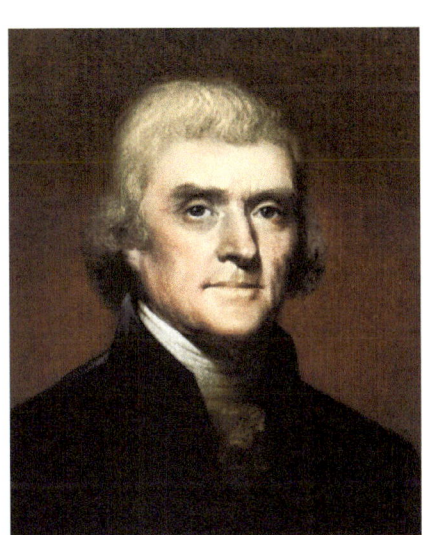

Photo 5.11   Thomas Jefferson (American Founding Father, the principal author of the Declaration of Independence, and the president of the United States from 1801 to 1809).

Source: Omikron/Getty Images

The Marijuana Paradox

From a health perspective, marijuana presents a paradox. It is effective for the treatment of illness, but it can also have negative health outcomes.

The use of cannabis as an herbal remedy and medicinal treatment has a long history. Cannabis has well-documented medical benefits for patients undergoing chemotherapy for cancer, chronic pain management, depression, anxiety, posttraumatic stress disorder, sleep problems, narcotic addiction, HIV/AIDS treatment, glaucoma, and gastrointestinal diseases (Kruger & Kruger, 2019). It even has antibacterial properties. A synthetic derivative of cannabis is helpful for treating nausea, vomiting, premenstrual syndrome, insomnia, and lack of appetite. Medicinal cannabis is also highly effective in cases of muscle spasticity, Parkinson's disease, multiple sclerosis, and spinal cord injury. It may be effective in treating adrenal disease, inflammatory bowel disease, migraine, fibromyalgia, and related conditions as well (Russo, 2004).

The use of marijuana in pain management extends to neurogenic pain (pain arising from the nervous system), asthma, and glaucoma (Grotenhermen, 2003). A study in California showed that people find it effective in the treatment of pain, muscle spasm, headaches, anxiety, depression, cramps, panic attacks, diarrhea, and itching. Others report using it to offset the side effects of other medications and to improve sleep, relaxation, appetite, concentration, and energy. Some even smoke pot for anger management (Reinarman, Nunberg, Lanthier, & Heddleston, 2011).

Many people report using marijuana as a supplement or substitute for pharmaceutical treatment (Kruger & Kruger, 2019). It is not yet clear how often medical professionals suggest or prescribe cannabis, but nearly half of the participants in one recent study reported that they did not discuss their cannabis use with their healthcare providers (Kruger & Kruger, 2019). The medical community may not yet embrace medical marijuana, but patients do. It is easy to wonder why marijuana is not more widely available, but many people have real concerns about its use.

The Health Risks

Marijuana is often labeled a "gateway drug," a drug that leads to the use of more dangerous drugs, especially in adolescence. It has the "disreputable status of being the most popular illicit drug in the United States" (Gonzalez, 2007; Meier & White, 2018). There is some support for this argument. For example, rats given doses of THC became more susceptible to the effects of nicotine; when taken together, the result is a greater risk of addiction to nicotine (Panlilio, Zanettini, Barnes, Solinas, & Goldberg, 2013). While smoking pot may precede the use of other drugs, overall, the link is inconclusive.

There are concerns about cognitive impairments as well (Fried, Watkinson, & Gray, 2005; Gonzalez, 2007). Persistent use of marijuana beginning in adolescence leads to lower neurological and intellectual functioning in midlife (Meier et al.,

2012). Regular marijuana use persisting into adulthood is associated with a significant drop in IQ by age 38, and the more frequent and continuous the use, the greater the impairments. There is also some evidence that pot smokers are more willing to engage in risky behavior. Although marijuana can cause acute intoxication—the "high" that pot smokers seek—the impairments in attention, memory, and decision-making ability outlast the high and can linger for days. Males showed greater cognitive effects than females (Crean, Crane, & Mason, 2011).

Cannabis use has been linked to *amotivational* syndrome, in which a person has a lack of interest in what is going on around them and prolonged periods of apathy (McGlothlin & West, 1968). While there is a stereotype that people "high" on cannabis have little motivation, the empirical evidence is mixed. This is, in part, due to the fact that most studies that have examined amotivational syndrome in pot smokers relied on self-reported lack of motivation. In a recent study, researchers recruited college students who used cannabis as well as someone they selected as an "informant"—someone who knew them well and spent time with them when they were high and when they were not (Meier & White, 2018). For undergraduates who used cannabis more than 52 days in the last year, informants reported that they showed more amotivational behaviors than those students who had used it less than that. This suggests that even after controlling for covariates such as depression and the use of other substances, cannabis-related amotivation is severe enough to be noticeable to others and to negatively impact one's life.

The neurobiological effects of marijuana have also been identified. THC travels to the CB1 and CB2 receptors in immune tissues and the central nervous system (Gonzalez, 2007; Munro, Thomas, & Abu-Shaar, 1993). In this way, cannabis affects the neurochemical signaling system that regulates the brain's reward pathways. Cerebral blood flow and brain metabolism both increase, especially in the cerebral cortex.

Marijuana use can become problematic. When it does, it is known as marijuana use disorder—an addiction, in severe cases. Marijuana use disorders are associated with dependence on the substance and withdrawal symptoms when the substance is not taken. Thirty percent of those who use marijuana have marijuana use disorder (Hasin et al., 2015). Like other SUDs, marijuana use disorder is marked by an inability to quit using the substance even when using it interferes with one's life and daily functioning. When people who are addicted to marijuana try to quit, they often experience irritability, restlessness, moodiness, sleep problems, decreased appetite or cravings, and, sometimes, various physical discomforts. Luckily, these withdrawal symptoms subside after the first two weeks. Marijuana use disorder, like other SUDs, is a brain disease.

The impact of marijuana use disorder can be seen in deficits in memory functioning and recall. Heavy pot smokers (more than five joints a week) may also show evidence of small declines in IQ (a four-point difference from other experimental groups), problems with immediate and delayed memory retrieval, and slowed information processing speed (Fried et al., 2005; Meier et al., 2012). Some evidence also shows that memory deficits may persist in pot smokers even when they are not intoxicated, although these deficits may be mild and transient (Gonzalez, 2007). This neurological evidence is novel and important, because it has identified the influences of cannabis on brain structure and functioning as well as cognitive and behavioral outcomes. Regular marijuana use in adolescence may also affect brain development, as demonstrated in animal models (Burston, Wiley, Craig, Selley, & Sim-Selley, 2010; Quinn et al., 2008; Rubino et al., 2009). Repeated long-term use may lead to a neurophysiological addiction to the substance.

Many important questions, however, remain unanswered. What differentiates those who become addicted to marijuana from other users? What are the effects on the brain of long-term cannabis use? When does cannabis protect brain functioning, and when is it harmful? Is cannabis so harmful that we should limit its medical use? Addressing these questions is crucial to helping us decide for ourselves where we stand in the debate on legalizing marijuana—and whether or not we should use it ourselves.

Thinking About Health

- ■ What factors do you think have influenced the changing public opinion on marijuana legalization?
- ■ Who smokes pot, and why?
- ■ Is pot smoking addictive?
- ■ What are the health consequences of marijuana?
- ■ If the issue of legalizing recreational marijuana came to a vote in your state, how would you vote?

Risky Sexual Behavior

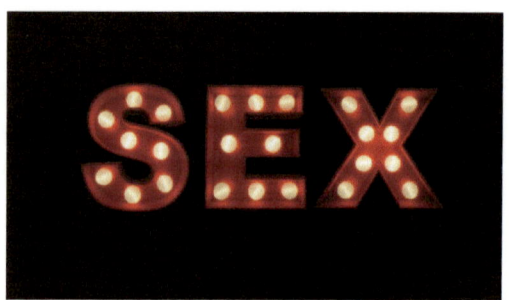

Photo 5.12   Franck Boston/Shutterstock.

High-risk sexual behaviors include early age of first intercourse, sex with multiple partners, sex with partners whose sexual history is unknown, sex without using a condom, and sex while under the influence of drugs or alcohol (Zietsch, Verweij, Bailey, Wright, & Martin, 2010). While these behaviors do not always have negative health outcomes, they pose a higher risk of STIs and unplanned pregnancy (**Photo 5.12**).

STIs and Unplanned Pregnancy

As we saw in Chapter 4, STIs are illnesses that are spread through human sexual behavior—including vaginal intercourse, anal intercourse, and oral sex. Further consequences of STIs include higher rates of genital and cervical cancers, pelvic inflammatory disease, infertility, and complications during pregnancy and childbirth. With higher rates of new infections and reinfection, STIs can be fatal (Fleming et al., 2019). Unplanned pregnancy, too, has many consequences—medical, psychosocial, financial, and mental (**Photo 5.13**) (Zietsch et al., 2010).

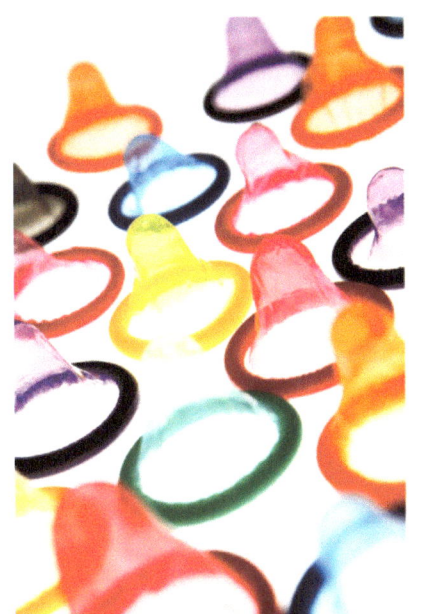 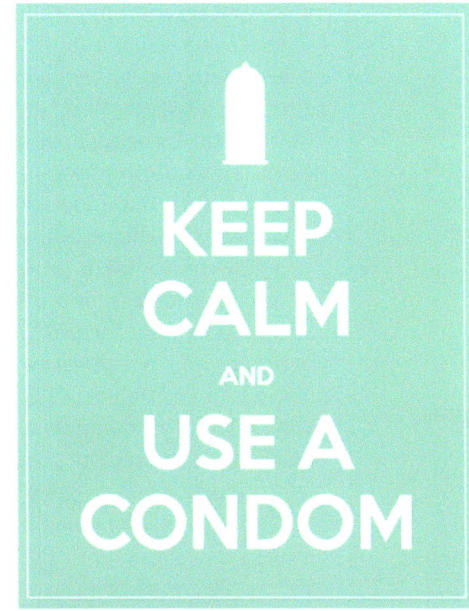

Photo 5.13   Using condoms and other forms of protection can help protect your health.

Source: Pederk/Getty Images (left) and Dragomer Maria/Shutterstock (right)

Causes of Risky Sex

What Explains Risky Sexual Behavior?

The evolutionary perspective on sex argues that people who have more sexual partners and more sexual experiences are more likely to pass on their genes to the next generation. Biological explanations suggest that early puberty and sexual maturation should be correlated with early risk-taking, especially in females (Belsky, Houts, & Fearon, 2010).

In modern society, cultural norms play a role. Half of all high school seniors report having had sexual intercourse (Kann et al., 2016). Adolescence, as we have seen, is a critical period in development that involves learning to make decisions about engaging in sex. Often that decision-making leads to risky sexual practices such as having multiple partners, inconsistent use of protection against STIs, and pregnancy. Among those teens who are having sex, 43% reported not using a condom the last time they had sex, and 14% said they had no method for preventing unintended pregnancy (Kann et al., 2016). In the United States, there are 19 million new cases of STIs each year, and they are most frequently diagnosed among people ages 15–24 (Eaton et al., 2012; Fleming et al., 2019).

There are also gender differences in sexual risk-taking. In their lifetimes, men tend to have more sexual partners than women, and they are more likely to engage in risky sexual behaviors such as intoxicated sex. Both biological and sociocultural factors may influence these gender norms. Paradoxically, research shows that sexual minority women (women who self-identify as lesbian, gay, or bisexual) and sexual minority men (men who identify as gay or bisexual, or who have sex with men) have increased risks for STIs and HIV, despite reporting using protection (Paschen-Wolff et al., 2019; Pérez, Gamarel, van den Berg, & Operario, 2018; Smith, Perrin, & Rabinovitch, 2018). Multiple sexual partners and the use of substances during sexual encounters may play a role. These findings require further research but underscore the role of social and contextual factors in negatively impacting the health outcomes of underrepresented minority groups.

Family environment, especially the absence of a father figure in childhood, also predicts adolescent promiscuity (Belsky et al., 2010; Draper & Harpending, 1982). Personality factors play a role—such as impulsivity, extraversion, psychoticism, and neuroticism. Risky sexual behaviors may also have a genetic component (Zietsch et al., 2010), although this predisposition has been shown to be mediated by family warmth and close sibling relationships (McHale, Updegraff, & Whiteman, 2012).

One study asked pregnant women between the ages of 15 and 19 for their own explanations for sexual risk-taking (King Jones, 2010). These young women reported social pressures. They spoke of wanting to "fit in" and of "partner pressure" in the form of promises or ultimatums. Friends were telling them how "good" it was, "building up the experience"; they also heard friends "making fun of virgins." Other women cited simple curiosity. An 18-year-old Hispanic woman said about having sex, "I was like, now I know how it felt so I don't have to have sex with anyone else." There was also the allure of "forbidden fruit." As one 15-year-old said, "My mom said don't do it, but she wouldn't tell me why not."

The influence of the media was also clear. The girls felt themselves flooded with the glamour of sex through TV, movies, music videos and lyrics, the Internet, and advertising. As one girl put it, "Kids sneak porn … and think, 'Oh, that's neat. I'll try that with my girlfriend.'"

Regardless of the drivers of sexual risk-taking, it is a very real health problem that has many negative health consequences. As we learned in Chapter 4, being assertive and open to having a conversation about protection can significantly reduce the risks of both STIs and unwanted pregnancy.

Social Media Behavior and Health

The influence of others on our own

Thinking About Health

- What drives risky sexual behavior, and what examples of risky sexual behavior do you see in popular culture?
- Who engages in risky sex, and why?
- Why is it so difficult to get people to practice safe sex?

Chapter Summary

In this chapter, we explored the most common health-compromising behaviors and how they relate to negative health outcomes. These risks are the antithesis of the health-enhancing behaviors we met in Chapter 4, and they can significantly affect health. The health risks are even greater because many of these behaviors tend to occur together. Adolescents engage in the most high-risk behaviors of any age group. Although many of the health risks of substance use share common neurological and psychological features as well as treatments, each is unique in some way. A common focus of the most current neurological research is the role of these health-compromising behaviors on the reward centers of the brain. The good news is that efforts to combat obesity and eating disorders are increasing, and the use of many substances is decreasing. Let's hope these trends continue.

KEY TERMS ▶ health-compromising behavior p. 143; problem-behavior theory p. 147; theory of triadic influence p. 147; levels of causation p. 148; Risk creep p. 148; social learning theory p. 148; brain disease model of addiction p. 149; comorbidity p. 149; dopaminergic system p. 151; substance use p. 151; psychoactive substance p. 152; substance use disorder (SUDs) p. 154; pharmacogenomics p. 160; people with alcohol use disorders p. 166;; alcohol use disorder p. 165; cirrhosis p. 166; Korsakoff's syndrome p. 166; fetal alcohol syndrome p. 167; alcohol myopia theory p. 167; marijuana p. 170; cannabis p. 170; THC (or tetrahydrocannabinol) p. 170.

CHAPTER 6

Understanding Stress

Learning Outcomes

After reading this chapter, you should be able to:

- **Define** *stress* and explain the person-environment interaction in the stress process.
- **Explain** why there is so much individual variability in how stress is experienced.
- **Outline** the biopsychosocial influences of stress and the ways that stress affects us physiologically, cognitively, and emotionally.
- **Compare** and contrast chronic stress, daily hassles, and life events.
- **Outline** the different theories that guide research on stress.
- **Identify** the ways stress affects health.

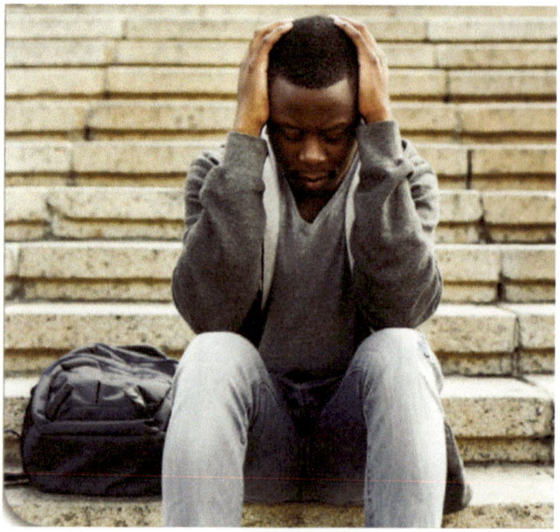

Photo 6.1   Prostock-studio/Shutterstock.com. Licensed material is being used for illustrative purposes only; any person depicted in the licensed material is a model

Halfway through the final exam, a student became noticeably distressed, got up, handed in his exam with only half of the questions answered, and left the room. Later that day, he came to my office. Jaylen was composed, but still clearly upset. He apologized for disrupting the exam, but that was the least of my worries (**Photo 6.1**).

Jaylen had come to the health psychology exam straight from the police station, where he had spent the night. The day before had started out well enough: He had gone to his girlfriend's house for a family dinner, and left the house around 11 P.M. As he was driving through the quiet streets of her gated community, he was stopped by the security guard on patrol. The guard, without even a greeting, pulled Jaylen from his car and demanded to know how and why he had entered the community. Trying to remain calm, Jaylen told the

DOI: 10.4324/9781032643090-6

guard that his girlfriend lived a few streets away and offered to call her family so that the guard could confirm his story. As Jaylen reached into his back pocket for his phone, the guard panicked and drew a handgun from his own jacket. With the gun aimed at his head, Jaylen raised his empty hands, his heart pounding in fear and anger. He had been coming to visit his girlfriend in this neighborhood for three months. He had encountered racism, prejudice, and discrimination all his life, and he had worked hard to rise above it. Nothing about this situation was right.

With the gun still drawn, the guard demanded to see Jaylen's license and vehicle registration. Cautiously, Jaylen extracted his wallet and license from his front pocket. He admitted that he was tight on money and had been unable to renew the registration on his car. Within minutes, the local police were called, Jaylen's car was towed, and he found himself being transported to the police station. Jaylen protested, suggesting that he was a victim of racial profiling—but the officers on duty did not appear particularly interested in his account. Jaylen spent hours at the station before anyone began trying to validate his claims. It was not until 5 A.M. that the police contacted his parents. Needless to say, Jaylen had not been able to study for the exam as well as he had hoped, and the stress of the experience had taken a toll on him.

And yet, despite the trauma of the night before, Jaylen had written exceptional responses to the exam questions that he had answered. He had worked hard during the course, and, upon completion of the exam, he earned a well-deserved A, as well as an A for the whole semester. The following month, I watched him graduate with honors.

A few weeks later, Jaylen e-mailed me, saying that he hoped to apply to graduate school in mental health counseling. He said that his experience with stress, combined with what he had learned in the health psychology course, had convinced him that he wanted to better understand the biopsychosocial processes involved in social marginalization and health disparities. Now, he wants to help others recognize how social determinants and stress might impact their own lives.

Jaylen experienced a staggering amount of stress in a short amount of time. All of us have experienced stress, and many life events and experiences are universally stressful, yet our individual circumstances significantly influence the stress we experience. Each of our experiences is unique. Although Jaylen felt fear in his encounter with the police, he endured, thriving after graduation. In fact, one could say that this experience changed him and gave his life a new purpose. Others are not so lucky—stress can have a negative impact in the short and long terms.

Stress can be a minor inconvenience, like forgetting the password to an important account, or a major life event, like the loss of a loved one or the birth of a child. We will also take a look at why experiences that affect humanity more globally like the COVID-19 pandemic affect people similarly and differently. How we experience stress, and how we cope with it, will determine its impact on our lives. In this chapter, we explore the different types of stressors, how they affect us, and what makes for successful adaptation to stress.

What Is Stress?

Stress is any negative emotional state accompanied by biochemical, physiological, cognitive, and behavioral changes aimed at removing, altering, or adjusting to its effects (Baum, 1990). As we will see in this chapter, stress is usually triggered by a situation or event in our environment. A situation or event that triggers stress is a **stressor**.

Stress is a biopsychosocial phenomenon. At its most basic level, stress is a physiological experience—that feeling of sweaty hands or a racing heart. Our physiological reaction is also influenced by psychological processes. We evaluate a stressor to decide whether it is a loss, a threat, or a welcome challenge, and much of our reaction is emotional. Finally, how we cope with stress depends on its social context. We often look for support from family, friends, therapists, school officials, or even political institutions. We will investigate all the components of stress in this chapter. (See **Figure 6.1** for a sneak peek at the different biopsychosocial components of stress.)

Acute and Chronic Stress

For Jaylen, stress came to a head on the day of his final exam. But even before spending that night in jail, he had lived for years with the strain of racial discrimination, financial challenges, and the pressure to get good grades and be successful in the future. Jaylen had been facing both dimensions of stress—*acute stress* and *chronic stress*.

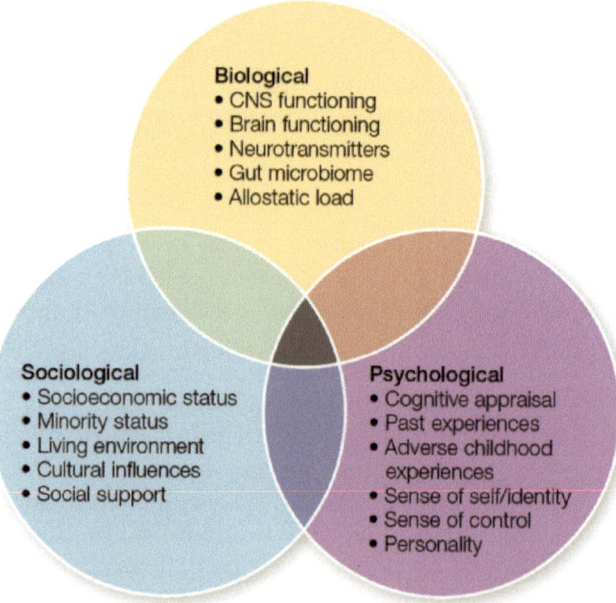

Figure 6.1   Biopsychosocial components of stress

The most common type of stress, **acute stress**, is rapid in onset and short in duration. For example, for those of us who fear roller coasters, riding the Twilight Zone Tower of Terror at Walt Disney World is a terrifying experience: the speeding ascent in pitch darkness, free fall, and a plunge more than 100 feet downward—only to be jerked back upward to open space, with the whole of the theme park visible below and everyone screaming throughout. For some people, this experience elicits nothing but sheer terror. The only way to "get through" the experience is knowing, on some rational level, that it will all be over in less than five minutes.

Acute stress is often sudden and unexpected. Consider the all-too-common experience of random acts of gun violence in the United States, which has recently been called an epidemic. Although acute stressors are abrupt and unexpected, we can expect, unfortunately, that their effects will last for a while.

Chronic stress, also known as *chronic strain*, is stress that lasts 12 months or more (McGonagle & Kessler, 1990). Think of a war zone, with bombs detonating randomly, constant fear and tension in everyone around you, and no sign of relief (Hoge et al., 2008). Or consider Detroit, Michigan in the United States—which, in 2024, was labeled the "most dangerous city in the U.S." because it had the most violent crime rate in the nation. There and in other cities in the United States, gun violence does not take the form of an acute, unexpected event—it is a constant. As one organizer of the Baltimore, Maryland Ceasefire movement said, "There's no such thing as post-traumatic stress in a lot of communities in America, because there's no 'post.' You don't get a chance to experience the aftermath before there's another trauma because of gun violence" (Weiland, 2018).

Yet, chronic stress can unfold silently, too. Think about what it's like to live with discrimination, economic hardship, an unhealthy relationship, an unsafe living or working environment, or a progressive medical disorder that has no cure. The unrelenting and uncontrollable nature of chronic stress makes it particularly damaging to health and well-being (Cohen, Glass, & Phillips, 1979; Juster, McEwen, & Lupien, 2010; Matthews, Gump, & Owens, 2001). In Jaylen's case, his experience with law enforcement the night before his exam was an acute stressor. The experience occurred in the context of a life-time of racial discrimination—a chronic stressor.

This is a major way of distinguishing stress: by how long it lasts. But not all stressors can be identified as acute or chronic; some are more complicated or ambiguous than that. Like gun violence, some stressors, especially those that accompany health problems, can have both acute episodes and ongoing chronic features (**Photo 6.2**).

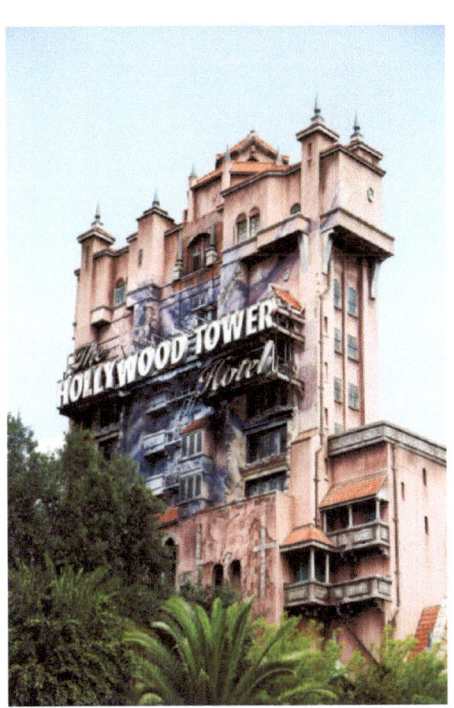

Photo 6.2   The tower of terror at Walt Disney World is an exciting thrill ride for some. For others, it is a source of acute stress

Source: Jeremy Pembrey/Alamy

Types of Stressors

Different types of stressors have different impacts. *Negative events* like a death in the family create greater psychological and physical distress than positive events, no matter how sudden and dramatic (Sarason, Johnson, & Siegle, 1978). *Ambiguous events* may also be stressful. When a situation is not clear or well defined, such as a puzzling medical symptom, energy must be spent trying to understand and respond to it. Compared with negative events, ambiguous stressors are harder to confront—and so may produce greater distress (Billings & Moos, 1984).

Around *the* World

Population Stressors

It doesn't happen often, but lately, there have been a number of events globally that have impacted large swaths of the world's population causing stress, burnout, and mental and physical health consequences. Population Stressors are stressors that can have lasting impacts on an entire population and leave many vulnerable to develop or experience worsening of their physical and emotional health problems (**Photo 6.3**).

Some examples of current population stressors are natural disasters, infectious disease outbreaks

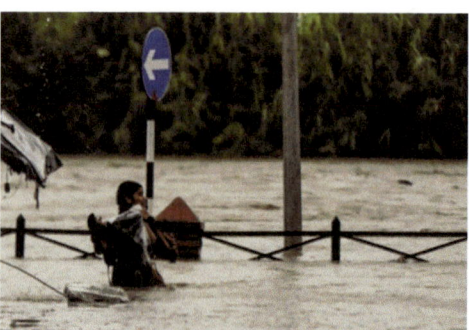
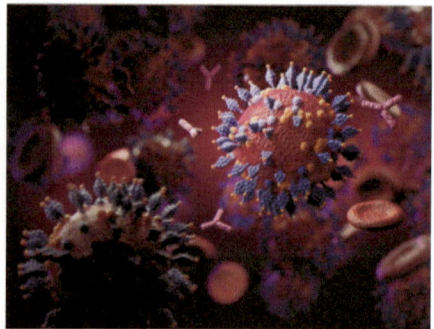
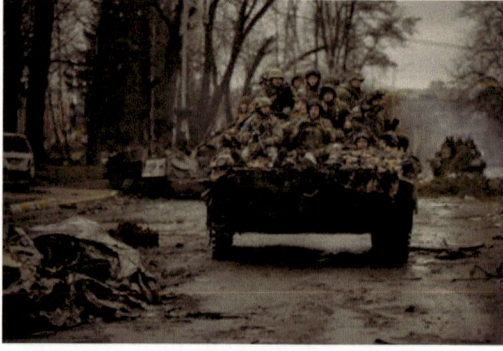

Photo 6.3   (a) Deadly floods in Nepal in September 2024; (b) Covid Virus; (c) War in Ukraine 2024

Source: (a) Reuters/Navesh Chitrakar; (b) Gov.UK; (c)Vadim Ghirda/AP

(like the COVID-19 pandemic), violence, conflict, and war. In the world, today population stressors include climate change, the ongoing wars in Ukraine and Gaza, gun violence in the United States. Population stressors are dangerous to people's health and wellbeing because they can create both acute and chronic stress and when people experience the highly salient stress in times of crisis it can deteriorate mental health and have both short and long term effects. Psychotraumatologists have shown that many population stressors can lead to clinically significant disorders years after the initial exposure (Weierstall-Pust et al., 2022). Research compared the effects of three recent population stressors, the COVID-19 pandemic, the war in Ukraine, and climate change. Findings showed that participants in the study were most concerned about the war, followed by climate change, and the ongoing incidence of COVID. The stress associated with the COVID-19 pandemic predicted current poor health, women and younger people were more affected by these population stressors than older people and men (Weierstall-Pust et al., 2022).

Growing psychological research shows that stress and poor mental health are consequences of climate change concerns. Some researchers suggest that as global warming progresses there will be an increase in the incidence and prevalence of mental and physical illnesses (Walinski et al., 2023). Vulnerable groups, including those with pre-existing mental health problems, children, adolescents, and older adults are especially at risk. And there is a very important role for health psychologists to play in researching and generating a greater understanding of how population stressors, including climate change, will impact health and well-being globally in the future.

Question:

What are some things that cause population stressors to be especially stressful for people?

Uncontrollable or *unpredictable events* are also generally perceived as more stressful (Thompson, 1981). Suppose, for example, that you are trying to concentrate on writing a paper for your philosophy class. If a fire alarm forces you to drop everything and evacuate, you will see events as outside your control, and they will feel more stressful. Conversely, even bursts of loud noise are less stressful if the listener can anticipate when the noise will come (Glass & Singer, 1972). Sometimes, the events we anticipate may be stressful because we get caught up in ruminating on what to expect (Wirtz et al., 2006). For example, imagine that you have a meeting with your boss next week to request a raise. The more you think about it, the more stress you may feel. Generally speaking, though, the more uncontrollable and unpredictable our stressors are, the more stressful they will feel.

Developmental Influences on Stress

From a developmental perspective, *life transitions* (such as graduating from high school, moving away from home, getting married, having children, or retiring) may also evoke stress (Moos & Schaefer, 1986). However, the stress will be diminished if that transition happens when we would normally expect it. *On-time* or *normative* events happen for most people in a culture at a similar point in a lifespan—such as the death of a parent when you're an adult. *Off-time* or *nonnormative* events do not—such as the death of a parent while you're still a child. Off-time events are often more stressful because they are unexpected and unpredictable; as a result, less social support may be available. Consider the untimely death of a spouse or partner in young adulthood. Think, too, of a woman who becomes pregnant while going through menopause. When events like these happen, a person may feel very alone. Those who have not had that experience at that point in time may not understand the extent of the stress.

In their development, some children may endure **adverse childhood experiences (ACEs)**, stressful or traumatic events such as physical, emotional, or sexual abuse, neglect, domestic violence, poverty, caregiver mental illness or substance abuse, or dysfunction in the home. Experiences of violence in the neighborhood, bullying at school, racism, and crime also contribute to childhood adversity. The more ACEs a child experiences, the greater the risk for negative mental and physical health outcomes due to the accumulation of toxic stress. Moreover, the stress of ACEs can lead to developmental disruption in the brain, causing impairments in memory and reasoning, attentional deficiencies, learning disabilities, emotional and self-regulation problems, and anxiety and depression. These early childhood experiences can also increase inflammation, compromise immune system functioning, and put children at risk for obesity, cardiovascular disease, and other health problems later in life (Hantsoo et al., 2019; Lapp, Ahmed, Moore, & Hunter, 2019; Nurius, Fleming, & Brindle, 2019; Rasmussen et al., 2019). Developmentally speaking, adverse childhood experiences create both acute toxic stress and a lifetime of health consequences.

Across the lifespan, events can be stressful if they affect something *central to our identity*, or our sense of self. Imagine a gymnast who is forced to retire because of a back injury, or an author who can no longer write after suffering a stroke. One way we can see the effects of stress through the lens of identity is in the context of acculturative stress. **Acculturative stress** is a unique set of stressors or cultural conflicts that people experience as they try to assimilate to a new culture (Berry, 1992). Recent world events and refugee crises have led to an upsurge in research on the impact of acculturative stress on refugees. A *refugee* is someone who flees his or her country of origin to escape violence, war, or persecution (United Nations High Commissioner for Refugees, 2016).

Typically, adaptation to a new culture poses challenges to one's identity and can create confusion, family conflict, and problems at work or school (d'Abreu, Castro-Olivo, & Ura, 2019). Acculturative stress in refugees, especially in children, has been linked to mental and physical health problems. Events are more stressful still when we are already *overloaded* with stress—for instance, refugees may escape wartime in their home countries, only to be confronted with the reality of a dangerous journey to a more peaceful destination. Taken together, understanding the various types of stressors and dimensions of stress can help us understand the factors that influence our appraisals of stress.

Thinking About Health

■ What is stress, and what are the different types of stress?

■ In your own life, what is a source of acute stress? What is a source of chronic stress?

■ What psychosocial factors influence the experience of stress?

The Biological Components of Stress

Stress is a biopsychosocial phenomenon. Let's look at each component in turn, starting with biology.

Stress is a physiological process. Most of our experiences come to us through our senses—through our eyes, ears, nose, and fingers. Sensory information travels directly to the brain, where it is immediately assessed for potential threat or harm. The brain determines the physical or behavioral response, which can happen without our awareness. The cognitive interpretation, or meaning of the sensation, is often processed after the response. The stress response may involve the whole body.

Imagine that you are driving to school. It is a sunny morning, your favorite music is playing, and you are feeling upbeat about the day. Then, in a split second, before you even realize what is happening, a truck swerves into the lane in front of you. As you hit the brakes, you begin to skid and fishtail, but you are able to pull the car safely to the side of the road. Your heart is beating so hard that it feels as if it will burst out of your chest. You may notice that you are breathing heavily, your hands are shaking, and there are beads of sweat on your forehead. Then your mind kicks in, and you realize how fortunate you are. Up ahead you see the accident that was caused by the truck's careless driving. Others were not so fortunate. You may grab your phone and call 911, you may get out and run to help, or you may be frozen in a state of shock. No matter what you're thinking, your body is likely to have responded before you had time to process the situation. This is how our bodies are designed to work in order to prepare us and protect us.

Central Nervous System Arousal

To understand the experience of stress, we must understand the parts of the nervous system. The **peripheral nervous system** is composed of sensory neurons and motor neurons. Sensory neurons receive information from our eyes, ears, mouth, nose, fingers, and skin, and motor neurons communicate this information to the muscles and glands. The **central nervous system**, which coordinates basic bodily functioning, is composed of the spinal cord and brain. This system transmits sensory information from the peripheral nervous system to the brain. It also transmits motor information from the brain out to the skeletal, muscular, and cardiac systems, and to the glands of the endocrine system. **Figure 6.2** illustrates this process.

The central nervous system regulates functioning through the **autonomic nervous system**, which monitors internal operations such as heartbeat and respiration, body temperature, and endocrine functioning. This system is largely involuntary and automatic, and it is controlled by the most primitive brain structures, the hypothalamus, and the medulla oblongata.

The autonomic nervous system has two subsystems involved in the stress response: the **sympathetic nervous system (SNS)** and the parasympathetic nervous system (PNS). The SNS is responsible for mobilizing the body in response to stress. Imagine that you are sitting quietly, deeply engaged in a book, when a friend sneaks up behind you and says, "Boo!" She startles you so much that you jump and let out a gasp, but then you both crack up laughing. Your reactions are the result of the SNS.

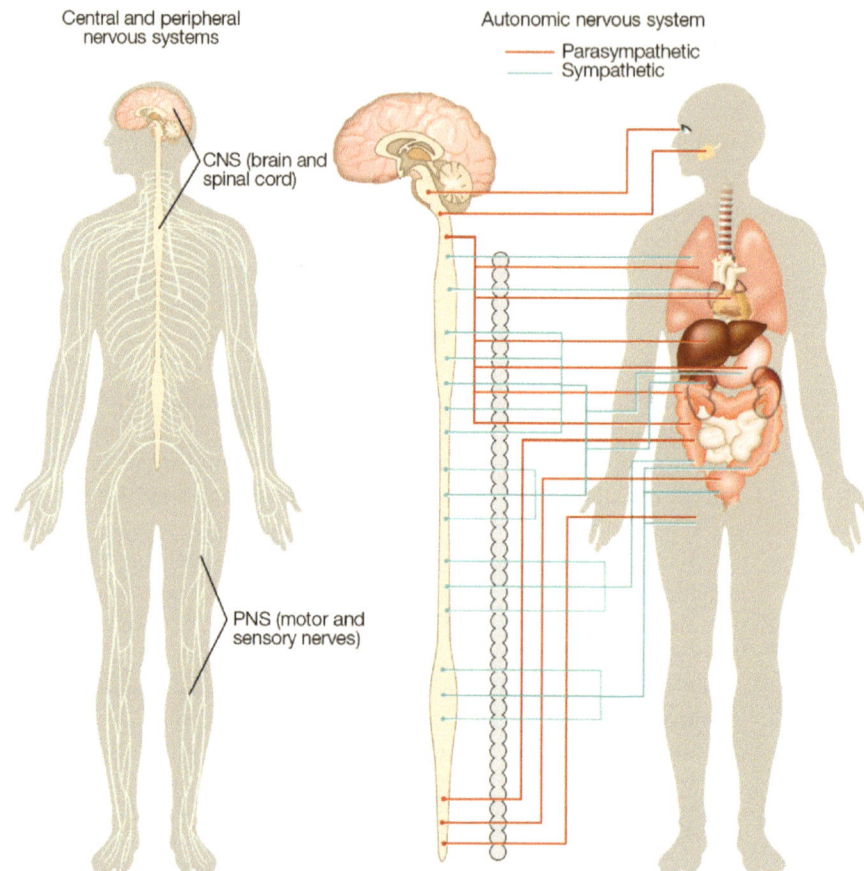

Figure 6.2   Peripheral and central nervous systems

When the neurochemical messages are carried by the SNS to the brain, they are processed in the **thalamus**, the relay station in the brain that interprets the message. If the message is pain, the thalamus relays the message further to the parietal lobe; an immediate appraisal of the threat might be relayed to the hypothalamus.

In our earlier example, while you are reading, your **PNS** is regulating your basic bodily functions and maintaining a steady state of equilibrium (or balance) called **homeostasis**. The moment your senses pick up a threat, the SNS sends neural impulses into the spinal cord and activates the preganglionic sympathetic neurons (neurons closer to the spinal cord) to release a neurotransmitter called *acetylcholine (ACh)*. Acetylcholine then stimulates further neurochemical activation and helps to transmit the nerve impulse up the spinal cord to the brain.

At the very same time, the SNS is activating postganglionic neurons to secrete catecholamines, hormones produced in the adrenal glands in response to stress, such as *noradrenaline (norepinephrine)*, which activates or excites some glands and muscles while inhibiting others. In this way, the SNS prepares the body to take action.

More specifically, noradrenaline stimulates the adrenal glands to produce *adrenaline (epinephrine)*, another stress hormone, which increases your heart rate, raises your blood pressure, and more: By dilating your pupils, it allows greater acuity in eyesight. By dilating the trachea and bronchi, it allows more oxygen into the bloodstream. Adrenaline also helps to convert glycogen in the liver to glucose, giving you more energy, and it shunts blood away from the skin and to the skeletal muscles, where it promotes movement. Meanwhile, norepinephrine acts to increase heart rate and blood pressure, slow digestion, and inhibit the bladder, so that that energy can be diverted to the body's response to stress. As amazing as it may seem, all of these processes occur in the few milliseconds after you hear "Boo!"

The organization of the SNS and PNS can be seen in **Figure 6.3**.

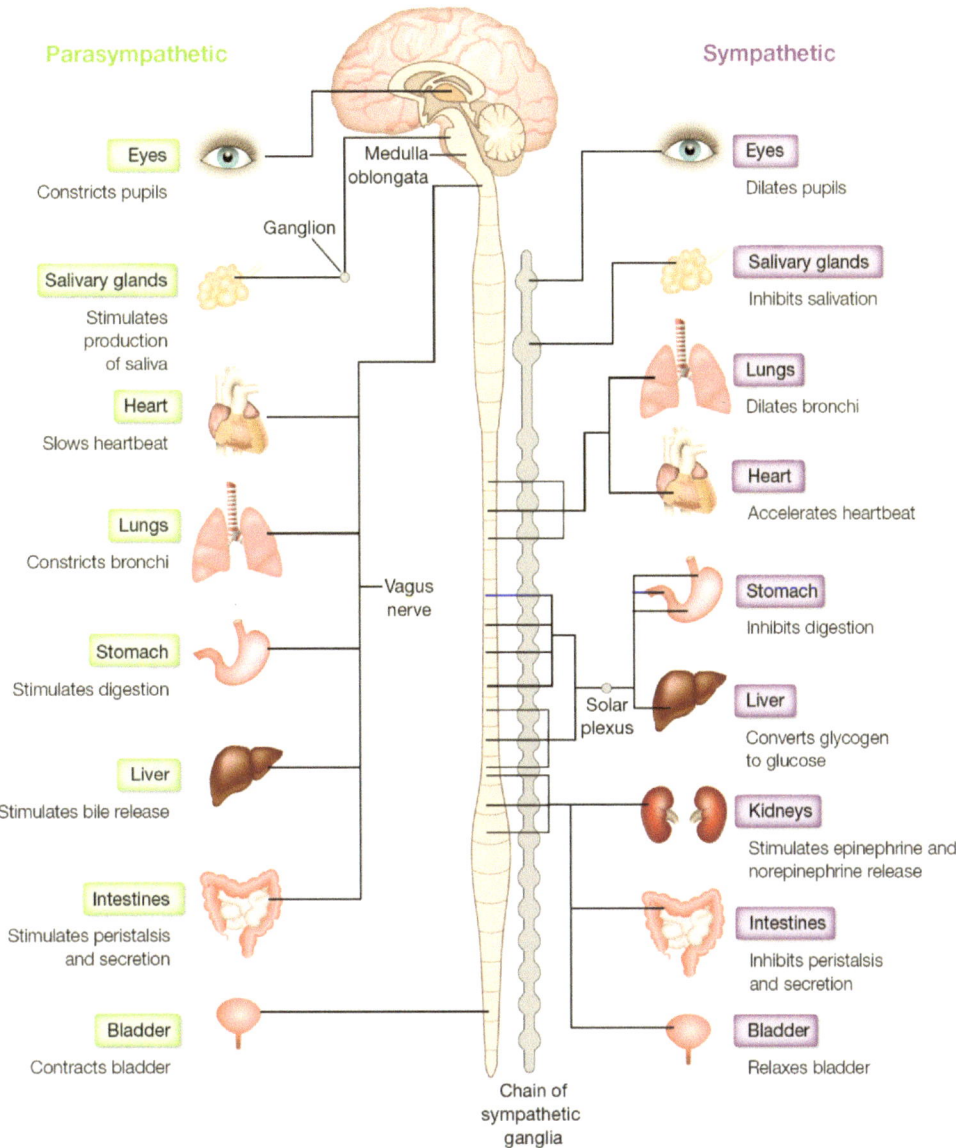

Figure 6.3   Parasympathetic and sympathetic nervous systems

Fight or Flight

The body's involuntary system of activation is evolutionarily advantageous because it allows the organism—whether that organism is you, a lion, or a koala—to protect itself against an external threat. This stress response, first observed by physiologist Walter Cannon in 1915, is found in many animals with a central nervous system (Cannon, 1932). Cannon called it the **fight-or-flight response** because it prepares the body to either attack the threat or run from it.

Once you have dealt with the threat, either by fighting it off or by running away to safety, the body starts to return to homeostasis. This process is guided by the PNS once the chemical message is activated from the brain. Neurotransmitters travel to all of the organs previously activated for fight-or-flight to reverse that state. Thus, the heart rate and breathing are slowed, pupils constrict, blood pressure slowly returns to normal, and digestion and intestinal functioning resume.

It should be mentioned that, since Cannon's groundbreaking research, other responses to stress have been uncovered. For example, some animals have a "freeze" response to threats from prey. The *fight-flight-freeze (F³) response* adds another dimension to the stress reaction—the fear response in which we are immobilized by our stress. The freeze response in animals and humans may provide time for the SNS to activate and energize the body to fight or flee. However, in some cases, the freeze response can be maladaptive, leading to heightened anxiety and helplessness (Roelofs, 2018).

Tend and Befriend

From an evolutionary perspective, males and females have adapted for different experiences, and these adaptations manifest in the stress response. Faced with the same threat, males and females may respond differently—males with the classic fight-or-flight, females with mutual defense and greater protection of offspring (Taylor & Master, 2011; Taylor et al., 2000). This **tend-and-befriend response**, first identified by Shelley Taylor and her colleagues, involves the release of *oxytocin*, a stress hormone that is also crucial in the female reproductive process (Taylor et al., 2006). In humans, oxytocin plays a key role in bonding between mother and newborn infant (Feldman, Weller, Zagoory-Sharon, & Levine, 2007; Jonas et al., 2008; Taylor, 2002), and it produces a sense of calm and relaxation during breastfeeding (Jonas et al., 2008). In both animals and humans, those with higher levels of oxytocin are found to be more relaxed (McCarthy, 1995), more nurturing, and more caring to others (Bales et al., 2007; Taylor et al., 2006). The tend-and-befriend response has been found in rat mothers separated from their pups (Meaney, 2001) and in sheep and deer when the herd is threatened (Kendrick, Lévy, & Keverne, 1992). Lactating monkeys showed less maternal behavior when their oxytocin production was chemically blocked (Keverne, Nevison, & Martel, 1997; Martell et al., 1995).

The tend-and-befriend theory is consistent with evolutionary explanations of behavior (Taylor et al., 2000). Females evolved to develop an additional behavioral stress response to protect, nurture, and comfort offspring and to ensure their survival. However, sociocultural influences have also contributed to and reinforced the gendered patterns of stress responses over time.

Although it has been thought that women are consistently more inclined than men to respond to stress by seeking out others (Luckow, Reifman, & McIntosh, 1998; Tamres, Janicki, & Helgeson, 2002), there is a good deal of evidence that, under stress, both men and women turn to others for protection and solace (Taylor, 2007). The tend-and-befriend response is additive to fight-or-flight, bringing social behavior more prominently into the stress process—because, of course, all humans are social beings (Taylor et al., 2000). In one double-blind study, men and women were randomly given either oxytocin or a placebo and then subjected to an experimental manipulation involving social rejection. Both men and women who had been given oxytocin demonstrated increased trust, more social support, and less distress after the social rejection (Cardoso, Ellenbogen, Serravalle, & Linnen, 2013).

Further evidence shows that the stress response is linked to higher levels of trust and trustworthiness in men (von Dawans, Fischbacher, Kirschbaum, Fehr, & Heinrichs, 2012), and that acute stress increases empathy and prosocial behaviors in both men and women (von Dawans, Ditzen, Trueg, Fischbacher, & Heinrichs, 2019). Here, again, we can see the stress response from a biopsychosocial perspective. We can also start to consider how prolonged, recurring, or chronic stress may be bad for our health.

General Adaptation Syndrome

Like Cannon, endocrinologist Hans Selye (1956, 1974, 1976, 1985) was intrigued by the stress response in animals. He observed that extreme heat or cold, insulin injections, and exercise-induced fatigue all produced stress. The animals he worked with all showed the same basic pattern of response or **general adaptation syndrome**. The fight-or-flight response, Selye argued, is only the first of three phases—the alarm phase, the resistance phase, and exhaustion.

The **alarm phase** is characterized by SNS arousal, which activates the adrenal glands (specifically, the medulla) to produce epinephrine and norepinephrine. The body's first response, the hormonal response, is the fight-or-flight response. This process is called *sympathetic-adrenomedullary activation* and can be seen in **Figure 6.4**.

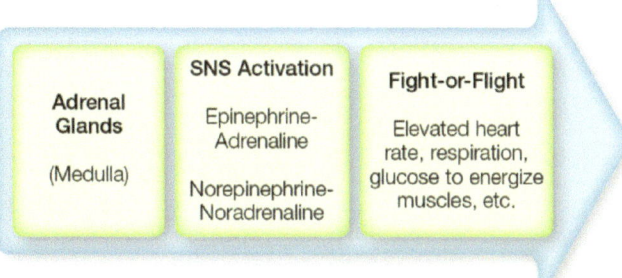

Figure 6.4   Alarm phase: sympathetic-adrenomedullary activation

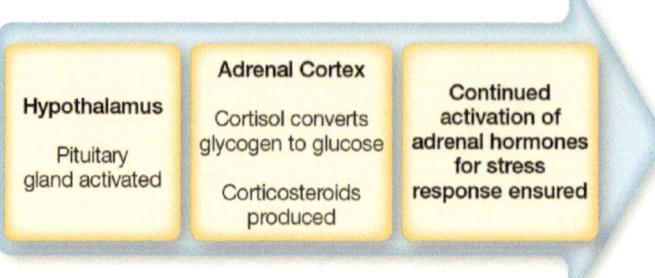

Figure 6.5   Resistance phase: hypothalamic–pituitary–adrenocortical axis

The longer the stressor is present, the more likely it is that the animal will move into the **resistance phase**, during which the organism tries to defend against or adapt to the stressor. As you can imagine, this stage requires a great deal of energy reserves. During resistance, SNS arousal begins to diminish, and the pattern of neurochemical communications changes. Here, the hypothalamus activates the pituitary gland, which then activates the adrenal cortex—known together as the *hypothalamic-pituitary-adrenocortical* axis (seen in **Figure 6.5**). The adrenal cortex produces the "stress hormone" called cortisol. *Cortisol* is responsible for converting stored glycogen into glucose for more energy. The adrenal cortex also triggers the release of glucocorticoids, hormones that regulate and mediate the stress response. The long-term production of cortisol has been linked to serious health problems, such as suppressed immunity, hypertension, and type 2 diabetes.

The final phase in the general adaptation syndrome is **exhaustion**. Over time, our reserves are worn down to such an extent that physiological damage begins. As an organism becomes depleted, exhaustion can lead to damage to internal organs. This exhaustion stage is characterized by the breakdown of physiological systems, leading to disease and sometimes death.

The accumulated wear and tear on the body is called **allostatic load** (Sterling & Eyer, 1988), and it can impair our ability to adapt to future stressors (see **Figure 6.6**). *Allostasis* refers to the body's process of maintaining homeostasis through change

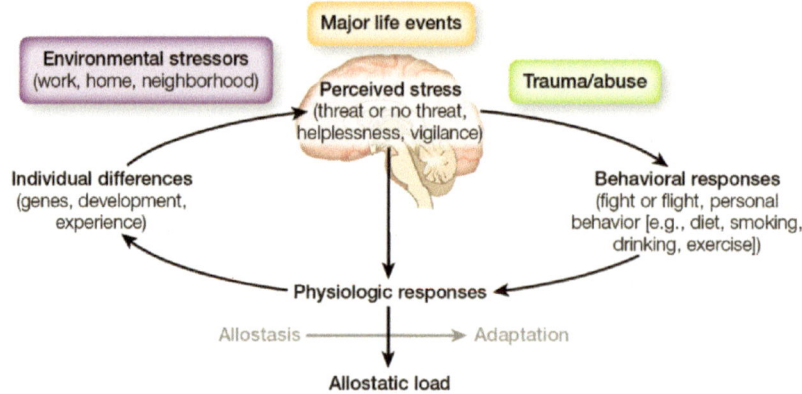

Figure 6.6   Allostasis and allostatic load

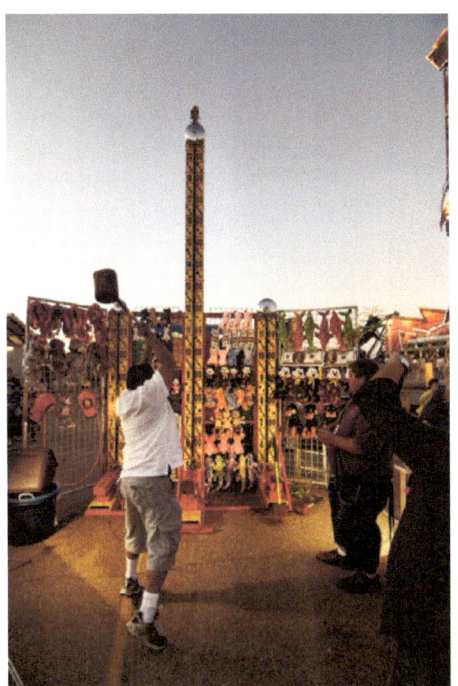

Photo 6.4   In the same way that physical strength varies from person to person, physiological reactions to stress are strong in some and weak in others

Source: Ryan McGinnis/Alamy

(Sterling & Eyer, 1988), and describes how the cardiovascular system adjusts in response to resting and active states. When we perceive a situation as stressful, our physiological and behavioral responses can lead to allostasis and adaptation. With time and the accumulation of excess exposure to neural, endocrine, and immune stress mediators, the allostatic load can build up and have adverse effects on our organs and our immune systems (McEwen, 1998; McEwen & Stellar, 1993).

Paradoxically, in short-term stress responses, the activation of the fight-or-flight response is adaptive—the immune response is critical for survival, and some studies even show that short-term stress can enhance immune system functioning. However, in the context of long-term or chronic stress, the resulting suppression of the immune system leads to adverse effects on health (**Photo 6.4**) (Dhabhar, 2009).

Individual Differences in Physiological Reactions to Stress

The physiological responses to stress are universal among humans—and similar in other species as well. Yet individuals may have a greater or lesser genetic predisposition to stress. Blood pressure, for example, is, in part, genetically based.

Physiological reactivity is the degree of change in the SNS and hormone production in response to stress. Think of High Striker, a game of strength often found at a carnival or county fair. There, you take a huge sledgehammer and swing it down with as much force as you can to see how high you can raise the lever. Some people have enough strength to reach and ring the bell at the very top; others, not so much. Individual degrees of arousal during stress are very similar.

Some people have very strong physiological reactivity, while the reaction of others may be quite minimal. Suppose your psychology instructor scans the classroom, making eye contact with each student, implying that he or she is about to pick someone to answer a tough question. Many students dread being called on in class. They may feel their heart rate quicken, "butterflies" in their stomach, and beads of perspiration on their foreheads. Nevertheless, there is always a student, hand high in the air, who enjoys being called on. This student's physiological reactivity to that particular stressor is lower than it is for other students.

Specifically, four factors contribute to an individual's response to stress (Uchino, Smith, Holt-Lunstead, Campo, & Reblin, 2007; Williams, Smith, Gunn, & Uchino, 2011; Williams, Suchy, & Rau, 2009):

1. The *amount of exposure*. Generally, there will be a greater reaction to a frequent, intense, and prolonged stressor. For example, someone who lives with chronic, unavoidable stress will have higher physiological reactivity.

2. The *magnitude of reactivity*, or amount of physiological arousal. When startled by a snake, one person may have only a mild reaction; another may have a full-blown panic attack.

3. The *rate of recovery*, or how quickly the PNS returns the body to homeostasis. The quicker one's body returns to normal, the less impact the stress will have.

4. The ability to *replenish resources* after stress. Someone who is thoroughly depleted by stress will feel the effects of stress longer.

Although all these factors depend on individual differences in nervous system functioning, one important way for everyone to replenish resources is through sleep (Smith & Baum, 2003). We have already seen the importance of sleep in Chapter 4. Just six days in a row of compromised sleep patterns can put one at risk for the common cold (Irwin, Mascovich, Gillin, & Willoughby, 1994). In a study of healthy older adults, sleep disturbances predicted mortality from all causes (Dew et al., 2003). Sleep also affects both the risk of experiencing stress and the ability to adapt to or manage stress. Chronic insomnia, or an ongoing inability to fall asleep and stay asleep, is often a result of ongoing stress (Shankar, Koh, Yuan, Lee, & Yu, 2008). Lack of sleep can be a stressor in itself as well (McEwen, 2006).

Frontiers of Research on the Biology of Stress

New research on the biology of stress reveals that both acute and chronic stress can impact brain structure and functioning—for better and for worse. When the body releases cortisol, it can trigger a reallocation of brain resources that impacts adaptation to the stressor. This shift can be beneficial and allow the person to adapt successfully to changing environmental conditions. In one study, participants were assigned stressful tasks (challenging mental arithmetic problems, immersing one's foot in freezing water for 3 minutes) that have been shown to induce both subjective and physiological stress responses. Brain function was measured before and after the stressful tasks using fMRI, and stress responses were assessed through the collection of cortisol levels from saliva samples. Findings showed that acute stress alters default brain processing, reallocating neural resources and allowing individual stress reactivity to promote adaptation (Zhang et al., 2019).

Research on the brain's role in stress may also reveal opportunities to offset stress. Another recent study showed that **transcranial magnetic stimulation (TMS)** of the prefrontal cortex reduced the negative emotions experienced during a stressful event (Smits, Schutter, van Honk, & Geuze, 2019). TMS is a diagnostic and therapeutic technique in which a noninvasive electric pulse is used to stimulate and change the magnetic field within brain regions (see **Figure 6.7**). TMS has been shown to be effective in treating a wide variety of neurological and mental health problems. Someday, we may all have our own personal TMS devices to offset stress.

Furthermore, as we learned in Chapters 2 and 4, the microbiome is critical for health. Emerging links between gut microbiota and stress show promise for understanding how stress-related disorders may develop and how best to treat them (Kelly et al., 2015). In particular, early evidence suggests that stress negatively impacts gut microbiota, which can influence and modulate brain development, function, and behavior through the immune, endocrine, neural,

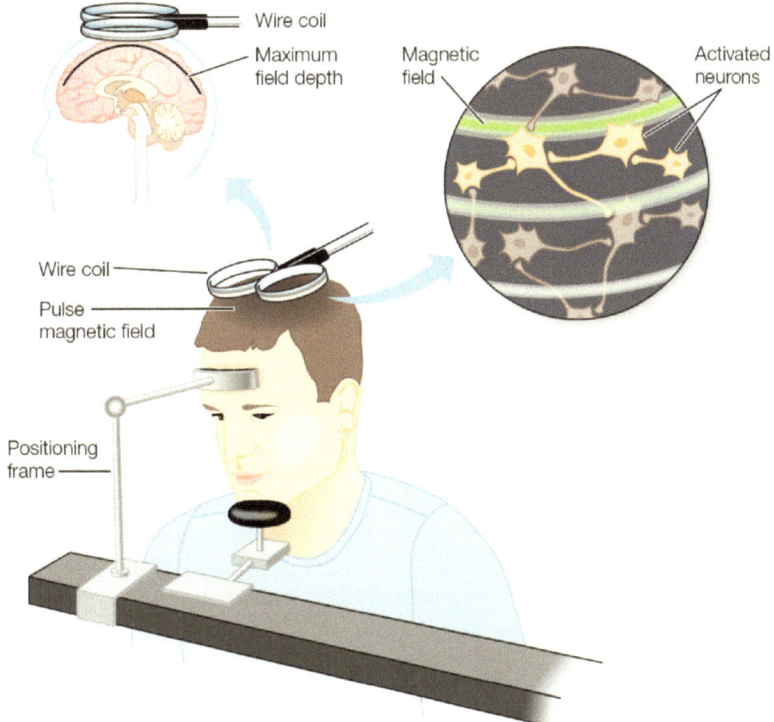

Figure 6.7   Transcranial magnetic stimulation

and metabolic systems, leading to disease (Kelly et al., 2015; Tetel, De Vries, Melcangi, Panzica, & O'Mahony, 2018). Research shows that there is a direct link between stress, gut health, and the development of stress-related disorders (Zhang et al., 2023). Evidence shows that stress leads to the release of cortico-tropin-releasing factor (CRF) which disrupts the gastrointestinal system leading to the disruption of the balance of gut microbiota which in turn increases the risk of gastrointestinal diseases (Zhang et al., 2023). Several stress-related disorders—from irritable bowel syndrome to colitis—are directly related to disruptions of gut microbiota. The impact of stress on the microbiota-gut-brain axis may have far greater impacts on the body as well. Overall, the biology of stress is a flourishing area of research that is subject to change and advancement.

Thinking About Health

- How has the fight-or-flight (or freeze) response influenced your behavior during a stressful event? How has the tendency to tend-and-befriend ever influenced your experience of stress?
- What is allostatic load, and how does it relate to the physiology of stress?
- What is physiological reactivity, and how would you characterize your own?
- What new areas of stress research intrigue you the most?

The Psychosocial Components of Stress

All of the phases of the body's response to stress are mediated by the psychosocial context. How an individual perceives or interprets a stressful encounter is crucial to how it is experienced.

The Person–Environment Fit

Like beauty, stress is often in the eye of the beholder. Some situations are stressful for almost everyone, such as the death of a loved one, a violent crime, a natural disaster, or living in a war zone. Other situations are only as stressful as they are interpreted to be. For some people, changing jobs or changing schools is stressful, while for others it is a welcome challenge. For some, moving to a new house is stressful, while for others, it is the chance for a new start. A divorce can be devastating—or a relief from years of anxiety, arguing, and abuse. Even the holidays can be a major source of stress due to social obligations to family and friends, the economic strain of travel and gift-giving, or simply expecting so much of ourselves. It is important to remember that even things we consider positive, like the birth of a baby or a new relationship, can cause stress. Think about the stress associated with being in college—the deadlines, social pressures, excitement, and lifestyle challenges. Is college stressful for you? Take the Undergraduate Stress Scale in **Table 6.1**.

Copy the "stress" rating number into the last column for any item that has happened to you in the last year, then add the numbers.

Event	Stress ratings	Your items
Being raped	100	
Finding out that you are HIV-positive	100	
Being accused of rape	98	
Death of a close friend	97	
Death of a close family member	96	
Contracting a sexually transmitted disease (other than AIDS)	94	
Concerns about being pregnant	91	
Finals week	90	
Concerns about your partner being pregnant	90	
Oversleeping for an exam	89	
Flunking a class	89	
Having a boyfriend or girlfriend cheat on you	85	
Ending a steady dating relationship	85	
Serious illness in a close friend or family member	85	
Financial difficulties	84	

Table 6.1   The college undergraduate stress scale   *(Continued)*

Event	Stress ratings	Your items
Writing a major term paper	83	
Being caught cheating on a test	83	
Drunk driving	82	
Sense of overload in school or work	85	
Two exams in one day	80	
Cheating on your boyfriend or girlfriend	77	
Getting married	76	
Negative consequences of drinking or drug use	75	
Depression or crisis in your best friend	73	
Difficulties with parents	73	
Talking in front of a class	72	
Lack of sleep	69	
Change in housing situation (hassles, moves)	69	
Competing or performing in public	69	
Getting in a physical fight	66	
Difficulties with a roommate	66	
Job changes (applying, new job, work hassles)	69	
Declaring a major or concerns about future plans	65	
A class you hate	62	
Drinking or use of drugs	61	
Confrontations with professors	60	
Starting a new semester	58	
Going on a first date	57	
Registration	55	
Maintaining a steady dating relationship	55	
Commuting to campus or work, or both	54	
Peer pressures	53	
Being away from home for the first time	53	
Getting sick	52	
Concerns about your appearance	52	
Getting straight As	51	
A difficult class that you love	48	
Making new friends; getting along with friends	47	
Fraternity or sorority rush	47	
Falling asleep in class	40	
Attending an athletic event (e.g., football game)	20	
Total		

Source: Data from Renner and Mackin (1998).

Note: Of the 12,000 U.S. college students who completed this scale, scores ranged from 182 to 2571, with a mean score of 1247. Women reported significantly higher scores than men, perhaps because most of the students used in pretesting the items were women. This being the case, items that are stressful for women may be overrepresented in the scale.

Table 6.1 The college undergraduate stress scale (*Continued*)

What explains these differences in stress? It comes down to how we interpret both the stressor and the changes within us: *The experience of stress is determined by how it is perceived.* We are constantly monitoring our environment and responding to things that happen around us. When we encounter something that threatens to exceed our capacity to manage it, we are likely to perceive it as stressful. Conversely, when our resources fit the demands of the stressor, we will have less stress. In sum, stress depends on the **person–environment fit**, or how the experience of stress is perceived (Lazarus & Folkman, 1984; Lazarus & Launier, 1978).

Think back to Jaylen, who overcame a highly stressful experience to fulfill a goal. His experience, though devastating and challenging, created an opportunity for growth, leading to his decision to attend a graduate program. Not everyone would have handled the stress he experienced that night the same way. Not many of us would have the fortitude to come to an exam after a night of hardship. Would you?

The Cognitive Appraisal of Stress

As we have seen, people differ in their physiological reactions to stress, but how do they differ psychologically? We assign meaning to our experiences, especially those that we perceive as stressful. We take in information from our environment, process it, interpret it, and decide how to respond to it. The process involves cognition and emotion.

The **transactional model of stress** describes this ongoing and reciprocal interaction between the person and the environment (Lazarus & Folkman, 1984). This interaction occurs within the person–environment fit, and explains the cognitive appraisal process that gives meaning to stress and the coping efforts to manage it. The model has guided over 35 years of research and helped to uncover many of the factors that influence one's experience of stress. In this model, no experience is stressful, in itself. Rather, we experience stress when we assign meaning to the stressor and judge for ourselves that it is likely to exceed our resources. A potentially stressful experience has three phases—primary appraisal, secondary appraisal, and reappraisal.

How we "frame" an event in our minds is the **primary appraisal** process. In the transactional model, it can take one of three forms:

- We see *harm* or *loss* if the stressor has damaged us in some way.
- We see a *threat* if we anticipate harm or losses.
- We see a *challenge* if the stressor offers the possibility for mastery, growth, or personal gain.

Suppose your girlfriend calls to tell you that you two should "just be friends." You may appraise this as harm or loss and feel depressed. Now suppose instead that she texts you to say, "We need to talk." If you suspect that she is going to dump you, you will feel a threat. The difference is subtle but important. In one case, something has already happened and cannot be undone. On the other, something may yet happen in the future. Finally, suppose that, after you get off the phone, you instead see time apart from her as an opportunity to catch up on your own interests. The event has become an opportunity for growth. Recent research shows that people who often perceive stress as a threat are more likely to experience problems that affect their mental and physical health and wellbeing whereas those who often perceive stress as a challenge do not (McLoughlin et al., 2023).

In **secondary appraisal**, the individual decides what can be done to deal with the stressor—to reduce, neutralize, or get rid of it. Part of the process involves assessing the costs and benefits of taking action. How might that coping strategy affect the outcome, including personal goals and constraints? Another part is assessing what resources can be used to counter the stressor. These resources can be internal or external, such as thoughts, actions, additional information, economic resources, social support, or religion.

There are vast individual differences in secondary appraisal. Imagine that you are sitting with your friends next to a window in a restaurant. Outside, it is snowy, and the side-walks are slippery. You watch as several people walk down the street, encounter a patch of ice, slip, and fall smack on their bottoms. How do different people react to this same situation? Some stand, laugh, and brush themselves off. Some walk away, looking angrily down at the ice that tripped them. And some look so embarrassed that they might cry. (Chapter 7 explores in greater detail the individual differences in how people cope with stress, including the health outcomes associated with stress management.)

The last phase in the transactional model is **reappraisal**, the ongoing evaluation of one's efforts and ability to cope. Less adaptive strategies for managing stress can lead to the intensification or prolonged experience of stress. If we see that our efforts are not ameliorating the stressor or reducing the distress, though, we may decide to try something different.

Individual Differences in Appraisal

Evidently, individuals differ in their cognitive and emotional perceptions of stress. The differences arise from many things, such as personality, age, and social context. For example, a work deadline or a visit from family is, in itself, a neutral event. However, once an individual *perceives* the event as negative and potentially damaging or threatening, the event will be more stressful. Those who experience daily hassles as stressful have a personality that makes them particularly vulnerable. Stuck in a traffic jam, one person may pound her fist on the steering wheel, while another person happily sings along to his music. It all comes down to individual interpretation.

The perception of events as stressful has a direct influence on our neurochemical responses. Physiologically, we respond differently based on our appraisals. When people perceive they do not have control over what happens to them, it can increase the production of catecholamines (Brosschot et al., 1998; Peters et al., 1999). Blood pressure is higher when the threat is high (Maier, Waldstein, & Synowski, 2003). Generally, it is easier to cope with situations that we perceive as challenges than with those we perceive as potential harms or threats, and these situations have more positive emotional and physiological effects (Maier et al., 2003; Skinner & Brewer, 2002).

A classic experiment illustrates the influence of the appraisal process (Speisman, Lazarus, Mordkoff, & Davidson, 1964). This study manipulated the information people had before an event to see whether that information shaped their perception of the event. The participants, college students, were randomly assigned to one of four groups. Each group was presented with different "framing" information and then shown a film depicting a painful tribal ritual in which adolescent boys were subjected to genital mutilation with a blunt instrument.

One group, the *trauma* group, heard a narrative describing the trauma of the event, the danger, and the boys' pain and fear. Another group, the *excitement* group, heard a narrative describing the willingness, excitement, and joy experienced by the boys and their families as they went through this esteemed rite of passage. The third group, the *scientific* group, heard a narrative describing the event from a detached, scientific perspective, observing the cultural artifacts portrayed. Finally, in the *control* group, participants were given no description of what they were about to view. Who do you think felt the most stress? If you guessed the trauma group, you are correct. This group had a significantly greater physiological reaction to watching the film and reported the film to be significantly more distressing than other groups (**Photo 6.5**).

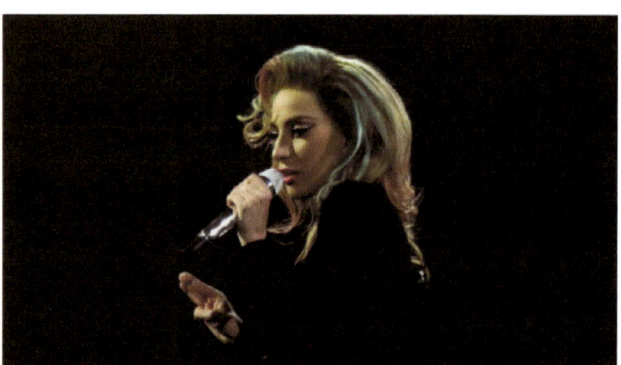

Photo 6.5   The unique social context of performing may alter how professional musicians, such as Lady Gaga, appraise and experience stress

Developmentally speaking, one's age creates a context that may influence the perception of stress. Age is not just a number but when stressed, a state of mind. Stress makes older people feel their age or even older than they actually are, but for young people a very stressful day can make them look and feel older (Lee and Neupert, 2024). Recent research shows that on days when younger adults (those between the ages of 18 and 30) felt high levels of stress, they reported feeling less in control of their lives than they usually did, and this related to looking and feeling older. This study also showed that young people are facing historically high levels of stress for their age (Lee et al., 2024). In later life, a sense of control is especially important for well-being and longevity (Aldwin, 1991; Frazier, 2000; Langer & Rodin, 1976). Yet many age-related changes, such as living with a chronic illness, present stressors that are outside of one's control (Frazier, 2000). In these situations, mental health outcomes like depression may result from the way in which the perception of control influences how people appraise and cope with stress (Aldwin, 1991; Frazier, Newman, & Jaccard, 2007). Here, the developmental context of age interacts with personality to influence appraisal, coping, and health outcomes.

Finally, the social context is an important influence on how individuals experience stress. Think of how performers may play through the stress of pain and injury in crucial moments. Musician Lady Gaga, who suffers from fibromyalgia (see Chapter 8), first began experiencing chronic pain while on tour in 2013. In spite of the fact that she endured a torn joint and "huge breakage" of her hip over the course of a nearly year-long tour, Gaga ensured that "nobody knew"—not her fans, nor her staff—until the pain reached a critical point. In an interview about the incident, Gaga admitted that she did not want to disappoint her fans, but "the surgeon told me that if I had done another show I might have needed a full hip replacement" (Iredale, 2013). How might Gaga's appraisal of this stressful situation have been different if her social context did not involve the pressure of performing?

The Stress Generation Hypothesis

Stress is a part of life, but some people feel more stress than others. Is it solely a matter of appraisal? The **stress generation hypothesis** suggests that people may in fact *create* negative life experiences because of their personality and behavior (Bodell et al., 2012; Safford, Alloy, Abramson, & Crossfield, 2007). Depressed people, for example, may seek reassurance so often that they invite negative feedback and deepen their depression (Davila, 2001; Giesler, Josephs, & Swann, 1996; Hammen, 2005; Joiner & Metalsky, 2001).

It becomes a vicious cycle. First, negative life events increase depression, and then depression increases the risk of negative life events (Ramana et al., 1995; Safford et al., 2007). Personality factors here can include hopelessness (Hammen, 1991; Joiner et al., 2005; Simons, Lorenz, Wu, & Conger, 1993), sociotropy (a strong need for acceptance from others), a strong need for autonomy (Daley et al., 1997; Nelson, Hammen, Daley, Burge, & Davila, 2001; Shih, 2006), and poor social skills (Segrin, 2001). How does your psychosocial context influence your experience of stress—and how do you, in turn, influence that psychosocial context?

Thinking About Health

■ How does the person–environment fit explain how we perceive and respond to stress?

■ Examine a stressful event in your life. According to the transactional model of stress, what were the three phases of your appraisal of this event?

■ How do individual differences influence perception and reaction to stress?

Social and Cultural Influences on Stress

Everyone faces stress. Indeed, there is evidence that basic human emotions are universal (Averill et al., 1994; Ekman & Davidson, 1994). We can all imagine the experiences of starving people in Somalia, unmoored tsunami survivors in Japan, war-torn families in the Middle East, or homeless families in Chicago. However, our time and place, and our political landscape, religion, age, and gender, all shape our personalities, our sense of self, and our experiences in the world.

Stress Around the World

Even today, many African and Pacific Island cultures have a rite called *scarification*, which marks the passage from childhood to adulthood. Depending on the tribe, it may involve cutting, branding, piercing, or removing flesh. For cultures in which scarification is the norm, adolescents who undergo it achieve honor and status. Children look forward to it, yet the painful process may still cause great stress and anxiety.

Geography and ethnicity, however, are hardly the whole story of the experience of stress. Cultural orientation also affects our reaction to stress, and certain types of orientation can extend across different ethnic groups. An *individualist orientation* refers to a belief in the independence of self from others (Hofstede, 1980; Triandis, 1995). This cultural orientation is characteristic of economically stable societies. In individualistic societies, the emphasis is on self and personal development. In contrast, a *collectivist orientation* emphasizes interdependence and shared goals. It sees individuals as part of larger groups, such as family and society. In a study of Arabs and Jews in Israel (Lavee & Ben-Ari, 2008), both ethnic groups contained individuals with individualistic and collectivist orientations. Individualistic people's life satisfaction is highly influenced by daily stressors, whereas collectivistic people's satisfaction within the family is influenced by daily stressors. Different societal orientations can influence the type of stress we feel and how we experience it.

However, there are cross-cultural similarities as well. In one study, college students from four different countries (the United States, Germany, India, and South Africa) rated the stressfulness of life events such as the death of a close family member or friend, serious illness, parental divorce, financial problems, problems with parents, and poor grades. Regardless of the country of origin, there was significant cross-cultural agreement about the stressfulness of these life events (McAndrew, Akande, Turner, & Sharma, 1998). The effects of stress on health are similar, no matter where you live.

Stress and Health Disparities in the United States

Both around the world and within the United States, the effects of stress can lead to health disparities. African Americans, when compared with white Americans, have higher morbidity and mortality rates at every age (Jackson, Knight, & Rafferty, 2010). Average life expectancy is lower for African Americans (70 years) than whites (77 years) and the average life expectancy of black men, in particular, is lower still (66 years). Death from cardiovascular disease is twice as likely for black women than white women (Jackson et al., 2010). Black women with lighter skin experience less stress and fewer negative health outcomes than women with darker skin (Uzogara, 2019). Why? One reason may be greater stress.

People from underrepresented, minority backgrounds experience discrimination, racism, racial profiling, stereotypes, and microaggressions on an ongoing and regular basis. **Microaggressions** are common, subtle, verbal, behavioral, or environmental indignities that can be direct or indirect, or intentional or unintentional; regardless, they communicate hostile, derogatory, and preju-diced beliefs toward a minority individual or group (Dickerson et al., 2019; Yeo, Mendenhall, Harwood, & Huntt, 2019). Like the racial profiling that Jaylen experienced, the experience of daily microaggressions can take a toll on mental and physical well-being. And in children from minority backgrounds, microag-gressive experiences can create ACEs.

Health disparities among gender minorities are also common. On a regu-lar basis, LGBTQ adolescents face outright discrimination and direct experi-ences of bullying, as well as subtle microaggressions, such as anti-gay slurs (Munro, Travers, & Woodford, 2019). Non-binary gendered people, and those who are transgender, also experience high levels of microaggression, harassment, discrimination, and stress (Pulice-Farrow, McNary, & Galupo, 2019). Overall, the LGBTQ community may be more vulnerable to the stress of victimization, discrimination, substance abuse, and suicide (Mereish, O'Cleirigh, & Bradford, 2014). The ongoing stress contributes to the health disparities that we see between sexual minorities and majority groups (la Roi, Meyer, & Frost, 2019).

Other examples of health disparities in the United States include living in densely crowded, crime-prone inner cities with little opportunity for advance-ment—doubtless, a chronic source of stress. Education is a key factor as well. People who do not have a high school diploma experience more stressors, including reduced earnings and lower socioeconomic status (Almeida, Neupert, Banks, & Serido, 2005; Lantz, House, Mero, & Williams, 2005). Unfortunately, in the United States today, there is still an appalling climate of silence and inac-tion in the face of the daily stressors—hatred, bigotry, injustice, and oppres-sion—faced by socially marginalized people (Sue et al., 2019).

Stress Across the Lifespan

Researchers began to study the effects of stress in children and younger adults only recently. Before the 1970s, childhood was assumed to be relatively stress-free. But as we have seen, ACEs cause toxic stress that can influence health for a lifetime.

Now, we also know that nearly 90% of college students experience high lev-els of stress, leading to poor academic performance, physical illness, anxiety, depression, high-risk behaviors such as substance use, and suicidal behaviors. However, those who have good social support networks fare better and enjoy better mental health (Wei, Heppner, & Mallinckrodt, 2003). So, the next time you begin to feel overwhelmed, try seeking out an empathetic friend. Often just talking about your concerns can give you a greater sense of control and help you master your stress. Also remember: You are not alone. Almost all college students are stressed. Finding a way to create balance in your college life is one of the most important challenges you will face.

Later in life, there is also stress. Older people may feel the effects of their own aging, and they may watch as their friends relocate to institutions, become debilitated, and die. Elderly people may also find themselves caregiving for chronically ill partners. The stress of caregiving has been found to negatively impact one's own health (Hooker, 1992). And when social factors such as ethnicity are thrown into the mix, the health consequences of stress can be even greater (Rote, Angel, Markides, & Hill, 2019).

> ## Thinking About Health
>
> ■ What are the social determinants of stress?
> ■ Why do health disparities in perceived stress exist?
> ■ What are the developmental influences on stress?
> ■ What accounts for the unique stress that college students experience?

Measuring Stress

How has research on stress changed over time? You might think that stress is greatest for those who experience the greatest number of stressful events. For years, many stress researchers thought the same way. The more objectively stressful an event appeared they assumed, the more likely it was to elicit stress. Today, we are more likely to look not only at the events alone but also at how people perceive them. Is there a way to measure stress, in order to understand the differences in perception? To answer, we need to look at how life events, daily hassles, and uplifts all change a person's life.

Stress and Life Events

Just as we can distinguish between acute and chronic stress, we can talk about two kinds of stressors—*life events* and *daily hassles*. **Life events** are events that significantly affect one's life. The event itself may be stressful, but the stress is magnified by how much one has to adjust to it. Take divorce: A divorce usually comes after a prolonged period of marital discord, very possibly putting chronic strain on both partners. It also may require negotiating child custody and separating belongings, finances, friends, and lifestyles. Compare this event with a vacation. It may involve dealing with all sorts of stressors, such as packing, arranging for pet care, and adjusting to a new place for a while. Although each of these events may be stressful, they differ in the amount of life change that they require. Early stress research focused on identifying the life events that were most stressful and how they affected peoples' lives.

For many years, the most well-known and widely used measure of stress was the **Social Readjustment Rating Scale (SRRS; see Table 6.2)**—a list of life events that may be stressful (Holmes & Rahe, 1967), from the death of a spouse (highest on the list) to minor traffic violations (lowest). The higher up on the list, the greater the change an event creates in one's life. Divorce is number two on the list, while a vacation is next to last. In this model, the more

Sampling of Top Life Event Stressors and Their Life Change Value

1. Spouse's death (100)

2. Divorce (73)

5. Death of someone in your family (63)

Lower-Ranked Life Event Stressors and Their Life Change Value

33. Change in school or college (20)

41. Vacation (13)

42. Christmas holiday (12)

Source: Information from Holmes and Rahe (1967).

Table 6.2   Life events and their change values

events on the list that a person experiences in a year, the more stress he or she is likely to experience.

The SRSS was not just an important assessment tool—it also helped develop what we mean when we say *stressor*. Still, the SRRS has serious limits, because it does not take into account individual or cultural differences. Take, for example, number 42 on the list: Christmas. For starters, not everyone celebrates the holiday. For some people, it is a festive time for family and friends. For other people, it is a very stressful time of crowded shopping malls and lonely meals at home.

There is actually very little agreement about what constitutes a stressful life event. Most researchers agree that the death of a child or spouse, sexual assault, and receiving a diagnosis of impending death are major stressful life events, but it is less clear what makes other life events stressful—there is plenty of individual variability (Cohen, Murphy, & Prather, 2019). Stressful life events vary by the extent to which they impact a person's sense of self, as well as by socialized gender roles, stages of life, and social and economic resources (Cohen et al., 2019). All of these factors can mediate the impact of stressful life events on health.

Americans and Malaysians have very different attitudes about breaking the law, romantic love and relationships, personal habits, financial security, religious activities, and work (Woon, Masuda, Wagner, & Holmes, 1971)—and every other culture has its own set of attitudes as well. The SRRS cannot measure these cultural influences on the appraisal of stress, either.

Stress and Daily Hassles

Early approaches to measuring stress had another weakness: Sometimes it is not major life events that pose the greatest health risks—we may suffer as much or more from the stress we experience each and every day (Bolger, DeLongis, Kessler, & Schilling, 1989; Brantley et al., 2005). The stress of daily hassles not only relates to poorer health (DeLongis, Coyne, Dakof, Folkman, & Lazarus, 1982) but also worsens symptoms that already exist (Peralta-Ramirez, Jiménez-Alonso, Godoy-García, & Pérez-García, 2004).

Daily hassles are the minor events in day-to-day life that trigger negative emotions. They include having a frustrating commute, waiting in line, receiving bills in the mail, interacting with an unpleasant sales clerk, or being criticized by your partner. In contrast, **uplifts** are the little things in life that trigger positive emotions: a phone call from a friend, a compliment, or Buy One, Get One Free Day at your favorite bakery. Evidence shows that uplifts can help offset daily hassles.

There is a complex interaction among life events and daily hassles. The cumulative effect of daily hassles may be more detrimental than life events. However, they can also exacerbate the stress of major life events (Serido, Almeida, & Wethington, 2004). Other research shows that when dealing with a major life event, daily hassles may actually be less stressful because you pay them less attention (McGonagle & Kessler, 1990). Again we see that individual experiences of stress have everything to do with the perception and interpretation of events.

The **Hassles and Uplifts Scale** measures the stress associated with daily hassles and uplifts (DeLongis, Folkman, & Lazarus, 1988; Kanner, Coyne, Schaeffer, & Lazarus, 1981). Common hassles include concerns about weight, too many things to do, and the health of a family member. Common uplifts include completing a task and relating well to a spouse or lover. More hassles and fewer uplifts not only lead to worse health and more stress-related symptoms (Bolger et al., 1989; Brantley et al., 2005); they can make existing illnesses worse as well (Peralta-Ramírez et al., 2004).

In discussing the transactional model of stress earlier, we came to understand the importance of peoples' perceptions in the experience of stress. One of the most widely used assessment tools today is the **Perceived Stress Scale** (Cohen, Kamarck, & Mermelstein, 1983). This scale taps into perceptions of stress in terms of feelings of lack of control, unpredictability, and overload. Higher levels of perceived stress related to negative health outcomes (Cohen et al., 1983). For example, the rapid sociocultural change among tribal peoples of the eastern Himalayas is leading to greater perceived stress and can account for the rising risk of cardiovascular disease, even after controlling for lifestyle (Sarkar & Mukhopadhyay, 2008). And perceived stress increases the negative effects of physical, sexual, and emotional abuse in women suffering from fibromyalgia (Smith et al., 2010). Perceptions of stress are important influences on health and well-being.

Earlier in the chapter, we learned about new developments in stress research. While self-report measures of stress are still being used, we have moved to examine biomarkers and genetic and psychoneuroimmunological factors in order to better understand how the experience of stress can lead to poor mental and physical health outcomes. Let's now look at some of those outcomes.

Thinking About Health

■ In which situations would different measures of stress be most useful?

■ Determine which stressors in your life are life events and which are daily hassles, and identify your most meaningful recent uplifts.

■ Assess your own stress using the College Undergraduate Stress Test.

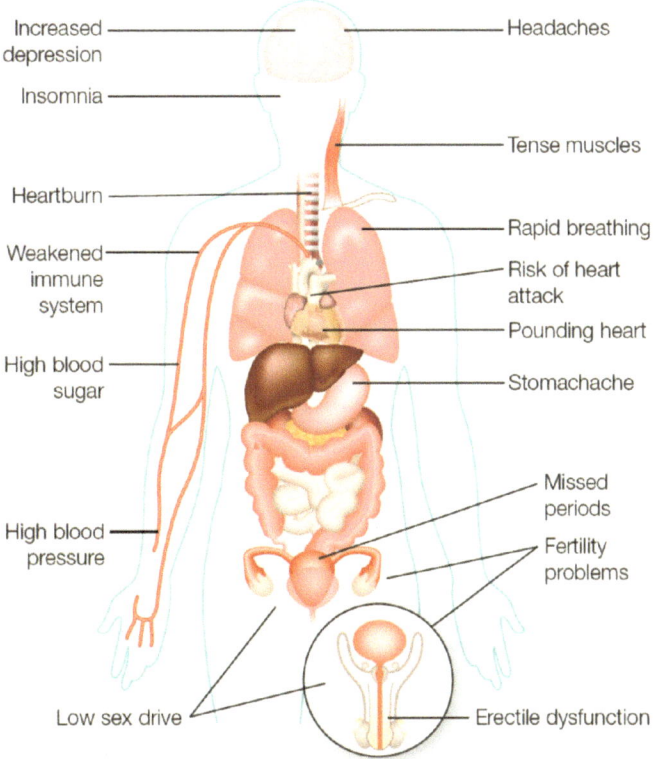

Figure 6.8   The impact of stress on physical health

Source: Information from the American Institute of Stress (2018)

Stress and Physical Health

Stress can make us sick. Under stress, we can become exhausted and depleted, making us vulnerable to acute illness, such as the common cold and flu. If stress is chronic, we become more vulnerable to heart disease and cancer as well. Stress relates to blood pressure, hypertension, body fat, and obesity. Not everyone becomes sick as a result of stress, but there is a common pattern that we will explore here. **Figure 6.8** shows the possible short- and long-term bodily reactions to stress.

The Wear and Tear of Stress

Stress acts first through the cumulative wear and tear on the body and its immune system, or allostatic load. Stress simply wears us out.

As the allostatic load increases, there can be decreases in immunity, a lessened ability to regulate cortisol production, less variability in heart rate, elevated epinephrine levels, and other long-term health consequences (McEwen & Stellar,

1993). The higher the allostatic load, the higher the likelihood of death in the following year (Karlamangla, Singer, & Seeman, 2006). Hassles and life events both correlate with negative health outcomes, hassles more so than life events; the effects of uplifts are not nearly as clear (DeLongis et al., 1982; Gortmaker, Eckenrode, & Gore, 1982; Holahan, Holahan, & Belk, 1984; Zarski, 1984).

There is ample evidence that stress makes us sick. In one study, researchers exposed adults to a strain of influenza virus (Cohen, Tyrrell, & Smith, 1991). Sure enough, those who were under greater stress were more likely to become ill, especially those experiencing chronic, severe stress (Cohen et al., 1991, 1998). People who were sleep-deprived prior to their exposure to the virus were more likely to get sick as well (Cohen, Doyle, Alper, Janicki-Deverts, & Turner, 2009).

Of course, just as people vary in how they respond to stress, they also vary in how stress affects their health. For example, an upbeat attitude may reduce the impact of stress on illness (Cohen et al., 2009).

Stress affects our health both directly and indirectly. The *direct effects* of stress can be seen in the changes that occur in our body that make us more vulnerable to disease. The *indirect effects* can be seen in the greater risk that results from health-compromising behaviors. Let's look at each effect in turn.

Direct Effects: Physiological Mechanisms As we will see in Chapter 9, *metabolic syndrome* refers to a group of risk factors (such as high blood pressure, high blood sugar, high cholesterol, and central obesity) that cluster together to elevate the risk of coronary artery disease, stroke, and type 2 diabetes (Kyrou & Tsigos, 2009). Stress directly affects metabolic syndrome.

Metabolic syndrome is rising in the United States, especially with the increasing rates of obesity. Metabolic syndrome is the link between stress and chronic heart disease, hypertension, diabetes, and stroke (Everson et al., 2001; Henderson & Baum, 2004; Johnston, Tuomisto, & Patching, 2008; Manuck, 1994). Chronic stress is a contributor to metabolic syndrome and chronic inflammation in the circulatory system and arteries, another factor in heart disease and diabetes (Tamashiro, Sakai, Shively, Karatsoreos, & Reagan, 2011).

Stress also leads to *immunodeficiency*, in which the immune system is unable to fight infection (Segerstrom, 2007). When your immune system is impaired or weakened, you are said to be *immunocompromised*. Developmentally, the young and the old are especially vulnerable (Johnston-Brooks, Lewis, Evans, & Whalen, 1998; Seeman, Singer, Rowe, Horwitz, & McEwen, 1997; Segerstrom & Miller, 2004). As children grow, their immune systems are developing antibodies to fight exposure to pathogens. In later life, with the accumulated wear and tear on the body and the development of age-related physical frailties, the immune system becomes vulnerable. Regardless of age, however, a high allostatic load can lead to illness and a greater risk of death (Karlamangla et al., 2006).

Our immune system protects us from invading pathogens. Stress reduces crucial enzymes that destroy invading pathogens and mutant cells, allowing damaged DNA to begin to replicate (Glaser et al., 1985; Kiecolt-Glaser & Glaser, 1986). Those who are stressed produce greater amounts of interleukin-6 and other neurochemicals that can weaken immunity, making them vulnerable to "diseases of adaptation" such as high blood pressure, ulcers, asthma, and a compromised immune system (Selye, 1946). The result is any number of health problems, from the common cold to cancer (Sarafino & Smith, 2011).

Indirect Effects: Stress and Behavior Stress also affects our behaviors. For example, a man with job-related stress may feel the need for a drink on the way home. Over time, drinking after work becomes a problem, affecting his work performance, his relationships, and his health (see Chapter 5). Stress can indirectly affect health through behavior.

People who are under a great deal of stress tend to engage in risky behaviors (Weidner, Kohlmann, Dotzauer, & Burns, 1996; Wiebe & McCallum, 1986). They consume more high-fat foods, get less exercise, and consume more alcohol (Baer, Garmezy, McLaughlin, Pokorny, & Wernick, 1987; Cartwright et al., 2003; Gupta & Jenkins, 1984; Herold & Conlon, 1981; Ng & Jeffery, 2003). Sleep impairments and distractions due to stress make people more vulnerable to accidents and injury (Johnson, 1986; Quick, Quick, Nelson, & Hurrell, 1997). Stress can also interfere with health-enhancing behaviors, such as a healthful diet and exercise (Sarkar & Mukhopadhyay, 2008). Under stress, exercise is often the first thing to do.

Stress is also related to smoking. Adolescents who try nicotine for the first time are more likely to have greater self-reported stress than those who refrain (Wills, 1985). For those who smoke, stress provokes the desire to smoke and increases nicotine consumption (Heslop et al., 2001; Metcalfe et al., 2003). Conversely, when smokers are prevented from smoking, their stress may actually increase (Gilbert & Spielberger, 1987). For smokers who have quit and weaned themselves from nicotine, a highly stressful situation can cause relapse (Carey, Kalra, Carey, Halperin, & Richard, 1993).

One possible explanation for links between health-compromising behaviors and stress comes from **tension-reducing theory**. Some risky behaviors, such as smoking, drinking, or drug use, may reduce stress. People report that they drink alcohol because it reduces tension (Cappell & Greeley, 1987). A stressful encounter at work or at home generates tension, and thus drinking may alleviate the discomfort (Heslop et al., 2001; Metcalfe et al., 2003; Violanti, Marshall, & Howe, 1983).

Stress can indirectly affect health through our behaviors, whether we actively engage in health-compromising behaviors or whether, when under stress, we are unable to practice health-enhancing behaviors. Each of these situations can lead to negative health outcomes.

Thinking About Health

■ What are the mechanisms through which stress affects our physical health?

■ How has stress directly and indirectly affected your physical health?

Stress and Mental Health

We have seen the toll of stress on our bodies. However, stress has a significant effect on mental health as well. It can lead to depression and other mental illnesses, but also to reactions that are at once emotional and physiological. Psychophysiological disorders are illnesses caused, to some extent, by psychological factors. As we see next, they include such debilitating disorders as *migraine headaches* and *posttraumatic stress disorders*. The *diathesis–stress model* is helpful in understanding stress-related disorders.

Psychophysiological Disorders

Psychophysiological disorders result from the interaction between psychosocial and physiological processes. Although inherently unpleasant, they are an excellent example of the biopsychosocial model of health.

Emotional distress and physiological reactions to stress have been implicated in a number of psychophysiological disorders. Some affect the digestive system, such as ulcers, irritable bowel syndrome, and inflammatory bowel diseases such as Crohn's disease and ulcerative colitis. *Ulcers* develop under high stress when too much stomach acid is produced and too little is reabsorbed. This is the effect of ongoing SNS arousal. The acids cause lesions in the lining of the stomach, which then become infected with bacteria. Ulcers are very painful and can be quite debilitating.

Asthma is a psychophysiological disorder of the respiratory system. In this condition, the bronchial tubes become inflamed and coated with mucus, leading to breathing difficulties, coughing, and wheezing. An asthma attack can be scary; one may feel unable to breathe. Stress can exacerbate asthma by sensitizing and heightening reactions to allergens in the environment. Asthma and asthma attacks are related to adversity during childhood, stressful family dynamics, and deficits in social support (Chen, Strunk, Bacharier, Chan, & Miller, 2010; Miller, Rohleder, & Cole, 2009; Scott et al., 2008).

Stress also contributes to *rheumatoid arthritis*, an autoimmune disorder involving stiff and inflamed joints and surrounding tissues (Parrish, Zautra, & Davis 2008). Stress can also aggravate *dysmenorrhea*, or painful menstruation accompanied by nausea, headache, and dizziness (Calhoun & Burnette, 1983; Ju, Jones, & Mishra, 2013). Hives, eczema, and psoriasis—skin disorders involving dry, flaking, cracked skin and rashes—can all be attributed in part to stress.

Another common stress-related disorder is the dull, unrelenting pain of *tension headache*. A tension headache involves disruptions in the central nervous system, which cause muscular contractions in the head and neck. This tension may be caused by stress.

Both tension headaches and migraines may be exacerbated by stress. A **migraine headache** is a debilitating, recurrent headache that results from a cascade of neurochemical changes. The process begins in the brain when the levels of a neurochemical called serotonin drop. This triggers the release of neuropeptides—chemicals that travel to the outer layer of the brain (the *meninges*)—and cause blood vessels there to dilate. The pressure and pain from these inflamed blood vessels on nearby nerves can last for hours.

Migraines may be *unilateral*, affecting only one side of the head, or *bilateral*, affecting both sides of the head, and are typically accompanied by dizziness, nausea, vomiting, or an increased sensitivity to light and sound. One-third of migraine sufferers experience an *aura* just before the pain. It may be flashing or shimmering light, numbness or tingling, a strange smell, or disrupted speech. More common in women (25%) than men (8%), migraines generally begin in young adulthood. Some patients have migraines up to once a month or more, followed by periods that are pain-free (Dalessio, 1994). Migraine is diagnosed after a complete physical and neurological examination, often including brain imaging. Although they are still not fully understood (Hildreth, Lynm, & Glass, 2009), migraines appear to have both genetic and environmental causes—one of which is stress (Hildreth et al., 2009).

The experience of having migraines can be stressful, too. A patient may live in dread of the next attack, never knowing when it will occur. Those who get migraines have higher distress and worse self-reported health, experience higher levels of depression, and consume more medications than people who do not have migraines (Jiménez-Sánchez et al., 2013). Mental health is also affected, as migraines are related to anxiety, panic attacks, depression, obsessive-compulsive disorder, obesity, and movement disorders, and maybe a risk factor for eating disorders (Brewerton & George, 1993; Pesa & Lage, 2004). Everyone gets headaches from time to time, but a migraine is not just another headache.

Decades of research show the many ways that stress and health affect one another. Almost any acute or chronic illness is exacerbated by stress. As we can see, there is an ongoing, reciprocal relationship between physical and mental health when it comes to stress.

The Diathesis-Stress Model

Stress, especially chronic stress, plays a direct role in mental health (McGonagle & Kessler, 1990). A major stressful life event precedes 80% of cases of major depression (Hammen, 2005). Stress in childhood relates to major depressive disorder, personality disorder, and other mental illnesses in adulthood (Weber et al., 2008).

The **diathesis-stress model** states that biological risk factors combine with stressful life events to cause illness. The greater the stress, the greater the likelihood of psychopathology. Although developed to explain the origins of *mental* illnesses, like schizophrenia (Bleuler, 1963; Rosenthal, 1970; Steptoe & Ayers, 2004), the model also suggests how *physical* health problems develop (Monroe & Simons, 1991). Specifically, in the context of a predisposition, vulnerability, or risk, stress can trigger a future episode or relapse of a mental or physical condition (Harkness, Bruce, & Lumley, 2006; Mazure, 1998; Monroe & Harkness, 2005). The diathesis-stress model is particularly helpful in understanding one of the most devastating outcomes of extreme or chronic stress: posttraumatic stress disorder (**Photo 6.6**).

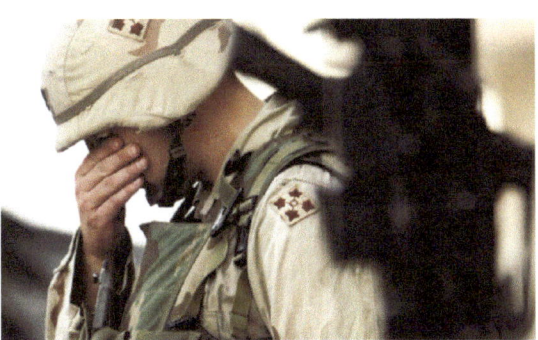

Photo 6.6 A traumatic event, such as The Stress of Combat, can cause PTSD

Source: Joe Raedle/Getty Images

Posttraumatic stress disorder (PTSD) is a psychological disorder that results from an extremely stressful event, an experience filled with fear, helplessness, or horror (Lamprecht & Sack, 2002). The symptoms linger for months or even years after the event. PTSD is commonly diagnosed in people who have survived war, terrorism, assault, rape, domestic violence, kidnapping, being held hostage, or natural disasters. Firefighters, urban police officers, and rescue workers all have a higher incidence of PTSD than people in less stressful occupations (McCarroll, Ursano, Fullerton, Liu, & Lundy, 2002; Mohr et al., 2003). PTSD is found in 7% to 8% of American adults and is experienced twice as often by women (10.4%) than by men (5%) at some point in their lives (National Center for PTSD, 2016). With more and more male combat veterans returning from war zones, the gender difference may be evening out. Living with racism and discrimination can lead to PTSD too. African American and Latinx adults who experience these aggressions develop PTSD at higher rates than white adults. The course of the PTSD may be worse as well (Sibrava et al., 2019).

The diagnostic criteria for PTSD have recently been revised (*DSM-5*; APA, 2013). PTSD used to be considered an anxiety disorder but now falls under the Trauma- and Stressor-Related Disorders category. This is an important change and one that may destigmatize the diagnosis and treatment of this disorder. PTSD is now diagnosed when an individual has a history of exposure to a traumatic event and experiences a specific cluster of symptoms, including intrusion, avoidant symptoms, negative alterations in mood, and increased arousal. In a **traumatic event**, a person is exposed to or threatened with death, serious injury, or sexual violence (directly, as a witness, or indirectly as a friend or loved one of a trauma sufferer). Professionals who are repeatedly indirectly exposed to trauma (first responders, emergency room personnel, clinicians) may also suffer.

Intrusion, or *re-experiencing symptoms*, is the feeling of re-experiencing the traumatic event as if it were still going on. These symptoms can include intrusive memories, nightmares, recurrent and distressing dreams, flashbacks, or mental and physical discomfort when reminded of the event. **Avoidant symptoms** are attempts to avoid anything associated with the past event, often a kind of numbness in response to trauma-related stimuli. Those with PTSD avoid people, places, things, thoughts, or emotions that could stir up memories. They may feel reduced interest in activities, a disconnection from those around them, a shortened sense of their future, and a limited range of emotions. They may indeed remember little or nothing of the event at all. **Negative alterations in mood and cognitions** are a set of symptoms that include problems with memory concerning the event; negative thoughts about oneself or the world; distorted self-blame or blaming others for the event; event-related, extreme emotions of horror, shame, or sadness that are difficult to shake; significantly reduced interest in pre-trauma activities; and a sense of isolation, detachment, and disconnect from others. Finally, the last cluster of symptoms is characterized by **increased arousal**, which is highlighted by being constantly "on edge," as well as by difficulty concentrating, an exaggerated suspicion of others, wariness or watchfulness, high irritability, outbursts of anger, difficulty falling and staying asleep, and a heightened startle reflex. PTSD can lead to other mental health disorders as well.

PTSD is a biopsychosocial disorder. It is likely that some people who develop PTSD have a genetic or biological predisposition related to the endocrine system, the immune system, and the release of neurochemicals like serotonin. This predisposition may heighten the reaction to a traumatic event and interfere with coping (Koenen, Stellman, Dohrenwend, Sommer, & Stellman, 2007). The sociocultural and political environment also provides a context for the development of the disorder (see the **In the News** feature).

In a meta-analysis including 2647 studies of PTSD, the majority focused on the trauma of war (Ozer, Best, Lipsey, & Weiss, 2003). However, the focus is now shifting to include racial and ethnic discrimination, environmental stressors, natural disasters, and terrorism. For many people, the world is growing scarier—and more stressful.

In the News

PTSD: From the War Zone to Facebook

With the wars ongoing in Ukraine, Gaza and elsewhere globally, the involvement of young men and women in the military is increasing, and the psychological impact of war is a growing problem. The incidence of PTSD is around 20% for those who witness or experience a trauma. The morbidity of PTSD is increasing because more people worldwide are caught in conflict and war. Globally, in 2019 nearly 230 million adults who survived a war experienced PTSD but the number is probably higher because of the increase in global conflicts since then and because many people do not seek treatment. Nearly 7% of U.S. veterans experience symptoms consistent with PTSD but this rate is much higher for female veterans (13%) than males (U.S. Department of Veterans Affairs, 2024), and many have turned to alcohol, other substances, or suicide.

But PTSD can be found in other contexts, as well. For example, in 2017, the *Wall Street Journal* identified "the worst job in technology" as those held by content managers in online settings such as Facebook and YouTube (Weber & Seetharaman, 2017). These managers, tasked with finding and removing inappropriate content on the web, spend their days weeding through thousands of videos of hate speech, sexual exploitation and rape, torture, and violent attacks, murders and suicides, and other gruesome content. In 2018, several content moderators at Facebook filed a lawsuit in California alleging their experiences of PTSD and psychological trauma resulting from exposure to this content, and that Facebook should have done more to protect them. This case was settled in 2020 when Facebook agreed to pay $52 million dollars in damages to moderators who developed PTSD on the job.

Unfortunately, PTSD in the workplace is not uncommon. Police officers, firefighters, EMTs, health care professionals (especially emergency room personnel), journalists, and those on the front lines of traumatic events may all experience PTSD. There has been a huge increase in PTSD in medical and healthcare personnel due to the global pandemic as well. Increasingly, we are seeing that not just Internet and social media content moderators, but also train drivers and traffic controllers, and even employees at banks, post offices, and stores, can experience PTSD related to work conditions (Skogstad et al., 2013). Many mental health problems, especially PTSD and depression, go unrecognized and untreated. In a world filled with trauma—whether on the battlefield or online—how can we ensure that all employees and all people receive the help that they need?

Question: How does the diathesis-stress model help us understand PTSD in the workplace?

Thinking About Health

■ What health problems have been identified as stress-related disorders?

■ How does stress affect your mental health and that of your family and friends?

■ What is PTSD, and how does this disorder influence the lives of those who have it?

Chapter Summary

As Benjamin Franklin said, nothing is certain but death and taxes—but he ought to have added stress. All of us will have stress throughout our lives. In this chapter, we saw that the experience of stress is shaped by how it is perceived, and there are great individual and cultural differences in that perception. Armed with several theories of the stress process, we explored its physiological impact, how stress is measured, and the physical and mental health outcomes of stress. A certain amount of stress is a part of life, but how one perceives and copes with it can make the difference between discovering an opportunity for growth and developing negative health outcomes. We will continue to examine stress and how we cope with it in Chapter 7.

KEY TERMS ▶   Stress p. 180, Stressor p. 180, Acute stress p. 181, Chronic stress (or *chronic strain*) p. 181, Adverse childhood experiences (ACEs) p. 184, Acculturative stress p. 184, Peripheral nervous system p. 185, Central nervous system p. 185, Autonomic nervous system p. 185, sympathetic nervous system (SNS) p. 185, parasympathetic nervous system (PNS) p. 185, Thalamus p. 186, Homeostasis p. 186, Fight-or-flight response p. 188, Tend-and-befriend response p. 188, General adaptation syndrome p. 189, Alarm phase p. 189, Resistance phase p. 190, Exhaustion p. 190, Allosta tic load p. 190, Physiological reactivity p. 191, Transcranial magnetic stimulation p. 192, Person–environment fit p. 196, Transactional model of stress p. 196, Primary appraisal p. 196, Secondary appraisal p. 197, Reappraisal p. 197, Stress generation hypothesis p. 199, Microaggressions p. 200, Life events p. 202, Social readjustment rating scale (SRRS) p. 202, Daily hassles p. 203, Uplifts p. 204, Hassles and Uplifts Scale p. 204, Perceived Stress Scale p. 204, Tension-reducing theory p. 207, Psychophysiological disorders p. 208, Migraine headache p. 208, Diathesis-stress model p. 209, Posttraumatic stress disorder (PTSD) p. 210, Traumatic event p. 210, Intrusion (or *re-experiencing symptoms*) p. 210, Avoidant symptoms p. 210, Negative alterations in mood and cognitions p. 210, Increased arousal p. 210

CHAPTER 7

Coping With Stress

Learning Outcomes

After reading this chapter, you should be able to:

- **Define** *coping* and the different styles of coping.
- **Compare** and contrast coping strategies that relieve stress with coping strategies that are often used, but that are not necessarily beneficial.
- **Describe** the biopsychosocial factors that influence how we cope with stress.
- **Explain** how coping is measured.
- **Describe** the various ways we can improve how we cope with stress.

Gwendolyn was 84 years old when she was transported to the hospital with respiratory symptoms. Her son had the same symptoms as did almost everyone in their family. They had all attended an inter-faith talk by a visiting Aman at the tri-faith religious campus near their home. Gwen remembers that there had been a few people coughing and sneezing nearby but she assumed it was the seasonal cold or flu. It was when both she and her son began to experience difficulty breathing that she became concerned. Her family insisted she got to the emergency room. Once there they asked a bunch of questions and gave her some breathing and blood tests and admitted her. She began to feel really stressed when she learned that no one was allowed to visit her and that all hospital staff were suited up in protective clothing and masks just to come in to check her vitals on the machines she was hooked up to. They had immediately put her on a ventilator to assist with the breathing and she had an IV for antibiotics, fluids, and nutrition. She had COVID-19. But it was March of 2020 and the United States was just figuring out what this new virus that was spreading like wildfire throughout the country was all about. Gwen was even more stressed when she found out that her son had been hospitalized and was in the room right next to her in an even worse condition than she was. Because of her age, medical personnel were quite concerned about her wellbeing. She ended up in the hospital for 2 months. Luckily her son was discharged after a few weeks. When Gwen was finally discharged she was very weak having been in bed for two months. She had to go to a rehabilitation facility for an additional 3 weeks to regain her strength to walk and eat on her own. She also had to get used to

DOI: 10.4324/9781032643090-7

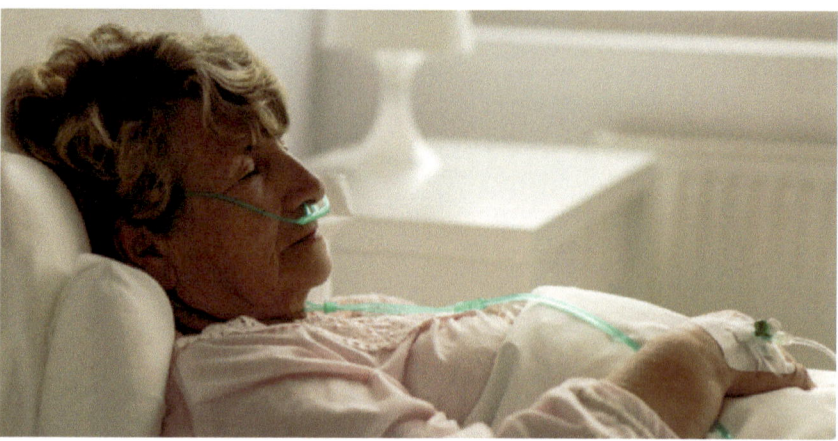

Photo 7.1

the fact that she was going to have to have supplemental oxygen for the rest of her life. This was overwhelming and distressing. Especially because as a child Gwen had had polio and had experienced depression during the time when she was very ill. She also had physical disabilities still as a result of her childhood illness. Her current health problems brought up a lot of stress from her childhood. Gwen was wondering how she would be able to maintain her home, walk her dog, enjoy her active social life playing mahjong and bridge, and taking learning in retirement classes with her friends. How was she going to get from place to place lugging this oxygen tank with her? For Gwen, this period was very stressful and depressing. She felt like her independence and her ability to live on her own were threatened (**Photo 7.1**).

Much to everyone's surprise, Gwen adjusted very well to her new limitations. Her cheerful demeanor, resourceful thinking, and social support made the transition home and to a life with a disability much easier for her. She found that her anxiety levels went down when she found an active way to tackle whatever problem she faced. For example, since the oxygen tank was heavy she had someone build a ramp for each of the doors of the house so she could roll it in and out when she walked the dog. She discovered that she could have groceries delivered and she decided that having someone come in and help her prep for meals for the week that she could then heat and serve would allow her to avoid the strenuous task of cooking. Sometimes Gwen would still be overcome with sadness for the loss of her old life, but so many people were dying of COVID-19. She had lost several friends and family to the virus. That put things in perspective for her and she would shift her thinking to the positive—she was still alive, she was seeing her grandchildren more because they came over often to help, and her friends loved her and suggested that they play mahjong, bridge and have book club at Gwen's house! She has now been living with disability and the long-term effects of COVID for four years. Sometimes she cannot believe that this happened but she often commented to her niece that she appreciated the silver lining of having long COVID and living with disability was the realization of the value of the relationships in her life. Gwen also often commented that she was "lucky" and that her heart went out to those less fortunate than she.

Gwen's story is a story of coping with chronic stress. As you read this chapter and learn about how people cope, keep Gwen's story in mind. What types of coping strategies did she use? How might you apply these strategies to your own life? How can you find meaning and opportunities for growth in the face of adversity?

We all experience stress differently, and we all differ in how we cope with it too. The resources you can draw on, from both within and around you, determine how much of an impact stress will have on your health and your life. Anticipating how you might cope with situations like Gwen's can help you identify those resources. What is the crux of the problem in Gwen's case? How did her experience change over time? What would you do if you were in her shoes?

In Chapter 6, we learned about how we perceive and experience stress—and the tremendous individual variability in our experiences. Now, we explore how people cope with stress and what strategies are beneficial to health. There is no correct way to cope with stress; the key is finding what works for you.

What Is Coping?

Stress is part of the human experience. As we saw in Chapter 6, everyone experiences stress at some point in life, and its effects are largely determined by how we perceive and appraise it. Yet the same process of assessing the situation and one's resources is essential to figuring out the best way to change, manage, adapt to, or eliminate the stressors. In other words, it is essential to coping.

Coping with stress is what we do to deal with it—our efforts to avoid or lessen threat, harm, or loss, or to reduce the experience of distress. Technically, coping represents what psychologists have called our "constantly changing cognitive and behavioral efforts to manage specific external and/or internal demands that are appraised as taxing or exceeding the resources of the person" (Lazarus & Folkman, 1984). Coping is a goal-directed process in which our emotions, thoughts, and behaviors are aimed at resolving the causes of stress and managing our emotional reactions to it (Compas, Connor-Smith, Saltzman, Thomsen, & Wadsworth, 2001; Lazarus, 1993). When we feel stressed, we strive to reduce the feeling, because, most of the time, stress does not feel pleasant.

The Many Dimensions of Coping

There are many forms of coping and many theories to explain it. Moreover, there are vast individual differences in which types of coping work, and which do not (Compas et al., 2017). Part of the puzzle of studying coping lies in figuring out why different approaches vary in their effectiveness. **Coping efficacy**, or the effectiveness of a coping strategy, varies across individuals, situations, and time. In this chapter, we look at how different factors influence coping, but we can already see something crucial: Coping has many dimensions.

There are many effective ways to cope, including using one's skills and competencies, available social support, and material or financial resources. Coping also includes efforts to adapt and re-establish a sense of equilibrium in the

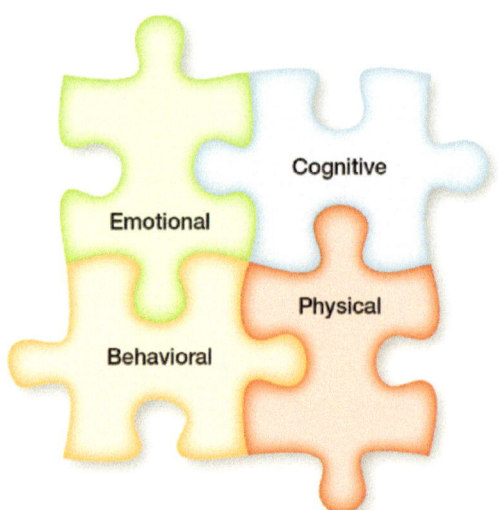

Photo 7.2   There are numerous ways to cope with stress, all varying in efficacy. These are just a few pieces of the puzzle

face of stress. Successful coping involves regulating one's attention, emotions, and behaviors. Often it involves willpower, delay of gratification, social and cognitive problem-solving, and help-seeking (**Photo 7.2**) (Zimmer-Gembeck & Skinner, 2011).

Successful coping may protect us and prevent long-term negative health outcomes. Unsuccessful coping may actually magnify rather than diminish the effects of stress. It can thus be either adaptive or maladaptive, leading to greater competence or greater dysfunction (Zimmer-Gembeck & Skinner, 2011). Examples of adaptive coping include confronting our problems, making realistic appraisals, recognizing and changing unhealthy emotional reactions, and working to offset adverse effects associated with a stressor. Examples of maladaptive coping include denial and alcohol and drug use. Once we know what coping approaches are available, we can teach others how to cope more effectively.

A Biopsychosocial Perspective

What determines whether someone copes well with stress? What determines whether poor coping will lead to negative health outcomes? In part, it has to do with our biological makeup. From a biopsychosocial perspective, our responses to stress are aimed at preserving equilibrium. At the cellular level, our immune system attempts to maintain homeostasis in the face of stress. At the hormonal level, the endocrine and limbic systems are involved in restoring balance.

As we saw in Chapter 6, genes, physiology, and neurochemistry all influence how we experience stress. Some people react more to stress than others, and some choose coping strategies that are less effective. For example, people who are highly reactive may respond to stress with anger (Herrald & Tomaka, 2002). Those who are highly avoidant may turn to self-medicating with drugs or alcohol. People who use escapism and avoidance as strategies to cope may turn to online videogames leading to problematic online gaming and Internet Gaming Disorder (Ko, 2014; Melodia et al., 2020).

Your gender may also determine the coping style you are most likely to use. Research has shown that men, on average, tend to use more active strategies: They focus on solving the problem at hand. Women, on average, tend to rely more on emotional regulation, such as venting, seeking social support, positive reappraisal, and self-blame. This tendency in women may relate to levels of the hormone *oxytocin* and gender role socialization (see Chapter 6). In one study, women who were prone to using emotion-oriented coping strategies were given a nasal spray of oxytocin. The spray reduced their anxiety and stress (Cardoso, Linnen, Joober, & Ellenbogen, 2012). Recent research shows that oxytocin not only offsets stress but also improves social cognition (Flanagan et al., 2019). In fact, oxytocin nasal spray was used in conjunction with psychoeducational coping skills training and found to be especially helpful for those who have

PTSD or substance use disorders (Back et al., 2023). Seeking social support or affiliation is a basic human coping response. The tendency may originate in our neurochemistry, but we become socialized through early life experiences (Taylor, Way, & Seeman, 2011).

In addition to the biological roots of coping, psychological influences also appear. Coping can be seen as a personality trait when the same strategy is used across different situations. Suppose, for example, that your friend laughs and makes silly jokes whether she burns her finger, argues with her boss, or learns that she has skin cancer. You could conclude that she copes with stress with humor and that this is part of who she is. Other coping styles include confrontation, behavioral disengagement and denial, and self-blame.

Recall from Chapter 4 the five major personality traits—neuroticism, extraversion, openness to experience, agreeableness, and conscientiousness. People who are high in neuroticism tend to experience negative emotions, and they also use more emotion-focused coping and avoidance (Barańczuk, 2019). In contrast, people high in extraversion, conscientiousness, and openness use more active coping and problem-focused coping, while people high in agreeableness use more active coping and humor (Roesch, Wee, & Vaughn, 2006). Whether coping is a personality trait or just intimately intertwined with personality, there are consistent and predictable links between personality and coping.

Coping Across the Lifespan

Developmentally, coping strategies evolve across the lifespan. Coping strategies are learned early in life, through an individual's relationship with parents or caregivers and the environment. Especially in childhood and adolescence, stress presents a significant and widespread risk factor for psychopathology, so learning how to manage it effectively is important (Compas et al., 2001; Grant et al., 2000). For children, a positive parenting style (such as support and acceptance) coupled with a sense of control leads to active and effective coping. Conversely, a negative parenting style (such as neglect and rejection) leads to more dysfunctional coping over time (Vélez et al., 2014). The way children cope with stress can influence future mental and physical health (Compas et al., 2017).

A critical part of learning to cope well with stress is learning to regulate and manage one's emotions, a developmental process that unfolds throughout childhood. Parents play an important role in shaping how children master emotional regulation, whether in responding to their children's efforts to do so or in modeling how to manage emotions (Power, 2004). In the aftermath of the Southeast Asian tsunami in December 2004, for example, many children relied on their parents for guidance and protection. Some kids wanted to talk about it, some sought information and comfort, and some showed increased attachment behaviors. Although all children relied on their parents for protection and guidance, and most expressed comfort in being with their parents, needs and coping strategies varied according to age. Older kids were engaged in more self-soothing behaviors, while younger kids sought more soothing from their parents (Jensen et al., 2014). In many contexts, whether it is the aftermath of trauma, transition to primary school, conflict with peers, dysfunction in the family, or illness, emotional regulation is critical for successful coping.

Just as children grow cognitively and socially, their coping skills develop and change as well. In a study of 7- to 12-year-old children who experienced bullying and social rejection, those who became angry most often showed aggressive coping. Those who experienced sadness tended to use ruminating coping styles and dwell on their hurts. In contrast, young adults tended to withdraw socially, avoiding situations in which they might be exposed to rejection (Watson & Nesdale, 2012).

Worldwide, children were especially negatively impacted by the COVID-19 pandemic. For young children school closures, restrictions in activities, and social distancing were especially disruptive and negatively impacted their well-being. In a study of Spanish children aged 3–12, there were age differences in the types of strategies kids used to cope with pandemic-related stressors (Domínguez-Álvarez et al., 2020). This research shows that for younger children parents' views, whether they were fearful for the future or conveyed resilience, were important for whether or not they coped in an active and engaged way or whether they were disengaged. Higher contextual vulnerability was problematic for younger as opposed to older children.

The transition to adulthood, too, is marked by many challenging changes: individuating from parents and family, becoming more independent, and experiencing new social settings, including living on one's own. As we age from young adulthood into midlife, problem-focused and meaning-focused coping increase, as does seeking social support. In adults older than 65 years, age-related social rejection (social exclusion due to age-related life circumstances, such as retirement or limitations in physical functioning) is magnified, often leading to poorer cognitive coping abilities, compromised social functioning, higher levels of loneliness, and lower life satisfaction (Cheng & Grühn, 2014; Chow, Au, & Chin, 2008). We can see, then, that throughout the lifespan, both social support and finding meaning in stressful encounters are linked with less stress and better adaptation (Leipold, Munz, & Michéle-Malkowsky, 2019).

Still, by adulthood, we generally have our own unique approach to managing stress. That approach likely encompasses many different strategies—which may or may not be effective, depending on the situation. Think back to Gwen at the beginning of this chapter. How does she deal with her recollections of her childhood illness and disability? What advice would you give on adaptive coping strategies for managing her current disability?

The social context, including the presence of other people and social norms, also dictates how we cope. For example, suppose that you are involved in a car accident. If the other drivers involved are calm, rational, and problem-focused, it is likely that you will remain calm as well. However, if the other drivers are yelling and pointing fingers, you may also become hostile and defensive. The social influences on coping can also be seen in athletes. An adult man is not expected to throw a temper tantrum in line at the grocery store or in the conference room. Watch a baseball game, however, and you will see adult men throwing gear on the ground, shouting at referees, and stomping off the diamond after a bad call. Context dictates how we cope, too (**Photo 7.3**).

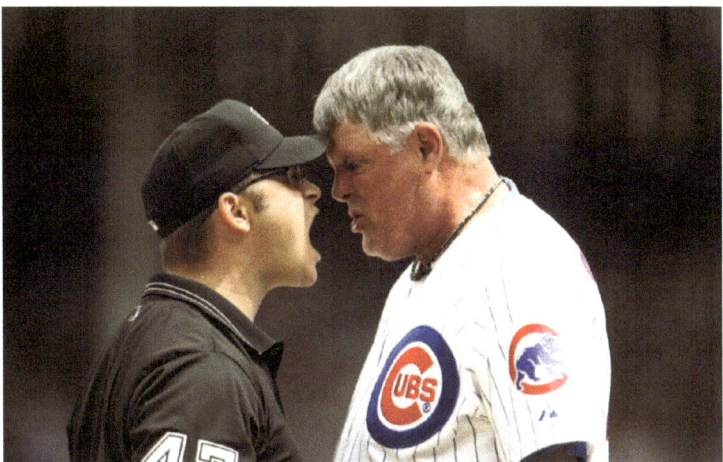

Photo 7.3   The social context often dictates our coping strategies. This coach and official feel comfortable yelling at each other on the baseball field; would they feel the same way in another setting, such as a quiet restaurant?

Source: Ron Vesely/Getty Images

It is important to remember that biology, psychology, and social tendencies do not act alone. Rather, they interact to determine how we respond to stress. To understand this interaction, we look next at different types of coping.

Thinking About Health

■ What constitutes effective coping, and how does coping change across the lifespan?

■ Consider an event that caused you stress as a child. How did you cope with the event then? How would you cope with it now?

Types of Coping

Some coping efforts are *voluntary*—we choose how to respond (Compas et al., 2001). For example, you may take a deep breath before having blood drawn at the doctor's office. Other coping efforts are *involuntary*. These automatic or non-conscious responses happen without thought (Skinner & Zimmer-Gembeck, 2007). For example, you may immediately tense up when you receive a text from someone that says, "I have bad news."

It is often quite difficult to tease apart voluntary and involuntary responses, because so many of our reactions occur without obvious thought. We may initially choose to respond in a certain way, but, over time, our response may become automatic (Carver & Connor-Smith, 2010).

However, what exactly are we choosing? One model of coping compares strategies by what they aim to regulate—the *problem* of the stressor itself or the *emotions* it elicits. Another model looks instead at whether we try to address, or *engage*, the feelings of stress or to *avoid* them. And yet another model questions personal views, as some people attempt to find *meaning* in a deeply stressful event. Finally, *proactive coping* encompasses trying to plan for events before they occur.

Recall Gwen's struggles. As you read the next section, ask yourself what coping strategies she has used. She—and every person—will continue to encounter stress over the course of a lifetime. Which coping strategies would help her the most?

Problem-Focused and Emotion-Focused Coping

When we addressed the differences between men and women, we introduced two styles of coping: problem-focused coping and emotion-focused coping (Lazarus & Folkman, 1984). **Problem-focused coping** aims at reducing, removing, or redirecting a stressor. In problem-focused coping, the person focuses on the problem and attempts to grapple with it. For example, if the company you work for encounters financial troubles, you may start working harder, so that you are less likely to be let go. Or you may seek additional training to make you more marketable while you look for a new job. **Emotion-focused coping**, however, is aimed at regulating and managing the feelings triggered by stress. Emotion-focused coping may include expressing feelings (crying, yelling, or venting), self-soothing (relaxing or seeking social support), self-blame and recrimination, dwelling on the distress (rumination), trying to emotionally distance oneself (avoidance, denial, or wishful thinking), or trying to put things in a less stressful perspective ("seeking a silver lining"). If your position is eliminated, you may complain to your friends that your boss had no clue how hard you worked. Alternatively, you may try to put off thinking about the situation by going out drinking. Or you may think that the loss is for the best, because now you can pursue your dream of being an entrepreneur.

Choosing the Best Fit: In the early years of coping research, it was thought that problem-focused coping was better at relieving distress than emotion-focused coping. As we have seen, men tend, on average, to be more action- or problem-focused, whereas women are more focused on emotional regulation. The problem with this line of thinking is that it leads to the conclusion that women cope less well than men. This finding has not been supported. Now, we understand that each person, regardless of gender, may use problem- or emotion-focused coping, and often both strategies are used simultaneously. In fact, they complement each other. If you approach a stressful situation with a plan of action, it may reduce your anxiety. In turn, effective emotion-focused coping diminishes emotional distress, leading to better problem-focused coping (Carver & Connor-Smith, 2010).

Could problem- or emotion-focused coping work better in some situations than others? According to the **matching hypothesis** (also known as the *goodness of fit* model), it helps to tailor the coping strategies to the type of stressor (Christensen, Benotsch, Wiebe, & Lawton, 1995; Frazier, 2000; Lazarus, 1993; Park, Armeli, & Tennen, 2004). In this model, problem-focused strategies work best when you can actually change something about the situation, while emotion-focused strategies work best when you can only deal with distress. It is a matter of what you can control.

Think about living with a debilitating chronic illness. Parkinson's disease, as you may recall from Chapter 2, is a chronic, progressive neurological disorder that leads to increased physical dysfunction and immobility. Symptoms range from muscular tremors, rigidity, and difficulty handling personal care to mental confusion, sleep disturbances, and sexual dysfunction. In this context, problem-focused strategies (like seeing a doctor for more effective medications, or undergoing physical therapy to help with walking) might work best for the stress associated with physical symptoms (Frazier, 2000). Emotion-focused strategies (such as accepting the reality of the disease and sharing fears with others) may address the emotional discomfort. Evidence shows that patients have more positive outcomes when they tailor the coping strategy to the type of stress—physical, cognitive, or emotional. When it comes to problem-versus emotion-focused coping, it helps to be flexible, and to be aware of what can and cannot be controlled. Knowing this, how would you suggest that Gwen cope with her disability?

The matching hypothesis essentially suggests that there is a fit between the situation and our coping strategies. The better the fit, the better we cope. It is adaptive to fit our coping strategies to the controllability of the situation and stressors. Within the context of the worldwide COVID-19 pandemic, ongoing racial trauma, climate change anxiety, wars, and divisive politics around the world, U.S. college students have had a lot of stress to grapple with on top of the regular stress of college (e.g., the academic demands, financial concerns, interpersonal issues). Because of the combination of these unprecedented stressors, many college students felt unsure how to cope (Wang et al., 2020). When students focused on the aspects of the stressor that they were able to control (e.g., studying for an upcoming exam), they felt less stress (Person & Frazier, 2024).

The coping literature grew out of initial research on problem-focused and emotion-focused coping. Today, there are many other ways to conceptualize how we cope with stress.

Engagement and Disengagement Coping

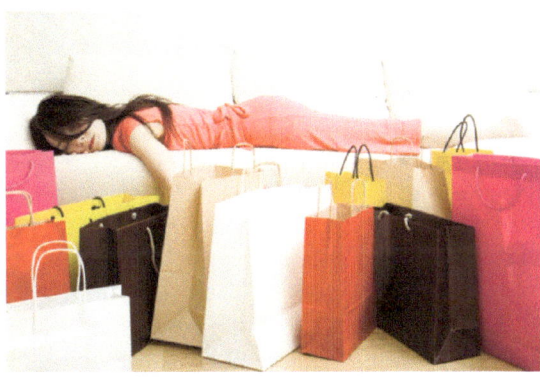

Photo 7.4 "Retail therapy" is a specific method of coping that people use to deal with stress. We know that this strategy is related to disengagement

Source: Image Source/Getty Images

Engagement coping, or *approach coping*, aims at actively managing the stressor and the ensuing emotions. Related to engagement is **proactive coping**, or *anticipatory coping*, which takes place before the stress occurs and helps to offset or prepare for it. It is nearly always problem-focused. Think of the steps that pregnant mothers take to prepare for a baby—researching, redecorating, and taking prenatal or birthing classes. As you know from Chapter 6, even the joyful event of the birth of a child can be stressful (**Photo 7.4**).

Disengagement coping, or *avoidance coping*, aims instead at escaping a perceived threat, by distancing oneself from the stressor and its related emotions (Carver & Connor-Smith, 2010; Moos & Schaefer, 1993; Skinner, Edge, Altman, & Sherwood, 2003). Disengagement is directed primarily at avoiding feelings of distress or pretending that the stress does not exist. This coping strategy includes cognitive disengagement (such as denial, procrastination, or escapist thoughts), behavioral disengagement (such as sleeping, drinking, or taking drugs), and distractions such as video games. "Retail therapy" is essentially avoidance coping.

As you can imagine, disengagement is not a very effective coping strategy. It can be especially problematic if the stress needs attention. Imagine ignoring a phone call from the doctor after a blood test. If medication or other treatment is necessary, then disengagement could put you at serious risk. Paradoxically, disengagement strategies may actually increase thoughts about the stressor, adding to anxiety (Carver & Connor-Smith, 2010; Najmi & Wegner, 2008). Although there are times when disengaging might give you a break from the stress, over time, it is an ineffective way to manage distress.

Meaning-Focused Coping

In **meaning-focused coping**, people do not attempt to change the situation or reduce the distress associated with it, but, rather, to find meaning in it. They ask questions about the situation and themselves (Collins, Taylor, & Skokan, 1990; Frazier & Schauben, 1994; McIntosh, Silver, & Wortman, 1993): "Why did this happen to me?" "How will this change my life?" "What does this situation mean?"

Meaning-focused coping can strengthen relationships and social networks, enhance one's personal resources, and lead to new and better ways of coping (Folkman, 2008). It can bring about cognitive or intellectual changes, strengthen self-reliance and self-understanding, and deepen empathy and altruism. Ultimately, it can lead to new goals, values, and priorities. Finding a silver lining, a renewed passion for life, or a deeper relationship with a loved one can help in coping with stress.

This model of coping distinguishes two levels of meaning (Park, 2007, 2008; Park & Folkman, 1997). **Global meaning systems** include your core beliefs about the very nature of the world. Think of them as your "worldview." You might, for example, believe that "things happen for a reason."

The **appraised meaning** of an event focuses instead on the specific stressor as a loss, threat, or challenge. It includes causal explanations for why the event occurred—such as God's will, coincidence, or self-blame. In this model, people under stress feel a discrepancy between their global beliefs and their appraised meaning of the event. Facing that discrepancy can be difficult emotionally. Our entire future may start to feel out of control. People can resolve the problem by changing either level of meaning. They are essentially "working through" the event (Creamer, Burgess, & Pattison, 1992).

Meaning-focused coping may be especially important in situations that affect one's sense of self. These situations can include acute life events, such as a natural disaster, or long-term circumstances, such as chronic illness. (The **Around the World** feature provides an example of how a long-term circumstance and an acute life event can lead to meaning-focused coping.) One study examined posttraumatic stress in victims of the 2008 Great Sichuan earthquake in China.

The survey was sent to adolescents whose school collapsed. Many lost family members, friends, teachers, and classmates. Students who used meaning-focused strategies were better adapted and had fewer mental and physical health problems. They even reported feelings of personal growth rather than loss alone (Guo, Gan, & Tong, 2013).

Humor and Religion in Coping: Often, meaning-focused coping relies on humor to discover new understandings and positive feelings. Gwen's story is one example of how humor can lighten the darkest situations. Another way to find meaning in a situation is through the lens of faith.

Religion has been defined as "a search for significance in ways related to the sacred" (Pargament, 1997). *Religiosity* is the belief in a divine power and generally involves worshipping that power. *Spirituality*, a related idea, is the belief in an ultimate purpose or meaning in life, such as a higher calling to love and compassion (Troutman-Jordan & Staples, 2014). Religion usually involves an organization or institution, while spirituality does not. Both have been found to influence how we cope with stress.

Although beliefs and practices differ from religion to religion and from person to person, some theorists see religion as an outgrowth of a human need to understand the most complex and deepest of problems (Park, 2007, 2008). It can influence how we think about the world and our role within it. Although religion has not always been a popular topic in psychology, recently it has become a hot area of research. The results are striking: For those to whom religion is important, religion is strongly related to better physical and mental health, psychological well-being, and resilience in the face of adversity (Oman & Thoresen, 2007; Park, 2005). Simply believing in a benevolent God can help in coping.

Spirituality, too, has been found to provide solace (Kelly, 1995). Take, for example, the spirituality of Native Americans. For them, humor is part of a long-standing spiritual tradition and is a powerful healing force in their lives (Garrett, Garrett, Rivera, & Roberts-Wilbur, 2005). According to Native American Clyde Hall, "Anytime you laugh about something, it shatters it. Then it doesn't have any power over you" (Thompson, 1995). Native American humor can be used to dissolve tension, manage potential conflict, or subtly convey an important message. Through stories, anecdotes, witty one-liners, and teasing, as well as songs, dance, art, and other symbolism, the spiritual humor in Native American culture is a way to cope with personal and collective adversity and has been found to relate to psychological well-being and health (Bennett & Lengacher, 2006; Kuiper & Nicholl, 2004; Svebak, Kristoffersen, & Aasarød, 2006).

Religious beliefs play a part in the appraisal process. Some might believe that a stressful event occurred because God was providing an opportunity for growth, testing their belief, or exacting punishment (Park, 2007, 2008). For example, following the September 11, 2001, terrorist attacks, many people turned to religion to make sense of what had happened, perhaps in part because the terrorists themselves framed their attacks in terms of religion (Nielsen, 2002). Religion can also provide a supportive social network of clergy and faith-based communities. Religiosity and spirituality, including humor, can be very beneficial for emotional adjustment, physical health, and well-being (Troutman-Jordan & Staples, 2014).

Around *the* World

A Village in Pakistan

In 2009, Taliban fighters were terrorizing areas of Pakistan. An 11-year-old girl in the Swat Valley named Malala Yousafzai spoke out against the Taliban's belief that girls and women should not be educated. She spoke of her passion for education and her dream to become a doctor someday (Walsh, 2012; Yousafzai & Lamb, 2013).

Three years later, masked gunmen returned to her village, took the 14-year-old girl off the school bus, and shot her in front of her classmates for defying the Taliban and speaking out for freedom of expression and against the injustice of subjugating girls and women. Malala was shot in the head and neck, and a bullet lodged in her brain. The event shocked the world, and people everywhere followed her fight to survive. Her miraculous recovery became a symbol of courage, bravery, and world peace (Walsh, 2012; Yousafzai & Lamb, 2013).

In 2013, on her sixteenth birthday, she was finally given a voice. Malala spoke to the United Nations about freedom from oppression, calling on world leaders to ensure that all children everywhere were able to get an education. She received several standing ovations and was a recipient of the 2014 Nobel Peace Prize. In her memoir, she tells how she found the courage to stand up for what she believed in, and she has continued to speak out for "a global struggle against illiteracy, poverty, and terrorism." All it takes, she says, is "one child,

one teacher, one book, and one pen to change the world" (Walsh, 2012; Yousafzai & Lamb, 2013).

Her story captures the essence of coping through finding meaning. In her own words, "The terrorists thought that they would change my aims and stop my ambitions … but nothing changed in my life, except this: weakness, fear, and hopelessness died. Strength, power, and courage were born" (Yousafzai & Lamb, 2013). Malala Yousafzai is a model of not only successful coping but also of hope for those whose oppression cannot be heard (**Photo 7.5**).

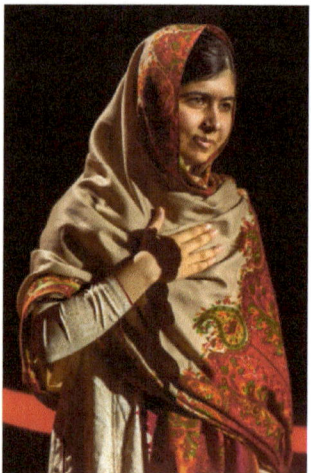

Photo 7.5

Source: Nigel Waldron/Getty Images

Question:

How is Malala's story an example of meaning-focused coping?

Life in college can be very stressful. Research on how college students cope with the many sources of stress in their lives shows that problem-solving or problem-focused strategies are linked to better mental and physical health, and negative emotion-focused strategies—specifically avoidance—are linked to poorer mental and physical health outcomes (Yun, Kim, & Awasu, 2019). Emotion-focused strategies such as acceptance and positive reframing, though, are generally beneficial for college students. As we saw with Gwen, humor, too, can lighten the proverbial load. When students studying social work were surveyed, faith or spirituality was also found to mediate the effects of stress on coping (Yun et al., 2019). This suggests that a person's faith can improve their overall ability to cope, all things being equal.

Thinking About Health

■ In what situations have you used problem-focused coping? In what contexts have you relied upon emotion-focused coping?

■ How well do you think that engagement and disengagement coping strategies work in the short and long terms?

■ Consider an instance in which a friend or family member used meaning-focused coping. How did their global meaning system differ, if at all, from their appraised meaning of the particular event?

■ Which methods of coping did Gwen use in her story?

Influences on Coping

Almost all the coping strategies that we have discussed can be beneficial—though some are clearly not. Behavioral disengagement or denial can be harmful when the stressor needs immediate attention. Similarly, a coping strategy will be most beneficial when it is combined with other strategies and is tailored to the type of stressor one faces. Recall from Chapter 6 that the most stressful events are unexpected and unpredictable. Trying to manage a problem that is outside of one's control may lead only to greater distress. To dwell on emotions when a problem demands action is also not productive.

Whatever the stressor, efficacy varies across the globe, because different people live within different contexts and with different resources. As we see next, these include situation, personality, how we compare ourselves with others, social support, and ethnicity and culture.

Situation and Disposition

Coping can be a response to a specific situation; this is called **situational coping** (or *state coping*). When we talk of coping strategies, we are speaking of situational coping. Alternatively, some people tend to rely on a consistent and stable strategy across many situations, which is **dispositional coping**. When we ask what a person generally does in a stressful situation, we are assessing dispositional coping. If we see that coping is stable over time and across situations, then we are more likely to attribute it to the person. In contrast, if people adapt their coping, we are more likely to see them as responsive to the situation. Which approach best explains coping styles? As we will see, the jury is still out.

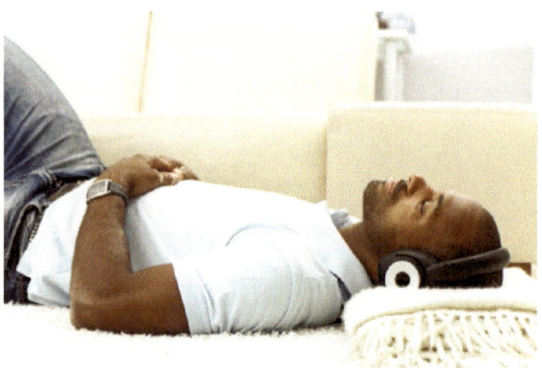

Photo 7.6 There are many ways to cope with stress. Do your coping methods vary by situation (situational), or are they mostly consistent over time (dispositional)?

Source: StockLite/Shutterstock

Certain situations require certain types of situational coping. Consider the stress of discrimination. Ninety-six percent of black college students reported experiencing racism or discrimination in the previous year, and 95% of them found these experiences stressful (Brown, Phillips, Abdullah, Vinson, & Robertson, 2011). These students tended to cope better when parents and teachers spoke with them about racism and how to respond. Some common techniques are relying on ethnic pride, practicing faith, and talking with family and friends (**Photo 7.6**) (Bynum, Burton, & Best, 2007; Hudson et al., 2016).

Other researchers looked specifically at *forbearance coping*, a common strategy used by ethnic minorities to minimize or conceal problems or concerns in order not to trouble or burden others (Wei, Liao, Heppner, Chao, & Ku, 2012). They found that, for Latinx students, forbearance coping could be a risk factor for lower persistence and less commitment to finishing college (Hernández & Villodas, 2019). Facilitating open dialogues about experiences of discrimination helps those who feel challenged to persist despite the additional stressors they face in college. Unfortunately, experiencing discrimination can lead to health-compromising behaviors, such as substance use, as a way to relieve stress (Carver & Connor-Smith, 2010; Gerrard et al., 2012). Understanding how best to handle situational stress can help students to persist.

Do people really have their own "styles" of coping, and do these matter? A longitudinal study of schoolchildren found that girls generally use the same techniques across stressful encounters. Boys were less predictable, especially when they used avoidance coping in the first case (Kirchner, Forns, Amador, & Muñoz, 2010). More generally, knowing what a person does may not always predict what they will do next (David & Suls, 1999; Penley, Tomaka, & Wiebe, 2002). That said, with age, people are generally able to determine what kinds of coping approaches are helpful and tailor them to the situation (Koolhaas, De Boer, Buwalda, & Van Reenen, 2007).

Personality

Coping may itself be an aspect of personality. Some personality traits appear to influence how people cope with stress (Vollrath, Torgersen, & Alnæs, 1995). As we have seen, these traits can be either biologically based or influenced by learning and socialization.

One such trait is neuroticism. Recall that people who are higher in this "Big 5" trait are more likely to experience such negative emotions as anxiety and depression (Costa & McCrae, 1987). When faced with stress, those high in neuroticism are more likely to report stress symptoms. They also report a greater number of stressful life events and tend to use more maladaptive strategies, such as emotional and behavioral disengagement, wishful thinking, escape-avoidance, and emotional venting, to cope with them (Costa & McCrae, 1987). They may also be more prone to drinking heavily (Malouff, Thorsteinsson, Rooke, & Schutte, 2007).

Clearly, people who tend toward negative emotions may not cope with stress as effectively. People with a *type D personality* (or *"distressed" personality*) tend to experience negative emotions and do not easily express their feelings (see Chapter 9). They show greater *negative affect* (NA) but are *socially inhibited* (SI). That combination can be damaging both mentally and physically (Ferguson et al., 2009; Kupper, Gidron, Winter, & Denollet, 2009; Mommersteeg, Kupper, & Denollet, 2010; Yu, Chen, Zhang, & Liu, 2011). Type D personality has been linked to higher rates of cardiovascular disease, hypertension, and high blood pressure—as well as greater morbidity and mortality in cardiac patients (Martin et al., 2011). Type D people report a poorer quality of life and sense of well-being. They also tend to use emotion-focused coping strategies such as self-blame, avoidance, and social isolation (Yu et al., 2011). Otherwise, healthy undergraduates who had a type D personality showed more stress, more burnout, and a higher risk of health problems (Martin et al., 2011; Polman, Borkoles, & Nicholls, 2010; Williams & Wingate, 2012).

Positive emotions have the opposite effect—better coping, better health, greater well-being, and longer life. **Optimism** is the tendency to look on the bright side of things, and the belief that one will experience good outcomes in life (Scheier & Carver, 1992; Scheier, Carver, & Bridges, 1994). It helps buffer the negative impact of stressful life situations and offset depression (Carver, Scheier, & Segerstrom, 2010; Goodin, Bier, & McGuire, 2009; Ramírez-Maestre, Esteve, & López, 2012). Optimists appraise situations as less stressful, use more problem-focused coping, and seek more social support (Conversano et al., 2010). They tend to be more persistent in their coping as well (**Photo 7.7**).

"Don't Worry, Be Happy." This catchy little tune by Bobby McFerrin could be the theme song for optimists. In biological terms, optimism leads to lower levels of the stress hormone cortisol (Polk, Cohen, Doyle, Skoner, & Kirschbaum, 2005), increased immunity (Segerstrom & Sephton, 2010), and greater resistance to the common cold (Cohen, Doyle, Turner, Alper, & Skoner, 2003). In patients undergoing coronary bypass surgery, those who were optimistic had a faster rate of recovery (Scheier et al., 1989). Optimism may also lead to better mental and physical health by promoting a healthy lifestyle (Conversano et al., 2010; Geers, Wellman, Seligman, Wuyek, & Neff, 2010). For example, Gwen's current feelings of optimism bode well for better coping, greater adaptation, and less stress in the future.

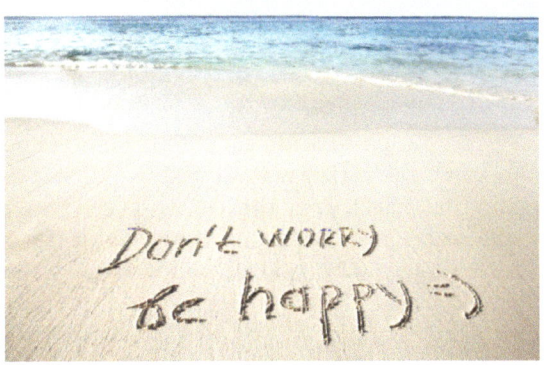

Photo 7.7   Positive emotions, like optimism, lead to better coping

Source: Ditty_about_summer/Stutterstock

Personal Control and Social Comparison

People with a sense of **personal control** tend to see what happens to them as directed by them, rather than as a matter of fate or chance (Rotter, 1966). This belief is associated with lower levels of distress and better coping. Of course, that may not always be the case. After all, according to the matching hypothesis, when the ability to control a situation is low, problem-focused strategies may actually increase distress. However, when one *can* exert control and *choose* to engage, the benefits are clear.

Although optimism has a strong genetic foundation, a positive outlook can be learned—and personal control can be taught. We will learn how to improve coping at the end of this chapter.

How we appraise stress depends on what we see in those around us. **Social comparison** is the process of comparing ourselves to others (Festinger, 1954). These comparisons can help us gain perspective on the challenges we face (Bauer & Wrosch, 2011).

Suppose, as your history professor hands back the exams, you see that the person sitting in front of you got a 94, and the person sitting next to you got a 68. You got an 80. Although you had hoped you'd do better, you quickly think, "At least I didn't get a 68." And, you think, "Next time, I am going to study more and do better than a 94. I know I am smarter than that!"

Sometimes we make *downward* social comparisons to those worse off than us (like the student who got a 68) to protect self-esteem. We might think of downward comparisons as a form of emotion-focused coping (Tennen, Affleck, Armeli, & Carney, 2000). At other times, we make *upward* social comparisons to those we see as accomplishing more (like the person who got a 94), and this motivates us to work harder and to cope more effectively. We may also compare ourselves to how we were in the past, to see how far we have come and what we have accomplished, which is called *temporal comparison*.

Social comparisons are common in the face of threats to health. For some chronically ill patients, seeing others who are worse off can make them feel better about their state of health (Wood, Taylor, & Lichtman, 1985), while seeing those who are perceived as doing better and coping well can give hope and provide a role model. It can help simply to imagine someone less fortunate (Taylor, 1983). Breast cancer patients who make downward comparisons adjust better psychologically (Wood et al., 1985). Downward comparisons also lower the rates of hospitalization and mortality among older adults who face limited control over their health (Bailis, Chipperfield, & Perry, 2005). Social comparison is an important strategy for caregivers, as well, and for those in support groups for chronic illness.

Social Support

Social support is the perception that we are cared for, that others are available to help, and that we are part of a strong social network. Having a sense of support and having people with whom you can share your experiences act as a buffer against stress and relate to positive health outcomes and well-being. Social support is both a resource for coping and a way for people to cope with stress.

Seeking social support can be either problem- or emotion-focused. Social support itself can be *emotional* or emotion-focused: When you are stressed, your mother or best friend will be there to listen to you vent and nurture you. It can also be *informative*: Faced with a diagnosis of Parkinson's disease, for example, you might seek others who understand the disease and who can help you navigate the diagnostic and treatment process. Social support can also be *tangible*, such as financial assistance in times of need. **Tangible support** (or *instrumental support*) is problem-focused in nature. Last, social support can be *invisible*. Yes, invisible: We can benefit from the help of others "behind the scenes" without even knowing it (Bolger & Amarel, 2007). Invisible social support is often motivated by a selfless motivation to help another. For example, imagine a woman who suffers from migraines triggered by loud, noisy, congested, or smoky environments. Perhaps her boyfriend will make their social plans to avoid those settings—most of the time, without her even being aware that he did. Another example is donating clothes to help those in need. The recipients do not know who donated, only that there are people out there who care.

How is social support protective? Decades of research show that close social bonds are beneficial for health and well-being (Cohen & Wills, 1985; Wittig et al., 2016). The **direct effects hypothesis** suggests that having more social support leads to better health *regardless* of stress levels. The **buffering hypothesis** suggests instead that social support forms a "buffer" that minimizes the negative effects of stress. There is solid evidence to support both theories (Cohen & McKay, 1984; Penninx et al., 1997). Having friends is protective, and so is having a variety of different social networks. However, when you really need someone to talk to, having someone close to you who cares really matters. For example, for LGBTQ adolescents, having the social support of peers, teachers, and especially parents increases self-esteem, lessens depression, and leads to better mental and physical health outcomes in response to stress (Watson, Grossman, & Russell, 2019).

The way we seek social support is changing. Think of Gwen's situation at the start of this chapter. Peer support, especially in the context of dealing with the stress of major life events such as pregnancy, divorce, disability or chronic illness, bereavement, or substance use disorder, can be crucial. It does not matter who the others are so long as we feel that we are not alone. Quality time with others over the Internet or messaging friends can combat depression and increase self-esteem (Shaw & Gant, 2002), especially for women (Teoh, Chong, Yip, Lee, & Wong, 2015). Many studies show the benefits of online social support networks for providing emotional and informational support. Engagement in these support networks relates to better outcomes, especially in medical contexts (**Photo 7.8**) (Mehta & Atreja, 2018).

Today, online social networks (social media) are an essential part of our daily lives. In particular, social media is beneficial to college students for conveying useful information, connecting with friends and family far away, and engaging in social activities (Alt, 2018). There do appear to be some downsides to these networks, however. **Fear of missing out (FOMO)** creates feelings of anxiety that exciting or interesting things may be

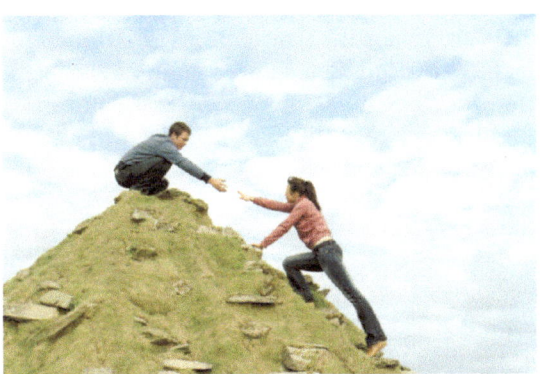

Photo 7.8   Social support takes many forms: emotional, informative, tangible, and invisible. What kind of support do you offer to others?

Source: Winder & Wiehahn/Getty Images

happening elsewhere that you are not part of, and is usually caused by exposure to social media. FOMO is related to social comparison processes and competition with others, and undermines the positive, socially supportive aspects of online networks. In college students, FOMO is linked to poor adjustment to college and may impact perceptions of social support through social media engagement (Alt, 2018). The bottom line is that social support networks are positive for coping with stress—until opportunities for social comparison through the platforms lead to stress themselves. One recent study showed that people who identify as male are at higher risk of addictive social media use than females and that FOMO is more prevalent among males as well (Brailovskaia et al., 2023). Given the connection among social media usage and elevated FOMO, these results suggest a vulnerability for men. An interesting study arose out of the unprecedented and unpredicted social network outage that happened on October 4, 2021 (Eitan & Gazit, 2023). This event, caused by a severe technical service failure at Meta (previously known as Facebook), created a worldwide "outage" lasting over six hours. This outage affected billions of people and created varying levels of stress for those who were not able to access their social media accounts. Researchers jumped on this event to study the effects of stress and FOMO. What they found was that while many people, especially men, experienced FOMO, many others experienced JOMO (or the joy of missing out!). This suggests that a break from social media can be an adaptive way to cope.

Overall, on and off the Internet, having friends increases our sense of self-worth and helps us feel that we are a good person to be around. And on a practical level, our social network gives us information, advice, guidance, an opportunity to express our emotions, and other types of assistance when we need it. It is comforting to know that we have people we can turn to in times of need.

Yet, social support is not beneficial in the same way for everyone. There are both individual and cultural differences. For example, overwhelming evidence suggests that social support benefits women more than men (Reifman, Luckow, & McIntosh, 1998). Women are called on more frequently than men to provide social support, they receive more social support than men, and they are more satisfied with the social support they receive. Women provide support to both men and women in their social networks, but when they seek social support, women, especially unmarried women, seek it from other females. Men tend to receive most of their social support exclusively from their spouses (Gurung, Taylor, & Seeman, 2003). There is a downside, though. Many women experience stress when there are interpersonal problems within their social network. In addition, developmentally, there is a winnowing of the social network with age, and both elderly women and men have smaller social networks and fewer people to call on for social support. Nevertheless, these gender patterns in coping should sound familiar. Remember the *tend-and-befriend response* we discussed in Chapter 6: The benefits of social support for females relate to the production of oxytocin.

Culture

As we saw in Chapter 6, culture can influence how stress is appraised, interpreted, and experienced. Culture can also influence how we cope with stress (Kuo, 2013). There are cultural differences in how people cope and what is socially accepted as a way of coping (Chun, Moos, & Cronkite, 2006), and this variability can be seen across national, racial, and ethnic groups.

We already encountered one major distinction, between collectivism and individualism, in Chapter 6 (Markus & Kitayama, 1991; Triandis, 2001). *Collectivist cultures* highlight the inextricable connectedness of people to one another, whereas *individualistic cultures* emphasize an individual's separateness or independence from others (Yeh, Arora, & Wu, 2006). These cultural orientations may influence one's sense of self, which in turn shapes behaviors, thoughts, emotions, and motivations (Markus & Kitayama, 1992; Waid & Frazier, 2003).

In collectivist cultures, people see themselves as part of a larger group—such as a family, ethnic group, or nation—and they put the needs and values of the group ahead of their own. They see people as depending on one another, and they believe that the group is only as strong as the interdependence among the people in it. Individualism, on the other hand, is found in cultures that value independence, autonomy, personal control, and self-reliance. Individualists give value to personal goals over group goals.

People from these different cultural orientations cope with stress differently (Chun et al., 2006; Kuo, 2013; Yeh & Inose, 2002). **Collective coping**, or *communal coping*, is aimed at engaging, relying on, and seeking advice from others in meaningful, purposeful, and culturally consistent ways. It considers the well-being of others as important when dealing with one's own stress (Moore & Constantine, 2005), and it gives weight to the values of forbearance, fatalism, family, and authority figures. Coherence is also important. In the highly collective Bedouin Arab culture, for instance, coherence with one's group and one's place in life provides an anchor in the midst of stressful and dangerous political events (Abu-Kaf & Braun-Lewensohn, 2019).

When it comes to emotion-focused coping, collectivism is more likely to lead to acceptance and resignation, cognitive reframing, focusing on the positive, and detachment or avoidance (Kuo, 2013). Collective coping also relies more heavily on religion, spirituality, and ritual (Fischer, Ai, Aydin, Frey, & Haslam, 2010). The Western tradition of seeking help from a stranger, such as a psychologist, may be seen as inappropriate from a collectivist perspective (Yeh et al., 2006).

Individualistic coping, in turn, tends to be approach-based, problem-focused, and aimed at exercising personal agency to deal with stress. Individualistic cultures do not emphasize the role or significance of others in coping. Coping is seen as autonomous and self-directed.

Traditionally, Asian, South American, and some African cultures are seen as collectivist, while the U.S. and Western European cultures are individualistic. Collective coping is prominent in Asian nationals, Asian Americans/Canadians, African Americans/Canadians, and to a lesser extent Latinx Americans (Kuo, 2013). For example, Asian Americans who had lost a loved one in the terrorist attacks of September 11, 2001, tended to seek comfort from family, other Asian Americans, or those who went through the same experience of loss. They were more likely to display forbearance and fatalism (Yeh et al., 2006). African Canadians who experience discrimination often use spiritual-based and ritual-based coping strategies (Joseph & Kuo, 2009), while African Americans cope by giving and receiving social support to other group members or through religion (Constantine, Alleyne, Caldwell, McRae, & Suzuki, 2005).

Ethnic Identity and Acculturation Another cultural factor that may influence how people cope is their ethnic identity. **Ethnic identity**, which begins to develop in childhood, consists of the cultural characteristics that are part of a person's concept of self. It influences one's sense of belonging to an ethnic group within a larger society (Phinney, Lochner, & Murphy, 1990). Ethnic identity is also a strong predictor of mental health and a buffer against stressors, especially for adolescents (Dubow, Pargament, Boxer, & Tarakeshwar, 2000) and those from ethnic minority groups (Spencer & Tinsley, 2008; Vera et al., 2011). For example, Jewish adolescents reported experiencing stress associated with religious and social practices such as learning the Torah for their Bar Mitzvahs (for boys) and Bat Mitzvahs (for girls). In these ceremonies, a Jewish child comes of age and is recognized as responsible for their own actions. Although this is, for most, a joyous occasion, it requires a great deal of studying in preparation.

Those who used coping strategies and resources associated with their ethnic group had better outcomes (Dubow et al., 2000). Korean American college students who had a strong and positive ethnic identity were buffered from the stress associated with discrimination (Lee, 2005). In Latinx adolescents, too, there is a positive association between self-esteem, ethnic identity, and well-being (Hernández & Villodas, 2019; Umaña-Taylor, Vargas-Chanes, Garcia, & Gonzales-Backen, 2008; Verkuyten, 2010). In a recent study of Latinx college students, the experience of a hostile school environment led to lower persistence, but those who had a strong ethnic identity were more likely to seek social support to deal with microaggressions. This support helped students be more committed to finishing school (Hernández & Villodas, 2019).

Although many immigrants maintain a strong ethnic identity, they may also start to adopt the language, cuisine, dating preferences, and holiday celebrations of their new country (Berry, 1992). **Acculturation** is the process of learning about and adapting to a host culture. Some people who move to a new country acculturate quickly, whereas others maintain a great deal of their cultural practices and assimilate less. The choice can be challenging on many levels. Early research showed that greater acculturation leads to better mental health (Ball & Kenardy, 2002). However, there is growing evidence that maintaining key cultural ties and ethnic identity leads, in fact, to better mental health in the face of *acculturative stress* (**Photo 7.9**) (see Chapter 6; Torres, 2010).

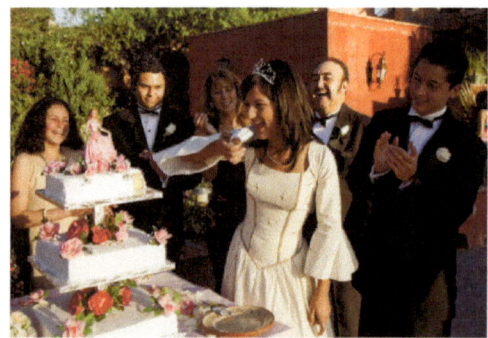 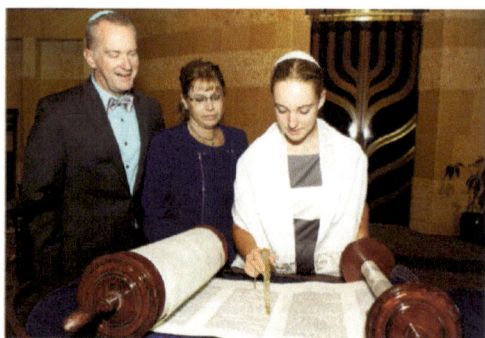

Photo 7.9   Ethnic identity can be a buffer against the stress of discrimination and microaggressions. Celebrations specific to one ethnicity or religion (such as a quinceañera [left] or a Bat Mitzvah [right]) are joyful and may have the added benefit of being protective against acculturative stress

Acculturation may come at the expense of the old culture (Roland, 1989), and trying to adapt may result in stress (Berry, Kim, Minde, & Mok, 1987; Torres & Rollock, 2004). This acculturative stress can take a lifelong toll on psychological adjustment, decision-making, career success, and health, resulting in higher levels of depression (Torres & Rollock, 2004). For Latinx, more time spent in the United States is associated with a greater likelihood of mental health problems (Finch, Frank, & Vega, 2004; Torres, 2010; Vega, Sribney, Aguilar-Gaxiola, & Kolody, 2004). In this *immigrant paradox*, Latinx who feel the pressure or desire to "fit in" with mainstream culture have higher rates of depression (Torres, 2010). Maintaining Latinx culture serves as a buffer. An active coping style can lessen the stress as well.

Thinking About Health

- How have different situations, your personality, and your sense of personal control interacted to affect your coping methods in times of stress?
- How does social support shape your experience of stress?
- How does culture influence coping?

Coping Outcomes

We may think our approach to a stressful situation is unique. As we have seen in this chapter, how we cope may even be a part of who we are. But we all share something in common: We can learn more effective coping strategies. However, to know what works best, we first need to know how coping is measured.

Measuring Coping

As we have seen, coping encompasses many diverse cognitive and behavioral activities (Coelho, Hamburg, & Adams, 1974), and many factors can shape coping—from the initial cognitive appraisal to personality factors, situational characteristics, cultural practices, and more. All this makes measuring coping quite a challenge. Still, there are many fruitful approaches.

Standardized coping inventories assess the thoughts or behaviors a person generally engages in when stressed. Interview protocols are designed to probe how people make meaning of their coping processes. Observational techniques have been used both in laboratory settings and in the natural environment to try to catch people "in the act" of coping. Coping has also been assessed in relation to other variables such as personality and defense mechanisms.

All these approaches are shaped by the **methods-foci approach** (Carver, Scheier, & Weintraub, 1989; Edwards, 1988; Folkman & Lazarus, 1980), which focuses on determining the methods or focus of one's coping efforts. Some questions on coping scales look at the coping strategies themselves. In a recent stressful event, such as an argument with a significant other, *how* did you cope?

Did you tackle the problem by gathering information, or did you try to avoid emotional upheaval by taking a nap or going to a movie? Other questions aim to assess the focal point of the strategies. For example, in a recent stressful event, did you try to change the stressful situation, or did you try to manage the emotional impact of the stressor?

One of the original methods-foci tools for measuring coping is the **Ways of Coping Checklist** (Aldwin, Folkman, Schaefer, Coyne, & Lazarus, 1980). This self-report measure asks people to think of a recent stressful encounter and answer a series of questions about what they did to deal with the stress. The Ways of Coping Checklist has been widely used to categorize coping efforts into problem-focused coping, emotion-focused coping, and seeking social support (Aldwin et al., 1980). Try to assign one of these categories to each example below:

- ■ "I fought for what I wanted."
- ■ "I bargained or compromised to get what I wanted."
- ■ "I blamed myself for what had happened."
- ■ "I kept others from knowing how bad things were."
- ■ "I listened to music."
- ■ "I talked to someone about the problem."

Another method for measuring coping is the **COPE scale** (Carver et al., 1989). This measure has 60 questions, with four items for each of the 15 subscales. For ease of use, a brief version of the COPE scale assesses 14 facets of coping (Carver, 1997): active coping, planning, positive reframing, acceptance, use of humor, turning to religion, seeking emotional support, seeking instrumental support, self-distraction, denial, venting, substance use, behavioral disengagement, and self-blame (see **Table 7.1**). Each question asks people to rate how they coped with a stressful event on a scale from 0 (*"I don't do this at all"*) to 4 (*"I do this a lot"*). People may be asked to think about how they generally approached a stressful event or about how they coped with a specific situation. This allows the assessment of dispositional coping (that is, coping as a trait) or situational coping (coping in response to a specific situation). This is important because, as we have seen, thinking of coping as a trait does not always reliably predict how people behave across different situations (Schwartz, Neale, Marco, Shiffman, & Stone, 1999). The COPE scale is an excellent instrument to assess coping because it allows both a broad overview of coping behaviors as problem-focused or emotion-focused, as well as more fine-grained analysis.

One problem with coping inventories is that they ask people to remember how they coped. Although many of us have good memories, our recollection of past events and experiences is often biased (Todd, Tennen, Carney, Armeli, & Affleck, 2004). Can you remember reliably how you coped the last time you received a low grade on an assignment—or when your plans for the weekend changed at the last minute? Daily reports of coping can be helpful, but it is hard to obtain reliable assessments "in the moment" as well. How people cope on a daily basis often differs from how they report they coped after the stressful encounter is over (Todd et al., 2004).

These items deal with ways you've been coping with the recent challenges in your life. There are many ways to try to deal with life's challenges. These items ask what you've been doing to cope with this challenge. Obviously, different people deal with things in different ways, but I'm interested in how you've tried to deal with it. Each item says something about a particular way of coping. I want to know to what extent you've been doing what the item says. How much or how frequently. Don't answer on the basis of whether it seems to be working or not—just whether or not you're doing it. Use these response choices. Try to rate each item separately in your mind from the others. Make your answers as true FOR YOU as you can.

1 = I haven't been doing this at all
2 = I've been doing this a little bit
3 = I've been doing this a medium amount
4 = I've been doing this a lot

1. I've been turning to work or other activities to take my mind off things.
2. I've been concentrating my efforts on doing something about the situation I'm in.
3. I've been saying to myself "this isn't real."
4. I've been using alcohol or other drugs to make myself feel better.
5. I've been getting emotional support from others.
6. I've been giving up trying to deal with it.
7. I've been taking action to try to make the situation better.
8. I've been refusing to believe that it has happened.
9. I've been saying things to let my unpleasant feelings escape.
10. I've been getting help and advice from other people.
11. I've been using alcohol or other drugs to help me get through it.
12. I've been trying to see it in a different light, to make it seem more positive.
13. I've been criticizing myself.
14. I've been trying to come up with a strategy about what to do.
15. I've been getting comfort and understanding from someone.
16. I've been giving up the attempt to cope.
17. I've been looking for something good in what is happening.
18. I've been making jokes about it.
19. I've been doing something to think about it less, such as going to movies, watching TV, reading, daydreaming, sleeping, or shopping.
20. I've been accepting the reality of the fact that it has happened.
21. I've been expressing my negative feelings.
22. I've been trying to find comfort in my religion or spiritual beliefs.
23. I've been trying to get advice or help from other people about what to do.
24. I've been learning to live with it.
25. I've been thinking hard about what steps to take.
26. I've been blaming myself for things that happened.
27. I've been praying or meditating.
28. I've been making fun of the situation.

To determine your score on each of the different coping styles, add your raw score on each of the two items together. The closer your score is to 8 on any subscale the more that coping style describes you.

Self-distraction, add items 1 and 19. Active coping, add items 2 and 7. Denial, add items 3 and 8. Substance use, add items 4 and 11. Use of emotional support, add items 5 and 15. Use of instrumental support, add items 10 and 23. Behavioral disengagement, add items 6 and 16. Venting, add items 9 and 21. Positive reframing, add items 12 and 17. Planning, add items 14 and 25. Humor, add items 18 and 28. Acceptance, add items 20 and 24. Religion, add items 22 and 27. Self-blame, add items 13 and 26.

Source: Information from Carver (1997).

Table 7.1   Brief cope scale

There are also other weaknesses with using checklists to measure coping. They may be hard to interpret and still harder to apply to real-life coping efforts. Nonetheless, decades of research have relied on these measures (Coyne & Gottlieb, 1996).

Recently, the power of the Internet has been harnessed to examine coping. One of the first studies to do this was conducted around the time of the devastating stress of the terrorist attacks of September 11, 2001 (Cohn, Mehl, & Pennebaker, 2004). In this longitudinal study of coping, participants used an online diary to record their thoughts, emotions, and behaviors. Researchers were able to examine their responses from two months before to two months after the terrorist attacks. Although there were some unique descriptive attributes expressing emotion and coping close to the time of the event, emotions, perceptions, and behavior all reverted to baseline over time.

Learning to Cope Better

Studies like these can be applied to help us learn to cope better. Remember that how we cope with stress is a result of the interactions among our biological predispositions, our personalities, our environment, and learning.

How do we know if we are coping effectively? One obvious way to tell is if we feel less stressed. More detailed answers will depend on the strategies we employ. Did we succeed in eliminating, reducing, managing, or adjusting to the stressor? Did we find an emotional balance, maintain a positive self-image, and maintain positive relations with others?

Recall that we tend to use the same coping strategies for the same stressor (Stone & Neale, 1984). And no matter what the stressor, we usually use the same combination of strategies (Tennen et al., 2000). However, that combination may not always be for the best. Coping with an acute, short-term stressor may require one set of strategies, while long-term stressors may require a different set. For example, once we cope with the shocking diagnosis of a chronic illness, we must still adapt to living with illness into the future.

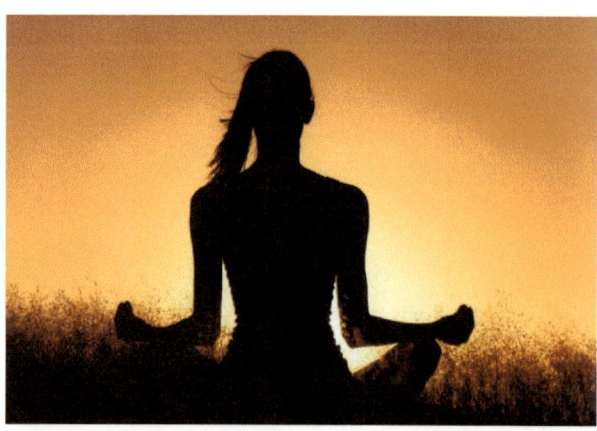

Photo 7.10   While planning out your day, dedicate a chunk of time to relaxation. A mindful approach to a stressful schedule increases the likelihood of successful coping

Source: KieferPix/Shutterstock

Some promising ways of coping include focusing on positive emotions, seeking meaning and benefits from the situation, emotional mindfulness, and finding ways to accommodate situations that cannot be changed (Carver & Connor-Smith, 2010). Many self-help and educational programs seek to enhance a perception of control. They are designed to help people gather and use information, be present and relaxed, and reframe events positively (Ludwick-Rosenthal & Neufeld, 1988). Think again about Gwen. Were any of her coping strategies unproductive, thus adding to her stress? (**Photo 7.10**)

Time Management, Exercise, and Relaxation: By now, you should be in a good position to think about how you cope with stress and what you can do to cope better. There are things that you can do to protect yourself against stress and to offset it. Looking for suggestions? Consider time management, exercise, and relaxation.

For a student, one of the most important ways to reduce stress is to practice good *time management* (Ruiz-Gallardo, González-Geraldo, & Castaño, 2016). That takes goal setting. Whether you are planning for tomorrow, next week, next month, or five years from now, thinking about the goals you wish to accomplish will help you set priorities, get things done, and be productive. Goals should be reasonable and obtainable. Having long-term goals can offset stress by keeping you focused on the "big picture." Try setting SMART goals, as illustrated in **Figure 7.1**.

Just as important is breaking things down into smaller steps to get you to your goal. On a daily basis, these steps are your "to-do list." You can write out your to-do list the old-fashioned way—or use one of the many apps that are available for list making. Ideally, you can fit your to-do list into a daily schedule. This allows you to anticipate when you will do things, allocate the appropriate amount of time for all the things you want to do, keep you on task and on time, and alleviate the distress of feeling disorganized. But the daily schedule should also include all the things that help you live a happy, healthy, and productive life. Be sure to set aside time for what matters to you—such as friends, listening to music, hobbies, watching TV, reading, and exercise.

In Chapter 4, we saw the health benefits of exercise. Regular exercise is also a great way to reduce stress and inoculate yourself against its negative effects (Sherwood, Smith, Hinderliter, Georgiades, & Blumenthal, 2017). Regular

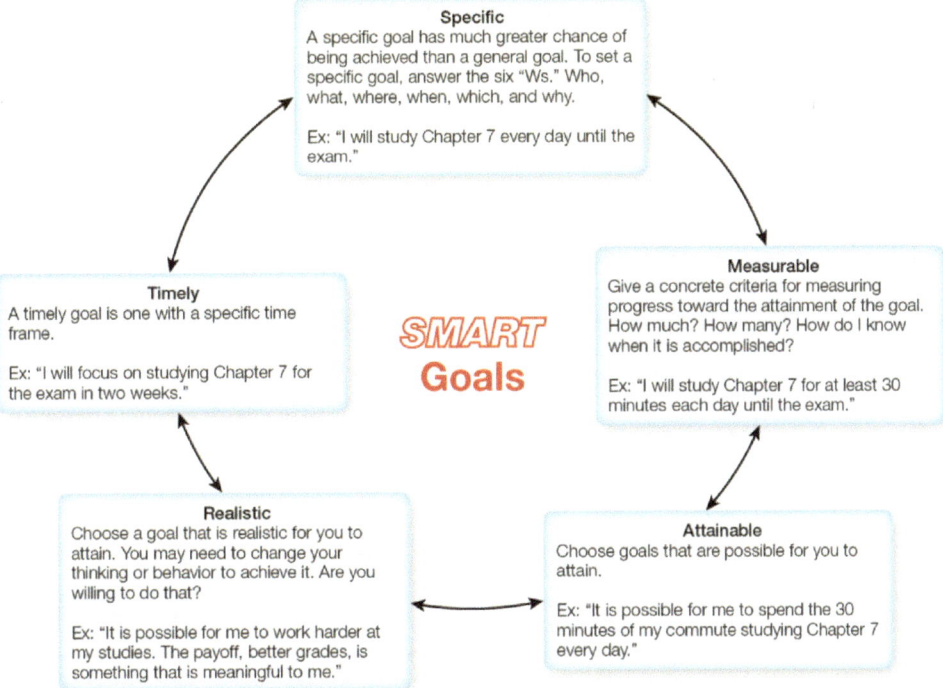

Figure 7.1   SMART goals

exercise increases intellectual functioning and personal control, strengthens your immune system, and acts as a buffer against health threats. It also elevates mood so that you feel more competent and self-confident, and have higher self-esteem. Among police officers and emergency response personnel, who must cope with a great deal of stress, those who were fit from exercising regularly experienced less stress and fewer stress-related health problems (Gerber, Kellmann, Hartmann, & Pühse, 2010). The next time you feel stressed about an upcoming exam, get some exercise.

Relaxation techniques that reduce arousal are also beneficial. Progressive muscle relaxation, yoga, guided imagery, and hypnosis have all been found to reduce heart rate, blood pressure, muscle tension, and lipid levels. They also reverse inflammatory processes. By calming the body and the mind, these techniques provide a feeling of control and calmness that can help you focus and cope more effectively. Meditation is beneficial as well. There are many methods for reaching a meditative state in which the mind is calm. Recent fMRI research shows that meditation causes beneficial changes in the brain, demonstrating its usefulness in coping with stress (Luders, Cherbuin, & Kurth, 2015).

Mindfulness is a mental state achieved by being aware of your thoughts, feelings, and bodily sensations at the moment (try the mindfulness exercise in **Table 7.2**). Mindfulness is important for coping because you have to first be aware that you are stressed, and then be aware of how your body responds as you attempt to

---

Holding: First take a raisin and hold it in the palm of your hand or between your finger and thumb. Focusing on it, imagine that you've just dropped in from Mars and have never seen an object like this before in your life.

Seeing: Take time to really see it; gaze at the raisin with care and full attention. Let your eyes explore every part of it, examining the highlights where the light shines, the darker hollows, the folds and ridges, and any asymmetries or unique features.

Touching: Turn the raisin over between your fingers, exploring its texture—maybe with your eyes closed if that enhances your sense of touch.

Smelling: Holding the raisin beneath your nose, with each inhalation, drink in any smell, aroma, or fragrance that may arise, noticing as you do this if anything interesting is happening in your mouth or stomach.

Placing: Now slowly bring the raisin up to your lips, noticing how your hand and arm know exactly how and where to position it. Gently place the object in the mouth, without chewing—just notice how it gets into the mouth in the first place. Spend a few moments exploring the sensations of having it in your mouth and exploring it with your tongue.

Tasting: When you are ready, prepare to chew the raisin, noticing how and where it needs to be for chewing. Then very consciously take one or two bites of it and notice what happens in the aftermath, experiencing any waves of taste that emanate from it as you continue chewing. Without swallowing yet, notice the bare sensations of taste and texture in the mouth and how these may change over time, moment by moment, as well as any changes in the object itself.

Swallowing: When you feel ready to swallow the raisin, see if you can first detect the intention to swallow as it comes up, so that even this is experienced consciously before you actually swallow the raisin.

Finally: See if you can feel what is left of the raisin moving down into your stomach, and sense how the body as a whole is feeling after completing this exercise in mindful eating.

Source: Information from Williams, Teasdale, Segal, and Kabat-Zinn (2007).

Table 7.2 Eating one raisin: A first taste of mindfulness

calm yourself. *Cognitive behavioral therapy (CBT)* is also beneficial for managing stress and coping well. Related to mindfulness, CBT is a short-term therapeutic approach focused on illuminating how a person's thoughts affect their emotions and behaviors. Once people are mindful of their maladaptive thoughts and behaviors, they can learn to modify them.

In the News

When No News is Good News

Terrorism, natural disasters, and mass shootings; sexual assault, child abuse, and maltreatment in detention centers; and widespread violence against racial, ethnic, sexual, and gender minorities—these are some of the upsetting topics that we see every day in the news. Yet nearly 20% of American adults monitor news and social media feeds "constantly" (American Psychological Association, 2017). While it is important to stay informed, exposure to these events can be highly distressing and lead one to feel anxious, sad, helpless, and threatened, whether one experiences the events firsthand or in the ongoing daily news cycle. For people who have experienced trauma, especially, the barrage of negative information in the news can be overwhelming and re-traumatizing, stirring up feelings of hopelessness, fear, and rage, and even a resurgence of PTSD symptoms. It is important to find ways to cope with exposure to traumatizing events and the news coverage that follows.

So, how can we strengthen our resilience? The American Psychological Association has offered guidelines for coping with distress, such as the trauma of exposure to a mass shooting. However, the following tips can help anyone facing a traumatic event:

■ Limit your exposure to the media. To reduce stress, cut back on how much time you spend watching the news, scrolling through social media feeds, and reading news stories, on paper or online. Disable notifications from news apps, and block notifications from news websites. Also be attentive to your children's and young relatives' exposure to the media and consider how you will answer their questions about traumatic events.

■ Discuss your fears. Ask for support from those who you know will listen to your concerns. Accept comfort and reassurance from loved ones. Remember that you are not alone.

■ Stay balanced. Resist becoming overwhelmed and pessimistic. Remind yourself of what is meaningful, comforting, and encouraging. Retain a healthy perspective on the world around you.

■ Take care of yourself. Eat well, sleep well, exercise, and avoid things that suppress or mask your feelings (e.g., substance use) in order to increase your ability to cope with stress. Maintain routines that allow you to practice healthful behaviors.

■ Be productive, for yourself and others. Helping others in times of need benefits the helper, too. Look for resources and volunteer opportunities in your community, or search for ways that you can help people affected by a particular incident.

■ Stay socially connected. Keep the lines of communication open to help maintain a feeling of normalcy. Support and be supported by friends and family, thereby reducing your stress and building resilience.

If you are having trouble coping with exposure to traumatic events, consider seeking help from a psychologist or other mental health professional. If your distress is acute, you feel that you cannot cope, or you are having thoughts of suicide, contact your university counseling center or the National Suicide Prevention Lifeline (1-800-273-8255) or online chat at **https://suicidepreventionlifeline.org/chat/**.

Question: How does the news affect your mental health on a daily basis? On a longer-term basis?

Information from the American Psychological Association Help Center (2019).

When mindfulness is applied in stressful situations, it helps with coping. For example, think about how stressful it must be for a new veterinary student to perform surgery on a live animal. When these students are taught mindfulness techniques, their stress decreases, their sense of calm increases, and they make fewer errors during surgeries (Stevens, Royal, Ferris, Taylor, & Snyder, 2019). Mindfulness can help with coping in any context—from school to work, from relationships to the news (see the **In the News** feature). We will explore more positive psychological tools to help us cope and adapt to life's challenges in Chapter 13.

Thinking About Health

■ How accurate and helpful do you find measures of coping to be, if at all?

■ Frame a goal through the lens of the SMART goals guidelines. How can setting SMART goals benefit you?

■ How do exercise and relaxation differ in their benefits? How are they the same?

Chapter Summary

With stress, there is an ongoing interaction between the person and the environment. Instrumental to this interaction is our coping: how we manage the stressor and alleviate the negative impact of stress. Coping is a biopsychosocial process. How we cope tells us about our personality, our development, our culture, and our physiology. Our degree of success is also important to our health. When we cope poorly, we may actually increase distress, with negative health outcomes.

We have looked at different theories of coping and at the different strategies we use to cope. We can see coping as problem-focused and emotion-focused, engagement or disengagement, meaning-focused or proactive, situational or dispositional, individual or collective. We have also seen how coping is measured and learned techniques for enhancing coping—especially in the stressful context of college. Such tools as time management, exercise, and relaxation can help us all cope better when faced with stress.

KEY TERMS ▶   Coping p. 215, Coping efficacy p. 215, Problem-focused coping p. 220, Emotion-focused coping p. 220, Matching hypothesis (or the *goodness of fit* model) p. 220, Engagement coping (or *approach coping*) p. 221, Proactive coping (or *anticipatory coping*) p. 221, Disengagement coping (or *avoidance coping*) p. 221, Meaning-focused coping p. 222, Global meaning systems p. 222, Appraised meaning p. 222, Situational coping (or *state coping*) p. 225, Dispositional coping p. 225, Optimism p. 227, Personal control p. 227, Social comparison p. 228, Tangible support (or *instrumental support*) p. 229, Direct effects hypothesis p. 229, Buffering hypothesis p. 229, Fear of missing out (FOMO) p. 229, Collective coping (or *communal coping*) p. 231, Ethnic identity p. 231, Acculturation p. 232, Methods-foci approach p. 233, Ways of Coping Checklist p. 234, COPE scale p. 234, Mindfulness p. 238

CHAPTER 8

Symptoms and Pain

Learning Outcomes

After reading this chapter, you should be able to:

- **Explain** the individual differences in symptom recognition.
- **Describe** how mental representations of symptoms are formed.
- **Outline** the reasons for delay in seeking treatment.
- **Explain** the concept of nociception and how we experience and measure pain.
- **Define** the different types of pain and pain disorders.
- **Identify** pain control and treatment techniques and evaluate their effectiveness.

The pain started with a bad toothache. Natalie needed a root canal procedure, which alleviated the pain for a short time, but then the pain came back worse than ever, along with dizziness and nausea. Natalie's dental surgeon told her just to "wait it out." She did—and pain has been her constant companion for 20 years (**Photo 8.1**).

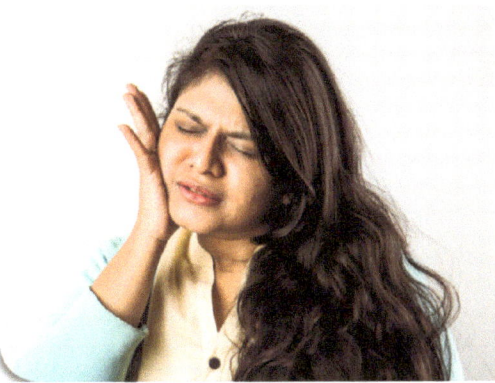

Photo 8.1   Licensed material is being used for illustrative purposes only; any person depicted in the licensed material is a model

In time, doctors found a culprit in nerve damage, which did not show up on X-rays. A "cocktail" of medications dampened the pain, but it had side effects, including fatigue, forgetfulness, and double vision. Natalie could not drive, except for very short trips, and she had to pace herself in every way. Even listening to music or holding a friendly conversation intensified the pain.

On the outside, Natalie appeared normal, but the pain changed her life. It felt like a dagger had been permanently plunged into the right side of her face. Although Natalie was a psychotherapist who loved her work, she had to give up her practice and lost her income. Her relationships suffered as well. Longtime friends noticed the change, but others saw only a quiet person with little energy. Natalie tried experimental neurosurgery, as well as

DOI: 10.4324/9781032643090-8

acupuncture, herbal remedies, and even the laying on of hands, all without success. Despite extraordinary medical care and a supportive family, she struggled with everyday activities, her plans for the future, and her very sense of self.

Finally, her pain specialist suggested that she add a narcotic to her medication cocktail. Lo and behold, relief! Now most days she is pain free, and it is impossible for her to imagine going back. Still, fatigue lingers, and so does a deep suspicion. From the start, her neurologist advised her against narcotics, because of the risk of addiction. Doctors may prescribe narcotics when there is no legitimate medical need, and patients may abuse them. Narcotic prescriptions may put physicians at risk even when they act responsibly, and some have had their licenses suspended for prescribing them. Natalie herself has been accused of lying, neuroticism, and intending to sell drugs to others—a criminal offense. Her chronic pain cannot be felt or understood by others.

Fortunately, Natalie is now receiving care at the pain-control center of a major metropolitan teaching hospital. It has been a 20-year journey, and she is happy for the emotional and medical support that she has received, and for her newfound quality of life. She accepts that pain is part of her life, and that she must do whatever it takes—no matter how challenging—to live as free of the pain as possible.

Natalie's story illustrates the number-one reason that people seek medical help: pain. Pain has come to be considered the "fifth vital sign" taken by health practitioners to assess our basic bodily functions. (The other four are body temperature, heart rate, blood pressure, and respiration.) Although there are a few rare conditions in which people feel little or no pain, pain is all but universal to humanity.

What is pain? And how do we recognize pain and other symptoms of disease or injury as serious and needing attention? As Natalie's story makes clear, the experience of pain is not just physical; it is emotional and cognitive as well. How we interpret our symptoms is part and parcel of how we register pain, seek help, and manage disease. In this chapter, we explore how people recognize pain and symptoms, what prompts them to seek treatment, and why pain is the most significant symptom we experience.

Recognizing Symptoms

Before we delve into the topic of pain, we must first explore the process of experiencing symptoms, and discover what drives people to seek medical care.

Close your eyes. Focus on the sensation of the air you are breathing in through your nose. Pay attention as you exhale. Do you sense that the air is cooler as it comes in and warmer as you breathe out? Does focusing on your breathing cause you to feel a tickling sensation inside your nose? Does attending to your breathing make you want to breathe more deeply? As you concentrate on breathing, do you begin to sense other physical and physiological states? (Is your throat dry? Is your waistband too tight? Are you becoming aware of how tired you feel?)

This simple mindfulness exercise has many positive benefits and is commonly taught to help people manage stress and pain (Owens et al., 2018; Zeidan et al., 2011). It can make you aware of the sensations occurring in your body at any given time.

Interoception

Interoception is the sensation and perception we have of our bodies physically, physiologically, and viscerally. Interoception influences our mood, emotions, and sense of well-being. It is our sense of the physiological state of the body; it is how we represent our bodies to ourselves. Interoception encompasses the sensory stimuli that come in through your senses (sight, hearing, smell, taste, and touch), as well as those that are internally generated (temperature, kinesthetic sense, pain, and balance).

You probably know what it feels like to have a blistering headache, to touch a cotton ball, and to taste a piña colada jelly bean. Right now, you are calling up these specific experiences from memory. The sensation is in memory because you experienced it in the past, but the experience *in the present moment* is interoception. In the brain, an interoceptive neural network monitors the emotional, visceral, and sensory processes (Critchley & Garfinkel, 2017; Pollatos & Herbert, 2018). These processes, honed through evolution, allow us to survive. They alert us when something is wrong. And they are essential to symptom recognition.

Although interoception may help us become aware of our bodies, most people are not very good at perceiving their internal states and their symptoms. Certainly, the stronger the sensation, pain, or discomfort, the more likely we are to perceive it. However, our own assessments of our heart rate, breathing, and nasal congestion are still highly unreliable (Pennebaker & Epstein, 1983; Rietveld & Brosschot, 1999).

We may not be very good at perceiving *external* symptoms either. For example, skin lesions can be a symptom of *melanoma*—skin cancers requiring immediate treatment. However, when it comes to potential melanomas, as opposed to normal freckles and moles, the chance of most people correctly identifying them is only one out of three (Danialan, Gopinath, Phelps, Murphy, & Grant-Kels, 2012). Given that skin cancer is the most common type of cancer, not being able to identify a potentially lethal skin lesion is dangerous (**Photo 8.2**).

Differences in Awareness

Some people are more aware than others of the sensations going on in their bodies. And some have higher thresholds for pain and discomfort. People also differ in when they consider a symptom as cause for concern. Think of the various ways people respond to having a bad cold. Some people take to their beds and rest, feeling absolutely dreadful. Others take over-the-counter medications and soldier on. The individual differences in the experience of symptoms are vast.

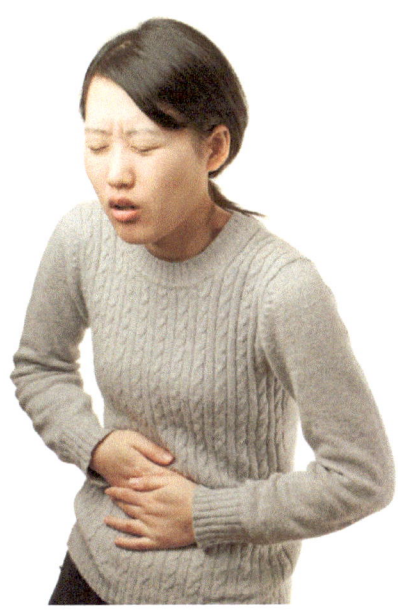

Photo 8.2 Our interoception is not foolproof. We may not realize the extent of our discomfort until we are in significant pain

Source: Gang Liu/Shutterstock

Why the differences? Several factors can influence symptom awareness: *personality, the situation, mood,* and *stress.*

We have already seen the huge role of personality in health experiences and behaviors. Recall from Chapter 4 that neuroticism is a tendency toward negative affect and a pessimistic outlook—and it is clearly linked to a higher awareness of symptoms, greater reporting of symptoms and treatment seeking, and fear that a symptom points to a serious disease (Feldman, Cohen, Doyle, Skoner, & Gwaltney, 1999). One aspect of neuroticism is *illness anxiety disorder,* or the excessive preoccupation and worry about health and illness (American Psychiatric Association, 2013). People who are high in illness anxiety often become alarmed at a new and unexplained symptom, no matter how minor, and become convinced that they have a serious medical condition (see Chapter 12). Illness anxiety, though not common in the general population (ranging from 1.3% to 10%), appears more often in people who are likely to visit doctor's offices and medical clinics. Although it was long thought that women are more prone to illness anxiety, the data do not support this: Men are just as likely to worry excessively about their health and symptoms. There are, however, understandable generational differences. Older people are more likely to report health concerns than younger adults, but many older adults have legitimate health problems to be concerned about.

Illness anxiety disorder is only one example of the *attentional differences* in symptom recognition (Feinstein & deGruy, 2011; Greenberg, Braun, & Cassem, 2008). And those differences may depend on our situation. When we are fully engaged in our activities, we are less likely to notice symptoms than when we are bored (Pennebaker & Epstein, 1983). When our attention is devoted to things that are exciting, interesting, or demanding of attention, we have less free time to think about our bodies.

Mood also affects the recognition of symptoms. When we are in a good mood, we tend to feel healthier, even when we are ill. In turn, when we feel angry, anxious, or depressed, we are more likely to report symptoms. In fact, people in a bad mood are more likely to feel pessimistic about their health and about the effectiveness of treatment (Leventhal, Hansell, Diefenbach, Leventhal, & Glass, 1996).

Stress and anxiety, too, can highlight symptoms or discomfort. This may not just be a function of awareness—chronic stress may actually increase symptoms and make us more vulnerable to illness. (Recall from Chapter 6 that prolonged stress depletes the immune system.) Stress alone may lead to an increased heart rate, breathing difficulties, gastric distress, fatigue, sweating, and palpitations—and any of these can be misinterpreted as signs of illness. Thus, stress can complicate awareness of symptoms. In contrast, after a diagnosis of a chronic condition like cancer, positive affect—especially optimism—can significantly enhance management of symptoms and illness (Taber, Klein, Ferrer, Kent, & Harris, 2016).

Thinking About Health

■ How does interoception influence your perception of your health?

■ Think about the last time you hurt yourself or felt ill. What factors influenced your awareness of pain and discomfort?

Interpreting Symptoms

How, then, can we best recognize and interpret symptoms? Just as individual differences can contribute to the awareness of symptoms, several factors can influence how we interpret a symptom once we have noticed it. These factors start with our earlier experiences of a symptom or illness and come to include our full range of expectations and experiences—in what psychologists have called the *illness perception model* and *confirmation bias*.

Prior Experience

If you have past experience with a symptom, you are in a better position to know whether it is serious. For example, you may recognize chest pain as the symptom of a heart attack if you have had one before. You will more easily recognize that uncomfortable sensation of pressure, squeezing, burning, or fullness under the breastbone in the center of the chest.

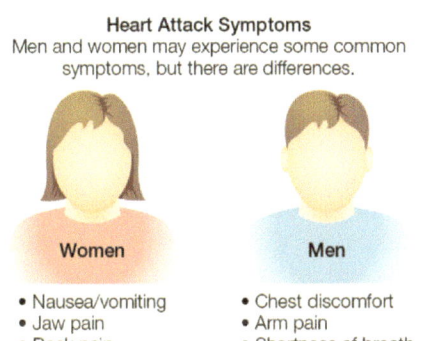

Heart Attack Symptoms
Men and women may experience some common symptoms, but there are differences.

Women
- Nausea/vomiting
- Jaw pain
- Back pain

Men
- Chest discomfort
- Arm pain
- Shortness of breath

Figure 8.1 Differences between men and women in symptoms of heart attack

Yet many people are slow in seeking treatment when symptoms arise, because they wrongly attribute them to something else, like stomach problems. Women are more likely to experience chest pain prior to heart attack than are men, but they have to recognize it as serious in order to seek treatment. Men and women who have no known risk of heart disease have experienced chest pain, dismissed it as indigestion, and not sought needed medical attention (see **Figure 8.1** for some differences in the way symptoms manifest themselves). That is one reason heart disease is the leading cause of death in the United States today.

Yes, chest pain can point to other problems. But when people are uninformed about the risks, they are more likely to misdiagnose the symptoms. Conversely, once you have had an experience, you know better how to interpret it. As we see next, this change in our expectations is at the heart of the illness perception model (Elwy, Yeh, Worcester, & Eisen, 2011; MacGregor & Fleming, 1996).

The Illness Perception Model

If you are feeling healthy, you may not expect a symptom to be serious, and you may disregard it. On the other hand, if you are feeling vulnerable to illness, you may not. The **illness perception model** (see **Figure 8.2**; Elwy et al., 2011;

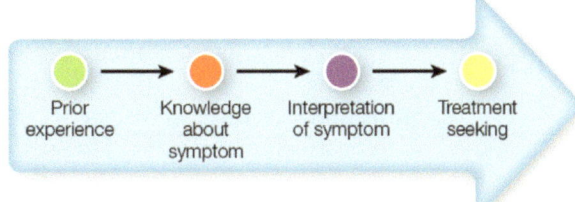

Prior experience → Knowledge about symptom → Interpretation of symptom → Treatment seeking

Figure 8.2 Illness perception model

MacGregor & Fleming, 1996) says that, first, expectations (what we think might happen) influence our focus on sensations (what we are feeling). Second, commonplace symptoms may well grow more intense to confirm our expectations. In short, the pain is consistent with our fears. This is especially likely in a boring situation, of low external stimulation, coupled with increased internal attention and an increased focus on the body (Pennebaker, 1994; Petersen, van den Berg, Janssens, & Van den Bergh, 2011).

Our entire social cognitive process influences how we perceive, interpret, and experience our health. When we experience a sensation and assign meaning to it, or *label* it, we are making attributions. The attribution is guided by the full range of our experience (Petersen et al., 2011). One factor is *environmental attribution*: If people in your class are coming down with strep throat and you are feeling tired, you may attribute your symptoms to what is going around. Information about the prevalence of an illness will shape how likely we are to become ill and our perception of the severity of our symptoms (Jemmott & Magloire, 1988).

Age, too, is a factor: When older people experience hip pain, they may attribute it to arthritis, whereas a teenager might attribute it to overexercise. Similarly, if a young woman often experiences premenstrual cramping, back pain, and fatigue, she is more likely to attribute those symptoms to her period than to the stomach flu. Again, past experiences shape our attributions.

Once we have identified and labeled our symptoms, we start seeing other signs to confirm our attributions. **Confirmation bias** (Kahneman & Tversky, 1973; Olson, Roese, & Zanna, 1996) is the tendency to favor information that confirms our beliefs. If you have interpreted your symptoms as a cold, you will probably interpret new feelings as symptoms of a cold, too.

Another common example is *insomnia*—difficulty falling asleep and staying asleep, nighttime waking, or poor-quality sleep. Between 6% and 15% of the adult population suffers from insomnia, especially under stress. It can occur by itself or in conjunction with other emotional or physical conditions (San & Arranz, 2024). Sleep disturbances, as we saw in Chapter 4, can be detrimental to health and well-being by increasing the risks of accidents, depression, anxiety, and substance abuse (Breslau, Roth, Rosenthal, & Andreski, 1996; Sivertsen, Harvey, Pallesen, & Hysing, 2015). Insomniacs, too, illustrate confirmation bias: They often overestimate how long it took them to fall asleep and underestimate how much time they actually slept. They also subjectively experience poorer-quality sleep than objective indications suggest. They may even report that they were awake when their brain waves demonstrate they were sleeping (Harvey & Tang, 2012). Moreover, insomniacs' misperceptions recur night after night. Once they have been diagnosed with insomnia, any information they take in about their sleep only serves to confirm how poorly they are sleeping.

Confirmation bias suggests that we see what we expect to see. And while it can lead to mislabeling symptoms, illnesses, and well-being, it can also be used to a patient's advantage. For example, if a dentist tells you that filling a cavity will be painless, you may only feel some pressure, and you are more likely not to experience pain at all.

Gathering Information About Symptoms

As we have seen, part of what influences what we perceive and interpret of our symptoms is what we know about illness. We glean this knowledge from our direct experiences, from what we learn from others, and from commonly held beliefs. Through these channels, we form *cognitive representations* of illness— what we picture, imagine, and experience. These representations, or *schemas* (Leventhal et al., 2011), shape how we perceive symptoms, how we experience illness, and whether we seek treatment for it.

One common schema is the distinction between acute illness, chronic illness, and cyclic illness. *Acute illness* has a short duration and few long-term consequences. Usually we think of acute illnesses as caused by bacterial or viral agents. An example of an acute illness is conjunctivitis (pink eye). *Chronic illnesses* are those that have a long timeline, must be managed, and may not be cured. Examples of chronic illness are age-related hearing loss, heart disease, cancer, and Alzheimer's disease. *Cyclic illnesses* are those that come and go— with flare-ups, marked by occasionally debilitating symptoms, and remission. Examples include herpes, migraines, and premenstrual syndrome. Some diseases can fall into more than one category. Rheumatoid arthritis, for example, is a chronic illness, although its symptoms are cyclic. Unfortunately, over time, each period of acute symptoms may last longer. In the late stages of illness, patients may never be without discomfort.

Schemas like these are at the heart of one model of illness. The *common-sense model of illness* (Leventhal, Leventhal, & Contrada, 1998; see Chapter 3) involves four factors that influence how we think about an illness:

- *Illness identity*: The label we place on the disease ("I think I have the flu.")
- *Cause*: Our thoughts about the underlying pathology and cause of the disease ("I have an upset stomach because I ate spicy food.")
- *Timeline*: Our conceptions of the prognosis, or how long the disease will last ("A cold means three days of getting sick, three days of being sick, and three days of getting better.")
- *Consequence*: Our thoughts about the seriousness of the disease, how it will affect our lives, and what its outcomes will be ("I'll miss a few days of school, but I'll be fine by next week.")

Our common-sense ideas provide guidance in the face of unknown symptoms (Petrie & Weinman, 2012). However, they may not be all that detailed or accurate. Typically, people perceive rare illnesses as more severe than common ones. Moreover, people who hold inaccurate models of illness may be less likely to seek treatment or to practice preventive health behaviors, putting themselves at greater risk. For example, if an older woman has no past experience of irregular mammogram results and no family history of breast cancer, she may mistakenly assume that she does not need to have regular mammograms.

Our common-sense models also influence our adherence to treatment and how we live with a diagnosis once we have one (Hekler et al., 2008). Ideally, we rely on credible sources of accurate information (Brooks, Rowley, Broadbent, & Petrie, 2012). When our models are consistent with those of our healthcare providers, our interpretation of symptoms, management of illness, and prognosis for future health are at their best. Most people, however, gather information from family, friends, coworkers, their social network, or the media as well. Our *lay referral network* is an informal network of people who offer their own interpretations of our symptoms (Freidson, 1961).

An outgrowth of the illness perception model and the common-sense model of illness is the Illness Perception Questionnaire (IPQ; Weinman, Petrie, Moss-Morris, & Horne, 1996), a measure that assesses our representations of illness. This scale is useful for understanding people's emotional, cognitive, and behavioral responses to symptoms, as well as their coping efficacy and treatment compliance (Kristoffersen, Lundqvist, & Russell, 2019). The next time you feel sick, take the IPQ in **Table 8.1** (Weinman et al., 1996) and learn about how you interpret your symptoms (Broadbent, Petrie, Main, & Weinman, 2006).

Delay in Seeking Treatment

Delay in treatment seeking can be life-threatening. Early diagnosis and treatment are crucial for conditions from cancer to heart disease. More than 795,000 Americans have a stroke each year, and 130,000 of them will die from it (CDC, 2015a). Of those, 50% die before reaching the hospital. Many others experience rashes, shortness of breath, radiating pain in the chest, skin lesions, seizures, severe headache, dizziness and fainting spells, and diarrhea or gastric distress for months without seeking treatment.

There are many reasons why someone may not seek treatment for serious symptoms (Andersen, Cacioppo, & Roberts, 1995). We have already seen how misinterpretation can lead to not recognizing the severity of symptoms. The time it takes to decide that a symptom is serious is called **appraisal delay**. **Illness delay** refers to the time it takes to interpret the symptoms as an illness and to seek medical treatment. The time between deciding to seek treatment and actually making an appointment is **behavioral delay**. Finally, **medical delay** is the time between making the appointment and receiving treatment from medical professionals.

Sociocultural Differences

Gender and sociocultural differences strongly affect both symptoms and delays. Although women tend to be more aware of sensations and symptoms and are more likely to go to the doctor than men, they tend to wait longer to go to an emergency room than men. Disturbingly, 20–30% of women delay seeking medical help for at least three months after noticing symptoms of breast cancer, for instance (Burgess et al., 2008). At the same time, women tend to have lower thresholds for pain than men do (Fillingim, 2000). This lower pain threshold may be due to gender role socialization and the cultural expectation of men to endure more pain (Alabas, Tashani, & Johnson, 2013; Robinson, Gagnon, Riley, & Price, 2003). Hormones and neuroanatomy may also play a role. One study showed greater activation in regions of the brain in women when subjected to painful stimuli (Fillingim, 2003). More women, and the elderly, also suffer from chronic pain (Melzack, 2001).

Illness Identity (core symptom list)

(Please indicate how frequently you now experience the following symptoms as part of your [illness].)

Ratings: all of the time, frequently, occasionally, never

Pain	Fatigue	Upset stomach
Nausea	Stiff joints	Sleep difficulties
Breathlessness	Sore eyes	Dizziness
Weight loss	Headaches	Loss of strength

We are interested in your own personal views of how you now see your (illness). Please indicate how much you agree or disagree with the following statements about your illness.

Ratings: strongly agree, agree, neither agree nor disagree, disagree, strongly disagree

Cause

A germ or virus caused my illness.

Diet played a major role in causing my illness.

Pollution of the environment caused my illness.

My illness is hereditary—it runs in my family.

It was just by chance that I became ill.

Stress was a major factor in causing my illness.

My illness is largely due to my own behavior.

Other people played a large role in causing my illness.

My illness was caused by poor medical care in the past.

My state of mind played a major part in causing my illness.

Timeline

My illness will last a short time.

My illness is likely to be permanent rather than temporary.

My illness *will* last for a long time.

Consequences

My illness is a serious condition.

My illness has had a major consequences on my life.

My illness has become easier to live with.*

My illness has not had much effect on my life.*

My illness has strongly affected the way others see me.

My illness has serious economic and financial consequences.

My illness has strongly affected the way I see myself as a person.

Control/cure

My illness *will* improve in time.

There is a lot which I can do to control my symptoms.

There is very little that can be done to improve my illness.*

My treatment will be effective in curing my illness.

Recovery from my illness *is* largely dependent on chance or fate.*

What I do can determine whether my illness gets better or worse.

* = Reversed Scoring.

Source: Reprinted by permission of Taylor & Francis Ltd. From "The illness perception questionnaire: A new method for assessing the cognitive representation of illness," by John Weinman, Keith J. Petrie, et al. Psychology and Health 11(3), 1996.

Table 8.1   The illness perception questionnaire

Many cultural differences in symptom recognition and interpretation exist. (The **Around the World** feature investigates different societies' recognition of pain, for instance.) The question of which symptoms of menopause are universally experienced is one example. Some common symptoms are depression, moodiness, hot flashes, night sweats, back and joint pain, fatigue, and headache. Classic Western biomedicine attributes these symptoms to hormones. Yet Japanese women tend to report fewer symptoms (11%) than Chinese or North American women (25%; Shea, 2006), and Asian women may attribute more of the same symptoms to psychological causes (Chun, Enomoto, & Sue, 1996). As another example, a large-scale study of Europeans (including people from France, Austria, Germany, Italy, Poland, Russia, Spain, the Netherlands, and the United Kingdom) age 14–98 revealed that chest pain was the only symptom of heart attack recognized by more than 50% of the participants (Mata, Frank, & Gigerenzer, 2014). Within the United States, symptoms of heart attack typically differ across racial backgrounds (Lee et al., 1999), and African Americans are more likely to delay seeking treatment (Lee et al., 1999).

Social determinants such as financial constraints and limited access to quality health care contribute to cultural differences, which often delay treatment seeking and lead to poorer outcomes. For instance, in ovarian cancer, the most deadly gynecological cancer for women, there are disproportionately higher mortality rates among African American women (Mullins et al., 2018). Compared to European Americans, African Americans also experience more symptoms of chronic pain, sleep disturbances, posttraumatic stress disorder, and depression (Green, Baker, Sato, Washington, & Smith, 2003). Unfortunately, financial constraints have been found in medical delay in elderly people, regardless of cultural background as well (Tan et al., 2019).

Pain is the most compelling symptom that drives people to seek medical attention. Recognizing a symptom, like pain, as serious is a complex and multifaceted process. It begins with interoception, or attention to sensations and perceptions, but also involves experience and what we already know. The illness perception model and our common-sense cognitive representations of illness help to explain this complexity.

Around *the* World

Why Do Americans Experience More Pain?

If pain is in the brain, then the experience of it should be universal, right? Wrong. Apparently, Americans perceive and experience pain differently from people elsewhere in the world (Blanchflower & Oswald, 2017). In response to this question—"During the past four weeks, how often have you had bodily aches or pains: never, seldom, sometimes, often, or very often?"—nearly 34% of Americans said they have pain "often or very often." This is a significantly higher percentage than that of any other country (see **Figure 8.3**). In Australia and Great Britain, the closest "pain" competitors, the average is around 30%. In the Czech Republic, self-reported aches and pains are at a low 8.5%.

What could be causing this difference? While it is important to account for the impact of culture and language on how people think and talk about pain, the overabundance of aches and

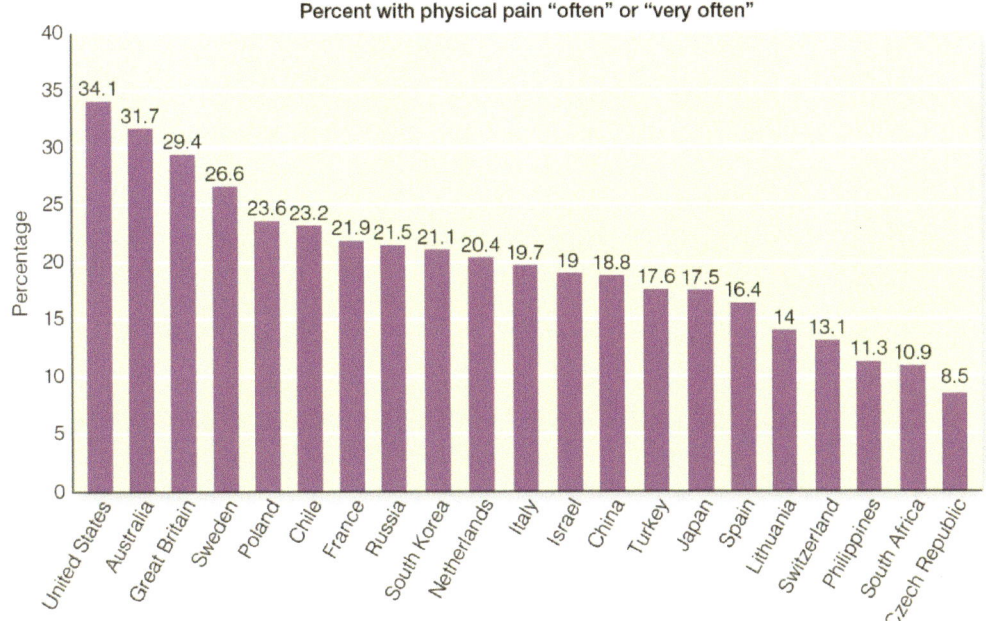

Figure 8.3   Percentage of people who experience physical pain "Often" or "Very Often," by country

Source: Data from ISSP Research Group (2015)

pains that Americans report may result from higher rates of obesity and other physical health problems, comorbid mental health problems such as depression and anxiety, and, paradoxically, a higher dependence on prescription pain medications. Reliance on pain medications may heighten awareness of aches and pains. Over time, people may grow dependent on or tolerant of these medications, meaning that the medications become less effective at managing pain.

Question:

What aspects of U.S. culture may lead to greater experiences of pain? How do comorbid mental and physical health problems lead to greater pain?

Thinking About Health

■ How do prior experiences and sociocultural influences account for differences in symptom recognition?

■ Consider the last time you were ill or in pain. How can you apply the illness perception model and the confirmation bias to your own experiences of symptoms or pain?

■ How does the common-sense model of illness help us understand how people respond to symptoms?

What is Pain?

Pain is a signal. It helps us protect ourselves and survive. Any stimulus that triggers pain receptors can jolt the body into fight or flight—and ensure survival.

Pain is universal, but its expression is not. It is found across nearly all species and is hard-wired into the survival mechanism of all animals. Aside from people with rare disorders in which they feel no pain (called congenital insensitivity to pain), everyone experiences pain. However, once again, individual, biological, contextual, psychosocial, and sociocultural factors all influence the perception of pain.

The Cost of Pain

Pain is the most common medical complaint (Blake, 2019; Fishman, 2007; King & Fraser, 2013; Párraga & Castellanos, 2023) and leads people (such as Natalie, at the start of this chapter) to seek medical treatment more than any other symptom. Roughly 80% of medical visits are motivated by pain (Gatchel, Peng, Peters, Fuchs, & Turk, 2007), and more than 50% of patients with recent injury or surgery report severe to intolerable pain (King & Fraser, 2013; Lipman, 2005). Problems with surgery and trauma can account for up to 25% of the burden of long-lasting chronic pain, affecting one in five adults (King & Fraser, 2013). Natalie's experience attests to this. Extreme pain is associated with many conditions, including multiple sclerosis, cancer, HIV/AIDS, chronic obstructive pulmonary disease, and end-stage organ failure. As we shall see, chronic pain is also a disorder in itself. Nearly 100 million adults in the United States have severe or chronic pain (Gaskin & Richard, 2012).

Pain, especially prolonged pain, can come to overshadow all other aspects of life. It can overwhelm our emotional and physical functioning, sense of self, relationships with others, work, ability to function in society, and our ability to derive meaning from life. Natalie's experiences are an example of how one's life is changed by enduring chronic pain. Chronic pain patients have higher rates of depression and anxiety, and are at greater risk for fatal and nonfatal suicide attempts (Ilgen, 2018). Interestingly, pain carries different weight for the patient and the practitioner. For the practitioner, pain is a symptom of an underlying medical condition. For the patient, the pain *is* the problem. It is what people fear most about illness, medical procedures, dying, and death (Cherny & Foley, 1996).

However, pain is not simply a problem: It *is* a symptom of an underlying medical condition, and no symptom of injury or illness is more important. Its presence increases the odds that a patient will seek timely help, and it guides medical professionals in diagnosis and treatment.

Pain, as we will see, has an enormous impact on society and an enormous cost. At any given time in the United States, more than one third of the population is suffering from pain that requires medical care, and millions of these people end up disabled by their pain (Sherman, Turk, & Okifuji, 2000). The cost of treating chronic pain is $635 billion each year in the United States alone—more than the annual costs of treating cancer, heart disease, and diabetes (American Pain Society, 2014; Gaskin & Richard, 2012). That cost includes treatment, but also missed days of work (anywhere from $11.6 to $12.7 billion), lost hours of productivity (adding up to as much as $96.5 billion), and lower wages (up to $226.3 billion). Americans spend $2.6 billion a year on over-the-counter pain relievers such as Advil, Motrin, aspirin, and Tylenol, plus another $14 billion on prescription pain medications (Krueger & Stone, 2008).

A Subjective Sensation

The scientifically accepted definition of pain is "an unpleasant sensory and emotional experience associated with actual or potential tissue damage, or described in terms of such damage" (International Association for the Study of Pain, 2017). Pain is "whatever the experiencing person says it is, existing whenever he says it does" (Lascaratou, 2007; McCaffery, 1972). However, because pain is a subjective, private sensation, the sensations experienced as pain can vary from person to person and over time.

Pain can be dull and aching, sharp and piercing, pounding or throbbing. It can be *localized*, so that it feels as if it is coming from a specific place. Or it can be generalized and *diffuse*, as when your whole body aches from the flu. Generally, pain from an external impact, such as a stubbed toe, will most often be localized, while pain originating from internal damage or processes, such as fibromyalgia (a disorder affecting the muscles and soft tissues), is often felt as diffuse.

Pain is universal, and all languages have expressions that are uttered in pain. *"Ow"* or *"ouch"* is the sound that most native English speakers use when they experience pain, *"Ay"* is what they say in Lebanon, *"Ahhh"* in Cantonese, and *"Autsch"* in German.

Regardless of the utterance, we know what it feels like when we stub our toe, and we have all experienced different types of pain. Take this description by Fernando Cervero (2012) of one boy's journey through life:

> A three-year-old boy has just fallen off a swing in a playground. He has injured his knee, the skin is torn, and there is a little blood coming from the wound. He cries and cries, because it hurts a lot. His mother gives him a big hug, washes the wound, and applies a little antiseptic. She knows that it is nothing serious and that it will happen again anyway…. The boy will quickly learn that pain is an essential part of life. There will be more scrapes and grazes from playing in playgrounds, falls from bicycles, perhaps even a broken bone. There will be visits to dentists, surgical procedures, injections, and muscle aches. As he grows into adolescence, a girl will break his heart and a different form of pain, invisible but no less real, will also make him cry. Later in life he will suffer from arthritis, heart disease, and perhaps cancer. Physicians will tell him again and again that he must learn to live with his pain. By the end of his life he will have endured a great deal of pain with dignity and resilience. He will know very well that pain is inevitable.

Feeling No Pain

Imagine feeling no pain … even when pricked with a pin or touched with an ice cube. In the rare inherited disorder called congenital insensitivity to pain with anhidrosis (CIPA), there is a complete lack of pain perception, and the nervous system prevents the sensation of pain, heat, cold, and any other sensation transmitted by nerve fibers (Indo, 2012; Shaikh et al., 2017). Patients who have this condition do not feel pain, do not perspire, and may also not be able to feel when they need to urinate. They cannot distinguish between hot and cold and are at constant risk of injuring themselves because, as we know, pain is adaptive to survival. See the **In the News** feature to learn more about the pros and cons of one woman's pain-free existence.

Because of this unique condition, administering pain control like anesthesia during surgery can be problematic (Oliveira, Paris, Pereira, & Lara, 2009). Several studies have reported cases of patients with CIPA having surgical procedures without anesthetics. However, there is still variability in just what they can feel, and some surgical procedures that may not cause pain are still very unpleasant. Surgeons will thus most likely provide anesthesia anyway (Oliveira et al., 2009).

In the News

The Woman Who Feels No Pain

Imagine what it would be like not to know that you'd cut yourself—that is, until your significant other says, "Honey, you're bleeding." Cuts, burns, and even bone fractures have caused no pain for 72-year-old Jo Cameron of Scotland. In fact, birthing a baby without pain medication felt like "a tickle" to Jo (Murphy, 2019). Why? Jo has a previously unidentified genetic mutation that has allowed her to live an essentially pain-free life. She also does not experience anxiety, and cuts and burns do not leave scars (**Photo 8.3**).

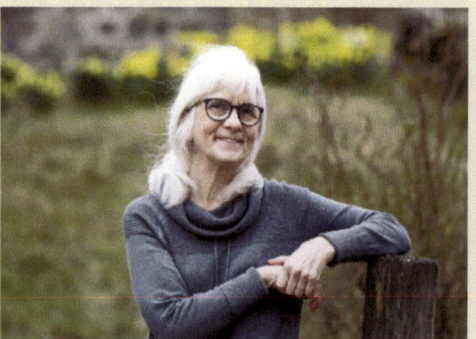

Photo 8.3

Source: Peter Jolly/Shutterstock

Although scientists have been studying people with genetic mutations for painlessness for nearly 100 years, Jo's condition is a new discovery, and has great potential to change the way pain is treated. The gene identified in Jo's condition is called the FAAH-OUT gene. Although all humans have this gene, Jo's DNA has caused the front of the gene to be removed—along with, presumably, the genetic code for pain. By investigating Jo's case, scientists are hoping to further our knowledge of pain relief via gene therapy. Given the urgent need for less addictive pain medications, new research is crucial.

You might think that never experiencing pain or anxiety is a good thing, but Jo's condition does have some down-sides. For one, she is more forgetful than most people, and she frequently loses her train of thought and misplaces her belongings. She also has never experienced the "adrenaline rush" that makes life so exciting. Most important, she does not have the evolutionary advantage of pain—for instance, she did not know that one of her hips had nearly completely degenerated until walking became difficult. Fortunately, when Jo refused pain medication during her recovery from hip surgery, the same astute doctor that treated her referred her to researchers, realizing that her approach to pain was out of the ordinary. And who knows? This simple referral, and the discovery of Jo's genetic mutation, may help shape the future of research into nonaddictive pain treatment.

Question: What are the pros and cons of living a life without pain?

Thinking About Health

■ What is your definition of pain?

■ What is the cost of pain?

■ Why is pain a private experience?

The Physiology of Pain

The experience of pain is adaptive: It protects the organism by bringing tissue damage into conscious awareness. On an unconscious level, the sensations of your body are being processed all the time. You are likely to become aware of some of these sensations when you injure yourself. Yet, other sensations do not make it into your conscious awareness. Think of an athlete continuing to play through the pain of an injury. What determines which sensations are processed as pain?

If you touch a hot stove, a reflex causes you to draw your finger back immediately to protect it from further injury. And to make sure you don't make that mistake again, the brain produces an unpleasant experience—pain—to condition you to be wary of hot stoves in the future. The process arises from interactions among multiple systems, and it is modulated by emotion and cognition (Schwartz & Krantz, 2018). As we shall see, it begins with the sensory neurons in the skin, called *nociceptors*, before traveling through nerve fibers in accordance with the *gate control theory* (Wall, 1978). This process involves emotional and cognitive factors as well as sensory ones.

Nociceptors

The sensation of pain almost always originates from tissue pressure or damage. This is called *organic pain* because it originates in the damaged tissue. Examples of organic pain include a sprained ankle, a broken bone, a burned finger, a migraine headache, a strained back, or childbirth.

Let's start at the beginning. You accidentally touch a hot stove. Immediately, **nociceptors**, or sensory neurons, in the skin pick up the signal from your finger and transmit that information to synapses in the spinal cord—in an area called the *substantia gelatinosa* of the *dorsal horn*, which runs the length of the spinal cord.

What kind of information do they transmit, and how? Nociceptors transmit different kinds of sensory information, including temperature (heat and cold), mechanical damage (say, a cut in the skin), or chemical irritants (such as toxin from a spider bite). The signal, depending on which fiber it comes in on, is either sent up to the brain for further processing, or not. If the pain signal is urgent, it will be transmitted to the brain, and the brain will send an immediate response (remove your hand from the hot burner!). The messages *to* the brain travel along the **afferent pathway**, and the messages *from* the brain travel along the **efferent pathway**.

The Gate Control Theory of Pain

Why are some signals processed, and others not? The **gate-control theory of pain** (Melzack & Wall, 1967; Wall, 1978) proposes that in the dorsal horns of the spinal column there is a "gate mechanism." But how does this gating mechanism work?

You have nociceptors throughout your body—in your skin, muscles, glands, and organs. These receptors pick up sensations as they occur. From there, all sensory information is carried on nerve fibers to the spinal cord. Two types of nerve fibers transmit pain signals to the brain (see **Table 8.2**). **A-delta fibers** are relatively thick fibers responsible for rapidly transmitting intense or sharp or stinging pain. A-delta fibers respond to heat, cold, and pressure. Smaller **C-fibers** are slow nerve fibers that transmit dull, aching, and chronic pain. Both are *afferent* nerves.

A-delta fibers are **myelinated**, or surrounded by a protein sheath that protects them, but C-fibers are not. Myelination is important because the protection it provides allows fibers to transmit messages more quickly. A-delta fibers are likely to process the immediate pain from injury. As that sharp, stinging pain shifts to a continuous throbbing, it begins traveling along the C-fibers. Hours after that first scalding "ouch" from pressure, pinch, cold, or burn, you still have an annoying and continuous reminder of the injury (Schwartz & Krantz, 2018).

The dorsal horn acts as a gate as well as a circuit. Input that is *not* painful closes the gate, blocking transmissions to the brain. Pain messages traveling on the A-delta or C-fibers open the gate so that information can get to the brain. Once the gate is open, such pain messages travel the spinal column and pass through the brain stem, where they may again be modulated. The brainstem inhibits or muffles pain signals by producing the body's natural analgesic, called *endorphins*.

Next, messages from the A-delta fibers reach the thalamus and cerebral cortex, while the duller pain traveling along the C-fibers first travels to the hypothalamus and limbic system. The hypothalamus, as we have seen, is indicated in the stress response, and the limbic system regulates our emotions. In each case, the anterior cingulate cortex in the prefrontal lobe is linked to both the emotional and cognitive elements of the pain experience.

Other fibers in our skin and organs do not carry pain stimuli, but they do help inhibit stimuli. That is why, when you scratch somewhere near a bug bite, it may stop the itching. Your scratch acts as **counterirritation**: It activates the

Type of fiber	Characteristics	Pathway	Pain signal
A-delta fiber	Myelinated, large fibers	Afferent (to the brain)	Fast sharp pain
C-fiber	Unmyelinated, small fibers	Afferent (to the brain)	Burning, dull, or aching pain
A-beta fiber	Myelinated, large fibers	Afferent (to the brain)	Touch, mild irritation

Table 8.2 Types of nerve fibers and their characteristics

thicker *A-beta fibers*, which are decoded as less urgent and close the gate, preventing the message from reaching the brain. In **stimulus-produced analgesia**, an electrical current blocks pain by stimulating the A-beta fibers in much the same way.

The experience of pain is also modulated by brain chemistry. As pain is processed in the central nervous system (CNS) (the spinal cord and brain), it is simultaneously regulated by our body's built-in pain relievers. **Endogenous opioids**, such as endorphins, are neurotransmitters produced in the CNS and the pituitary gland, and they modulate input from the nociceptors in two ways. First, they block calcium influx into the cells. Second, they open the potassium channels in cell membranes (Al-Hasani & Bruchas, 2011). By changing the electrical charge of the cells, they control the transmission of pain impulses into consciousness (Garland, 2012). In this way, they act as naturally produced analgesics. Drugs like morphine bind to the same receptors in the brain, as we shall see.

More Than Injury: The Neuromatrix

The gate can respond to other factors as well. *Physical factors* that may open the gate include the extent of the injury and of physical activity. *Emotional factors* that may open the gate include anxiety, stress, depression, and tension. *Cognitive factors* include attention and boredom. Think of a visit to the dentist. Having your teeth cleaned can be painful, but you know that your dentist is not trying to hurt you, so you submit in order to make your mouth healthy and your smile bright. Because you know the benefits of enduring the dental pain, gating may mute the pain (Davis, Taylor, Crawley, Wood, & Mikulis, 1997). The three factors—physical, emotional, and cognitive—provide input into a dynamic system called the neuromatrix.

The **neuromatrix** (Melzack & Katz, 2004) is a neural network in the brain that synthesizes and integrates information from the senses, along with cognitive and emotional states. It includes specialized areas of the somatosensory cortex, but is distributed over the entire forebrain. We can think of the neuromatrix as an ever-spinning sphere, taking the input from associated brain regions and churning out a **neurosignature**, a distinct pattern that activates systems for pain recognition, motor responses, and emotional reactions.

The two take-home messages are these: First, the experience of pain occurs in the brain and nowhere else (Cervero, 2012). Despite the critical filtering function of the dorsal horns in the spinal column, you experience pain as a function of brain processes. Second, the personality, social, and cultural factors that influence the experience of pain work at the cognitive level.

As you can see in **Figure 8.4**, the neuromatrix is based on cognitive, emotional, and sensory input, and a neurosignature is created that shapes the output. The sensory component is what helps you to recognize a pain sensation. This component is directly linked to nociception and the detection of injurious or harmful stimuli. Evolutionarily speaking, it is the oldest pain function, associated with the ability to sense danger and to produce a fight-or-flight response.

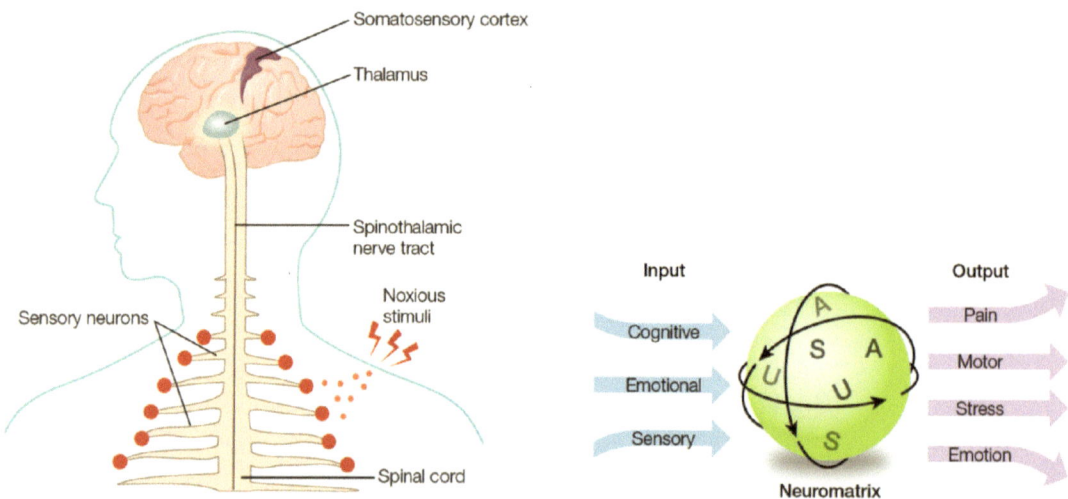

Figure 8.4   Neuromatrix theory of pain. Left to right: a diagram of the neuromatrix model; an illustration of the neuromatrix theory of pain

Source: Information from Melzack (2005)

Probably most animals have this pain experience, but certainly vertebrates and complex invertebrates do (Cervero, 2012).

The second component, the emotional component, is the reaction to the *"Ouch!"* Our heightened emotions make us cry, raise our heart rate and respiration, and make us want to be free of the pain. Primates, dogs, cats, and other higher vertebrates probably have an emotional experience to pain.

The third component of pain, the cognitive component, is uniquely human. Not only do we feel pain and show an instinctive aversion to it, we also worry about the pain we feel (Cervero, 2012). When we are in pain, we want to know why, how it will affect us, how serious it is, and when it will go away. It is the cognitive component of the pain experience that transforms pain into suffering (Cervero, 2012). It is these inputs in various combinations that create the neurosignature and shape the multifaceted experience of pain.

The New Thinking on Pain

You have probably heard the saying, "No pain, no gain." The reality is, "No *brain*, no pain." Pain cannot exist without the brain. Recent research has revised the idea that pain messages are "sent" to the brain, in favor of the view that they are "brain-generated." As we will see in the next section, it is also now widely accepted that chronic pain can rewire the brain. Patients who suffer from chronic pain show structural changes in several brain regions, including the insula, cingulate cortex, prefrontal cortex, somatosensory cortex, and cuneus as well as some subcortical structures like the amygdala and thalamus. The longer the pain lasts, the more it reorganizes the cortical structures of the brain (Torrecillas-Martínez, Catena, O'Valle, Padial-Molina, & Galindo-Moreno, 2019). These structural changes may be influenced by **neurogenic inflammation**, a localized inflammation of the peripheral nervous system (PNS) and the CNS. Neurogenic inflammation is triggered by the activation of nociception, and can be found in illnesses such as asthma and psoriasis (Ji, Nackley, Huh, Terrando, & Maixner, 2018). This pain process is characteristic of acute pain and may explain the clinical disorder of chronic pain.

Other new research ties the gut microbiome to pain. The microbiota-gut-brain axis we learned about within the context of stress in Chapter 6 has been implicated in the experience of pain and pain syndromes as well (Yang et al., 2019). Signaling along the axis allows the brain to shape motor, sensory, autonomic, and hormonal functions within the gastrointestinal track. And, in turn, the gastrointestinal tract modulates brain function for the pain response. **Figure 8.5** shows how this process works in the experience of *visceral pain*, or pain from the internal organs.

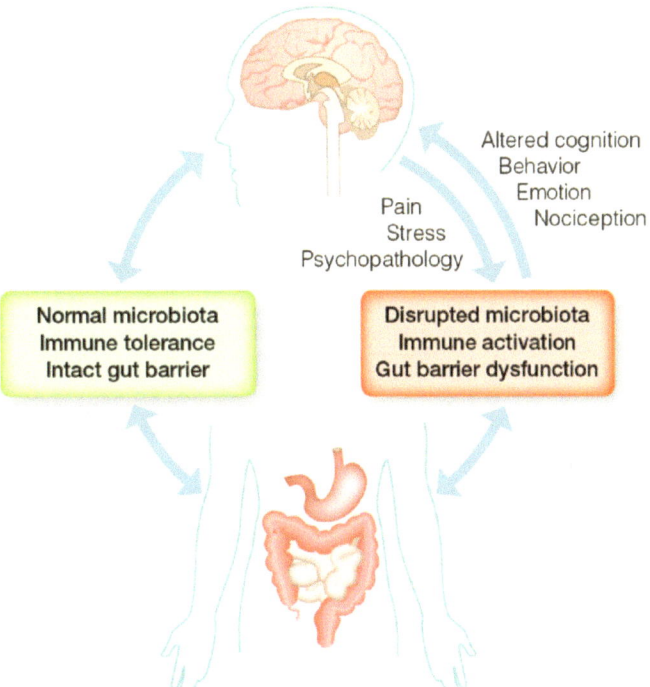

Figure 8.5   Pain response in the microbiota–gut–brain axis

Source: Information from Quigley (2018)

Thinking About Health

■ How do the gate control theory and the neuromatrix model explain how pain is processed?

■ What aspects of pain would you be interested in researching in order to increase our understanding of pain?

Types of Pain

Pain is most often experienced as acute or chronic. Both the intensity of acute pain and the long suffering of chronic pain can take over someone's life. As one patient cried out, "There are two kinds of pain: mine, which is always real, and yours, which is nothing but a lot of complaining" (quoted in Cervero, 2012).

Acute and Chronic Pain

Acute pain is the pain you feel upon injuring yourself. Like an acute illness, acute pain is generally intense but short term and temporary. A broken bone is most painful right after the break. The pain lessens over time, as the bone begins to heal, and the swelling and bruising in the tissue around it begin to subside. The pain associated with a surgical or dental procedure is also acute, as is the pain associated with the flu or a stomach virus. Acute pain can cause anxiety or depression; it can enter all aspects of a person's life. Still, acute pain tends to dissipate in a matter of minutes, hours, days, weeks, or months, leading to no lasting problems.

Chronic pain is unrelenting, continuing day after day for more than 6 months. Like acute pain, it can begin with an injury, but it does not so easily lessen in response to treatment or time. And the longer it lasts, the more of a psychological impact it has. Sufferers, like Natalie at this chapter's outset, often feel helpless, especially when medical treatments do not alleviate the pain. Moreover, the psychological distress can complicate diagnosis and treatment, magnifying the sensations of pain and pain-related behaviors (Bair, Wu, Damush, Sutherland, & Kroenke, 2008; Burns et al., 2008). There are different types of chronic pain; see **Table 8.3**.

Acute pain and chronic pain involve different areas of the brain. Although many higher brain regions are involved in the processing of pain, acute pain is associated with the anterior insular cortex and the anterior cingulate cortex. In functional magnetic resonance imaging (fMRI) research, these two areas of

Type of pain	Characteristics	Examples
Chronic benign	Lasts 6 months or longer Unresponsive to treatment May vary in severity May involve different muscle groups	Chronic lower back pain
Recurrent acute	Acute episodes Pain-free periods in between Episodes recur over 6 months or more	Herpes Migraine headaches Myofascial pain syndrome Trigeminal neuralgia
Chronic progressive	Lasts longer than 6 months Increases in severity over time	Typically associated with a degenerative disease (arthritis) or malignancies (cancer)

Table 8.3   Types of pain and their characteristics

the prefrontal cortex light up when a subject's forearm is subjected to a painful application of heat. In contrast, and as we have seen, chronic pain can literally change your brain (Cervero, 2012). In imaging studies, patients with chronic lower back pain showed a reduction in the gray matter of the thalamus (an important area for sensory processing) as well as a reduction of gray matter in the prefrontal cortex (areas associated with cognitive and emotional processing of pain). These same patterns of loss of gray matter are seen in patients suffering from neuropathic pain, fibromyalgia, migraine, and irritable bowel syndrome. Overall, we can see changes in brain structure and function in the transition from acute to chronic pain (Guo, Wang, Sun, & Wang, 2016).

In addition to structural changes, there are biochemical alterations in the brains of these chronic-pain patients as well. There is a reduction in the levels of both serotonin and dopamine, the neurotransmitters in the brain's reward systems. We still do not know whether the structural changes lead to the development of chronic pain, or whether chronic pain leads to structural changes in the brain. Nevertheless, someday we may diagnose chronic pain with an fMRI, much as we diagnose heart disease with an electrocardiogram.

Pain can often linger, or even worsen, after surgery, as it did for Natalie. Sometimes the surgery itself seems to trigger chronic pain. For example, many adult men undergo surgery to repair an *inguinal hernia*—a protrusion of the abdominal cavity into the groin. However, chronic pain after surgery is found in up to 54% of these men, and 30% still have chronic pain one year later (Poobalan et al., 2003). Although risk factors for acute pain immediately after surgery include a younger age, the type of surgical repair, and higher body mass index, an individual's personality again plays a part (Powell, Liossi, Moss-Morris, & Schlotz, 2013). Those with an optimistic attitude toward the surgery and a higher sense of control over the pain seem to do best.

The body's response to pain can also make the difference. After an automobile accident, for example, someone might compensate for the pain of broken ribs with a posture that puts added pressure on the neck and shoulders (Flor, 2012; Glombiewski, Tersek, & Rief, 2008). The very attempt to suppress the acute pain can then lead to chronic pain (**Photo 8.4**) (Flor, 2012).

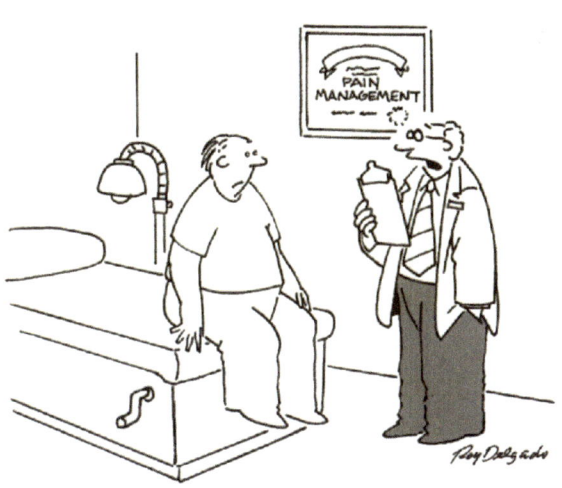

" Have you tried enjoying the aches and pains ? "

Photo 8.4   "Have you tried enjoying the aches and pains?"

Source: Roy Delgado

Living with Chronic Pain

Chronic pain is pervasive. In 2021, more than 20.9% of U.S. adults (51.6 million people) have experienced chronic pain (Rikard et al., 2023). Seventy to 85% of Americans suffer from chronic back pain at some point in their lives (Oz, 2011). For nearly 7% or 17 million adults the pain is "high-impact" and results in substantial restrictions of their lives and daily activities (Rikard et al., 2023). High impact pain is highest in non-Hispanic indigenous Americans and those who identify as bisexual. One of every 10 people have migraines, and more than 14 million people (including children) experience migraine on a near-daily basis (Migraine Research Foundation, 2016). Arthritis pain is also pervasive. Osteoarthritis affects 27 million Americans, and rheumatoid arthritis affects 1.3 million Americans (Barbour et al., 2013).

Patients with chronic pain are four times more likely to suffer from anxiety and depression (Lohman, Schleifer, & Amon, 2010). They may also have lower pain thresholds (Sherman et al., 2004), and may develop maladaptive ways to cope with the pain and the impact it has on their lives. They may magnify their distress and amplify their pain (Tennen, Affleck, & Zautra, 2006), or they may turn to wishful thinking and withdrawal (Severeijns, Vlaeyen, van den Hout, & Picavet, 2004). Because chronic pain is harder to relieve, sufferers are more likely to seek treatment than patients with acute pain.

Living with chronic pain can disrupt all aspects of a person's life. Like Natalie, many people with chronic pain may have to give up their professional goals and income, which, in turn, exacerbates the pain (Rios & Zautra, 2011). Leisure activities may fall by the wayside. Those with chronic pain may feel the dilemma of having to depend on others, but not wanting to be a burden, causing relationships to suffer (Smith, 2003). As sleep, self-esteem, and quality of life decline, patients may also suffer from chronic fatigue. Over time, they may develop an entirely new lifestyle around their pain. Even if the pain is successfully treated or subsides, the emotional and behavioral changes may remain.

Referred and Psychogenic Pain

Pain takes many forms. **Referred pain** originates from tissue damage, but is experienced in another part of the body. An example is the experience of pain running up the left arm during a myocardial infarction (heart attack). How can that be?

One explanation is that the pain signals from the site of injury are carried to the spinal cord, where they converge with information coming from elsewhere. For example, many people who have a gallbladder attack experience pain in the right shoulder and back. The sensory fibers from the gallbladder enter the spinal cord, as does stimulation along the pathways from the skin. The two signals get confused.

Psychogenic pain may not originate in damaged tissue at all, but rather psychological processes. Some stress headaches, queasy stomachs, or muscle cramps can be caused by tension, anxiety, worry, or depression. Medical examinations may not be able to determine the source of the pain, but it is real for those who suffer from it.

Neuropathic Pain

In **neuropathic pain**, the nerve fibers themselves become damaged and begin to send incorrect signals to the pain centers of the brain. This can result from disease or from damage to the PNS. In an epidemiological survey of a small U.S. community, 9.8% of people had been diagnosed with neuropathic pain (Yawn et al., 2009).

There are three types of neuropathic pain: *neuralgia, causalgia,* and *phantom limb syndrome.* Each originates from some initial trauma, injury, disease, or surgery, but the pain persists long after that initial cause has healed. The pain may even intensify over time and spread to different locations of the body.

Neuralgia is characterized by intense, and often sudden, episodes of extreme pain. Patients typically describe it as severe, sharp, superficial, piercing, or burning. For example, the International Association for the Study of Pain defines the pain of trigeminal neuralgia (spasms of the facial muscles) as "a sudden, usually unilateral, severe, brief, stabbing, recurrent pain in the distribution of one or more branches of the fifth cranial nerve" (Zakrzewska, 2002). Attacks like these can be brought on by such everyday activities as eating or chewing food, talking, brushing teeth, or washing one's face. Some neuralgia can emerge as a result of viral infections such as shingles (*herpes zoster*).

Causalgia, or *complex regional pain syndrome,* is recurrent, episodic pain that results from severe trauma, such as gunshot and stab wounds, burns, frostbite, surgery, muscular injections, and blood drawing, and such illnesses as diabetes, stroke, or multiple sclerosis. The pain persists long after the wound, if any, has healed. Causalgia most often affects the upper extremities, usually the hand. The patient will experience burning pain, muscle spasms or weakness, coldness in the extremities, slowed hair growth, and brittle or cracking nails. In time, the skin may turn pale, shiny, and blue, accompanied by limited joint movement and muscle loss.

As many as 60–80% of people who lose a limb experience *phantom limb syndrome,* sensations in the limb that is no longer there. People who have had a breast, tooth, or eye removed may experience this phenomenon as well. The pain can be intense and debilitating (Sherman, 1994). Phantom limb pain is usually intermittent, experienced as tingling, itching, burning, aching, or cramping, and can increase with anxiety and stress. Twenty-two-year-old Kristy Mason lost her right arm just below the elbow at the age of 18 when she blacked out and fell onto the tracks ahead of an incoming train. The wheel of the train severed her arm. In her phantom limb, she says that she feels "my fist clenching, my fingernails digging in. I can see the hand isn't there but the sensation is so realistic."

What accounts for phantom limb pain? The best explanation is that the brain has a representation of the limb before the loss, and that neural representation does not fade after. One study used fMRI to measure changes in blood flow during brain activity (Makin et al., 2013). The study asked hand amputees, people born without a hand, and two-handed people to move

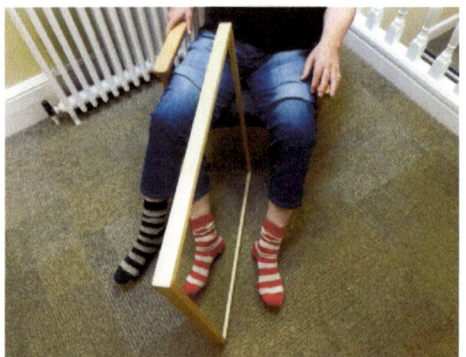

Photo 8.5   This person is demonstrating V.S. Ramachandran's therapeutic mirror box, which has proven helpful in treating phantom limb pain

Source: Annegret Hagenberg

their hands while inside the scanner. Amputees with phantom pain had the same brain activity during movement as people with two intact hands.

One promising treatment for phantom pain is the mirror box (Ramachandran & Rogers-Ramachandran, 1996; Ramachandran, Rogers-Ramachandran & Cobb, 1995). This therapy uses the mirror image of the remaining limb to replace visual input from the missing limb. As the patient unclenches the actual fist, the image tricks the brain into thinking that the phantom limb is releasing its tension, too (**Photo 8.5**).

Thinking About Health

■ How do the types of pain differ?

■ What are the difficulties experienced by those who live with chronic pain?

■ What experiences of referred and psychogenic pain have you had in your own life?

■ If you or someone you know has experienced neuropathic pain, how has the pain shaped your or their life?

Measuring Pain

Although the *experience* of pain is what drives people to seek treatment, physicians are most often concerned with identifying a *cause* for the pain. And that begins with measuring and assessing pain. But how? For a physician, a "throbbing" pain may have different implications than a "continuous dull ache." That, however, is only a start.

Think about it: If a patient has a dark mole with irregular boundaries that's increasing in size, skin cancer is easy to diagnose. If the patient presents a fever, a sudden sore throat, yellow blisters in the back of the throat, and difficulty swallowing, strep throat is clear. What if the patient complains of severe pain below the ribs that comes in waves and fluctuates in intensity? It may take the physician a bit of exploration to come to a diagnosis of kidney stones. Visceral pain is often challenging to diagnose. The questions facing researchers are even harder.

Tools for Measuring Pain

The most widely used tool to describe and measure pain is the McGill Pain Questionnaire (Melzack & Torgerson, 1971). This questionnaire allows patients to provide their doctor with a good description of the quality and intensity of the pain they are experiencing, and it draws on the vast language that we have to

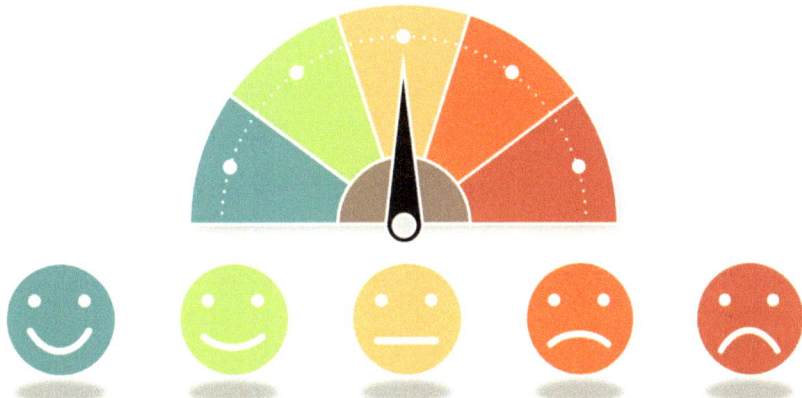

Figure 8.6   Example of a FACES Pain Rating Scale

describe pain (Melzack, 1975). Pain is assessed along several dimensions. The sensory dimension includes information on the location, intensity, quality, and pattern of the pain. The affective dimension assesses the emotions associated with the experience of pain (fear, depression, anxiety). The cognitive dimension probes the overall appraisal of pain. Finally, the behavioral dimension looks at the actions that aggravate or alleviate the pain. Research has shown that the measure is highly reliable, and, in fact, patients with the same pain syndromes choose the same words to describe their pain (Melzack, 1975). This questionnaire has been translated into many languages and should be administered in the patient's native language.

Other pain measures do not require language proficiency and are widely used with children. The Wong-Baker FACES Pain Rating Scale is one example (Wong-Baker FACES Foundation, 2009). Variations on the Wong-Baker faces (see **Figure 8.6**) are often presented with numeric ratings that help people to quantify their pain. This tool is now widely used in healthcare settings, with nurses and doctors asking patients to use the faces as a barometer of their pain over the course of their hospital stay.

In addition to describing pain, patients often look like they are in pain or respond with pain-related behaviors when the sore spot is touched. Walking with a limp, a wincing look, and saying "*Ouch* "when touched are all clues to what hurts. Medical professionals can use our pain behaviors as a diagnostic tool. An example of a pain behaviors assessment measure, seen in **Table 8.4**, is the Checklist of Nonverbal Pain Indicators (**Photo 8.6**) (Feldt, 2000).

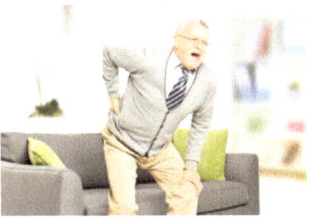 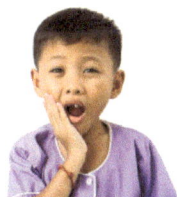 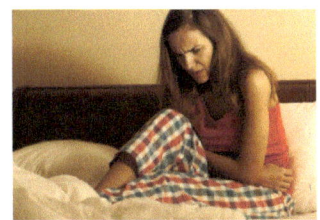

Photo 8.6   Pain is often observable. It can also be determined via self-report, such as questionnaires and scales, and behaviors, such as touch

Instructions: Observe the patient for the following behaviors both at rest and during movement.

Behavior	With movement	At rest

1. Vocal complaints: nonverbal (sighs, gasps, moans, cries)
2. Facial grimaces/winces (furrowed brow, narrowed eyes, clenched teeth, tightened lips, jaw drop, distorted expressions)
3. Bracing (clutching or holding onto furniture, equipment, or affected area during movement)
4. Restlessness (constant or intermittent shifting of position, rocking, intermittent or constant hand motions, inability to keep still)
5. Rubbing (massaging affected areas)
6. Vocal complaints: verbal (words expressing discomfort or pain ["ouch," "that hurts"]; cursing during movement; exclamations of protests ["stop," "that's enough"])

Subtotal Scores

Totals

Scoring: Score a 0 if the behavior was not observed. Score a 1 if the behavior occurred even briefly during activity or at rest. The total number of indicators is summed for the behaviors observed at rest, with movement, and overall. There are no clear cut-off scores to indicate severity of pain. Instead, the presence of any of the behaviors may be indicative of pain, warranting further investigation, treatment, and monitoring by the practitioner.

Source: Information from Feldt (2000) and Horgas (2003).

Table 8.4   Checklist of nonverbal pain indicators

The Elusive Meaning of Pain

We are still teasing apart the mystery of pain. Neuroscience is shedding light on what is going on in the brain, but pain is always both a physiological and a psychological process. When we experience pain, we imbue it with context and meaning, both of which influence the experience.

We have seen how personality, emotions, and social factors influence pain perception. A physician named Henry Beecher directly observed these factors during World War II. Beecher compared soldiers wounded in battle and civilians he treated after the war. Once off the battlefield and in the relative safety of the military hospital, many soldiers were euphoric—even those with severe injuries. Knowing that they would most likely be discharged and sent home, they displayed disregard for their injuries and experienced less pain than would have been expected given the extent of tissue damage (Beecher, 1946). Only 32% of these soldiers requested morphine for pain relief. In contrast, civilian patients undergoing routine surgical procedures displayed the opposite pattern—more than 83% of those with relatively minor tissue damage and pain requested pain relief (Beecher, 1956).

For the wounded soldiers, pain meant being alive and an end to battle. For civilian surgical patients, pain meant the beginning of a lengthy recovery. "There is no simple, direct relationship between the wound per se and the pain experienced," Beecher observed. "The pain is in very large part determined by other factors, and of great importance here is the *significance* of the wound" to the patient (Beecher, 1959, 165; cited in Morley & Vlaeyen, 2010). Beecher concluded that there was no dependable relationship between the extent of the wound and the pain experienced. Rather, the magnitude of suffering is primarily determined by *what pain means to the patient* (Beecher, 1956).

Thinking About Health

- Which methods of measuring pain are most useful for healthcare providers?
- How can Beecher's research on pain be applied, both on and off the battlefield?

Treating Pain

When we are in pain, the most immediate concern is ending the pain. If it is a headache, muscle strain, or gastric distress, we usually go to the medicine cabinet and see if there is something there that we can take. *Pain management* or *pain control* includes any effort to relieve or lessen the pain.

Pain control comes in many forms. Analgesics range from aspirin to narcotics. These act at different locations in the CNS to block the pain signals from being processed in the brain. Drugs for anxiety and depression also chemically alter the experience of pain. Surgical pain control involves lesioning the fibers conducting pain signals to the brain, but it is extreme and risky. Electrical stimulation of the spinal column can close the gate against pain signals. Psychosocial pain control includes exercise, which has the most scientific support, and biofeedback and relaxation techniques.

Pharmacological Treatments

By far, the most common method for treating pain comes in the form of a pill. Pain medications are used to relieve the discomfort associated with injury, disease, surgery, or other causes. **Table 8.5** lists some of the many *analgesics*, or drugs used to treat pain.

Common over-the-counter pain medicines include acetaminophen (Tylenol) and nonsteroidal anti-inflammatory drugs (NSAIDs; aspirin, Aleve, Motrin). Acetaminophen relieves headaches, fever, and other common aches and pains, but does not reduce inflammation. NSAIDs reduce inflammation as well, so they are good for arthritis. These analgesics will help with everything from the common cold to tennis elbow, from toothaches to muscle sprains. Some kinds of pain medications work better for some types of pain, and what helps take away *your* pain may not work for your best friend.

Prescription pain medications are prescribed by a physician or medical specialist. The drug and dosage are carefully considered, based on the patient's age, weight, medical history, and needs. Morphine, sold under nearly 100 different trade names, is a derivative of opium and is a very powerful opioid analgesic

Drug class	Drug name	Treatment	How it works
Nonsteroidal anti-inflammatory drugs (NSAIDs)	Aspirin, ibuprofen, naproxen	Available over the counter for everyday aches and pains: headaches, coughs and colds, sports injuries or muscle spasms, arthritis, menstrual cramps.	Acts as an analgesic that also brings down inflammation and swelling.
Corticosteroids	Cortisone, prednisone, methylprednisolone	Prescribed by a medical professional. Administered locally by injection, eye drops, ear drops, skin creams, or orally. Can be used for musculoskeletal injuries, lupus, rheumatoid arthritis.	Decreases inflammation and reduces the activity of the immune system (white blood cells).
Opioids (narcotic analgesics)	Codeine, Vicodin, Demerol, morphine, OxyContin, Percocet	Prescribed by a medical professional. Used to treat serious pain from surgery, injury, or chronic pain.	Modifies pain messages in the brain. Binds to opioid receptors in the brain, spinal cord, and other areas. Reduces or mutes pain messages to the brain.
Muscle relaxants	Soma, Flexeril, Valium	Prescribed by a medical professional. Used to treat back pain and muscle spasms.	Reduces the muscle tension that accompanies pain through sedation in the CNS.
Anti-anxiety drugs	Xanax, Valium, Atavan, Klonopin	Prescribed by a medical professional. Used to treat anxiety and pain.	Reduces anxiety, relaxes muscles, and helps the patient cope with discomfort. Relieves anxiety and pain by slowing down the CNS.
Antidepressants	Amitriptyline, amoxapine, desipramine, imipramine	Prescribed by a medical professional. Traditionally used to treat major depression but can be beneficial in chronic pain.	Reduces pain message transmission in spinal cord. Blocks the absorption (reuptake) of neurotransmitter serotonin in the brain.
Anticonvulsant drugs (anti-epileptic drugs)	Topamax, Trileptal, Tegretol, Lyrica	Prescribed by a medical professional. Traditionally used to treat epilepsy and epileptic seizures, but have been found to reduce neuropathic pain.	Thought to relieve the pain of neuropathies by stabilizing nerve cells. Suppresses the excessive firing of neurons.

Source: Information from WebMD.com (2017).

Table 8.5   Types of drugs, what they treat, and how they work

(and narcotic) drug. Morphine is a potent pain reliever because it works swiftly and acts directly on the CNS. It works like the endogenous opioids, and it is highly effective for treating severe pain. Morphine is given to patients undergoing surgery and postoperatively for pain management. It is also used to treat some chronic and severe pain conditions, such as cancer-related pain.

The Narcotics Controversy The use of narcotics to control pain is controversial, as we saw with Natalie at the start of the chapter. Many patients in extreme pain are thus left undermedicated because the most effective pain control drugs—narcotics—are not prescribed. For example, imagine the survivor of an automobile accident who suffers perforated lungs, broken ribs, and a fractured femur. Or imagine a patient diagnosed with lung cancer that has metastasized to the liver and bones, or an HIV-positive parent of five who has just been diagnosed with tuberculosis.

These cases have much in common (King & Fraser, 2013). First, their conditions are *global* health problems and priorities. Second, these people are all likely to experience a great deal of pain. More than 5 million cancer patients, 1 million terminal HIV/AIDS patients, and nearly 1 million trauma patients worldwide have little or no access to treatment for their pain—and these are conservative estimates (King & Fraser, 2013; WHO, 2009b). Given the growth and aging of the world's population, the burdens of chronic diseases like HIV/AIDS will only grow, as will the prevalence of untreated pain (Taylor, 2007).

There is a growing conviction that freedom from unnecessary pain is a basic human right, and that the extent of untreated or undermedicated pain in the world today represents a "global health catastrophe" (King & Fraser, 2013). Current pain medications are highly effective and, in high-income countries, readily available and affordable. In fact, opioids are so widely effective that they have been on the WHO Model Lists of Essential Medicines since 1986 (WHO, 2017e). Yet inequities in the availability of pain medication are well-documented, both within the United States and around the world (King & Fraser, 2013).

What lies behind this global epidemic? Pain management is not just a medical issue, but is also subject to national and international law. Because most opioid pain relievers are narcotics, they are heavily regulated. Illicit narcotics (such as opium and heroin) and drugs used for medical and scientific purposes (such as morphine and codeine) are all regulated—and for two reasons.

First, pain medications are often sold on the black market, where they become a significant part of the illicit drug trade. Second, under certain circumstances, morphine and other narcotic pain relievers are addictive. Users may "doctor shop" (illegally deceive multiple doctors to receive overlapping prescriptions) to feed their drug dependence. Like heroin, morphine use can lead to *tolerance*, which means that higher doses are needed to relieve pain as the body becomes habituated to the drug. Rush Limbaugh, the conservative talk show host, has been addicted to OxyContin and other painkillers. Actress Nicole Richie, rapper Eminem, and actor Charlie Sheen also have sought treatment for dangerous addictions to painkillers.

Because of the legal scrutiny they face, many physicians are cautious and concerned about prescribing pain medication, even when their patients may, in fact, need it. Careful patient supervision can ensure that a prescription is being used as dictated and that the patient is safely medicated. A physicians' advisory board also provides training to help identify and protect against illegal drug seeking. Doctors learn about the possibility of patients' illegally sharing drugs or carrying pain medications without proper identification; the risks of prescription pain medications; street gangs that steal patient medications and identities to get prescriptions; and the need for patients to sign an agreement that they understand the law.

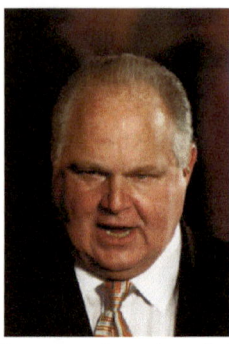 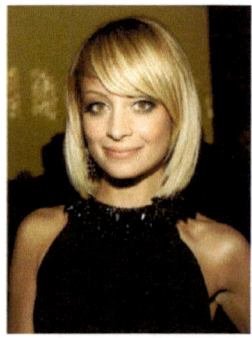 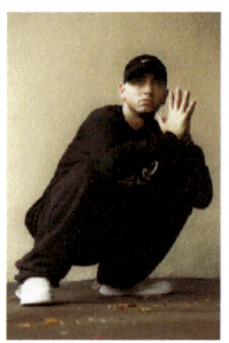 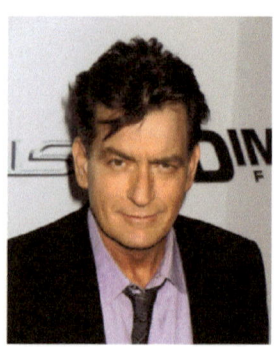

Photo 8.7   A number of celebrities have been addicted to pain medication (left to right: Rush Limbaugh, Nicole Richie, Eminem, Charlie Sheen)

Source: left to right: AP photo/Ron Edmonds, KMazur/Getty Images, Gary Friedman/Getty Images, and Jettrey Mayer/Getty Images

The good news is that several factors can actually prevent true addiction. When rats are forced into addiction to morphine and then given enough space, good food, companionship, areas for exercise, and opportunities to mate and raise litters, many overcame their addictions and chose not to ingest the drug (Xu, Hou, Gao, He, & Zhang, 2007). The same may be true of humans (**Photo 8.7**).

Human patients in acute pain, too, are less likely to overmedicate while in proper medical settings (Citron et al., 1986). **Patient-controlled analgesia** allows the patient to control the flow of pain relief, usually morphine, through an intravenous line. The patient can determine when to dose to get immediate relief. In men hospitalized with severe cancer pain, their morphine use declined over two days (Citron et al., 1986; Tyler, 1990). Patients in severe pain may initially use more medication, but they also get the pain relief they need quickly (Hudcova, McNicol, Quah, Lau, & Carr, 2006). In sum, when morphine is used for only a short time, abuse should not be a concern.

Surgical Pain Control

Although it has a long history, surgical pain control is still a radical approach. It involves severing (or lesioning) the pain fibers that transmit the pain messages to the brain. Surgery may be done along the pathway from the nociceptors to the spinal cord or between the spinal cord and the brain. There are other surgical techniques as well. For example, heat can be surgically applied to the trigeminal nerve, glycerol rhizotomy involves injecting glycerol to kill nerve fibers and disrupt pain transmission, and stereotactic radiation therapy involves using computer-guided radiation to destroy targets of pain transmission in nerves. These procedures are risky and in many cases do not lead to lasting pain relief (Turk & Winter, 2005). Natalie, for instance, tried an experimental neurosurgery procedure, and was devastated when the pain returned after surgery. There may be significant side effects as well, including numbness, paralysis, and phantom limb syndrome. Surgery can actually worsen chronic pain by further damaging the CNS. It is also expensive.

One method of surgical pain control does not involve severing nerve fibers. *Synovectomy*, used to treat chronic arthritic pain, involves removing inflamed membranes found in the joints. Thus far, it is the only surgical procedure with a solid track record for relieving pain.

Sensory Pain Control

As we learned, pain signals must pass through the dorsal horn of the spinal column. Some signals open the gate, and others close it. Counterirritation, like scratching just next to a bug bite, aims to close the gate and to block out pain signals.

More generally, *counterirritation* involves a competing stimulation to inhibit pain. Even a mild electrical current can close the gate against the pain in another location (North, Kidd, Farrokhi, & Piantadosi, 2005). **Spinal cord stimulation** places electrodes where pain signals enter the spinal cord. It is an effective treatment for a wide range of conditions, including pain from failed back surgery, heart disease (angina pectoris), diabetes, and peripheral nerve damage. This technique has been shown to inhibit pain and improve quality of life for chronic pain sufferers (de Vos et al., 2014).

In another experiment, subjects were given mild electrical stimulation to evoke a nociceptive response—the trigger for pain. At the same time, they placed a foot in an ice bath. The counterirritation of the cold water dulled the pain of the electrical stimulation (Piché, Arsenault, & Rainville, 2009). The researchers could even identify the brain regions affected—the somatosensory cortex, the anterior cingulate cortex, and the amygdala (**Photo 8.8**).

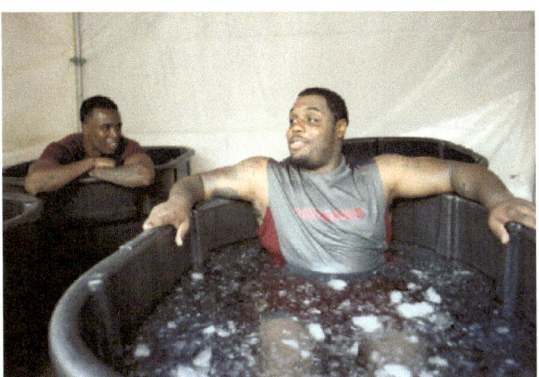

Photo 8.8 *Cryotherapy*, an ice bath, is among the most effective, inexpensive, and simple ways to manage sports injuries (Algafly & George, 2007). Ice baths reduce inflammation and swelling, and they significantly reduce pain. It is not just a matter of counterirritation from the extreme cold. Ice water also dampens the conductance of pain messages in the nerve fibers (Algafly & George, 2007). This photo from July 2012 shows two football players in ice baths

Source: The Washington Posr/Getty Images

Psychological Pain Control

Pain is a biopsychosocial process. The physical, cognitive, and emotional response to pain shapes our experience of it. No wonder that biofeedback, relaxation, and exercise are all useful in coping with pain.

Biofeedback allows patients to gain more control over such normally involuntary functions as heart rate, skin temperature, and blood pressure. It can prevent or treat migraine headaches, chronic pain, high blood pressure, and incontinence. Biofeedback involves *operant*, or behavioral, conditioning: by learning to harness the power of the mind, one can gain more control over pain.

In a typical biofeedback session, electrodes on the patient's skin emit a sound, a flash of light, or an image of the bodily function to be brought under conscious control. That function could be heart rate, blood pressure, breathing, or sweating. The patient then practices deep breathing, muscle relaxation exercises, or guided imagery. Eventually, the patient will be able to evoke the pain relief by practicing this alone.

Neurofeedback, a form of biofeedback, teaches patients to gain control over their brain states while monitoring biofeedback from the brain. Electroencephalography, a kind of brain wave monitoring, is used to examine brain abnormalities or unusual electrical activity. Electrodes on the scalp detect electrical charges from the firing of the brain cells and can be displayed in real time on a computer.

In neurofeedback training sessions, patients are taught to monitor their brain waves and to adjust their breathing or heart rate to achieve more relaxed brain activity (Jensen et al., 2013). Unfortunately, neurofeedback has not been consistently and significantly successful in reducing chronic pain.

Relaxation Techniques: Patients may use relaxation techniques to cope with the discomfort of pain. Focusing on relaxing the muscles may dispel pain and tension, as in biofeedback.

Relaxation works by placing the body in a state of lowered arousal, so that the pain signals will be less intense. In a procedure called progressive muscle relaxation, patients are taught to focus on each area of the body, from the toes to the top of the head. They work their way up the body, tensing and then releasing the muscles in each region. This helps patients become aware of the tension in their bodies and to systematically release it. Though relaxation may be helpful when one is experiencing acute pain, it is less effective for chronic pain (**Photo 8.9**).

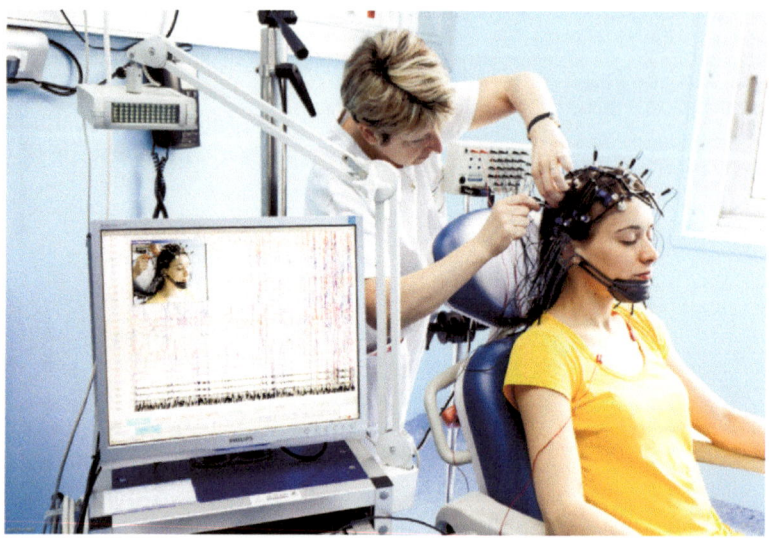

Photo 8.9   Neurofeedback, a form of biofeedback, trains patients to calm their brain activity to reduce pain. More scientific evidence is needed to determine its efficacy

Source: PHANIE AGENCY/Science Source

Mindfulness, which we learned about in the context of coping with stress (Chapter 7), can also be effective in managing pain. Research shows that people who are dispositionally mindful—having a tendency to be present in the moment—feel less pain (Zeidan et al., 2018). Similarly, mindfulness meditation has been found to be helpful in pain management. Pain and meditation seem to involve similar brain regions—those involved in the sensory, affective, and cognitive aspects of subjective experience (Cahn & Polich, 2006; Koyama, McHaffie, Laurienti, & Coghill, 2005; Zeidan et al., 2011)—and there is evidence that mindfulness meditation helps to close the gate on pain processing (Zeidan et al., 2011). When participants in one study were placed in an fMRI scanner and trained to engage in mindfulness meditation to reduce pain, both the intensity and the unpleasantness of pain were reduced, and relaxation increased (Zeidan et al., 2011). This empirical evidence suggests that mindfulness and mindfulness meditation may be very helpful for patients in pain.

The opposite of mindfulness might be distraction. Some research suggests that the distraction of playing video games dampens the pain experience (Gordon, Merchant, Zanbaka, Hodges, & Goolkasian, 2011). Interactive gaming may command attentional resources away from pain, though more research is needed to be able to explain the mechanisms of this effect (Gordon et al., 2011).

Exercise and Pain Control: Back pain, one of the most common problems in industrialized societies, can be effectively treated with a simple change in lifestyle: exercise! A focus on improving spinal flexibility reduces pain intensity and disability. Exercise can also improve conditioning, strength, and endurance. It also makes people feel good.

Pain sensitivity decreases after high-intensity aerobic exercise, such as running and cycling (Koltyn, 2002), and the pain reduction continues after exercise. Not only does exercise dampen pain throughout the body, but exercising the body part that is injured (when it is safe to do so) can also reduce the pain sensations in the injured area (Vaegter, Handberg, & Graven-Nielsen, 2014). Even isometric exercises (weight lifting or resistance training) can help. The more intense the exercise, the more the pain is reduced, though this effect is greater in women than men (Vaegter et al., 2014).

Exercise influences the pain modulation system in several ways. First, it helps remove the cytokines that promote inflammation. By reducing inflammation, it reduces pain. Second, exercise produces endogenous opioids, the body's natural analgesic, that numb the pain (as with "runner's high"). And exercise has been shown to increase levels of serotonin, dopamine, and noradrenalin, which elevate mood and reduce anxiety and depression (Mazzardo-Martins et al., 2010).

For patients with osteoarthritis, any exercise is beneficial. Osteoarthritis, a degenerative joint disorder, is the leading cause of disability worldwide, especially in the elderly (Tanaka, Ozawa, Kito, & Moriyama, 2013). A recent meta-analysis examined a wide range of exercises, including muscle-strengthening exercises (both non-weight-bearing and weight-bearing), balance exercises, aerobic exercise, and stretching and range-of-motion exercises. All were found to lead to pain reduction (Tanaka et al., 2013). Short-term interventions with non-weight-bearing exercises helped the most. Water aerobics is especially beneficial for all sorts of chronic conditions and pain (Field, 2012).

There are many other pain-control methods, from acupuncture to interpersonal therapy, and many have potential benefits. However, of all the psychosocial approaches, the one with the most current scientific evidence behind it is exercise.

Thinking About Health

■ Which pain-control techniques are most effective, and why?

■ Why do medical practitioners advocate for pain control?

■ What is your opinion on the narcotic pain-relief controversy?

Chapter Summary

Pain is the most important symptom that humans experience. Symptom recognition and pain are the major motivating factors in treatment seeking. In this chapter, we examined the myriad factors that influence symptom recognition and pain perception. We examined how pain is processed in the CNS and brain and how we respond physically, emotionally, and behaviorally to pain. There are two different types of pain—acute and chronic—and we experience them quite differently. Both can be debilitating and interfere with our daily functioning, but, over time, chronic pain can overtake and destroy a person's quality of life. We also explored the role of personality and sociocultural context in the expression and experience of pain. We examined the different pain-control techniques and the controversy surrounding narcotic pain control.

KEY TERMS ▶ Interoception p. 243, Illness perception model p. 245, Confirmation bias p. 246, Appraisal delay p. 248, Illness delay p. 248, Behavioral delay p. 248, Medical delay p. 248, Nociceptors p. 255, Afferent pathway p. 255, Efferent pathway p. 255, Gate-control theory of pain p. 256, A-delta fibers p. 256, C-fibers p. 256, Myelinated p. 256, Counterirritation p. 256, Stimulus-produced analgesia p. 257, Endogenous opioids p. 257, Neuromatrix p. 257, Neurosignature p. 257, Neurogenic inflammation p. 259, Referred pain p. 262, Psychogenic pain p. 262, Neuropathic pain p. 263, Patient-controlled analgesia p. 270, Spinal cord stimulation p. 271

CHAPTER 9

Weight and Eating Disorders

Learning Outcomes

After reading this chapter, you should be able to:

- **Define** obesity, weight, and eating disorders.
- **Describe** how the hunger satiety process works.
- **Identify** the biopsychosocial processes that lead to the development of obesity, weight, and eating disorders.
- **Outline** metabolic and neurologic systems and explain its links to obesity, weight, and eating disorders.
- **Identify** developmental, cultural, and individual influences on obesity, weight, and eating disorders.

Lola is almost 30 years old. For her whole life, she has struggled with her weight and body shape. Both of her parents carry excess weight. For most of that time, she has carried extra weight that causes her to be less able to take part in sports and leisure activities because she gets winded and easily fatigued. She has also experienced intermittent periods of anxiety and depression associated with her weight, her body image, and her sense of being a failure because she has been unable to change her weight or body shape for any length of time. Every time she has taken on a diet or fitness routine, she's achieved some changes but as soon as something stressful happens or she takes a break from a rigorous routine the weight creeps back up. She has encountered extremely hurtful and stigmatizing reactions from strangers, friends and family, employers, and even doctors. Her sense of self-worth and her visions of her future are tainted by these dehumanizing, discriminatory, and painful experiences. She feels that she is unlovable and has contemplated that life is not worth living. Those who care about her are worried about her. But even her therapist cannot help her change the way she feels about herself. In the last year, things have gotten really difficult for her and she has had other health complications as a result of gaining even more weight. Recent blood work revealed that she already shows signs of prediabetes and her doctor recommended that she try Ozempic, the new "miracle" weight loss drug. She has now been on Ozempic for six months and she has lost 40 pounds. She is eating a healthy diet and getting regular exercise and is beginning to feel good about herself and her

DOI: 10.4324/9781032643090-9

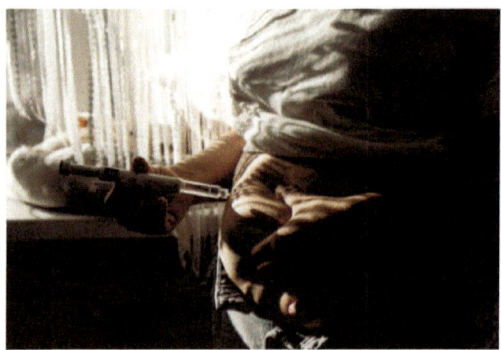

Photo 9.1

body. The weight loss has been helpful, and she is feeling physically healthier and growing stronger. However, Lola says that "being on this weight loss drug is a mixed blessing, because while I like the way I look and feel I don't like that my self-esteem is so tied to how I look, but I still hear the hurtful comments that people have made about my body. They don't disappear as the weight falls off and given my history, I am terrified that as soon as I stop taking this drug, I could go back to where I was weight-wise and emotionally and I don't feel like any of that is within my control." Lola also shared that only her therapist and her doctors know she is taking Ozempic because there is a stigma associated with losing weight that way as well. She feels like she just can't win (**Photo 9.1**).

Lola's situation is very complex and highlights all the topics we will cover in this chapter. First, she has a genetic predisposition to gain weight and her weight has been classified as obese and therefore puts her at risk for many negative mental and physical health outcomes. Due to the societal pressures on the "thin ideal" she has a deeply ingrained body dissatisfaction, and her self-esteem is tied to her appearance. The social stigma and discrimination she has experienced create stress and make her vulnerable to anxiety and depression, elevating her risk for exercise compulsion and eating disorders. The medical treatment to reduce her prediabetes and reduce her weight is great but brings a host of emotional risk factors in and of itself.

In this chapter, we will learn about the biopsychosocial factors that lead to weight gain, overweight, and obesity. We will also explore the many and varied health risks associated with overweight and obesity. Obesity is at epidemic proportions in the United States presenting a huge health challenge. There is a lot of pressure to lose weight and losing weight is healthy for many overweight people; however, weight loss can easily cross over from being balanced and healthful to being obsessive, compulsive, and pathological leading to eating disorders. This is a major health crisis as well because eating disorders are rising in all groups and are associated with higher rates of anxiety, depression, and suicide risk in those who have them.

One main goal of this chapter is to highlight the fact that obesity and eating disorders do not discriminate, anyone regardless of their age, gender, race, socioeconomic status, education level, or cultural background can develop either of these weight-related disorders. Therefore, we will take a diversity-affirming approach to understanding the societal influences on these disorders. It is also important to keep in mind that both obesity and eating disorders are intractable health problems that they are because of the social views that Western cultures have of bodies, especially women's bodies. Each of us has become socialized to view the ideal body through a lens that is socially constructed and often very much at odds with what is realistically attainable or healthy for us as individuals or as a group subjected to social pressure to adhere to an unattainable aesthetic. While we will look at how these sociocultural expectations came to be and how they affect us, we will ultimately advocate for body neutrality—the view that we can accept, appreciate, and come to respect our bodies for what they can do for us, not how they look. **Body neutrality** means that we focus on the functions of the body and remember that our bodies are just one part of us, not the totality, and they do not have to define who we are and how we feel about ourselves (Albers, 2018).

Consistent with the American Psychological Association we will avoid perpetuating weight stigma by using neutral terms that respect and affirm the dignity of people who are of lower or higher weight. Although it is important to understand the linkages among weight and health, it is important to remember that bias against people because of their body size, just like all other forms of bias and discrimination, weight stigma (or sizeism) leads to psychological distress and emotional suffering. Like that which Lola experienced.

Obesity

In Chapter 4, we saw the importance of a healthful diet, weight management, and physical activity for a long and healthy life. We discussed how maintaining a healthy weight can help us avoid disease and disability. The other side of this issue is unhealthy eating and a sedentary lifestyle, which put us at risk of having excess weight and increase the risk of early death. Some of these outcomes are modifiable through behavioral change and some are not.

Obesity is characterized by the accumulation of excessive body fat. It is a chronic disease that increases the risk of cardiovascular disease, high blood pressure, high cholesterol, metabolic syndromes, diabetes, cancer, sleep apnea, non-alcoholic fatty liver disease, and mental health problems. Having excess weight often leads to depressed mood and low self-esteem (Dziurowicz-Kozłowska, 2010). Even a 5–10% loss in body weight can significantly improve mental health and well-being.

From a biopsychosocial perspective, the health conditions of overweight and obesity are multifactorial and have many causes. Biological factors include neuroanatomy, neurochemistry, hormones, bacteria, and genetics; psychosocial and environmental factors include socioeconomic status, early feeding patterns, availability of high-quality foods, and emotional eating; and sociocultural factors include ethnic and cultural food choices. Overweight that leads to obesity represents a complex disease with many factors and devastating health outcomes. Obesity is a disease that is due, in most cases, to a combination of obesogenic environment, psychosocial factors, and genetic factors that predispose people to carry excess weight.

A Worldwide Epidemic

As we have seen, overweight and obesity are defined as an excessive amount of body fat that puts a person's health at risk. Although this was once considered a health problem only in high-income countries such as the United States, an

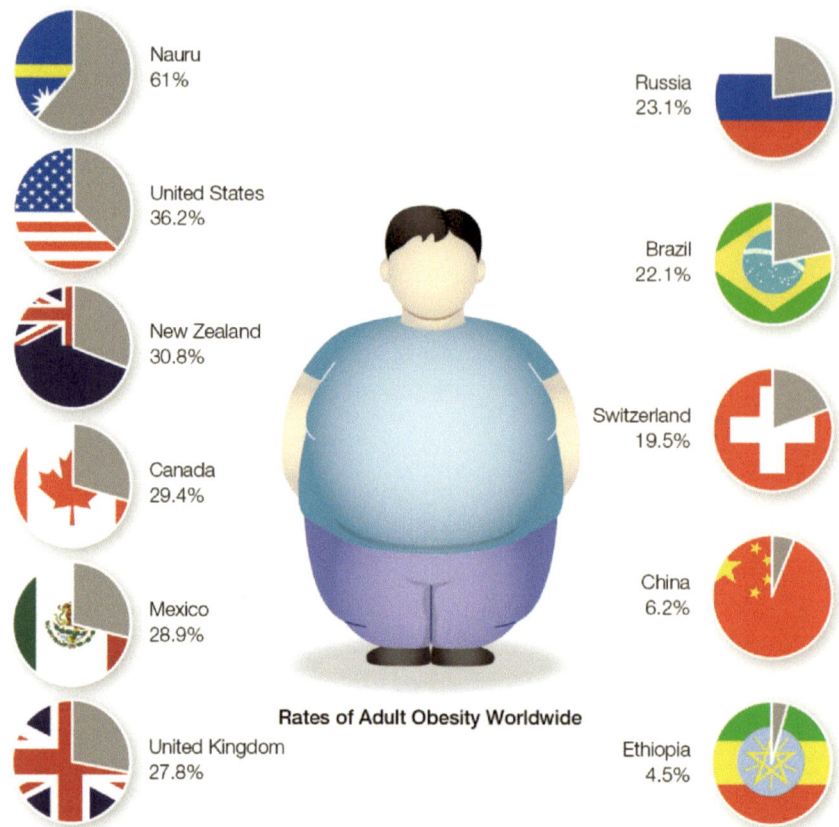

Figure 9.1   One out of every eight adults is overweight globally (2017).

obesity epidemic is on the rise throughout the world, especially in poor urban cities where cheap fast food has become easily accessible. (**Figure 9.1**).

Recent epidemiological data from the World Obesity Atlas 2023 shows that prevalence rates of 38% of the global population are overweight or obese (Chen et al., 2022). The population of people with overweight or obesity is projected to rise to 51% of the global population by 2035, but by 2030, 78% of adults in the United States will be in overweight or obese weight zones (Koliaki et al., 2023). Despite the fact that the World Health Organization declared that obesity was an epidemic in 1997, the escalating rise in obesity has been called "globesity" and is now one of the most critical public health challenges facing our global societies and health care systems (Koliaki et al., 2023). Epidemiological data also shows that women are more likely to have obesity as are those who come from socioeconomically disadvantaged racial and ethnic groups. People with lower levels of education are related to higher levels of obesity as well

Obesity in Childhood

The percentage of children with overweight and obesity is growing at an alarming rate. Globally, the World Health Organization has found that more than

390 million children aged 5–19 are overweight and 160 million live with obesity in 2022 (WHO, 2024e). Overall, 18% of children worldwide are at risk for the negative health consequences of obesity. And childhood obesity continues to rise.

Developmentally, childhood obesity adds to the risk of health problems across the lifespan. Obesity can disrupt nearly every system in the child's body, affecting the functioning of the heart and lungs; the growth of muscles and bones; the regulation of the endocrine system, hormones, kidneys, digestion, and blood sugar; and more. And obesity affects every aspect of a child's development. Infants who have obesity are significantly delayed in learning to crawl, walk, and talk compared with normal-weight infants. Earlier sexual maturation in girls is linked to excess body weight. Girls who are overweight can begin to develop breasts as early as age 8 and begin menstruation between the ages of 10 and 12, a trend that may lead to a greater risk of breast cancer in women (Steingraber, 2007).

The main causes of obesity in kids are the same as in adults—less physical activity coupled with increased consumption of high-calorie, high-fat, prepackaged, highly processed, and fast foods. However, the impact of excess weight is much greater in children, because the psychological and health consequences are lasting. For both boys and girls, adolescence is a vulnerable time, and excess weight may affect the individual for the rest of his or her life.

As with adults, obesity in children puts them at greater risk for many negative health consequences. Type 2 diabetes, a disease that used to develop only later in life, is now being seen in young children. High blood pressure, high cholesterol, metabolic syndrome, and heart disease, too, were once considered exclusively adult diseases, but now are becoming common in children with overweight and obesity (see Chapter 10). Again, the effects are lasting. Children with obesity have a 30–40% greater risk of heart attack and stroke later in life (Friedemann et al., 2012). Although parents may think that their children will just grow out of their "puppy fat," these children instead carry increased risks into adulthood.

The psychological and mental health consequences are just as devastating. Kids with obesity are more often teased, bullied, or rejected by their peers (Lumeng et al., 2010). A study showed that weight-related teasing is related to higher rates of anxiety, depression, and low self-esteem in children with obesity (Blanco et al., 2019). The authors raise concerns about the harmful effects of weight-related stigma for children and the alarming impact of bullying on children's quality of life (Blanco et al., 2019). Other research shows that when children with overweight and obesity experience teasing the impact on their self-esteem increases the likelihood that they will internalize weight biases (Fields et al., 2021). Children who are unhappy with their weight are also more likely to develop eating disorders and are at higher risks of substance abuse, depression, and suicide.

As we have seen, overweight and obesity are complex health problems in which developmental and biopsychosocial factors intersect, leading to long-term and debilitating health problems. Let's look more closely at some of these factors—they are key to the lifestyle and health changes that can offset disease.

The Biology of Obesity

As common and widespread as obesity is, the causes remain contested. Obesity may be influenced by many factors, including obesogenic environments, genetics, nutrition, and physical activity. Let's start with the biology of obesity.

In 1994, researchers in the laboratory of Dr. Jeffrey Friedman were studying genetically modified mice (Friedman, 2010). They noticed that morbidly obese mice had a genetic mutation that interfered with the production of the hormone leptin. When they injected these mice with leptin, the animals returned to normal body weight. This was an amazing discovery: The hormone leptin is made in fat tissue and is responsible for regulating weight and feeding cycles (Friedman, 2010). Leptin levels are monitored by the brain and influence energy levels and appetite. As we cycle through our daily rhythms, our bodies burn calories and use energy from fat; as fat stores decrease, the levels of leptin decrease, which signals the brain to trigger feelings of hunger. By eating, fat stores are replenished, leptin levels increase, and appetite is suppressed. So, the discovery of leptin's significance sheds light on how the body regulates energy, appetite, and weight, and has important implications for health conditions, like obesity and diabetes (**Photo 9.2**).

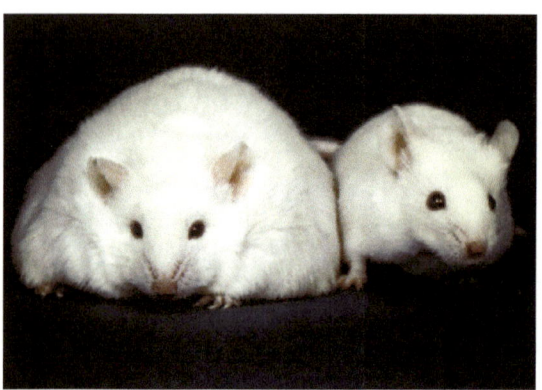

Photo 9.2   Scientists discovered how leptin affects weight when morbidly obese rats who were injected with the hormone soon returned to the weight of their average-sized peers (Friedman, 2010).

Source: SCIENCE SOURCE

Individuals with severe obesity have a genetic propensity to store excessive caloric intake as fat. Weight is between 40% and 75% genetically determined (Hall et al., 2022). Although over 400 different genes may be linked to the causes of overweight or obesity, only around 15 genes are involved in the regulation of eating and fat storage (Gutierrez-Aguilar, Kim, Woods, & Seeley, 2012). Still, an abnormality in a single gene can disrupt leptin pathways (Farooqi & O'Rahilly, 2005), leading to obesity.

With over 90% of its heritability still unexplained (Tam et al., 2019), cracking the genetic code of obesity has become a main goal of science. Each discovery in the field is important for several reasons. First, identifying genetic markers may lead to new drug treatments to treat obesity. Since obesity is linked with metabolic syndrome, diabetes, and many other negative health outcomes, preventing and treating it is important. Second, understanding the genetics of obesity can influence our perception of the problem. In 2013, the American Medical Association, a leading voice in public health policy, formally recognized that obesity is a disease (Hoyt, Burnette, & Auster-Gussman, 2014; Stoner & Cornwall, 2014). Defining obesity as a disease makes clear that the body is malfunctioning to create obesity (Hoyt et al., 2014). Seeing obesity as a disease with a biological origin could lead to greater acceptance and understanding of those who suffer from it.

On the other hand, explaining obesity in terms of physiological or genetic factors implies that weight is unchangeable (Hoyt et al., 2014). Could the discovery of the role of genetics in obesity actually stand in the way of successful behavioral change? If people believe that obesity is genetically determined, will they have less motivation to choose a healthy lifestyle? In one study, more than 72% of participants named lifestyle factors as the main cause of obesity, while only 19% cited genetics. However, those who said genes caused obesity were significantly less likely to adopt physical exercise and a healthy diet (Wang & Coups, 2010). In another study (Hoyt et al., 2014), people were randomly assigned to an experimental group that read an article published in the *New York Times* (Pollack, 2013) that discussed the American Medical Association's definition of obesity as a disease and the benefits of this definition, such as reduced stigma for obese individuals. The control group read a leaflet with basic information about weight management. Findings showed that there are potential costs to presenting obesity as a disease, not the least of which was reducing the importance placed on health-focused dieting and concerns for weight. People in the experimental group also made less healthy food choices (Hoyt et al., 2014). In sum, one's perception of the causes of obesity can influence one's behaviors.

There are several theories of obesity. The **Energy Balance Model** suggests that obesity is the result of excessive energy intake in relation to energy expended. When we take in more energy in the form of calories than we burn, the excess is stored as fat. This model proposes that the brain is primarily responsible for regulating body weight by regulating the integration of external signals from the environment with the body's internal signals from organs that control food intake. In the brain, the hypothalamus, basal ganglia, and brainstem work together with endocrine, metabolic, and nervous system signals to regulate food intake without our conscious awareness. Together, they monitor the body's changing energy needs and environmental influences. There may be a lot of variability in a person's day-to-day energy intake but the neural regulation of the body's energy balance is generally achieved over much longer time scales (Hall et al., 2022). The **Carbohydrate-Insulin Hypothesis** suggests that obesity results from the excessive intake of foods containing sucrose (table sugar) as well as high intake of high glycemic carbohydrates like white bread, white rice, potatoes, and cereals). When ingested these carbohydrates elevate blood glucose levels stimulating the response of insulin, which in turn causes glucose to enter the cells of the body where most of it is stored as fat. The **Protein-Leverage Hypothesis** proports that we have a nutritional need for protein and an appetite for foods that contain protein. However, because most available foods have high carbohydrate and low protein content, we tend to eat more to get sufficient protein. Our need for protein overrides the body's energy balance. Another model, **Seed Oil Hypothesis** argues that recently people have been consuming more foods that contain seed oils (e.g., soybean, safflower oils) high in polyunsaturated fats, and these energy-dense foods promote inflammation, oxidative stress, and obesity. Finally, the **Obesogen Model** (Heindel et al., 2024) argues that it is exposure to environmental chemicals (called obesogens), especially during critical developmental periods (e.g., in utero, early childhood), but throughout the life span that affects long-term metabolism by creating hormonal changes that lead to weight gain and obesity. Some researchers have argued that ultraprocessed foods are obesogenic because of the number of chemicals involved in their production. Consider food additives, preservatives, emulsifiers, and antioxidants, the chemicals used in the packaging of foods to enhance shelf-life, and many fruits and vegetables are treated with pesticides that are hard to remove. Foods in the ultra-processed Western diet are drenched in chemicals that over time can disrupt hormonal functioning and lead to obesity (Heindel et al., 2024). These are just a few of the theories being debated as causes of the obesity epidemic.

Given that the body has evolved to regulate energy intake and this process has been relatively stable, what has caused the recent upsurge in obesity worldwide? For some researchers, the answer is that the increase in the world's prevalence of obesity is due to changes in the food environment, such as the increased availability and increased marketing of high-calorie, energy-dense ultra-processed, inexpensive foods in larger portion sizes. These foods are higher in fat and sugar and lower in protein and fiber. As our diets have become higher calorie, it is argued that our energy balance has changed leading to higher rates of obesity. It has also been suggested that over time as people have shifted to jobs that require less physical activity, there has been less opportunity to expend energy leading to increased weight gain. The quality of the foods we eat, high fat, high sugar, and highly processed clearly affects the regulation of hormones and the gut microbiota also increasing the risk for obesity. Clearly, obesity is a multifactorial biopsychosocial disease.

Environmental Factors

Understanding the biological causes of obesity is crucial. Although people may have a genetic predisposition to obesity or an elevated risk due to changes in the gut microbiome, epidemiological evidence points to the significance of environmental factors (Stoner & Cornwall, 2014). Obesity has many causes, and our biological predispositions can be overcome by a healthful lifestyle (Anderson & Butcher, 2006; Leatherdale & Papadakis, 2011). It is important to remember that many people with obesity have no biological predispositions, but gain weight because of a complex interaction of different factors.

In Chapter 4, we discussed how food preferences can develop *in utero* and how early feeding patterns may shape eating behavior. We also discussed the roles of promoting an active lifestyle, healthy food choices, and family meals. The role of peers is also significant (Ogden, 2009; Salvy, de la Haye, Bowker, & Hermans, 2012). Most teens with overweight eat insufficient amounts of fruits and vegetables, consume an excess of sugar-sweetened soft drinks, are physically inactive, and watch excessive amounts of television. In a Canadian study of ninth and tenth graders, 21% were overweight or obese, and obesity was linked with less physical activity, more screen time, and little participation in varsity sports (Janssen, Katzmarzyk, Boyce, King, & Pickett, 2004; Katzmarzyk et al., 2013).

One growing environmental concern in the rising rates of obesity is the role of obesogenic environments. An **obesogenic environment** is an environment that contributes to weight gain and undermines weight loss (Andoy-Galvan et al., 2023), and some argue that these environments are driving the obesity epidemic (Powell et al., 2010; Swinburn et al., 1999). One way obesogenic environments promote overweight and obesity is through promoting unhealthy eating behaviors and physical inactivity (Schneider & Holzwarth, 2024). However, an obesogenic environment can relate to economic factors (such as the high costs of high-quality nutritious foods), political factors (the law requiring nutrition labels on foods, for example), physical factors (might be what's available in the environment like fast food or vending machines), and socio-cultural factors (refer to the beliefs, attitudes, and values that our social networks and communities place on eating and physical activity). Obesogenic environments vary in scale from large and institutional such as the healthcare system in one's country to the local level such as what is available in one's home, at one's school or at work.

We are all part of the **built environment**, the surroundings created by human beings. The built environment includes our neighborhoods, the architecture of the buildings, the presence of greenery and open space, the modes of transportation, and the proximity of shopping and restaurants. Innovative technology like geographic information systems on our smartphones can tell us the travel time to the nearest park or the preparation time for meals ordered via a delivery app. And, in fact, certain built environments can lead to obesity (Thornton, Pearce, & Kavanagh, 2011). When people have easy access to convenience stores with high-calorie, high-fat foods, it is easier for them to gain weight and harder to lose weight (Epstein et al., 2012; French, Story, & Jeffery, 2001). The good news is that changes in the built environment, like making green space and recreational facilities easily accessible, can promote healthier lifestyles, reduce obesity, and ultimately cut down on health risks (Epstein et al., 2012; French et al., 2001).

The social environment plays a huge role in shaping behavior. **Social learning theory** (Bandura, 1989) highlights the importance of the social context, the influence of others, and how these affect our own behavioral choices. Many kids with overweight have parents with overweight and peers with overweight; those around us directly influence the amount and type of foods we eat (Salvy et al., 2012; Vilhjalmsson & Thorlindsson, 1998). Peers also influence behavior through modeling, shaping self-image, and social pressure to conform to expectations. For example, children and adolescents who have social networks (including parents and classmates) that include people with overweight are more likely to underestimate their own weight and hold inaccurate ideas about what a healthy and appropriate weight is (Maximova et al., 2008). People with morbid obesity, regardless of age, tend to underestimate their weight (Carr & Jaffe, 2012). This presents a significant problem, because an inaccurate perception of one's weight may lead to a failure to take steps to reduce the risk of negative health outcomes.

Social contagion refers to the spreading of ideas, information, and behaviors through networks, much as an infectious disease spreads through a population. We can think of the obesity epidemic as, literally, a contagion. People are 57% more likely to have obesity if they have a friend who has obesity (Christakis & Fowler, 2007). The risks are greater, too, if a spouse or adult sibling has obesity (Christakis & Fowler, 2007; Hruschka, Brewis, Wutich, & Morin, 2011). Family, peer groups, schools, neighborhoods, and communities—all these contexts interact with one another and can lead to health-compromising lifestyles.

Psychological Consequences

We have looked at the factors that lead to excess body weight and the resultant physical health risks. More often overlooked, even by the medical community, are the psychological consequences of having obesity.

Although obesity has become more common, people with obesity are still stigmatized, devalued, and discriminated against (Asthana, 2012). And the stigma experienced by people who have excess weight is associated with higher rates of depression, body image disturbances, lower self-esteem, and psychiatric symptoms (Asthana, 2012). Children are especially vulnerable (Puhl & Latner, 2007). Obesity in kids relates to poor self-esteem, poor body image, social anxieties, anxiety disorders, sadness, loneliness, and depression (Harrist et al., 2016). It may not be the weight itself that leads to low self-esteem in children but, rather, the teasing from peers, the criticism or nagging from parents, and the belief that there is nothing they can do to change (Harriger & Thompson, 2012; Puhl & Latner, 2007).

Obesity is a risk factor for unsafe dieting, fasting, binging, purging, and the use of laxatives and diuretics (Harriger & Thompson, 2012; Thompson et al., 2007). Studies also show that women with obesity report more violence from intimate partners (Alhalal, 2018; Huang, Yang, & Omaye, 2011). People with a higher BMI and those who engage in binge eating also have a higher suicide risk (Pompili, Girardi, Tatarelli, Ruberto, & Tatarelli, 2006). Clearly, obesity correlates with significant psychological distress (Friedman & Brownell, 1995; Geller et al., 2019; Sutaria, Devakumar, Yasuda, Das, & Saxena, 2019).

Food Addiction: Like taking drugs, consuming delicious foods creates a rewarding feeling and stimulates reward centers in the brain. Specifically, **food addiction** refers to when certain foods lead to compulsive eating behaviors and become linked with stimulating the reward centers of the brain (Carter, Van Wijk, & Rowsell, 2019; Romer, Kang, Nikolova, Gearhardt, & Hariri, 2019). Food addiction is a behavioral addiction that leads a person to become reliant on the dopamine that is released when consuming foods. People with food addiction eat compulsively and are unable to control or stop their eating despite negative consequences. Food addiction has not yet been integrated into the Diagnostic and Statistical Manual of Mental Disorders (DSM 5) but it is gaining legitimacy throughout the medical and psychological community.

People become food addicted when eating releases the neurochemical dopamine into the *nucleus accumbens* through the mesolimbic (reward) pathway. Foods that are high in sugar and fat work similarly to drugs in the brain, potentially causing impaired decision making, compulsive eating, and loss of control over food intake (Lindgren et al., 2018). Food addiction has both genetic and neurobiological foundations and is consistent with the brain disease model of addiction. Moreover, food addiction may be a factor in both obesity and eating disorders (more on these later), shedding light on the biopsychosocial similarities among the risky behaviors we are exploring.

Treatments for Obesity

Treatment for obesity aims at weight loss and maintenance. The key is to balance the energy consumed (in the form of food and drinks) with the energy expended (in the form of physical activity). Greater nutritional knowledge can help.

For lifestyle changes to be effective, they must be achievable. Safe, steady weight loss can help people meet their goals and maintain that loss in the future. To lose 1–2 pounds per week, or 10% of body weight over six months, adults should cut their intake by 500–1000 calories per day. (For reference, for the average American woman [5'5" and 135 pounds], daily intake should not exceed 1200 calories per day.) Very low-calorie diets are dangerous and should be followed only under medical supervision. In fact, cutting calories too drastically can have the unintended effect of *caloric hoarding*: The body goes into "starvation mode" and does not burn the calories it takes in, actually stalling weight loss.

Other behavioral changes are often necessary as well. Someone trying to lose weight should avoid situations that might lead to overeating in the first place. Being aware of how environments can be obesogenic is helpful. Modifying the environment to avoid tempting foods will help too. So will building in prompts and incentives to eat healthfully and exercise regularly.

Social support from family and friends is beneficial. Commercial programs such as Weight Watchers provide many benefits, including social support, education about foods and exercise, diet assignments, and activities such as keeping a food diary (**Photo 9.3**) (Heshka et al., 2003).

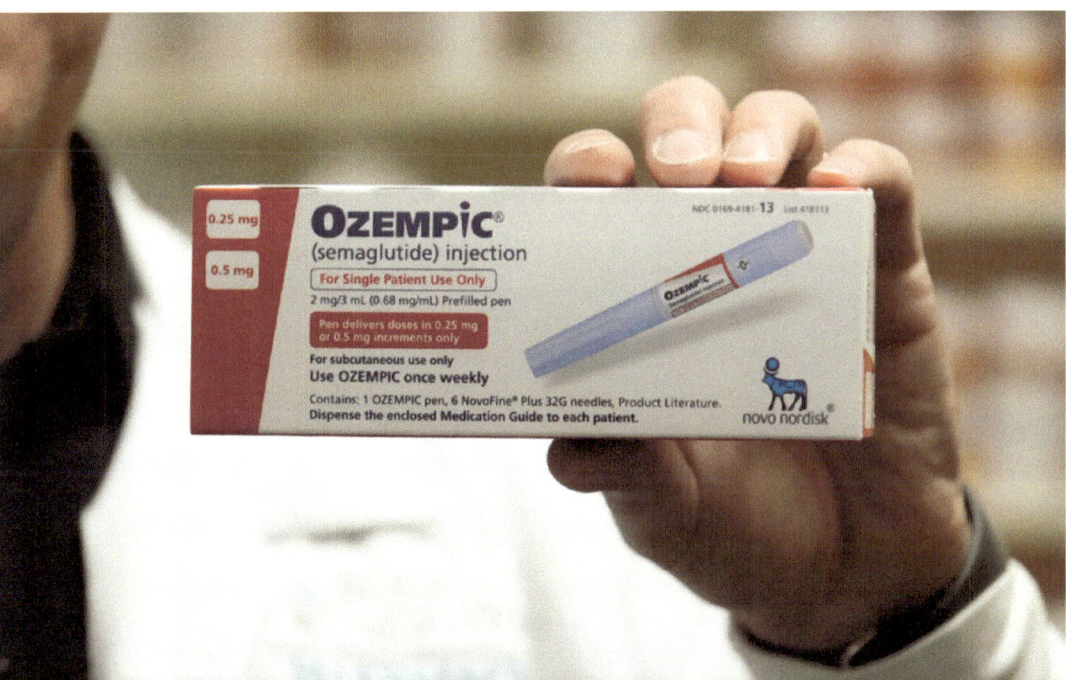

Photo 9.3   A pharmacist holds a box of the weight loss drug, Ozempic

When it comes to weight loss, there is no cure-all. Medications may be helpful for those who are unable to lose weight through lifestyle changes alone—especially for those with obesity. You may have been seeing headlines, news stories, and social media related to the drugs Ozempic, Rybelsus, and Wegovy. The most widely known is Ozempic (a peptide with the pharmaceutical name semaglutide) which has been touted for its off-label use as a weight-loss medication. Semaglutide was originally developed as a long-term treatment for type 2 diabetes. This drug is administered in an injection pen and dosed weekly at the start. It has the effect of slowing gastric emptying that helps people feel fuller after eating and it works to suppress appetite by influencing the brain regions responsible for cravings and hunger. The FDA has approved these drugs for the treatment of type 2 diabetes, and they can be prescribed for weight loss if a person has a body mass index of 30 or higher or if they have weight-related conditions. There are some potential side effects of taking these drugs and there is certainly a lot of social controversy surrounding them as well.

Many of the other weight loss medications can be dangerous. They may increase the risk of heart problems or liver disease, and several, such as sibutramine (trade name: Meridia), have been taken off the market because of dangerous side effects. Medications should be used in conjunction with physical activity and a healthy diet.

Weight-loss surgeries are another extreme form of treatment, used when the patient has a BMI of 40 or greater and all other treatments have failed. The most common surgery is gastroplasty, in which bands or staples are implanted to restrict the size of the stomach, limiting the amount of food and liquid it can hold. In another form of surgery, gastric bypass, the stomach is sealed, and a small stomach pouch is created around part of the small intestine, where normally most calories are absorbed. Although weight-loss surgeries can help morbidly obese patients, they have significant risks and unpleasant side effects. Lifelong medical supervision is essential.

Thinking About Health

■ What biopsychosocial factors lead to obesity?

■ In what ways have you experienced the pressures and temptations that can lead to obesity?

■ Why are children at such high risk for obesity?

■ What are the most effective treatments for obesity?

Eating Disorders

Eating disorders can be another consequence of not maintaining a healthy body weight and getting regular exercise. They are not just fads, phases, or lifestyle choices. **Eating disorders** are serious and potentially life-threatening eating behaviors that significantly impair emotional, physical, and social well-being (see **Table 9.1**). Eating disorders are characterized by dysfunctional eating

Anorexia nervosa	Bulimia nervosa	Binge eating disorder
Symptoms		
Resistance to maintaining a normal body weight	Recurrent episodes of eating large amounts of food, accompanied by a sense of loss of control over eating behavior	Recurrent episodes of eating large amounts of food accompanied by a sense of loss of control over eating behavior
Intense fear of weight gain or being fat while actually underweight	Inappropriate compensatory behaviors such as self-induced vomiting, laxative or diuretic abuse, extreme fasting, and compulsive exercise	Episodes feature at least three of these behaviors: eating fast; eating until uncomfortably full; eating large amounts when not hungry; eating alone due to embarrassment; feeling disgusted, depressed, or guilty after eating
Distortions of body weight or shape, undue concern for weight and shape in self-evaluation, and denial of the seriousness of low body weight	Extreme concern with body weight and shape	Feeling distressed about binging
		Binging episodes occur, on average, once a week for three months
Warning signs		
Dramatic weight loss	Evidence of binge eating, including the disappearance of large amounts of food in short periods or finding wrappers and containers from large amounts of food	Eating very quickly, eating beyond the point of satiety to the point of being uncomfortably full, or eating when not hungry
Preoccupation with weight, food, calories, fat grams, and dieting	Evidence of purging, including frequent trips to the bathroom after meals, signs and/or smells of vomiting, and the presence of packages or wrappers from laxatives or diuretics	Consumption of a large amount of food and calories, feeling embarrassed about eating, or eating alone
Frequent comments about feeling fat or overweight despite weight loss	Unusual swelling of the cheeks or jaw area	Feeling guilt or depression after eating
Anxiety about gaining weight or being fat	Calluses or lesions on the backs of hands and knuckles from self-induced vomiting	Feelings of self-disgust or shame
Denial of hunger	Discoloration or staining of teeth, chronically sore throat, acid reflux, or other gastrointestinal disorders	Excessive weight gain
Development of food rituals (eating foods in certain orders, excessive chewing, or rearranging foods on plate)	Rituals to make time for binge-and-purge sessions	
Consistent excuses to avoid meals or situations involving food		
An excessive, rigid exercise regimen despite bad weather, fatigue, illness, or injury; the need to "burn off" calories taken in	An excessive, rigid exercise regimen despite bad weather, fatigue, illness, or injury; the need to "burn off" calories taken in	
Withdrawal from friends and activities	Withdrawal from friends and activities	
In general, behaviors and attitudes indicating that weight loss, dieting, and control over food are becoming primary concerns	In general, behaviors and attitudes indicating that weight loss, dieting, and control over food are becoming primary concerns	In general, behaviors and attitudes indicating that weight loss, dieting, and control over food are becoming primary concerns

Table 9.1 Symptoms and warning signs of eating disorders

behaviors and a problematic relationship with food; they also have interactive biopsychosocial risk factors, so in many ways, obesity and eating disorders represent two extremes on the end of the same spectrum (Lee, Elias, & Lozano, 2018). Eating disorders are psychiatric conditions that typically emerge in adolescence and affect between 1 to 5% of the U.S. population, and 3.4% to 7.8% of the world's population (Galmiche et al., 2019). At subclinical levels, symptoms are referred to as **disordered eating** which occurs at a much higher rate than eating disorders. For example, during adolescence, 15% of boys and up to 30% of girls show signs of disordered eating (Breton et al., 2023). Disordered eating can be a precursor to clinical eating disorders.

Eating disorders are a biopsychosocial disease that emerges from the interaction among biological susceptibility (e.g., neurodevelopment, genes associated with body weight), psychological factors (e.g., personality, life experiences), and sociocultural and environmental factors (e.g., social standards of beauty and body shape).

What Are Eating Disorders?

Eating disorders are complex disorders with a biopsychosocial origin. They impact physical and psychological health and all the domains of a person's life and can have serious, chronic consequences for quality of life, productivity, and relationships (Patel, Tchanturia, & Harrison, 2016). Although eating disorders are developmental in nature, with the peak onset around 13–18 years old (Patel et al., 2016), the effects of eating disorders can last a lifetime.

Anorexia nervosa is a type of eating disorder that is characterized by self-induced starvation and excessive weight loss. **Bulimia nervosa** is a type of eating disorder characterized by cycles of binging and purging—typically involving self-induced vomiting, fasting, compulsive exercise, or abuse of laxatives and diuretics. People who suffer from bulimia feel out of control during a binge, when they eat well beyond the point of fullness. The purge is an attempt to manage or control the perceived damage done by the binge. Dieting and extreme concerns about body weight and shape are also prevalent. **Binge eating disorder** is similar to bulimia but without the purging. **Avoidant restrictive food intake disorder** (ARFID) is characterized by active restriction or avoidance of a specific type or quantity of food, but unlike anorexia nervosa, it is not accompanied by distorted body image or fear of weight gain. All these disorders feature extreme emotions, attitudes, and behaviors surrounding weight and food.

People die from eating disorders, more often than from any other psychological disorder (Andreeva et al., 2019; Castellini et al., 2023; Micali & Herle, 2023), making them one of the deadliest of all mental illnesses (Castellini et al., 2023). The emotional impact of these disorders can be devastating as well. The majority of teenagers with these disorders report significant cognitive, emotional, or social impairments. In the case of bulimia and binge eating disorders, especially, that can include plans for and attempts at suicide.

In the United States, an estimated 29 million people, or 9% of the U.S. population will develop clinically significant eating disorders at some point during their lives (Deloitte Access Economics, 2020). More than 15% of young women meet the diagnostic criteria for an eating disorder (Stice & Van Ryzin, 2019), and there is good reason to fear for the future. Girls as young as 6 years old begin to express concern about their weight and shape, and 40–60% of girls in elementary school are worried about becoming overweight (Cash & Smolak, 2011). Up to 10 million U.S. men will develop an eating disorder as well. Less than 6% of people with eating disorders are "underweight" and research shows that people with larger bodies are at the highest risk (Duncan et al., 2017; Lipsom & Sonnerville, 2019).

In "A Plea for Diversity in Eating Disorders Research," Dr. Georg Halbeisen and colleagues (2022) argue that because these disorders have historically been stereotyped as affecting the SWAG (skinny, White, affluent, girls) not enough progress has been made to understand the differences in the way eating disorders may emerge in other groups. All individuals regardless of gender, age, ethnicity, sexual orientation, or socioeconomic background can be at risk for eating disorders. The social determinants may present differences that need to be considered in the etiology, presentation, assessment, and treatment of the disorder. As a result, data are beginning to emerge that shows that eating disorders are rising in non-White women, men, people in middle age and later life, and across all income levels and geographic regions. **Table 9.2** highlights some of the groups for which eating disorders are rising and emerging as a serious mental health threat (Bazo Perez & Frazier, 2024; Bazo Perez et al., 2023; Hudson, Hiripi, Pope, & Kessler, 2007; Wade et al., 2011). For example, we now know that eating disorders are higher in Asian-American men, Black women, transgender and other sexual minority individuals than they are in White cis-gender women (Halbeisen et al., 2022).

BIPOC (Black, Indigenous, and People of Color)

*Similar prevalence to white peers but 50% less likely to be diagnosed, less likely to be asked about eating disorder symptoms than non-minority peers

*Asian American college students report higher rates of body dissatisfaction, negative attitudes toward obesity, greater restricted eating, purging, muscle building, and cognitive restrain than white or non-Asian BIPOC counterparts

Males

*25% of people with eating disorders are male

*Many men with eating disorders do not recognize symptoms as problematic because of the stereotype of eating disorders as a women's disorder

*Due to a lack of awareness in the patient and medical community, by the time males seek treatment their symptoms tend to be more severe

*Research shows that healthcare professionals often minimize symptoms of eating disorders in men

LGBTQ+

*Higher prevalence than heterosexual counterparts

*LGBTQ+ youth are up to 3 times more likely to have an eating disorder compared to straight peers

*1/3 of sexual minority adolescents report engaging in dangerous weight control behaviors in the last month, highest in gay and bisexual boys

*Over 75% of transgender college students who have eating disorders attempt suicide

*56% of transgender people with eating disorders do not believe their disorder is related to their physical body, but 32% of transgender people use eating disorders as a way to modify their bodies.

Table 9.2   Eating disorder statistics   (Continued)

Older adults

*71% of middle aged women aged 50 and over are currently trying to lose weight and nearly 80% said their weight/shape significantly impacted their self-esteem.

*41% of women over 50 have a present (13%) or past (28%) eating disorder symptoms.

*The rising rates of eating disorders in women over age 50 are likely related to the biopsychosocial changes associated with menopause

*Older adults (over age 65) experience age-related stress and life transitions that make eating disorders worse

People with larger bodies

*40% of girls who are overweight and 20% of boys who are overweight engage in disordered eating behaviors

*People of all ages who have larger bodies are at higher risk of unhealthy weight control behaviors

*People who experience weight stigma and discrimination are 60% more likely to die

Athletes

*Athletes report significantly higher rates of excessive exercise than non-athletes

*Athletes in weight-dependent sports including 77% of men and 80% of women report engaging in weight and diet-compensatory behaviors

*Female athletes have two times greater risk of eating disorders than male athletes

*Eating disorders in athletes are harder to detect due to sport culture, secretiveness, symptom presentation, and stigma associated with weight; similarly, athletes are less likely to seek treatment due to these factors

Military and veterans

*More than 16% of female active duty and veterans have eating disorders often combined with PTSD and sexual trauma

*Between 2017 and 2021 incidence of eating disorders among active-duty military personnel increased by 79%

*33% of female and 19% of male Veterans who served in Iraq and Afghanistan showed signs of probably eating disorders

*Body dysmorphic disorder is 5 times higher in military personnel than non-military personnel, with 22% of female service members and 13% of male service members affected

*Military service and the culture of military life, with its emphasis on fitness, the stress of combat exposure, and sexual trauma exacerbate eating disorder symptoms

---

Source: Data from National Association of Anorexia Nervosa and Associated Disorders (2024) Resources can be found at https://anad.org/

Table 9.2   Eating disorder statistics (*Continued*)

Gender and Eating Disorders: Eating disorders can develop in anyone, regardless of gender. Although eating disorders are more common in women, 43% of people with binge eating disorder, 30% of people with bulimia nervosa, and 20% of individuals with anorexia nervosa are men (Hay et al., 2015). Moreover, between 55% and 77% of those with "other specified feeding and eating disorder and 67% of those with ARFID are men (Eddy et al., 2015). More than 15% of gay men have an eating disorder (Feldman & Meyer, 2007; see the **Around the World** feature). Nearly 61% of LGBTQ+ adolescents reported having at least one symptom of disordered eating within the last year (Gordon et al., 2019) and 54% of LGBTQ+ adolescents have been diagnosed with a full-syndrome eating disorder at some point in their short lives (Trevor Project, National Eating Disorders Association, 2018). Research shows that adult sexual minorities were over two times more likely to experience food addiction compared to their heterosexual counterparts (Parker & Harriger, 2020).

These findings suggest that there is diversity in eating disorders and that the presentation may not be the same for different identity groups. Men are more likely than women to take steroids or other dangerous drugs in a quest to increase muscle mass. **Muscle dysmorphia**, a preoccupation that one's body is not lean or muscular enough (Bégin, Turcotte, & Rodrigue, 2019), can be a feature of eating disorders in both heterosexual and gay men (Waldorf, Vocks, Düsing, Bauer, & Cordes, 2019). Whereas men turn to excessive exercise to manage their weight, nearly one-third of adolescent boys skip meals, fast, smoke cigarettes, induce vomiting, or take laxatives (Neumark-Sztainer, 2005).

When considering eating disorders in historically non-typical groups such as in people who are non-White, ethnically diverse, older, or who are sexual minorities several theoretical models have been suggested. The minority stress model posits that individuals from sexual minority and gender minority groups result from unique stressors such as stigma and discrimination that result in the internalization of homophobia or the need to hide one's sexual or gender identity and these pressures increase the risk of the development of mental and physical health issues such as eating disorders. Research shows that people who are sexual and gender minorities are likely to perceive higher levels of stigma, shame, discrimination, and concealment of one's identity and that those experiences are linked to higher rates of eating disorder symptoms (Bayer et al., 2017; Parker & Harriger, 2020; Watson et al., 2016).

Around *the* World

An Athlete's Battle with Anorexia Nervosa

Tommy Kelly, a semiprofessional soccer player in Scotland, battled an eating disorder. Now, he wants to help others do the same (**Photo 9.4**) (Aitken, 2015).

Tommy had anorexia nervosa for 18 years. It ravaged his body and his mind. He spent three months in a coma, suffered two heart attacks, and nearly died. Nine months of hospitalization helped him to recover (Aitken, 2015).

How did things get so bad? Tommy didn't realize what was happening to him, and he had nowhere to turn for help. His family and friends knew that something was wrong, but they

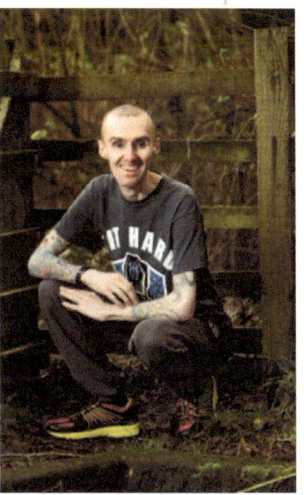

Photo 9.4

Source: Mirrorpix

didn't really understand what it was, even after a health emergency brought Tommy into treatment (Tulloch, 2016).

Now that he has recovered, he wants to share his story. He knows that eating disorders can be stigmatizing—especially because they are sometimes mistakenly seen as a problem only for women. Unfortunately, men are less likely to seek treatment, and their symptoms are less likely to attract the attention of loved ones. Slowly but surely, resources and support groups for people with eating disorders, male or female, are popping up all around the world. For Tommy, it feels good to be alive, to be healthy, and to be able to help others (Aitken, 2015; Tulloch, 2016).

Question:

What support would you recommend for a family member or friend if they were battling an eating disorder?

Males and females with eating disorders do share many of the same symptoms. Today, both sexes are bombarded by media images and social pressure to attain the thin ideal. Like females, males with eating disorders are likely to have a distorted body image, but the distortions differ between the sexes (Andersen & Holman, 1997; Pope, Gruber, Choi, Olivardia, & Phillips, 1997). Females see themselves as heavier than they are, whereas males often see themselves as smaller and want to "bulk up."

LGBTQ adolescents and young adults are also at risk for eating disorders (Gordon et al., 2019). In one study, nearly 70% of LGBTQ college students reported engaging in disordered eating behaviors. Social media, traditional media, LGBTQ-specific media, and family were all sources of the "body ideal" that created pressure and may have contributed to eating disorder symptoms (Gordon et al., 2019). This study highlights the importance for the medical community to recognize and promote eating disorder prevention and treatment programs that benefit all people. Regardless of the source, internalized disruptions in body image are a major psychosocial factor in the development of eating disorders.

Developmental Eating Disorders: Windows of Vulnerability

There are two developmental periods that create windows of vulnerability for eating disorders, especially in women. The first is in adolescence when female reproductive hormones (estrogen and progesterone) begin being produced in puberty leading to the development of secondary sexual characteristics such as breasts, and adipose tissue on hips, thighs, and buttocks. With these physical changes as well as the psychological and social changes that emerge during this time, the pressure on developing women is to be curvy and thin and the thin ideal is thought to be attractive to romantic partners. However, not all bodies develop in the socially valued way and many adolescent girls develop body image distortions that lead to eating pathology. That is one window of vulnerability for eating disorders. The second occurs when the reverse happens in women's middle-aged years. During the menopausal transition, those same hormones begin to diminish significantly. As estrogen stops being produced women stop having menstruation, and eventually, the ability to conceive children ceases. Menopause has three stages: premenopause—when hormone production becomes inconsistent and symptoms associated with this change begin to occur such as spotty periods, weight gain, and mood swings. The second stage, perimenopause, usually occurs for most women from economically stable countries around the age of 51, and this is when they have their last menstrual period. After they have gone for one full year without a period they are said to have entered postmenopause. Throughout the menopausal transition, there are many biopsychosocial changes that influence how a woman feels about her body. One of the most common physical changes in menopause is weight gain. The weight gain happens because when estrogen stops being produced metabolism slows and women's bodies begin to store energy in fat cells at a higher rate than they did previously. This, coupled with the Western emphasis on youth and thinness as a form of beauty, renders many middle-aged women feeling invisible and undesirable and can create a new form of body dysphoria. Women who have had eating disorders earlier in their lives are at the greatest risk for the re-emergence of eating disorders during this developmental period. However, there is evidence that for many women eating disorders develop for the first time during this developmental period. Either way, middle age is a crucial developmental window of vulnerability for eating disorders.

Later life (after age 65) when people are experiencing many age-related changes that may affect their senses, their lifestyles, social lives, and physical health their diet and eating patterns may change. In fact, eating disorders such as anorexia nervosa can occur when people lose the ability to smell and taste food, when they develop dementia and forget to eat, or when they lose close loved ones and are grieving. Recent research is showing how eating disorders emerge and manifest in older adults.

These are just some of the developmental changes that may influence a person's risk of developing an eating disorder.

The Biology of Eating Disorders

Eating disorders have complex causes, and it is impossible to disentangle them. Many people want to lose weight, but relatively few end up with an eating disorder. Although 60% of young women say they are dieting, only 10% go on to develop clinically diagnosed eating disorders (Neumark-Sztainer et al., 2006). Research has still not clearly identified the key factors that may put those 10% at greater risk for developing an eating disorder. We can, however, investigate from a biopsychosocial perspective.

Genes, biology, and temperament all interact with the environment to increase risk (National Alliance for Eating Disorders, 2024; Stice, South, & Shaw, 2012). Genetic factors explain between 50% and 80% of the variance in anorexia and bulimia (Kaye, Wierenga, Bailer, Simmons, & Bischoff-Grethe, 2013). However, there are more than 40 different genes involved in the regulation of psychosocial, emotional, and behavioral components of eating pathology. Patients with eating disorders are 11 times more likely to have a close family member who has an eating disorder (National Alliance for Eating Disorders, 2024). However, the actual genes or genotypes involved have not yet been identified.

Although the neural foundations of eating behaviors are still not fully understood, an interaction between the reward centers of the brain and the brain circuitry that regulates caloric intake is likely (Lee et al., 2018). The *hypothalamus* (which controls many bodily functions, including the release of hormones) is critical. In experiments with rodents, when the hypothalamus was damaged, anorexia developed (McClean & Redmond, 1988). There is some evidence that individuals with eating disorders may have altered responsiveness in the brain regions involved in appetite regulation (Kaye, Bailer, Frank, Wagner, & Henry, 2005; Steiger & Bruce, 2007; Stice, Yokum, Blum, & Bohon, 2010).

The **serotonin hypothesis** suggests that many people with eating disorders are unable to regulate the neurotransmitter serotonin (Akkermann et al., 2012; Díaz-Marsá et al., 2011). One useful index of serotonin functioning is the level of monoamine oxidase (MAO) platelet activity. This activity is at significantly lower levels in those with bulimia nervosa, although the causal relationship is still unclear. (The results are less conclusive in cases of anorexia nervosa.) Other research shows that the neurotransmitter dopamine (which works in the reward centers of the brain and motivates us to desire foods) may play a role as well. Dopamine activity is altered in people with anorexia and bulimia, but in opposing ways (Frank et al., 2012). It may influence the reward circuits differently in those with bulimia and in those with anorexia (Frank, 2015), explaining why bulimia is associated with binging, while anorexia is linked with starvation.

In addition to exploring the role of neurotransmitters, neuroimaging studies have identified some key brain regions that are involved in eating disorders. When healthy women and women who were recovering from anorexia were asked to focus on what they were experiencing in different body regions (their hearts, stomachs, or bladders), the region of the brain called the *insula* showed abnormal activity in the women with anorexia, suggesting that there may be an altered sense of interoception, or physiological awareness (Kerr et al., 2016). Neuropsychological research is pushing the frontiers of knowledge on eating disorders.

Psychosocial Factors

Many people report pressure to be thin. The **dual pathway model of eating disorders** identifies how psychosocial risk factors act together to predict the onset of eating disorders, especially bulimia nervosa (Stice, 1994; Stice, 2001; Stice & Van Ryzin, 2019). Specifically, the pressure to be thin and the pursuit of the "thin ideal" increase body dissatisfaction, leading to dietary restrictions, negative emotions, and, ultimately, unhealthy weight control behaviors. For example, binge eating is more likely in people with bulimia nervosa when they feel negative emotions (Zunker, Mitchell, & Wonderlich, 2011). Overregulation of eating, especially sweet foods, may actually increase the risk of binging (Stice et al., 2010). Other possible correlates include early childhood trauma and maltreatment, social isolation, parenting style, and cultural pressures. Eating disorders are also comorbid with depression and anxiety (Frazier & Hayes, 2019; Haynos, Roberto, & Attia, 2015; Pila, Murray, Le Grange, Sawyer, & Hughes, 2019), with some disordered eating behaviors resembling obsessive-compulsive symptoms (**Photo 9.5**).

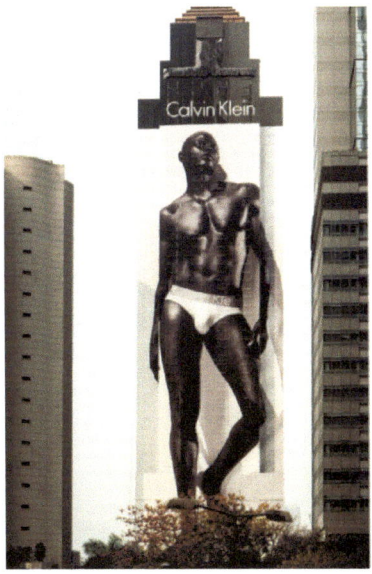 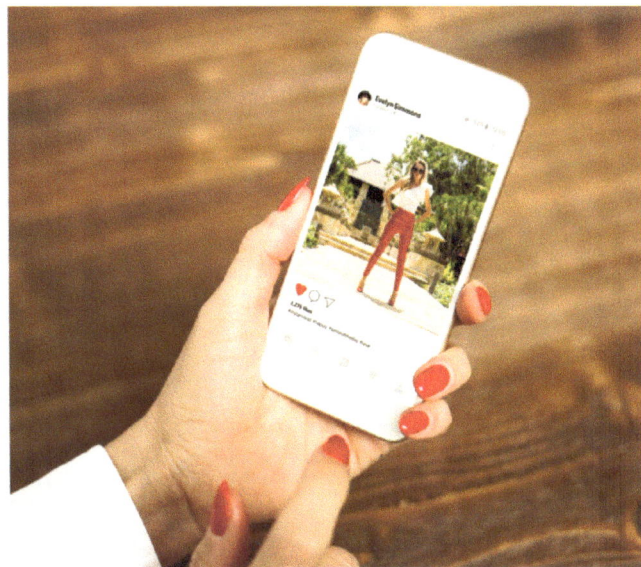

Photo 9.5   The way people perceive themselves is influenced by psychosocial factors, such as the media—whether on a billboard or on social media

Source: Kees Meselaar/Alamy (left) and Kaspars Grinvalds/Shutterstock (right)

In the News

Social Media and Eating Disorders

Social media is a ubiquitous part of our lives today. One of the most common and prevalent issues on social media concerns people's appearance and lifestyles. Research shows that social media can push people to engage in unhealthy eating behaviors, develop body distortions and low self-esteem, and that directly exacerbates eating disorders. Based upon life-threatening outcomes on exposure to social media, many platforms began monitoring and removing the most damaging content. However, that just drove postings underground with hashtags that conveyed content but eluded censorship. It is still out there and research using machine learning was able to analyze millions of

tweets to uncover troubling and harmful content related to eating disorders that were very easily accessible and often embedded within "safe" and "healthy" discussions of diet and exercise (Chu et al., 2024). There are sites and influences who are actually "pro-anorexia" and who actively promote and intensify highly toxic content that vulnerable groups are exposed to. Some experts have concluded that the friends people make on social media can actually make people's mental health worse! What may look like a discussion board on the latest diet craze (i.e., Keto, intermittent fasting) can morph quickly into an echo chamber for toxic eating disorder content. In 2023 the U.S. Surgeon General, Dr. Vivek Murthy, put out a social media and youth mental health advisory outlining the most current scientific evidence of the negative effects of social media on the mental health of young people. This was necessary because while 95% of teenagers use social media, 1/3 of all teens report they use social media "constantly." Take the experience of Sophie Szew, who said that when she was 10 years old she downloaded Instagram which led her down a life-threatening path to self-harm. "It started out just as images of very thin models but slowly it transitioned into content that I would describe as 'pro-ano' (i.e., pro-anorexia)" which encouraged eating disorders behavior, she said (CBS News, 2023). Due to this exposure and encouragement, Sophie developed an eating disorder and was hospitalized 13 times. By the age of 15 years old, it wasn't clear if she would survive, she was given two weeks to live. Luckily, her family and the medical community were able to turn things around and today Sophie is a senior at Stanford University in California. She has been called to testify in the Senate for legislation that would require closer monitoring of social media content to prevent these life-threatening outcomes for other youths.

Question: Have you encountered social media content that you think promotes eating disorders?

Personality and Eating Disorders

A host of personality traits have been indicated in eating pathology. Specifically, perfectionism, neuroticism, compulsivity, harm avoidance, dysphoria, low self-directedness, sensation-seeking, impulsivity, lack of persistence, and lack of planning all have been found to be linked to eating disorders. Personality and temperament may also predict the course of eating disorders and their treatment. People with eating disorders are often restrained, cautious, and perfectionist, and can be impulsive, dramatic, and easily emotionally aroused (Adan & Kaye, 2011). Negative emotions, the drive for thinness, poor awareness of one's internal functioning, a feeling of ineffectiveness, and obsessive-compulsive personality traits may all predispose an individual toward eating disorders (Lilenfeld, Wonderlich, Riso, Crosby, & Mitchell, 2006).

In a biopsychosocial fashion, some research suggests that personality may interact with the stress and hormonal fluctuations of puberty to increase the risk of eating disorders. Many personality traits are highly heritable, so the interactions among personality, genetics, and physiology are hard to tease apart. For example, one study found higher rates of eating disorders in people with borderline personality traits (Díaz-Marsá et al., 2011). Both borderline personality traits and eating disorders share a common mechanism in the dysregulation of serotonin.

In an effort to understand the interplay among personality and eating disorders, several theories have emerged. The **predispositional model** suggests that personality precedes and may elevate the risk of developing an eating disorder. This model assumes that personality is independent of eating disorders and that each has distinct causes, but personality vulnerabilities may predispose one to develop an eating disorder (Lyon et al., 1997). The **complication model** sees personality traits as arising from the eating disorder itself (Keyes, Brozek, Henschel, Mickelsen, & Taylor, 1950). Many people with eating disorders, especially anorexia, are extremely restrictive in their eating and may become more compulsive in personality as a result. This theory is supported by a landmark study of severely restricted eating (Keyes et al., 1950). Semi-starved participants came to exhibit many of the same symptoms and personality constructs as one another, and it was concluded that these characteristics arose out of starvation (Keyes et al., 1950). Finally, the **common cause model** proposes that there is some underlying factor, such as a genetic predisposition, that causes both personality traits *and* eating disorders to develop (Plomin, DeFries, & McClearn, 1990).

Even within the common cause model, there are three possible explanations. First, one can look for a *third variable* beyond personality or eating disorders. For example, childhood trauma may increase the risk of both borderline personality disorder and eating disorders (Lyon et al., 1997). Second, the *spectrum approach* sees personality and eating as two possible outcomes of a single cause (Lilenfeld et al., 1998). Last, the *pathoplasty model* suggests that an eating disorder and personality traits, once established, shape each other.

Eating disorders involve many interrelated factors, from genetics to parenting style and from cultural influences to traumatic experiences. Although the definitive answers about the causes are still unknown, biopsychosocial research on eating disorders is advancing. There is promising evidence that eating disorders begin with the reward centers in the brain (Weir, 2016). But the impact of psychological, social, and cultural forces is emerging from research exploring the growing impact of social media, which prompts us to compare ourselves with others (Thompson & Stice, 2001).

Treatment for Eating Disorders

Although large-scale efforts to prevent eating disorders are still limited, public awareness is growing. Over 82% of American adults understand that eating disorders are real illnesses; 85% think that treatment for eating disorders should be covered by insurance; and 70% would prefer that the media and advertisers use healthier, average-size people in their advertising campaigns (National Eating Disorders Association, 2010).

The very best treatment approach for eating disorders is a multidisciplinary approach that involves—at the very least—an eating disorders-trained therapist, a psychiatrist, a primary care physician, and a nutritionist (National Alliance for Eating Disorders, 2024). The immediate treatment goals for patients with eating disorders are adequate nutrition, reduced excessive exercise, and prevention of purging. Some patients may need to be hospitalized initially, especially if being severely malnourished or underweight is a concern. Psychotherapy and medications can be highly effective, but they should be tailored to individual needs. Typical treatment plans include medical care and monitoring; individual, group, or family psychotherapy; and nutritional counseling. Cognitive behavioral therapy can help patients focus on restructuring their disordered body image and maladaptive thought processes.

For anorexia or bulimia, antidepressants, antipsychotics, or mood stabilizers together with supportive psychotherapy are more effective than psychotherapy alone. Antidepressants such as fluoxetine (Prozac) may help patients with bulimia manage their feelings of depression and anxiety, improve eating attitudes, reduce binge eating and purging, and reduce the chance of relapse.

The Intersection of Obesity and Eating Disorders: Prevention and Intervention: To offset the potentially damaging body images of traditional and

1.   Reclaim health

Goal: Determine what influences you, and prioritize your health.

Benefit: Become the authority of your own body.

2.   Practice intuitive self-care

Goal: Eat and exercise intuitively, yet healthfully.

Benefit: Develop bodily wisdom and awareness.

3.   Cultivate self-love

Goal: Show compassion toward yourself and others, and discard criticism.

Benefit: Build your confidence and personal contentment.

4.   Declare your own authentic beauty

Goal: Enjoy living in your own skin.

Benefit: Behold beauty in yourself and others.

5.   Build community

Goal: Connect with others while modeling love and respect.

Benefit: Construct a community of body positive people.

Source: Information from The Body Positive (2016).

Table 9.3   The body positive model

social media, advocacy programs that employ cognitive reframing have appeared across the United States. The Body Positive Movement, a web-based program that provides training in reframing, is one example (see **Table 9.3**). According to the movement, there are thoughts and actions that can be practiced daily to develop a positive body image. Another example is the Dove Campaign for Real Beauty, which aims to build self-esteem and a self-defined appreciation of one's beauty.

These social advocacy programs can help people battling obesity deal with the stigma associated with their disease and can help those suffering from eating disorders reconcile what is real versus what is an unattainable standard of beauty. Although these programs are grounded in solid research, neither have been empirically tested to determine if they lead to changes in self-concept. But these efforts represent a good start to addressing a health-compromising issue at the societal level.

Thinking About Health

■ What are eating disorders, and who is at risk for developing them?

■ What biopsychosocial factors contribute to eating disorders?

■ If you have family or friends who suffer from eating disorders, how do the different models apply to their experiences?

■ What actions would you recommend be taken in order to address the problem of eating disorders at the national or global level?

KEY TERMS ▶ Energy Balance Model p. 281, Carbohydrate-Insulin Hypothesis p. 281, Protein-Leverage Hypothesis p. 281, Seed Oil Hypothesis p. 281, Obesogen Model p. 281, Obesogenic environment p. 282, Built environment p. 283, Social Learning Theory p. 283, Social contagion p. 283, Food addiction p. 284, Eating disorders p. 286, Disordered Eating p. 288, Anorexia Nervosa p. 288, Bulimia Nervosa p. 288, Binge Eating Disorder p. 288, Avoidant Restrictive Food Intake Disorder (ARFID) p. 288, Muscle dysmorphia p. 291, Serotonin hypothesis p. 294, Dual pathway model of eating disorders p. 294, Predispositional model p. 296, Complication model p. 296, Common cause model p. 297

CHAPTER 10

Cardiovascular Disorders and Diabetes

Learning Outcomes

After reading this chapter, you should be able to:

- **Define** cardiovascular disease (CVD) and other related diseases (such as diabetes).
- **Describe** how the cardiovascular system works.
- **Identify** the pathological changes that lead to the development of CVD and diabetes.
- **Outline** metabolic syndrome and explain its links to CVD.
- **Explain** the biopsychosocial factors that relate to CVD.
- **Identify** developmental, cultural, and individual influences on CVD.

At age 40, Shawn never imagined that he could be a stroke victim. But if his stroke was the wake-up call that he needed to live a healthier life, then, he realized, he was actually very fortunate that the stroke had not been worse (**Photo 10.1**).

It was an unexpected surprise for Shawn to wake up that December morning with numbness in his left foot. Shawn had several presentations scheduled at work that day, and he had finally fallen asleep around 1 A.M., after hours of preparation and anxious tossing and turning. The stress of a demanding sales job was wearing on him. It had been two months since he had found the time to exercise, and nearly a year since his last vacation. Recently, the pressure had grown so unbearable that he had relapsed into smoking, a habit that he hadn't indulged in since he was a teenager. His renewed smoking had spurred so many fights with his husband, Alex, that he had begun to drink more heavily as well, seeking an escape from the disagreements and the daily grind. The stress of it all had caused Shawn's health to fall by the wayside.

But that morning, Shawn was jolted back to reality. The sensation in his foot resembled the

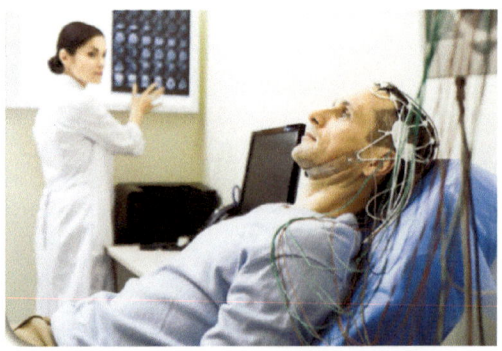

Photo 10.1 YAKOBCHUK VIACHESLAV/Shutterstock. Licensed material is being used for illustrative purposes only; any person depicted in the licensed material is a model.

DOI: 10.4324/9781032643090-10

"pins and needles" of lost circulation, only they did not go away when he tried to move his foot, nor when he got out of bed. Instead, the numbness spread, coursing up the left side of his body, until even his face felt flaccid and numb. It was at that point that he realized something was terribly wrong. He called frantically for Alex, who, seeing the severity of his symptoms, drove him to the emergency department.

At the hospital, the doctors took a scan of Shawn's brain. There, they found a small blood clot that had caused a stroke. Shawn's condition was serious, and the doctors were worried that he might have another stroke, so they admitted him to the hospital for observation. But Shawn was one of the lucky ones: After the numbness subsided, there was no long-term damage from the stroke, and he was permitted to go home. Before he was discharged, however, the neurologist gave him some blunt advice: quit smoking, check the excessive drinking, exercise daily, and, most importantly, find healthy ways to reduce stress. No one should reach the point where only a dangerous wake-up call can bring them back to a healthier reality.

Today, Shawn will tell you that he knew he needed to make lifestyle changes all along. In living a healthier, more balanced life, his work, marriage, and overall well-being have all improved. But why did it take such extreme lengths for these improvements to happen?

Cardiovascular disease (CVD) is very common. Many people have it and don't even know it! Shawn's story is just one example, and you may have family members or friends with stories like this one as well. One notable aspect of Shawn's story is how well he recovered. What do you think contributed to his recovery? What are the important take-home messages from this story?

Taken together, diseases that affect the heart and circulatory system are called **CVDs**. This is an umbrella term for a variety of diseases that affect the heart and blood vessels. (You may also hear terms such as *coronary heart disease, coronary artery disease,* or *cerebrovascular disease.*) Gaining an understanding of the risk factors for CVD is important because it is the leading cause of death in the world today. Over 20 million people died of CVD in 2021 and over 80% of those deaths occurred in low and middle-income countries (Di Cesare et al., 2024). Moreover, CVD is projected to account for more than 24 million deaths per year in 2030 (Benjamin et al., 2018). Many factors have contributed to the increased mortality associated with CVD including the COVID-19 pandemic. The COVID-19 pandemic has created another risk factor for CVD. Especially for those people with "long COVID" CVD risk a risk factor, comorbid condition, and a consequence of long COVID (Dennis et al., 2023). More important, CVD is preventable. One large-scale meta-analysis showed that 90% of CVD is attributable to modifiable risk factors (O'Donnell et al., 2016).

CVD is chronic, meaning that many people have to live with and manage their illness throughout their lives. It is also comorbid, which means that it is found in people with other physical and mental health problems. Take diabetes, for example. When not treated or managed, diabetes can lead to heart disease and stroke. In fact, the leading causes of death for people with diabetes are stroke and heart disease (Oakes, 2018). However, diabetes, too, can be managed through diet, exercise, and medications.

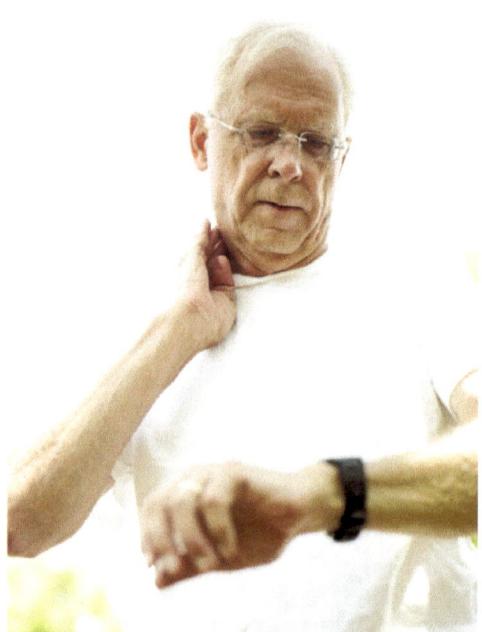

Photo 10.2   Can you feel your heart beating? Check your pulse by pressing gently against the side of your neck, to the side of your throat.

In this chapter, we explore the biopsychosocial and cultural factors that influence the development of different diseases of the cardiovascular system—including hypertension, metabolic syndrome, stroke, and diabetes. We shall see that these are, in part, diseases of modernization and lifestyle, and their management involves significant behavioral changes—and, as with Shawn, they require prompt attention. Although CVD is a global disease, millions of Americans have had their CVD discovered in time and successfully treated. Today, thanks to great advances in medical techniques and procedures, heart surgeries are routine and associated with high rates of successful recovery and long healthy lives (**Photo 10.2**).

The Cardiovascular System

We need to be familiar with the cardiovascular system in order to understand how disease develops. The **cardiovascular system** consists of the heart, blood vessels, and the blood, and it is the system responsible for transporting oxygenated blood and nutrients to all the cells in the body. It also transports hormones and neurochemicals and controls body temperature. Arteries carry oxygenated blood to the organs and tissues of the body, and veins carry it back to the heart. This cycle is called **circulation**.

Think of your cardiovascular system as a tree. Its "trunk" is the main artery (the *aorta*) that flows directly from the heart, branches into other large arteries, and then breaks out into smaller and smaller blood vessels all the way to the small capillaries in your skin. You can also think of it as two distinct but closely related systems, like a highway with northbound and southbound lanes. The system of arteries that bring oxygen-rich blood to the organs, tissues, and cells throughout the body are the southbound lanes. The northbound lanes are the veins that bring the oxygen-poor blood and waste products back to the heart.

The Heart

On average, an adult's heart beats 80 times per minute, 115,200 times a day. That is around 42 million times a year. Just imagine: If you live to the ripe old age of 80, your heart will have beat more than 3.3 billion times.

Gently press your fingers on the side of your neck, just to the side of your throat. Can you feel the pulsing of the blood through your artery? The beating of your heart sends the blood pumping through the system. Circulation begins when the heart relaxes between two heartbeats: Blood flows in from both the upper two chambers of the heart (the *atria*) into the lower two chambers (the *ventricles*). When the heart contracts, the ventricles pump the blood into the arteries. Again, the heart functions as a pump causing the circulation of the blood through the body.

The circulatory system works in conjunction with the *pulmonary* or *respiratory* system, which exchanges carbon dioxide for oxygen as we breathe. **Figure 10.1** displays this process. The left side of the heart (the *left ventricle* and *atrium*) brings in *oxygenated blood* from the lungs, through the major artery leaving the heart (the *aorta*) out to all the organs and tissues of the body. As it travels through the circulatory system, the blood brings oxygen to the organs and tissues and removes the waste and carbon dioxide. The blood returns to the right side of the heart into the *right atrium* and then through the *right ventricle*, which pumps the blood back into the lungs. There it releases the carbon dioxide and becomes oxygenated, and then the process starts again.

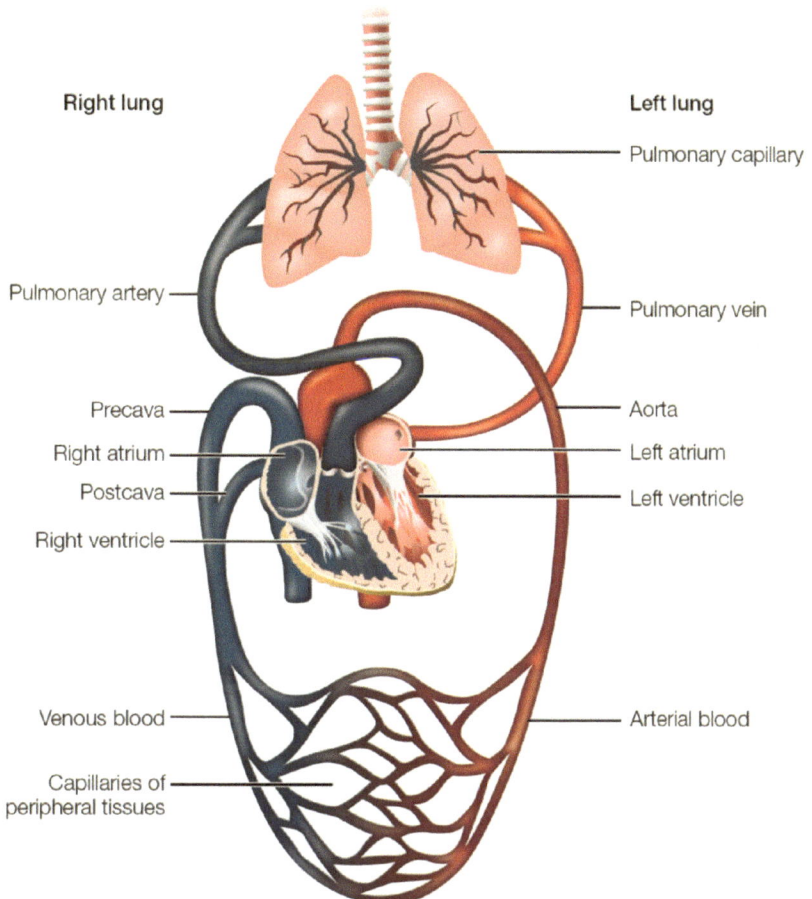

Figure 10.1   Blood circulation via the cardiovascular system.

Blood pressure category	Systolic mm Hg (upper number)		Diastolic mm Hg (lower number)
Normal	Less than **120**	and	Less than **80**
Elevated	**120–129**	and	Less than **80**
High blood pressure (hypertension) **Stage 1**	**130–139**	or	**80–89**
High blood pressure (hypertension) **Stage 2**	**140** or higher	or	**90** or higher
Hypertensive crisis (emergency care needed)	Greater than **180**	and/or	Greater than **120**

Source: Information from the American Heart Association (2024).

Table 10.1   Blood pressure chart

The Cardiac Cycle

The beating of the heart, or *cardiac cycle*, has two phases. The pumping of the heart is the **systolic phase**, as the heart muscles contract and blood is pushed out to begin its flow. Here blood pressure rises. The relaxing of the heart between pumps is the **diastolic phase**, during which blood pressure drops to its minimum. Worried that you may have high blood pressure? A *sphygmomanometer* measures the pressure in both phases—the systolic pressure on the blood vessels while the heart is beating and the diastolic pressure while the heart is at rest. Blood pressure readings always give a pair of numbers to indicate both pressures, and both are important to the health of your heart. For example, if you have your blood pressure taken, you might be told your pressure is "105 over 64."

In 2024, the American Heart Association guidelines for blood pressure changed. Specifically, the guidelines were lowered for the diagnosis of hypertension (high blood pressure). Normal healthy blood pressure is 120/80. However, Stage 1 hypertension is between 130–130/80–89; and stage two is now 140/90. In fact, 70–79% of men age 55 and older are now classified as having hypertension (Harvard Health Publishing, 2018). **Table 10.1** reflects the blood pressure categories defined by the American Heart Association (**Photo 10.3**).

Not all high blood pressure readings are signs of danger. When you are excited, stressed, or exercising hard, your heart rate and blood pressure also rise. Simply being in a doctor's office can increase your blood pressure, a result known as "white coat syndrome." The time it takes for the body to recover after bouts of high blood pressure and heart rate is, in fact, a good indication of overall health.

Yet people with a family history of high blood pressure or regular high readings may

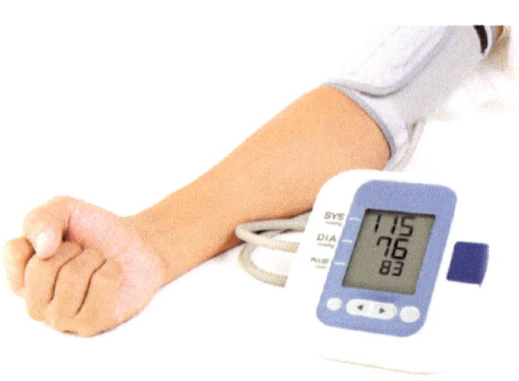

Photo 10.3   Measuring your blood pressure is a quick, easy way to be proactive about your health.

Source: ImpackPro/Getty Images

need to modify their lifestyle to bring pressure down. Over time, high blood pressure is an indication of strain on the cardiovascular system. If lifestyle changes are not successful, medication to control blood pressure may be prescribed. As we see next, these people may be suffering from CVD.

Thinking About Health

■ What was your latest blood pressure reading?

■ Before you read further, can you guess what factors might negatively affect the cardiovascular system's functioning?

What Is Cardiovascular Disease?

Diseases of the cardiovascular system begin to develop when plaques build up in the artery walls, diminishing the amount of blood that can flow through the arteries to the organs, tissues, and cells. In the early stages, this buildup is largely asymptomatic. Many people have CVD and are not even aware of it.

CVD can be a silent and deadly disease. Shawn, from our chapter opening story, is one example; Don is another. One Saturday morning, Don, a physically fit 42-year-old, was playing his usual weekly pickup basketball game with friends at the park. Don played sports regularly and even coached sports at the university level. Yet, he collapsed while going for a layup. The men on the court gave him CPR and called an ambulance, but they could not revive him. It was a devastating loss to family and friends, none of whom had suspected that his health had been at risk. It was only upon autopsy that the cause of death became known: Don had had a massive heart attack.

Lifestyle choices such as smoking, poor diet, and a lack of exercise can contribute to CVD, as we saw with Shawn. Other less visible risk factors include high blood pressure, inflammation, obesity, diabetes, and atherosclerosis. CVD has been called the "silent killer" because of the damage from ordinary lifestyle factors, none of which may show symptoms until the disease has progressed.

Atherosclerosis and Heart Attacks

Atherosclerosis is the buildup of plaques on the artery walls. A high-fat, high-calorie diet is a risk factor for the buildup of plaque. This buildup causes the blood to encounter more resistance, so systolic pressure will be higher. Eventually, if the coronary artery becomes too narrow and the blood flow too slow, the heart is deprived of oxygen and nutrients, a condition known as **ischemia**. Sometimes, ischemia can exist even without symptoms—already a very dangerous situation (**Photo 10.4**).

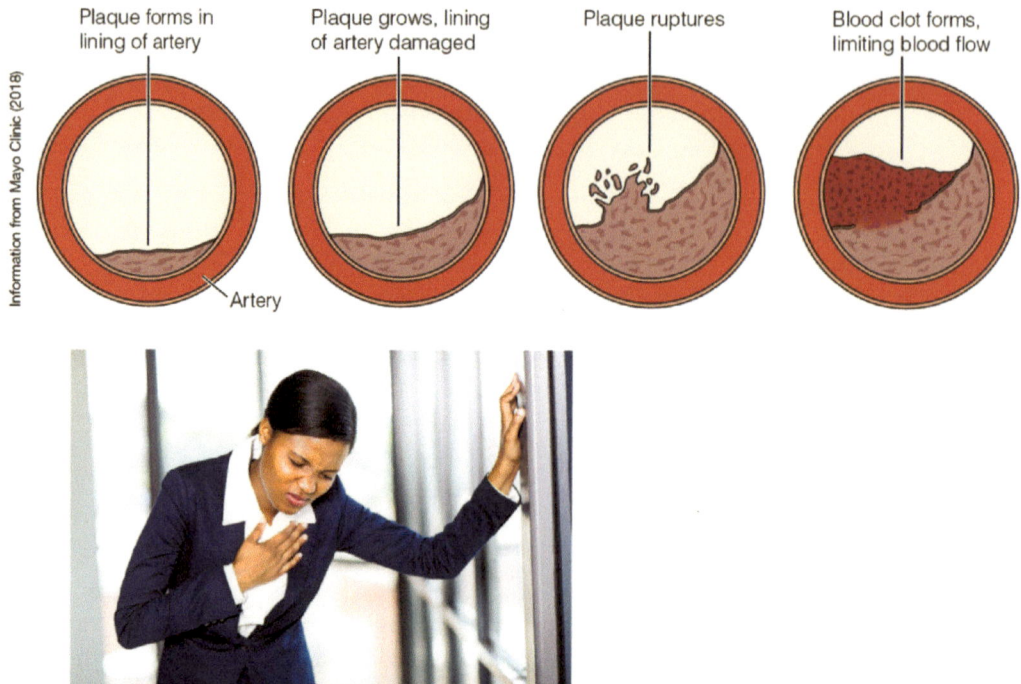

Plaque forms in lining of artery

Plaque grows, lining of artery damaged

Plaque ruptures

Blood clot forms, limiting blood flow

Artery

Information from Mayo Clinic (2018)

Photo 10.4   Atherosclerosis is the buildup of plaque on the artery walls (top). This buildup can lead to ischemia, a condition in which the heart is deprived of oxygen and nutrients. When ischemia persists, the lack of oxygen can cause angina pectoris (bottom), which is most often manifested as a crushing pain in the chest.

Source: Information from Mayo Clinic (2018) (top) and Michaeljung/Getty Images (bottom)

When ischemia persists, however, the lack of oxygen to the heart can cause the pain or discomfort of **angina pectoris**—a crushing feeling and shortness of breath. Angina is most commonly felt in the chest, but it can also appear in the arms, neck, jaw, or upper back. Angina is often felt during heightened emotional states (stress) or physical exertion. Sometimes, an ischemic attack is a single episode that resolves itself, with no permanent damage to the heart. However, in severe or prolonged ischemia, the heart muscle (or *myocardium*) begins to die, producing a **myocardial infarction**, or heart attack.

Stroke

Every year around the world 15 million people suffer a stroke. Of those five million will die and 5 million will be permanently disabled from the stroke (WHO, 2024f). Strokes are uncommon in people younger than age 40 but when they do happen they are associated with high blood pressure. A **stroke** results from disrupted blood flow to the brain, which causes cell death.

There are three types of strokes. **Ischemic strokes**, accounting for 87% of all strokes, result when blood flow to the brain becomes blocked (American Heart Association, 2017). This is the most common form of stroke and the kind that Shawn suffered from. In ischemic strokes, plaque breaks off and circulates through the arteries, where it encounters a narrowing in the artery leading to the brain. (If the plaque breaks off and blocks an artery that feeds the heart instead of the brain, a heart attack can occur.) **Hemorrhagic strokes** result from the rupture of a weakened blood vessel, which causes bleeding in the brain. These are less common than ischemic strokes. Only 13% of all strokes are hemorrhagic, but more than 30% of people who have a hemorrhagic stroke will die from it. The third type of stroke is also caused by a temporary clot blocking blood flow in the brain. **Transient ischemic attacks** (TIAs, or "mini-strokes") are brief episodes of neurological dysfunction due to ischemia, without acute obstruction of the blood supply. TIAs are warning signs of stroke. More than 50% of all people who experience a TIA will go on to have an actual stroke, usually within the first 48 hours of the TIA (Panuganti, Tadi, & Lui, 2019). TIAs are hard to diagnose since they are fleeting by nature. But they are often associated with a neurological deficit and speech disturbance of sudden onset. Sometimes, these symptoms will disappear in the aftermath.

After a TIA, future stroke risk can be assessed by an *ABCD² score*, an assessment tool that predicts short-term stroke risk (National Stroke Association, 2014). The score is designed to assess the risk of stroke within 2–90 days after a TIA by calculating and summing points for five factors:

A = Age	=> older than 60 years (1 point)
B = Blood pressure	=> greater than or equal to 140/90 mm Hg (1 point)
C = Clinical symptoms	=> focal weakness with the spell (2 points) or speech impairment without weakness (1 point)
D = Duration	=> a TIA lasting longer than 60 minutes (2 points) or a TIA lasting between 10 and 59 minutes (1 point)
D = Diabetes	mellitus (1 point)

In people who have had a TIA, an ABCD² score of 6 or 7 is 8% likely to lead to an elevated 2-day risk of stroke (National Stroke Association, 2014). The World Health Organization has said, "for every 10 people who die of stroke, four could have been saved if their blood pressure had been regulated (WHO, 2024g)." In people under the age of 65 40% are linked to cigarette smoking. Heart failure, heart attack, and atrial fibrillation are other risk factors.

A stroke often begins with sudden feelings of weakness or numbness in one half of the body. It is a medical emergency; treating a stroke as quickly as possible is crucial. Two million brain cells die each minute during a stroke, so every minute without treatment increases the risk of permanent brain damage, disability, and death (Saver, 2006).

Stroke: The Warning Signs Want a quick way to recognize the signs of a stroke? Think FAST:

F = Face	Ask the person to smile. Does one side of the face droop?
A = Arms	Ask the person to raise both arms. Does one arm drift downward?
S = Speech	Ask the person to repeat a simple sentence. Does the speech sound slurred or strange?
T = Time	If you observe any of these signs (independently or together), call 911 immediately.

Strokes can happen to anyone at any time, regardless of age, sex, or race, though more women than men have strokes each year. African Americans have double the risk of stroke than whites. Diabetes or a family history of stroke increases the risk, as does high blood pressure, high cholesterol, alcohol use, and smoking. Another risk factor is *atrial fibrillation,* in which the chambers of the heart don't beat the way they should. Rather, they either beat irregularly or too rapidly, causing a quivering (like a bowl of gelatin). Lifestyle changes and long-term medical management are then crucial.

Thinking About Health

■ If your family or the family of someone you know has a history of CVD, what actions have family members taken to offset the risks?

■ How would you react if you encountered someone experiencing a heart attack or stroke? How would you be able to tell what they were experiencing?

What Causes Cardiovascular Disease?

Risk factors for CVD include high cholesterol levels, increased blood pressure, inflammation, and obesity. There are genetic and cultural factors as well.

Good and Bad Cholesterol

Cholesterol is a waxy substance found in all the cells in the body; it comes from the foods we eat but is also made by the body. Cholesterol itself is not bad—our bodies create and use it to keep us healthy. However, too much cholesterol leads to health problems. When we consume foods that are high in cholesterol—such as meat, poultry, full-fat dairy products, and other animal products—the liver produces excess cholesterol, leading to higher cholesterol levels. Cholesterol is what builds up and forms plaque on the artery walls.

There are two types of cholesterol: "good" **high-density lipoproteins (HDLs)** and "bad" **low-density lipoproteins (LDLs).** LDLs are what build up in the artery walls, and a diet high in saturated fats and trans fats can lead to high cholesterol. HDLs, rather, act as scavengers by traveling through the bloodstream to remove the bad cholesterol from where it does not belong and taking it to the liver, where it is broken down and eliminated from the body. If your overall cholesterol reading is high (say, above 200), but your doctor says that your HDL/LDL ratio is normal, you may be fine (see **Table 10.2**). However, if your LDL level is too high, your doctor will probably

Total cholesterol level*	Category
Less than 200 mg/dl	Desirable
200–239 mg/dl	Borderline high
240 mg/dl and above	High

* Cholesterol levels are measured in milligrams (mg) of cholesterol per deciliter (dl) of blood.

Table 10.2   Cholesterol levels

suggest dietary changes and exercise to bring it down. If, over time, your cholesterol level still does not improve, you may need medication to control it.

Metabolic Syndrome

A cluster of five biochemical and physiological abnormalities commonly come together to increase the risk for heart disease, stroke, and type 2 diabetes (Saklayen, 2018). These five conditions are collectively called **metabolic syndrome:**

1. *A large waistline.* Excess fat in the stomach area presents a greater risk for CVD than fat in other areas of the body (see Chapter 4).
2. *High triglyceride level.* Triglycerides are a type of fat that circulates in the blood. After eating, your body converts the calories it didn't use for energy into triglycerides, which are stored in your fat cells and circulate in your blood. If you often eat more calories than you burn, especially calories from carbohydrates and fats, you may have a high triglyceride level.
3. *Low HDL.* A low HDL level indicates that the LDLs are not being sufficiently removed from the body and may be building up in the artery walls.
4. *High blood pressure* (or *hypertension*). High blood pressure, as we have seen, can indicate a buildup of plaque on the artery walls and a strain on the cardiovascular system.
5. *High fasting blood sugar.* This is often an early sign of diabetes as well as a risk for heart disease.

A person is given a diagnosis of metabolic syndrome when they have three of these conditions.

Metabolic syndrome has been around for a while but has only recently become an important indicator of cardiovascular risk (Franco et al., 2009) and mortality (Lewis, Rodbard, Fox, & Grandy, 2008). Alarmingly, a recent report showed that only 12% of American adults are metabolically healthy (Araújo, Cai, & Stevens, 2018). It has also been estimated that over one billion people worldwide have metabolic syndrome (Saklayen, 2018), related to the epidemic of obesity (Araújo et al., 2018). A person with all five factors of metabolic syndrome is twice as likely to develop heart disease and five times as likely to develop diabetes as someone without metabolic syndrome (CDC, 2011a, 2011b).

The syndrome has a genetic component: It runs in families and is also more common in African Americans, Hispanics, Asians, and Native Americans. In geographic regions of the United States with high Native American populations, the rates of metabolic syndrome are as high as 50% (Sinclair, Bogart, Buchwald, & Henderson, 2011). Metabolic syndrome is also associated with lower socioeconomic status, loneliness, depression, poor health, and increased use of healthcare services (Johnson, Riley, Granger, & Riis, 2013).

Developmentally, the risk of metabolic syndrome increases with age. Today, however, more than two-thirds of U.S. adolescents have at least one of these metabolic abnormalities that will carry into adulthood (de Ferranti et al., 2004). Metabolic syndrome is a significant international health concern, now, and for the future.

Hypertension

Hypertension, or high blood pressure, is diagnosed when blood pressure readings are consistently above normal. Because high blood pressure has no overt symptoms, most people do not know they have hypertension until they are tested. And like metabolic syndrome, many people suffer from it. Nearly half of all American adults have hypertension—that is more than 122 million people (Tsao et al., 2023). Another 30% of adults have elevated blood pressure levels, an indication of cardiovascular risk.

Eight out of 10 people who have a stroke for the first time have hypertension, and 7 out of 10 people who have congestive heart failure have hypertension (Go et al., 2013). African Americans develop hypertension at an earlier age than others, as do women, and African American women have a still-higher risk: 45.7% (Go et al., 2013). South Africa has the highest hypertensive rate among adults aged 50 and older in the world (Lloyd-Sherlock, Beard, Minucci, Ebrahim, & Chatterji, 2014), with potentially devastating consequences for health and well-being. Hypertension is also striking in low- to middle-income countries, where there is too little public awareness and medical help to combat the disease. Worldwide, hypertension puts 1 billion people at greater risk for heart attack and stroke, and 9 million die from its consequences each year.

Hypertension is an example of a biopsychosocial illness. It may have biological (genetic), environmental (stress), psychological (behavioral and lifestyle), and socioeconomic (income and education) causes (see **Figure 10.2**). In 95% of people with hypertension, there is no single identifiable cause (Dosh, 2002). That is, the biological, psychological, and social factors interact, and disease manifests. Like metabolic syndrome, hypertension tends to run in families, especially when it develops before age 40. However, a person with a genetic risk may not develop hypertension if he or she eats a healthy diet, exercises regularly, doesn't smoke, and manages stress well. Although it can be diagnosed at any age, high blood pressure is most commonly diagnosed in middle-aged adults.

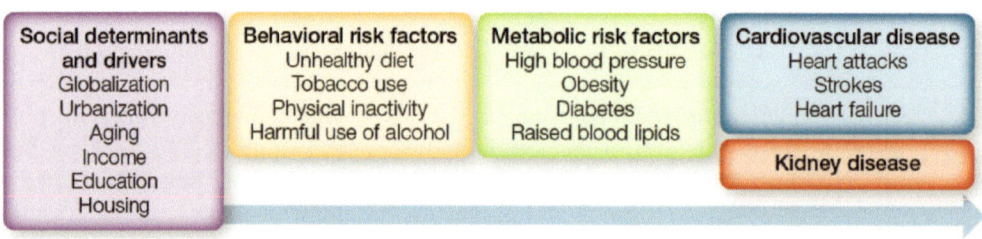

Figure 10.2   How hypertension leads to CVD.

Source: Information from WHO (2013)

High alcohol and high sodium intake are also associated with hypertension, as are low potassium and calcium intake (Carretero & Oparil, 2000).

Inflammation

Recently, inflammation has been implicated as another important driver of CVD. Low-grade chronic inflammation is involved in the development of plaques and can lead to ischemia prior to myocardial infarction. Thus, measurements of inflammation are critical biomarkers in tracking the onset and course of CVD.

Your immune system is designed to keep you healthy and fight off invading bacteria. It uses inflammation as a mechanism to destroy pathogens. In the 2000s, researchers discovered that high levels of inflammation that were *not* associated with an obvious immune response were related to increased chances of stroke or heart attack (Glynn, MacFadyen, & Ridker, 2009). In addition to irritating blood vessels, sustained low levels of inflammation in the body can trigger the formation or dislodging of plaques, contributing to all three types of stroke and heart attack.

Lifestyle changes such as quitting smoking, weight loss, and increased exercise can lower inflammation over time. A new body of research is also looking at pharmacological treatments for lowering inflammation. For example, the amount of inflammation present in the body at any given time can be measured in the blood via a protein called *C-reactive protein (CRP)*. Blood tests that measure CRP are now commonplace and can be used as an indicator of risk for developing cardiovascular problems. Whether through lifestyle or pharmacological interventions, targeting inflammation should be part of the first line of treatment for CVD (Moore, 2019).

Health Disparities in Cardiovascular Disease

Heart disease is the leading cause of death in the United States and worldwide today. In spite of medical advances, cardiovascular health inequities by geography, age, gender, race and ethnicity, and socioeconomic status persist (Mensah et al., 2019).

African American men and women, for instance, have a much higher rate of coronary heart disease, including heart attack and heart failure, than do other racial groups (Mensah et al., 2019). They are more likely to die prematurely because of heart disease as well. Sadly, 62% of black men, compared with 42% of white men, die before the age of 75 (Mensah et al., 2019). This same mortality disparity exists for stroke. A higher percentage of black women (39%) and men (61%) than white women (17%) and men (31%) die of stroke each year (CDC, 2011a). African Americans also have higher rates of hypertension, and it is more often left untreated as well (Mensah et al., 2019).

In the United States, Hispanics/Latinx have high rates of obesity, metabolic syndrome, diabetes, and heart failure, creating an elevated risk profile for CVDs (Mensah et al., 2019). Puerto Rican Americans have the highest rates of hypertension in the Hispanic groups, and Mexican Americans have the highest rates of untreated blood pressure (CDC, 2013). Those with low socioeconomic status, and those living in rural areas and the southeastern United States, have higher mortality rates as well (Go et al., 2013).

What causes these disparities? For one thing, inequities in society create barriers to good health and medical treatment. Minorities may also be less likely to seek treatment to control high blood pressure and other cardiovascular issues (CDC, 2010). Regardless of the cause, there is a great deal of research documenting health disparities in all aspects of CVD (Lee et al., 2019).

Disparities in the rates of premature deaths due to heart disease and stroke are a call to action for health psychologists. Although recent research suggests that socioeconomic influences may outweigh biology in explaining health disparities in heart disease risk (Vaughan et al., 2019), the interactions between adverse environmental and economic stress, coupled with psychological and biological challenges, make teasing apart social determinants quite difficult. Understanding the risk factors, motivating behavioral change, and developing evidence-based interventions to help reduce risks and increase healthy lifestyle choices are crucial and will all go a long way to reducing these disparities.

Changing Patterns of Cardiovascular Disease

Most of what we know about CVD today comes from large-scale studies. The Bogalusa Heart Study, for example, began in Louisiana in 1972 under the direction of Dr. Gerald Berenson, a Bogalusa native and pediatrician who was deeply concerned about the number of children who were developing risk factors for CVD. The higher risk factors in minorities raised a red flag as well.

The study began as a cross-sectional study during the 1973–1974 school year, but it became a longitudinal study that is still active today (Berenson et al., 1992, 1998). The study found clear links between childhood obesity, high blood pressure, high levels of lipids in the blood, and deaths from CVD (Freedman, Khan, Dietz, Srinivasan, & Berenson, 2001). Childhood obesity also predicts adult obesity, again highlighting the importance of early prevention and treatment (Freedman, Mei, Srinivasan, Berenson, & Dietz, 2007). The study also underscores health disparities in CVD. Recent longitudinal research from the study, for instance, shows that adolescence is a crucial window for the development of diabetes and CVD later in life (**Photo 10.5**) (Zhang et al., 2019).

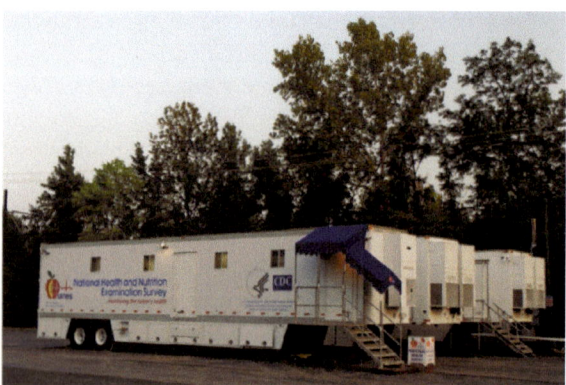

Photo 10.5 The NHANES uses mobile research units such as this one to learn as much as possible about disease, locally, regionally, and nationally.

Source: CDC/National Center for Health Statistics

Another large long-term study, the National Health and Nutrition Examination Survey (NHANES), began in the 1960s. Each year, the National Center for Health

Statistics, an arm of the CDC, has added nearly 5000 people to the study, representing a diverse sample of Americans. The study looks for links between lifestyle, heredity, and environmental risk factors for disease. For example, a history of kidney stones raises the odds of developing CVD, especially for African Americans (Glover, Bass, Carithers, & Loprinzi, 2016), while patients with diabetes who experience depression are at greater risk of complications from their disease (Wang, Lopez, Bolge, Zhu, & Stang, 2016). And a more recent longitudinal study of NHANES data showed that overweight and obese people who were able to maintain long-term weight loss were able to reduce their metabolic risk profile considerably (Olson et al., 2019).

But the NHANES does not just uncover risks for disease—it also points to prevention. For example, physical activity and strength-building exercise reduce the odds of metabolic syndrome, which we know is a precursor for CVD (Dankel, Loenneke, & Loprinzi, 2016; Olson et al., 2019). Patterns like these can help guide us to a healthier future.

These longitudinal studies are important for demonstrating how CVD changes over time. They also highlight the developmental nature of the disease, showing how early health and lifestyle choices shape health outcomes later in life. Thus, instilling optimal health behaviors and wellness from an early age is crucial.

Thinking About Health

- If you or someone you know has ever had their cholesterol measured, what did the results tell you about your or their health?
- What are the different biopsychosocial factors that lead to changes in the cardiovascular system?
- What factors shape health disparities in CVD, both in the United States and around the world?

Preventing and Treating Cardiovascular Disease

CVD, from hypertension to heart failure, is preventable, and early action is key to avoiding death and disability. Eighty percent of heart disease, stroke, and type 2 diabetes can be prevented by changing or eliminating behavioral risk factors (Habibović et al., 2018).

As Dr. Tom Frieden, former director of the Centers for Disease Control and Prevention, said, "It is heartbreaking to lose just one patient to a preventable disease or injury…. [F]ar more than a hundred thousand deaths each year are preventable" (from CDC, 2014b).

Preventing Cardiovascular Disease

As we have seen, predictors of CVD include hypertension and high levels of "bad" cholesterol. Doctors work with patients to recognize predictors and to enable changes in lifestyle. These efforts can be especially important for groups at risk.

The first step to better prevention is knowing your genetic risk profile. Free health checks (such as blood pressure monitoring machines in grocery stores, pharmacies, and fire stations) or health fairs where people can have their CVD risk factors assessed can help, as do annual visits with primary care physicians. The health benefits of screening programs for CVD are numerous (Hansen et al., 2019).

In one recent clinical trial called Do CHANGE, patients with CVD were recruited and randomly assigned to a "care as usual" (control) group or a lifestyle intervention (experimental) group. The experimental group was provided with monitoring tools (e.g., Fitbits) and underwent a behavioral change program designed to break maladaptive habits in favor of beneficial ones, like exercise, good sleep, and eating well. The intervention lasted three months. Although the data are still being analyzed, early results are promising and expected to show long-term, sustainable behavioral change and positive outcomes for those with CVD (Habibović et al., 2018).

Another recent review of the literature showed the benefits of harnessing smartphones and wearable technology for heart-healthy behavioral change. Overall, and as we saw in Chapter 3, devices that allow patients to monitor and track their physical activity promote better adherence to physical activity guidelines and can lead to reductions in CVD-related mortality and morbidity (Feldman et al., 2018). The **In the News** feature explores this idea further.

CVD risk can be lowered with medications as well. Medications can help not only by directly lowering blood pressure and cholesterol levels but also by increasing a patient's tolerance to exercise. Long-term medical management is also important and requires regular doctor visits. Unfortunately, often those who are at the greatest risk for CVD are the least likely to adhere to medical treatment plans. Perhaps due to a scarcity of resources—whether financial or medical—a lower socioeconomic status is related to lower adherence and higher mortality rates from CVD (Lee, Park, Park, & Kim, 2019).

If someone you know is at risk for CVD, be sure that they see a medical professional. Recognizing the signs of CVD—via health screenings, wearable technology, or medical visits—and engaging in behavioral prevention are critical.

Heart Attack: The Warning Signs Knowing the warning signs of a heart attack can save lives. Yet, many people—more than 92% of respondents in a classic survey—recognize only one symptom of a heart attack: chest pain (CDC, 2008). In essence, only 27% of those surveyed knew all the symptoms and the importance of calling 911. Because nearly half (47%) of all sudden cardiac deaths occur outside a hospital, it is clear that many people do not act on early warning signs.

In the News

Can a Smart Watch Save Your Life?

Smart watches such as the Apple Watch—as well as the Withings Move ECG, iBeat Heart Watch, and more—could be very helpful for people who want to monitor their biorhythms and share that data with their physicians. Wearable technologies may also enhance the motivation to engage in physical fitness to monitor, manage, and offset heart problems (**Photo 10.6**).

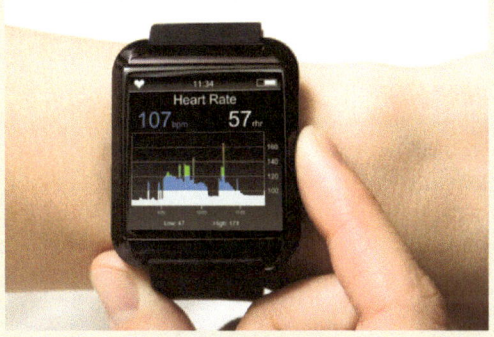

Photo 10.6

Source: Andrey_Popov/Shutterstock.com

While physicians do not unanimously agree on the benefits of wearables, one man credits his smartwatch with saving his life. Attorney Scott Killian reported in 2017 that his Apple Watch woke him around 1 A.M. with an alert from a third-party app called HeartWatch. The notification said that, while he was sleeping, his resting heart rate had spiked to 121 from a resting level of 49 beats per minute. The alert alarmed him, and he went to the emergency department as a precaution. At the hospital, his heart rate was still elevated, and the readings on the watch were consistent with those on the medical equipment. A blood test showed elevated enzymes, indicative that a heart attack was occurring. Further tests revealed that Scott had four blocked arteries, which required major heart surgery. Today, Scott credits his Apple Watch with saving his life.

The good news is that heart technology is available on all new Apple Watches and is being integrated into the hardware and software of the other leading wearable technologies, too. Someday, we may all be able to trust our health to our wearables.

Question: How would you benefit from wearing a health-tracking device? If you already wear one, what aspects are most valuable to you?

The following are the major warning signs of heart attack:

- chest pain or discomfort
- upper body pain or discomfort in the arms, back, neck, jaw, or upper stomach
- shortness of breath
- nausea
- light-headedness
- cold sweat

Increasing public awareness of these dangers can make the difference between life and death.

In a study across nine European countries, chest pain was the only symptom recognized by more than 50% of the participants, and as many as 8% of people could not list any symptoms at all (Mata et al., 2014). Only 51% of Europeans said they would call an ambulance when they thought someone was having a heart attack. Women and those who had higher levels of education were better at recognizing heart attack symptoms. And, as you might expect, older people (perhaps with more experience and awareness) were better at knowing the symptoms than younger people. Germans and Austrians were best at symptom recognition, while participants from Italy, Spain, Poland, and Russia identified the fewest symptoms.

Shawn's story—the story of someone with CVD that is not discovered until it has progressed—is common. Public education is needed to create better awareness if we want to save lives and prevent avoidable deaths from CVD in the future.

Treating Cardiovascular Disease

Once we know what contributes to CVD, we are better able to prevent it. How, though, can we treat it? It may take more than changes in lifestyle, and, again, early recognition is crucial. Shawn benefited from prompt attention, and his doctor's advice illustrated the options.

Stent catheterization involves inserting a small mesh tube into a blocked artery to allow the blood to flow through again. This surgery is now performed on nearly 1 million Americans per year. The stent can remain in place and support a weak artery. This procedure can be a lifesaver.

An **angioplasty** is a nonsurgical procedure that involves inserting a catheter with a balloon at the end into an artery. As it passes through the artery, the balloon inflates and presses the plaque against the arterial walls, diminishing the buildup to restore blood flow. In tandem, heart medications may be prescribed to maintain proper blood pressure and flow.

More radical is a coronary artery bypass graft surgery, a **heart bypass** procedure. This surgical procedure, which lasts from four to six hours, is common in cases of severe coronary artery disease, with more than 500,000 surgeries performed each year in the United States. There are two types of coronary artery bypass surgery: *on-pump* and *off-pump*. In on-pump bypass surgery, a six- to eight-inch incision is made through the sternum to give direct access to the heart. Then, the patient is connected to a heart–lung bypass machine (on-pump), which allows the blood to circulate throughout the operation. The patient's heart is then stopped while the surgeon performs the procedure—usually from 30 to 90 minutes of the four- to six-hour surgery.

In off-pump heart bypass surgery, the heart–lung bypass machine is not used, and the heart is not stopped. Instead, a section of the heart is stabilized so the graft can be done. Off-pump bypass is chosen when there is a concern of increased risk of complications from the heart–lung machine. In both types of heart bypass, the surgeon takes a vein or artery from another part of the body (often the leg) and uses it to make a detour (or graft) around the blocked area in the artery (hence, "bypass"). Up to four arteries can be bypassed in the same operation (called a quadruple bypass).

Recovery from a heart attack, heart surgery, or stroke is a challenging process that affects all aspects of a person's life. After a cardiac event, many patients are referred to **cardiac rehabilitation**, biopsychosocial programs that can help patients achieve meaningful, heart-healthy lifestyle changes. Guidelines suggest that cardiac rehabilitation programs involve educational components and psychological counseling as well as dietary and exercise promotion (Dalal, Doherty, & Taylor, 2015).

Thinking About Health

■ How can behavioral changes and increased public awareness help prevent CVD?

■ What are the treatment and rehabilitation options for patients with CVD?

Major Risks for Cardiovascular Disease

As we have seen, CVD most often stems from high blood pressure, in combination with high LDL cholesterol and poor lifestyle choices. Over half of American adults have at least one of these three risk factors (CDC, 2011a), and smoking alone is the number one behavioral risk factor. Other risk factors include diabetes, poor diet, obesity, a sedentary lifestyle, and excessive alcohol use. We have discussed the physiology of CVD, and now we will turn to the biopsychosocial risks of CVD.

Biopsychosocial Risks

Older people are more likely to develop CVD than younger people, and so are those with a family history of the disease. Aside from family history, sex, ethnicity, and age, however, the risk of CVD can be substantially reduced through preventive behavioral change.

Psychological risk factors, too, can increase the risk, and many of these are also modifiable. Risk factors include depression, anxiety, and low social support (Kupper & Denollet, 2007).

Major risk factors are factors that significantly increase the risk of heart disease. Some risks are not changeable. The more of these biological factors you have, the higher your risk:

■ *Age.* Eighty-two percent of people with CVD are 65 years old or older.

■ *Sex.* Males are at greater risk than females for heart attacks and tend to have them earlier.

■ *Family history.* Children of parents with CVD are more likely to develop it themselves.

■ *Race and ethnicity.* African Americans, Mexican Americans, Native Americans, and Native Hawaiians are at higher risk for CVD than whites.

As Shawn was informed at the start of this chapter, behavioral or lifestyle risk factors can be reduced by changes in lifestyle or medical treatment:

- *Tobacco smoke.* Smokers' risk of CVD is two to four times higher than non-smokers'. Smoking a pack per day increases the risk of heart attack by a factor of two. Even secondhand smoke increases risk in those who are exposed to it.
- *High cholesterol.* As cholesterol rises, so does the risk of CVD.
- *High blood pressure.* High blood pressure indicates that the heart is strained and at greater risk of heart attack and stroke.
- *Physical inactivity.* A sedentary lifestyle is a risk factor for CVD.
- *Obesity.* Excessive body fat, especially in the abdomen, increases the risk of CVD.
- *Diabetes.* Even when glucose levels are under control, diabetes is a risk for heart disease and stroke. If blood sugar is not controlled, the risks are even higher. More than 65% of people with diabetes die of some form of CVD.

These risk factors act *synergistically*—the more risk factors you have, the greater your risk of disease, disability, and death. For example, smokers who also have a family history of CVD are especially at risk. Similarly, being overweight increases the risk of diabetes, which is itself a risk factor for CVD. Losing even 10% of body weight can cut the risk.

Stress and Depression

Stress and physiological reactivity to stress are related to the development of heart disease. Both chronic stress and acute stress are linked to CVD, and so are anger and anxiety (Pulkki-Råback et al., 2009). Although this connection has been known for a while, in the last decade, the role of psychological factors has become more widely recognized as critical in the development of CVD. Even our relationships can influence the development of CVD (see the **Around the World** feature).

Hostility, anxiety, job stress, and depression can increase pulse and steroid levels, elevate white blood cell counts, and lead to poor lifestyle choices (Theorell, 2019). Stress elevates steroid and adrenaline levels that constrict blood vessels, raise blood pressure, and may damage the lining of the blood vessels, which can cause angina. Additionally, adrenaline can cause electrical disturbances in the heart as well as rupture the plaques that generate a blood clot, both of which can lead to heart attack or stroke.

Depression, in particular, seems to increase risk. In middle-aged women, high levels of depression predicted the risk of developing metabolic syndrome within the next seven years (Räikkönen, Matthews, & Kuller, 2002, 2007). In another study, a previous episode of depression made young women twice as likely to develop metabolic syndrome later on (Kinder, Carnethon, Palaniappan, King, & Fortmann, 2004).

Why? Depressed people are not likely to take good care of their health. Depression has been linked to a sedentary lifestyle, high intake of saturated fats, smoking, and heavy alcohol consumption (Carney, Freedland, Miller, & Jaffe, 2002; Franko, Striegel-Moore, Thompson, Schreiber, & Daniels, 2005; Pulkki-Råback et al., 2009). Another connection between depression and metabolic syndrome may be increased levels of CRP in the blood, which, as we have seen, indicates inflammation throughout the body. Evidence is mounting that high levels of CRP are linked to increased CVD, peripheral vascular disease (diseases that affect the blood vessels outside the heart and brain), and stroke (Dollard et al., 2015; Shoamanesh et al., 2015). Evidence is also emerging that inflammation may underlie the well-established links between depressive symptoms and cardiovascular risk (Kunte, Rentzsch, & Kronenberg, 2015). Otherwise healthy, depressed individuals with elevated CRP levels have a two- to threefold greater risk for CVD (Wium-Andersen, Ørsted, Nielsen, & Nordestgaard, 2013).

Around *the* World

A Bad Relationship Can Break Your Heart

"Only love can break your heart." True? Maybe not, but a bad relationship *can* lead to CVD (Joseph, Kamarck, Muldoon, & Manuck, 2014; Liu & Waite, 2014). A meta-analysis of studies across the United States, Russia, Denmark, Spain, Sweden, the United Kingdom, Canada, Israel, Japan, Finland, Greece, Turkey, Norway, and China has revealed that a poor-quality relationship may have a negative impact on health and well-being (Wong et al., 2018). Being divorced is associated with increased rates of coronary heart disease, while being widowed is associated with increased mortality after stroke (Wong et al., 2018). Worldwide, people who are not happy in their marriage have an 8.5 times greater risk of suffering a heart attack or stroke than those whose marriages are positive and filled with good feeling.

"Growing evidence suggests that the quality and patterns of one's social relationships may be linked with a variety of health outcomes, including heart disease," said Thomas Kamarck, one author of a study that found a link between unhappy relationships and heart disease (Joseph et al., 2014). In this study, researchers asked participants to report hourly on their feelings about their partners (for example, their agreeableness) and their relationship (for example, the level of conflict). Nearly 300 healthy, employed, middle-aged people took part over four days; all were married or in a close, long-term relationship. Those who had overall positive marital quality had fewer markers of CVD, such as arterial plaque, and those who rated their marriages negatively had greater signs and risk of heart disease. According to the study's lead author, the findings may have wider implications as well: "Biological, psychological, and social processes all interact to determine physical health." The effects are lasting, too; another study showed that even past marital discord is related to cardiovascular health (Donoho, Seeman, Sloan, & Crimmins, 2015).

Question:

How do you think that a past or current relationship has affected your cardiovascular health?

How does CRP lead to depression? One potential mechanism is that increased inflammation raises the levels of cytokines (small proteins involved in cell signaling), which leads to greater stress and depression. Although the role of inflammation is still not fully understood in depression, patients with high levels of CRP appear at increased risk for depression and, as we have previously explored, CVD.

Type A Personality

The risks of psychological distress for the development of CVD are well documented (Hamer, Kivimaki, Stamatakis, & Batty, 2012; Nicholson, Kuper, & Hemingway, 2006; Rumsfeld & Ho, 2005; Rumsfeld et al., 2003; Yu, Sánchez-Lozada, Johnson, & Kang, 2010). Psychological distress is a risk factor for recurring cardiac events, longer recovery from these events, and a higher risk of death from CVD.

The role of personality and stress in CVD has a long history. In 1959, two cardiologists, Drs. Meyer Friedman and Ray Rosenman, proposed that **type A personality** is a major risk factor for CVD. This personality, they argued, is characterized by competitive, hard-driving behavior, including a predisposition to interact with others in a hostile or aggressive way (Friedman & Rosenman, 1974). Excessive competitiveness, irritability, hostility, and a persistent desire for recognition are all hallmarks of type A people. People high in type A tend to be ambitious, high-achieving workaholics, who are rigidly organized, and "short fused"—or, overly sensitive and impatient. They may also be status-conscious and take on more tasks than they can handle.

From several decades of research, Dr. Friedman distilled the type A behavior pattern into three major symptoms: (1) free-floating hostility (which can be triggered by even mild incidents), (2) time urgency and impatience (which causes irritation and exasperation), and (3) a competitive drive (which cause stress and an achievement-driven mentality).

The *type B* behavior pattern is the opposite of type A, although many people have a mix of different traits. Type Bs are relaxed, tolerant of others, reflective, higher in imagination and creativity, and lower in anxiety. Type A traits appeared to double a man's risk of CVD when compared with a man who did not have these traits (Friedman & Rosenman, 1974).

The Friedman and Rosenman study (Friedman & Rosenman, 1974) turned out to have serious limitations. Its sample contained only middle-aged men, and research discrediting its findings has caused the theory to fall out of favor. However, continued research has sought to tease apart the role of type A personality in CVD. Of all the type A characteristics, hostility has gained particular attention. Hostility is seen as an emotional state charged with anger, aggression, antagonism, opposition, and defiance. Despite different empirical approaches to measuring hostility, research shows that—after controlling for age, sex, education, smoking, and health history—hostile people are twice as likely to die of heart problems than those who are low in hostility (**Photo 10.7**) (Wong, Sin, & Whooley, 2014).

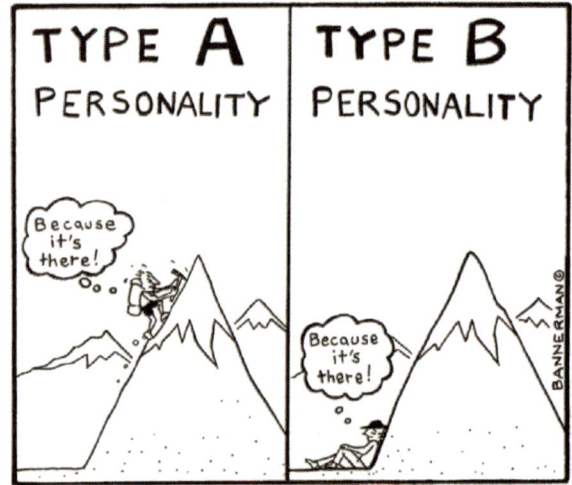

Photo 10.7   Think about how you would react to a difficult situation: Are you more of a type A or B personality?

Source: Isabella Bannerman

Type D Personality

Do you keep an eye out for trouble rather than pleasure? Do you get irritated by minor things, see the glass as half empty, have trouble making friends, and keep your feelings bottled up inside you? If so, you could be hurting your heart.

The decades of research on type A and CVD led to the realization that a tendency to experience negative emotions and stress more acutely is crucial to understanding the links between personality and CVD. Thus, researchers have begun examining type D personality in relation to CVD.

Individuals with **type D personality**, or *distressed personality*, are inclined to experience interpersonal difficulties that can affect health (Denollet, Sys, & Brutsaert, 1995), including negative affectivity and social inhibition. *Negative affectivity* is a tendency to experience negative emotional states across time and different situations. People with high negative affectivity experience dysphoria (a state of unease or dissatisfaction with life), tension, worry, a negative view of the self, and an attentional bias toward adverse stimuli. They see the worst in every situation. High negative affectivity is very similar to neuroticism, and people under more stress also report more somatic (bodily) symptoms.

Also linked to type D is high *social inhibition* (Bagherian-Sararoudi, Sanei, Attari, & Afshar, 2012). Inhibited individuals tend to repress or hide their negative emotions rather than express them, especially in social interactions. People high in social inhibition are driven by a need to avoid negative interactions with others, especially disapproval and conflict. They end up feeling insecure and socially distant from others (Asendorpf, 1993). They are also less likely to seek social support from others in times of stress.

Individuals with type D personality are more likely to experience negative emotions. They will also inhibit or restrain those emotions so that others do not respond to them negatively, even when they are feeling ornery, grouchy, and sad. Type D people are at an even greater risk for heart attack and death than type A people (Yu et al., 2011). Type D personality is characterized by a more marked stress response with higher levels of cortisol, excessive sympathetic nervous system arousal, and an imbalance leading to greater inflammation. Type D personalities are more likely to have other risk factors as well, such as anxiety, depression, irritability, low self-esteem, and less social support (Pedersen, van Domburg, Theuns, Jordaens, & Erdman, 2004). In a study of 286 men and women who had enrolled in a rehabilitation program because of a diagnosis of CVD, one-third was high in type D personality traits (Denollet, 1993). Eight years later, of those who had been high in type D traits, 27% had died of heart problems, compared with only 7% of those who had been identified as low in type D traits.

Since then, more research has demonstrated the dangers of type D personality: early death, increased risk of developing cardiovascular problems after a heart attack, poorer response to proven treatments for heart disease, and increased risk of sudden cardiac arrest (Condén et al., 2017).

If you are wondering how having a type D personality leads to heart disease, you are not alone. Research is ongoing, but it is likely that the cause is elevated blood pressure and other reactions to stress, along with a highly activated immune system, which leads to greater inflammation and thus more damage to the blood vessels and the heart.

Thinking About Health

■ How do different psychological factors influence cardiovascular functioning and the development of disease?

■ Which CVD risk factors are modifiable, and which are not?

■ Which type of personality do you have? How do you think your personality affects your cardiovascular health?

Diabetes

You may be wondering why diabetes is mentioned in a chapter on CVD. The reason is that obesity, diabetes, and CVD are intertwined. Diabetes can lead to a thickening of the arteries, a buildup of waste in the blood, and hypertension. Diabetes and hypertension share common pathways and may interact and influence each other, creating a vicious cycle of disease (Cheung & Li, 2012). They share many risk factors—such as poor diet, obesity, and a sedentary lifestyle—and both are end results of metabolic syndrome (Cheung & Li, 2012). Although interventions to reduce the risks of both CVD and diabetes focus on behavior modification and lifestyle changes, there are some disease-specific issues that make diabetes unique.

Diabetes is a disorder in the body's ability to regulate glucose, or sugar, levels in the blood. There are three types of diabetes (National Institute of Diabetes and Digestive and Kidney Diseases [NIDDK], 2017):

■ *Type 1 diabetes* results when the pancreas does not produce enough insulin. The body's immune system destroys the insulin-producing cells, which causes the pancreas to stop producing insulin. (See Chapter 10 for more information about type 1 diabetes.)

■ *Type 2 diabetes* results when the cells in the body do not respond properly to insulin. They are said to develop *insulin resistance*. As the need for insulin rises, the pancreas gradually loses its ability to produce sufficient amounts to regulate blood sugar.

■ *Gestational diabetes* occurs when pregnant women without a previous history of diabetes develop high blood glucose levels during pregnancy.

Type 1 diabetes usually develops early in childhood. It is managed through insulin injections. Type 2 diabetes may be managed with medications, including insulin, or through lifestyle changes. Until recently, although there is a genetic component, type 2 diabetes has been an age- and lifestyle-related disorder, primarily developing in midlife. However, with growing rates of obesity, it is being seen more often in childhood. Gestational diabetes usually disappears when the baby is born, but, during the pregnancy, the mother must be carefully monitored.

The Dangers of Diabetes

In all three types of diabetes, the hallmark is high levels of glucose in the blood. When glucose builds up in the blood instead of going to cells, it can cause the cells to be starved of energy, and, over time, this will result in cell death and organ dysfunction. High levels of glucose in the blood (called high blood sugar) produce such symptoms as frequent urination, increased hunger and thirst, fatigue, weakness, irritability, nausea, and fainting. If not treated, diabetes can cause serious complications from seizures, heart disease, stroke, kidney failure, foot ulcers leading to amputation, and blindness.

Occurrences of diabetes are on the rise, as of June 2024 the Centers for Disease Control and Prevention estimate that 422 million people around the world have diabetes (WHO, 2024g), 1.5 million deaths a year are attributed to it, and it is expected that 592 million people worldwide will have the disorder by 2035 (International Diabetes Foundation, 2015). Type 2 diabetes is highly correlated with obesity and CVD and is the most rapidly growing chronic illness today. As **Table 10.3** shows, in the United States almost 40 million people across all ages have diabetes, and 23% of them don't even know it (NIDDK, 2024). Diabetes was the seventh-leading cause of death in the United States in 2018, though this number is hard to determine since deaths may also be due to complications from diabetes (Heron, 2018).

Type 2 diabetes is associated with many other significant psychosocial effects. People with diabetes are at a higher risk for anxiety, depression, and psychological distress. Those with type 2 diabetes are particularly sensitive to stress

	Diagnosed diabetes		Undiagnosed diabetes		Total diabetes	
Characteristic	No. in millions (95% CI)[a]	Percentage (95% CI)[b]	No. in millions (95% CI)[a]	Percentage (95% CI)[b]	No. in millions (95% CI)[a]	Percentage (95% CI)[b]
Total	**23.0 (21.1–25.1)**	**9.3 (8.5–10.1)**	**7.2 (6.0–8.6)**	**2.9 (2.4–3.5)**	**30.2 (27.9–32.7)**	**12.2 (11.3–13.2)**
Age in years						
18–44	3.0 (2.6–3.6)	2.6 (2.2–3.1)	1.6 (1.1–2.3)	1.3 (0.9–2.0)	4.6 (3.8–5.5)	4.0 (3.3–4.8)
45–64	10.7 (9.3–12.2)	12.7 (11.1–14.5)	3.6 (2.8–4.6)	4.3 (3.3–5.5)	14.3 (12.7–16.1)	17.0 (15.1–19.1)
≥65	9.9 (9.0–11.0)	20.8 (18.8–23.0)	2.1 (1.4–3.0)	4.4 (3.1–6.3)	12.0 (10.7–13.4)	25.2 (22.5–28.1)
Sex						
Women	11.7 (10.5–13.1)	9.2 (8.2–1 0.3)	3.1 (2.4–4.1)	2.5 (1.9–3.2)	14.9 (13.5–16.4)	11.7 (10.6–12.9)
Men	11.3 (10.2–12.4)	9.4 (8.5–1 0.3)	4.0 (3.0–5.5)	3.4 (2.5–4.6)	15.3 (13.8–17.0)	12.7 (11.5–14.1)

Source: Data from CDC (2017d).

Table 10.3 Diagnosed and undiagnosed diabetes among adults in the United States

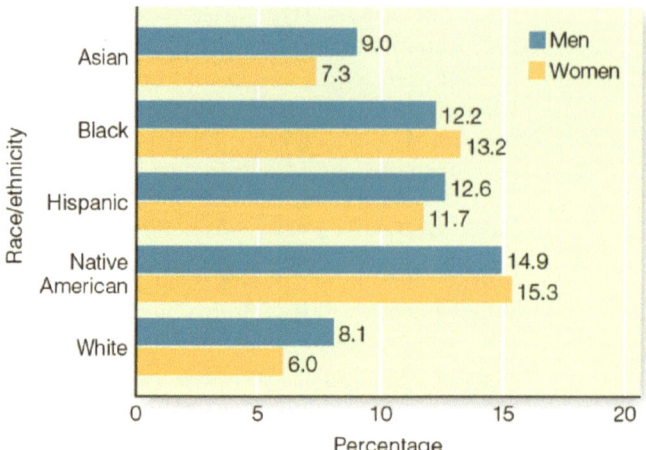

Figure 10.3   Diagnosed diabetes by race/ethnicity and sex among adults in the United States.

Source: Information from CDC (2017d)

(Halford, Cuddihy, & Mortimer, 1990), and stress can exacerbate insulin resistance, creating a vicious cycle. Cognitive functioning may be affected, especially memory and attention. Diabetics often experience sexual dysfunction, which can harm intimate relationships.

Diabetes is more prevalent in Native Americans and Alaskan Natives, African Americans, and Hispanics than in Asians and whites (see **Figure 10.3**). Among Hispanics, Mexican Americans and Puerto Ricans have the highest rates of diagnosis.

There are complex links between diabetes and CVD. Risk factors such as poor diet and a sedentary lifestyle increase the risk of metabolic syndrome, diabetes, and CVD (Cheung & Li, 2012). Between 2009 and 2012, 71% of people with diabetes had a blood pressure reading above 140/90 and were taking blood pressure medications (CDC, 2014c). Hospitalization for heart attack was nearly two times higher for those with diabetes, and those with diabetes are nearly two times more likely to die of heart disease. People with diabetes are also 1.5 times more likely to have a stroke. Although these links are difficult to tease apart, the take-away message is that diabetes may be underreported as a cause of death even when it is the underlying disease.

Diabetes and the Obesity Epidemic

As mentioned earlier, one alarming aspect of the obesity epidemic is the increasing number of children who are developing type 2 diabetes. Historically, type 1 diabetes was referred to as *juvenile-onset diabetes* because it was most common in children, while type 2 was called *adult-onset* because it was most common after age 65. With the drastic increase in overweight and obesity, the age of onset for type 2 diabetes—which is often caused by diet and lifestyle—is falling. Now, children are increasingly being given a diagnosis of type 2 diabetes (CDC, 2014c).

Type 2 diabetes in children is most often related to a strong family history of type 2 diabetes, poor glycemic control, and insulin resistance. The pathway for type 2 diabetes in children can begin early in life, with low birth weight and

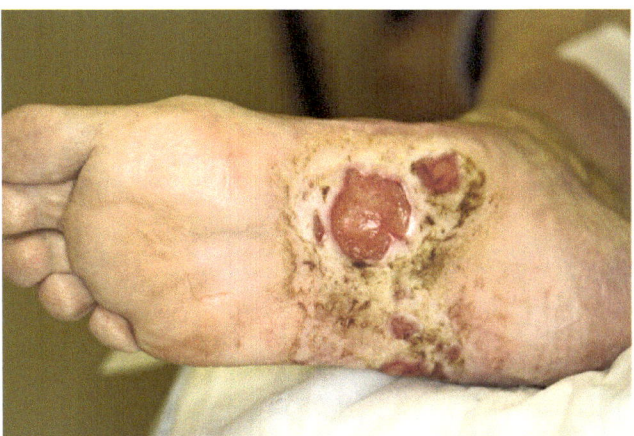 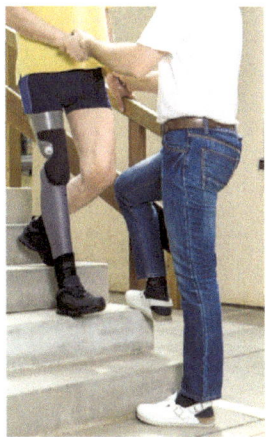

Photo 10.8   Complications from diabetes include foot ulcers (left), which can then lead to the need for amputation (right).

Source: ROBERTO RENNE-CASANOVA/Science Source (left) and Bleushi/Shutterstock (right)

poor early nutrition, and continue later with a sedentary lifestyle and poor diet (Bloomgarden, 2004). Children from lower socioeconomic brackets may be at greater risk (Goodman, Daniels, Meigs, & Dolan, 2007), especially if they are obese. In the United States, Native American children have the highest rates of diabetes—50.9% of children from the Pima Tribe in Arizona, for example, have the disease (Dabelea et al., 2014). Part of the problem with the growing incidence of type 2 diabetes in children is that it can take a while to be detected. Children often do not have many symptoms, or their symptoms are mild, and it can be hard to differentiate between type 1 and type 2 diseases within them. Nevertheless, the rates of obesity and diabetes are a growing public health concern (**Photo 10.8**).

Managing Cardiovascular Disease and Diabetes

Treatment for heart disease, stroke, and diabetes often includes medical attention, counseling or stress management, and dietary and lifestyle changes. The biopsychosocial approach of cardiac rehabilitation helps people adjust to illness, improves adherence to a new lifestyle regimen, and reduces the likelihood of future cardiac problems (Linden, Phillips, & Leclerc, 2007). One study of coronary heart disease patients tailored behavioral health education to gender-related stressors (Orth-Gomér, 2012). In spite of differing concerns, for both men and women, anxiety decreased over time, thanks to a combination of relaxation training, self-monitoring, and cognitive restructuring.

Cognitive behavior therapy (CBT) is highly useful for encouraging lifestyle changes and managing the emotional impact of being diagnosed with CVD or diabetes. Experiencing a major health event such as a stroke, heart attack, or surgery may create tremendous stress and emotional upheaval, and CBT is an important tool for reducing the risks of depression and the recurrence of cardiovascular problems. Several studies show the evidence-based value of CBT as a preventive measure, as a way to improve recovery and prevent recurrence, and as an effective means to manage the psychosocial impact of living with these chronic conditions (Gulliksson et al., 2011).

If patients have had a myocardial infarction or stroke, or if they have undergone coronary artery bypass surgery, they will often be hospitalized in a coronary care unit so their cardiac functions can be continually monitored. After discharge from the hospital, they may have to adjust to extensive cardiac rehabilitative therapy and lifestyle changes. Depression and anxiety are common reactions. CBT has been found to be effective at reducing depression in patients with heart disease, as have other collaborative or integrative approaches (Rollman et al., 2009).

One last, critical feature in recovery is social support. Specifically, the positive presence of loved ones is crucial for managing the anxiety of recovery (Kulik & Mahler, 1989). Especially when coping with the stress of surgery and cardiac rehabilitation, perceived familial support is key to positive outcomes (Cardoso-Moreno & Tomás-Aragones, 2017).

Thinking About Health

■ How are CVD and diabetes connected?

■ How are the risk factors for diabetes and CVD the same? How are they different?

■ How can diabetes and CVD be successfully managed, in the short term and the long term?

Chapter Summary

CVDs are diseases that affect the functioning of the cardiovascular system and are currently the number one cause of preventable death worldwide. Cardiovascular problems often start with conditions such as hypertension, high blood pressure, and high cholesterol and can progress to diabetes, stroke, congestive heart failure, or myocardial infarction. The pathological changes that occur in early CVD create a greater risk for more serious health outcomes. There are many important biopsychosocial risk factors of CVD, and cutting-edge research focuses on identifying and treating the predictors of disease, such as C-reactive protein levels and inflammation. Many risk factors can be modified through lifestyle changes, and much can be done to improve our overall health.

KEY TERMS ▶ cardiovascular disease (CVD) p. 301, cardiovascular system p. 302, circulation p. 302, systolic phase p. 304, diastolic phase p. 304, atherosclerosis p. 305, ischemia p. 305, angina pectoris p. 306, myocardial infarction p. 306, stroke p. 306, ischemic stroke p. 306, hemorrhagic stroke p. 307, transient ischemic attack p. 307, cholesterol p. 308, high-density lipoproteins (HDLs) p. 308, low-density lipoproteins (LDLs) p. 308, metabolic syndrome p. 309, hypertension p. 310, stent catheterization p. 316, angioplasty p. 316, heart bypass p. 316, cardiac rehabilitation p. 317, type a personality p. 320, type D personality p. 321, diabetes p. 322

CHAPTER 11

Psychoneuroimmunology and Related Disorders

Learning Outcomes

After reading this chapter, you should be able to:

- **Define** psychoneuroimmunology.
- **Describe** how the immune system works.
- **Outline** what happens when the immune system is compromised.
- **Explain** the interactions between the immune system and the central nervous system, and describe their combined influence on health.
- **Describe** how stress influences immunity.
- **Identify** and define different autoimmune diseases.
- **Describe** the various biopsychosocial influences on cancer and arthritis.

Meghan's problems began during a stressful year after her mother died, with debilitating fatigue and swollen lymph nodes (O'Rourke, 2013). Later, she found a strange rash on her arm and began to forget things. She became dizzy while eating. Before long, she had hives, migraines, a buzzing in her throat, numbness in her feet, and frequent viruses, including the Epstein-Barr virus (O'Rourke, 2013). "What," she kept thinking, "is wrong with me?" Her doctors were just as puzzled.

Laboratory results showed that Meghan's immune system was attacking her thyroid—a condition called Hashimoto's disease. Her doctor prescribed a thyroid medication and told her that she would feel better within 6 weeks. Instead, she felt worse. Her joints hurt, she had blistering headaches, she fainted, she itched uncontrollably, and she was so dizzy that even walking was dangerous (O'Rourke, 2013).

Eventually, Meghan tried a radical diet. She cut out all processed and chemical additives, gluten, refined sugar, and dairy products. She began exercising as well. After a few weeks, she began to feel better,

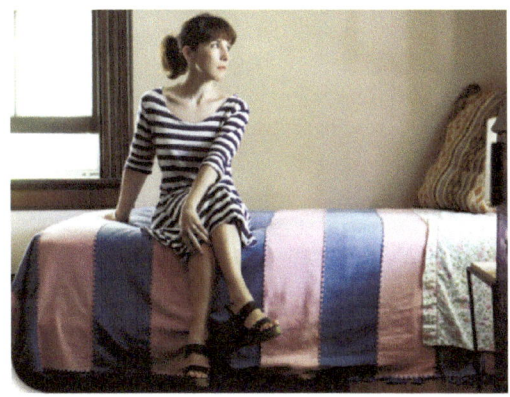

Photo 11.1

Mike McGregor/Contour by Getty Images

and her level of destructive antibodies was lower, but she knew that she would never fully recover. After several years of medical tests, doctor visits, and, finally, a diagnosis and treatment plan, Meghan's health had begun to improve. Now, she faces a new challenge—to avoid succumbing to the identity of a "'sick person,' as someone afraid of living." Meghan says, "The real coming to terms with autoimmune disease is recognizing that you are sick." Often, it is "not the kind of sick you can conquer"—but it can be successfully managed (O'Rourke, 2013).

Sometimes, what ails us is complex and difficult to tease apart, especially when different bodily systems are involved. Then, we have to bring together more of what we know about health and disorders, starting with the body's primary defense against illness: the immune system. And it is to our immune system that we now turn.

In this chapter, we explore the biopsychosocial and cultural factors that influence the development of autoimmune diseases, such as HIV/AIDS, cancer, arthritis, and diabetes. We look at how several different disciplines come together in order to understand how systems of the body interact—either to maintain homeostasis or to cause disease. This interaction is the subject of *psychoneuroimmunology*.

We will also learn more about the immune system and how an autoimmune disease develops. Some of these diseases primarily involve lifestyle, and their management involves significant behavioral changes. More generally, the study of these diseases is stimulating new research and understanding of the complex interplay between the biological, psychological, and social aspects of disease.

What Is Psychoneuroimmunology?

Psychoneuroimmunology is the study of interactions among the behavioral, neural, endocrine, and immune systems. It illuminates the connections between the brain and the immune system, and it shows how each system adapts in the face of illness and infection. Psychoneuroimmunology is a multidisciplinary field that joins specialists from immunology, endocrinology, neurochemistry, neurophysiology, pharmacology, psychiatry, psychology, and virology. Findings from psychoneuroimmunological research are important to medical specialists in many other disciplines, such as allergic and infectious diseases, oncology, and rheumatology as well.

Psychoneuroimmunology builds on an idea that has long influenced medicine and science: Our mental states influence our physical states and affect diseases and healing. In fact, the field emerged from novel approaches to exploring how stress and anxiety can affect a person's immune system and, ultimately, their health. In the 1970s, most doctors would have said that the immune system has no influence on other bodily systems. The landmark studies of Robert Ader showed otherwise. Ader, who coined the term *psychoneuroimmunology*, looked at the impact of environmental factors on rats (Ader, 1981). He found important interactions between the immune system and the central nervous system (Ader & Cohen, 1981).

The field has blossomed, and now hundreds of studies have explored how stress, hostility, and depression affect the immune system. Negative emotions play a role, too, in the development of premature aging, heart disease, some cancers, osteoporosis, arthritis, and delayed wound healing (Kiecolt-Glaser, McGuire, Robles, & Glaser, 2002). Happiness and other positive emotions, in turn, have a beneficial influence on health (Kiecolt-Glaser et al., 2002).

We now know that the immune and nervous systems act together. From stress to fever to cancer, the influence of one system on the other has evolved to help us sense danger and survive (Ziemssen, 2012). Moreover, the interplay between the brain and immune system is modulated by psychological factors, such as cognition, emotions, behaviors, and social support. Together, they influence both immunity and disease. How does this happen? To answer, we need to review the immune system and what it does.

Thinking About Health

■ In what ways do you think that the behavioral, neural, endocrine, and immune systems work together?

■ How might these same systems work against one another?

The Immune System

The immune system, your body's defense against infection and illness, is designed to prevent or limit infection. It protects the body from invaders and keeps it healthy. The immune system distinguishes between normal cells and unhealthy cells, targeting *pathogens* (such as bacteria and viruses), toxins, or parasites. Essentially, it tries to rid itself of anything that is unfamiliar. It does this by identifying a variety of "danger" cues, called **danger-associated molecular patterns** (DAMPs).

Usually DAMPs are **antigens**, substances on the surface of all cells, bacteria, viruses, or fungi. Antigens are most often proteins, but can also be other nonliving substances such as toxins, chemicals, drugs, or foreign particles. The immune system is programmed to recognize and destroy anything that contains foreign antigens. Your body recognizes its own antigens and learns that they are normal, and so it *usually* does not mount an immune response against them. However, as we shall see later in this chapter, some disorders do result from the system's attempts to destroy the body's own cells.

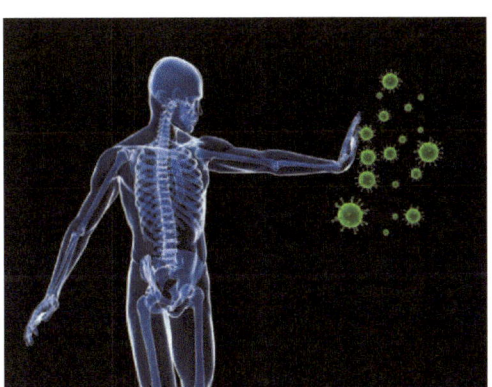

Photo 11.2   The immune system identifies danger-associated molecular patterns (DAMPs) and seeks to protect us from anything that contains foreign antigens.

Source: Sebastian Kaulitzki/Shutterstock

The Immune System at Work

The immune system is at work every day, fighting off infection. Consider just a few examples.

If you fall and skin your knee, a bit of dirt and debris might enter your body through the break in the skin. Your immune system will mount an attack to purge the invaders from the body while the skin

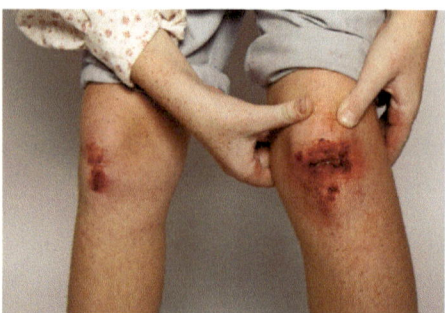 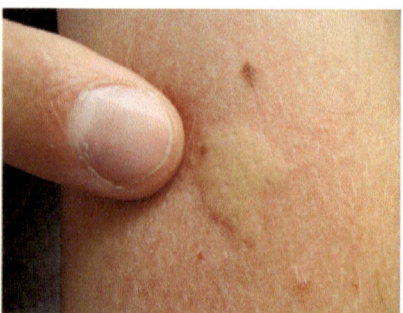

Photo 11.3   As soon as you are injured, your immune system goes to work fighting infection. If a scraped knee becomes infected, the immune system responds with inflammation and pus. If you receive a mosquito bite, the immune system responds with a welt (inflammation) at the site of the sting.

heals. If the immune system is not effective in thoroughly eliminating the dirt or bacteria, the wound might become infected, with symptoms of pain, inflammation, and pus. The inflammation and pus are signs that the immune system is fighting off the infection.

Another example of the immune system at work is the itchy welt that develops when you are bitten by a mosquito. This is a visible sign of inflammation, which the immune system uses to fight off the bacteria transmitted through the sting. We'll look more closely at inflammation later in this chapter.

Each day, too, we breathe in thousands of germs—both bacteria and viruses—that are floating around in the air. Most of the time, our immune system eliminates them without a problem. Occasionally, and especially if your immune system is weakened, you may not be able to get rid of the pathogens. A cold or the flu is evidence that your immune system failed to kill the germs, and feeling better is a sign that your immune system has battled the invader and won. The system may also react to harmless invaders, such as pollens, grains, and particles. The result is allergies, such as hay fever.

Another case of immune system failure is cancer. Occasionally, cells will change in a way that causes them to reproduce uncontrollably. If the reproduction error "gets by" the immune system, or if the immune system is not able to prevent reproduction, eventually a tumor will develop. The tumor is a mass of cancerous cells. An example of cancer is when melanocytes, cells in the skin, are damaged by the ultraviolet radiation in sunlight, causing skin cancers or melanomas to form. We'll look at cancer and how it can circumvent the immune system later in this chapter.

How the Immune System Works

The body uses several different kinds of immune response to protect and defend itself. **Innate immunity**, also called *nonspecific immunity*, is the immune response you were born with. It protects against antigens and keeps harmful agents from entering the body. Its first line of defense includes the skin, the cough reflex, sneezing, mucus (which traps bacteria and small particles), and stomach acid (which kills bacteria). Another type of innate immunity is fever, which the body mounts to destroy invading pathogens. This response is a chemical reaction, called *innate humoral immunity*.

Acquired immunity, or *specific immunity*, is not present at birth, but develops in response to an antigen. Acquired immunity develops when you are exposed to an infectious disease or are given a vaccination. Take, for example, measles, a highly contagious respiratory infection caused by a virus. It results in flulike symptoms and an itchy rash all over the body. However, having measles once results in lifelong immunity: Once you have had measles, you will never get it again.

Can we harness acquired immunity to prevent an illness like measles in the first place? We can, and we do. Now, most children are vaccinated against measles, so it occurs more rarely. There were just 372 cases in all of the United States in 2018 (Centers for Disease Control and Prevention [CDC], 2019c). But consider this: In the first seven months of 2019, 1123 individual cases of measles were reported—a tremendous increase. Why are measles cases increasing if vaccinations are available?

The reason is that some parents have chosen not to vaccinate their children—in spite of decades of data showing that all common vaccinations are perfectly safe and absolutely necessary for protecting the public against threatening diseases. These so-called *anti-vaxxers* avoid vaccines for different reasons, including religious grounds, suspicions that vaccines are unsafe, fears of negative health outcomes misattributed to vaccines, or a misguided desire for personal choice. Regardless of their reasons, anti-vaxxer parents put their children at risk of contracting highly contagious and serious diseases that they could otherwise protect against, and they put everyone else's children at risk, too. Each person who does not get vaccinated reduces the herd immunity of the population. **Herd immunity**, a resistance to contagious disease that develops if a sufficiently high proportion of a population is immune to the disease, can only occur when each member of a population is vaccinated.

Public health campaigns for vaccination provide evidence-based science to demonstrate the safety and efficacy of vaccinations—but, in the face of fake news and viral posts, are these campaigns enough? Recently, state and national governments have adopted harsher measures for combating anti-vaxxers. In New York and Germany, for instance, legislation has been drafted to fine parents who refuse to vaccinate their children. Legislative loopholes for public school vaccinations—such as exemptions due to religious and moral reasons—continue to evolve and be closed across the United States

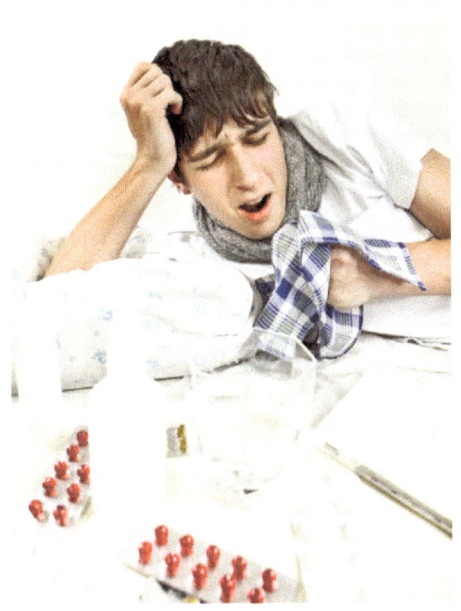

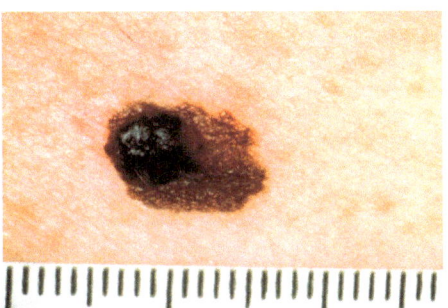

Photo 11.4 Unfortunately, the immune system is not infallible. Disease occurs when the immune system cannot sufficiently fight off or contain cellular changes or pathogens, resulting in conditions as varied as a cold (top) or a tumor (bottom).

Source: Sabphoto/Shutterstock (top) and the website of the National Cancer Institute (bottom)

as well (National Conference of State Legislatures, 2019). Vaccines work by triggering the immune response, using a small dose of the virus as an antigen. This single small dose can make a world of difference in the health of an individual and a population—but more on this in a moment.

Blood, too, has a role in the immune system. The immune system is made up of an army of defender cells—the *white blood cells*. A healthy person produces about 1 billion new white blood cells every day in the marrow of the bone. Blood also contains proteins and other chemicals, such as antibodies and complement proteins. Some of these blood cells work directly to destroy foreign agents in the body while supporting the immune response. For example, interferon prevents the replication of invading cells, while interleukin-1 creates fever to heat up and destroy the invader.

There are several types of white blood cells. **Macrophages** constantly patrol your body and destroy unfamiliar germs or cells. Macrophages circulate throughout the body and are often found in the spleen, liver, and connective tissue of the body. **Lymphocytes**, another type of white blood cell, are crucial to distinguishing your own body tissues and substances from those that are not part of your body. So-called *B lymphocytes* produce antibodies by taking a piece of DNA from the invading antigen and storing it for future recognition. *T lymphocytes* attack the antigens directly. They also release chemicals called *cytokines* that send signals that control the entire immune system. Together, B and T lymphocytes provide the immune system with its "memory" so that it can respond more quickly and efficiently the next time you are exposed to the same antigen. When you are vaccinated, or *immunized*, B lymphocytes form the antibodies to that virus. This is why once you have had measles or are vaccinated, you are immune to getting that illness again. Immunization is crucial to public and individual health.

Inflammation

Inflammation is the body's response to tissue damage. It comes into play when we suffer cuts, injuries, or burns, or are exposed to bacteria, trauma, or toxins. In each case, the body responds with increased blood flow to the damaged tissue, which increases body temperature and produces redness, swelling, and pain.

Inflammation unfolds as the damaged cells release chemical messengers, including *histamine*, *bradykinin*, and *prostaglandins*. Histamine increases blood flow to the injured or infected area, and the leakage of fluid and proteins into the tissues causes the redness and swelling. Swelling helps fight infection, too, by surrounding the foreign substance, keeping it from further contact with body tissues. The chemical messengers also attract a type of white blood cell, called *phagocytes*, that "eat" the germs, pick up dead and damaged cells, and remove them. Pus is the result of the dead tissue, dead bacteria, and live and dead phagocytes. The immune system also works to control its response, thanks to cytokines secreted by cells (see Chapter 4). *Pro-inflammatory cytokines* produce inflammation, while *anti-inflammatory cytokines* fight it.

Inflammation is essential for survival. It isolates the damaged area, mobilizes the immune response, and promotes healing. Yet inflammation can also be out of proportion to the threat—or directed toward the body's own cells. That over-reaction is *chronic inflammation,* and it can actually cause more damage. Allergies are a common example.

Thinking About Health

■ How has your immune system responded to health threats, whether viral or bacterial?

■ Why are vaccinations crucial to the health of both individuals and entire populations?

The Immune System and the central Nervous System

The immune system does not work alone. Psychoneuroimmunology ties the immune system and the central nervous system (CNS) together. Their communication goes both ways: The brain modulates the immune system to help fight off disease, while the immune system, in turn, affects how we feel and behave. Their interaction also explains how stress and chronic strain can make us more vulnerable to disease.

Working Together

At first glance, the CNS and the immune system work quite differently. The brain is the CNS command center. It sends and receives electrical signals along fixed pathways, much like an old-fashioned telephone switchboard.

In contrast, the immune system is decentralized, much like the U.S. Postal System (Sompayrac, 2015). Its organs are located throughout the body—the spleen, the lymph nodes, the thymus, and the bone marrow (as shown in **Figure 11.1**). They communicate directly through hormones and neurochemicals traveling through the bloodstream.

At the same time, the two systems are quite similar in how they handle signals. Each has both "sensory" elements, which receive information from the environment and other parts of the body, and "motor" elements, which respond. The immune system and the CNS also affect each other.

The brain modulates the immune system by hardwiring sympathetic and parasympathetic nerves (the autonomic nervous system) to lymphoid organs that make up the endocrine system (Ziemssen & Kern, 2007). As we learned in Chapter 6, hormones released by the brain during stress regulate the fight-or-flight response. In turn, the immune system modulates brain activity, affecting

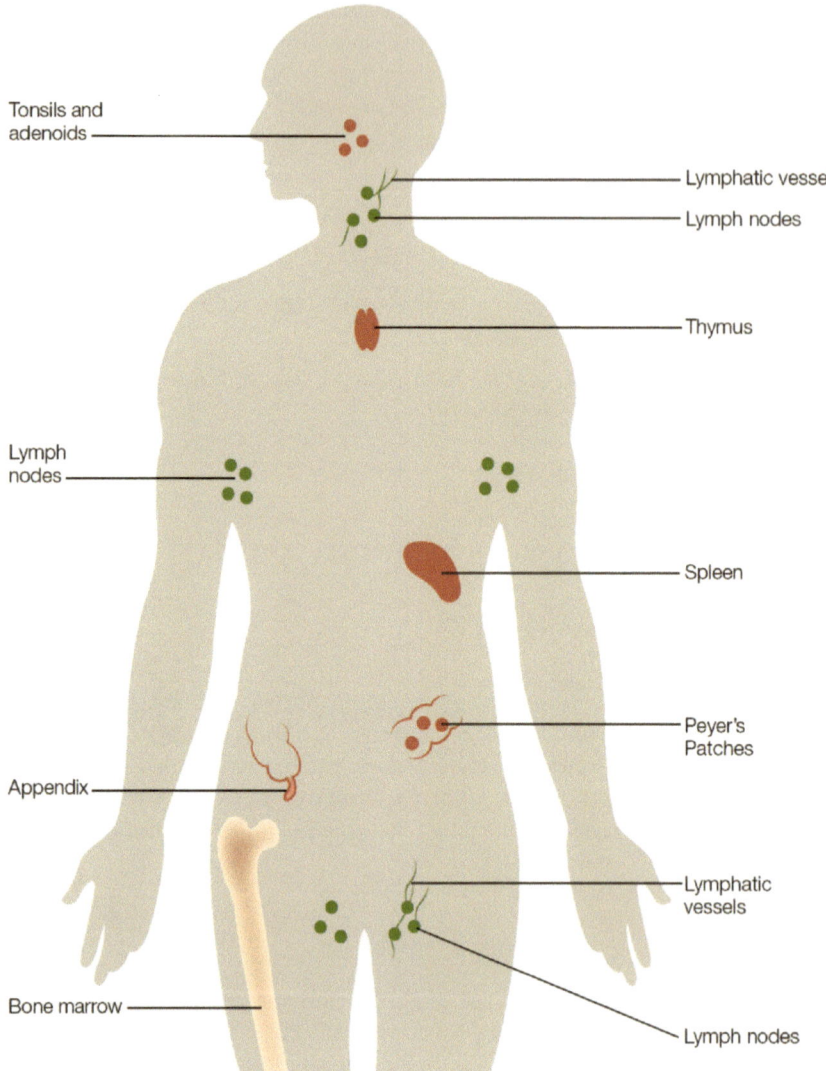

Figure 11.1   The Organs of the Immune System.

sleep, body temperature, and behavior. For example, when we are fighting off a cold, we may feel fatigue, irritability, and loss of appetite.

Stress and the Immune System

Strong evolutionary forces have forged the connection between stress and immune functioning (Segerstrom & Miller, 2004). Stress triggers a response to threats, and the immune system works to help the body repair wounds and to prevent infections. Together, these responses are adaptive and increase the chances of survival (Segerstrom & Miller, 2004). Yet, as we know, stress can be bad for health as well.

Stress increases the risk of disease, from the common cold to cancer, by suppressing the immune system (Adamo, 2012; Glaser & Kiecolt-Glaser, 2005; Turpin et al., 2019). This happens not just in humans (Glaser & Kiecolt-Glaser, 2005), but in all animals (Adamo, 2012). Stress makes us more susceptible to infection, makes infections worse, and delays wound healing. It can also diminish a person's response to vaccines and reactivate viruses. Recent research shows, for example, that perceived stress is directly associated with the incidence of sexually transmitted infections (Turpin et al., 2019), such as when, after a stressful episode, blisters appear in people who have herpes. Yet, the full impact of stress on health is still being uncovered.

How does stress affect the immune response? For one thing, stress increases the production of proinflammatory cytokines, which are associated with many age-related diseases. More generally, the CNS modulates the immune response through a complex network of neurochemical and hormonal signals (Segerstrom & Miller, 2004). Two likely pathways are the hypothalamic-pituitary-adrenocortical axis, which we learned about in Chapter 6, and the autonomic nervous system. Negative emotions and events activate these pathways and provoke the release of pituitary and adrenal hormones. All cells in the immune system have receptors for these hormones—which include adrenaline and noradrenaline (called *catecholamines*), adrenocorticotropic hormone, cortisol, growth hormone, and prolactin (Glaser & Kiecolt-Glaser, 2005).

The hormones activated in the stress response may affect health in two ways. First, they may bind directly to receptors at the surface of the cell and thereby change the immune response, creating a vulner-ability to disease. Second, these hormones may affect immune functioning by dysregulating the production of cytokines, interferon-γ, interleukin-1, and tumor necrosis factor—all of which have an impact on the functioning of cells and tissues in the body, and ultimately weaken immunity. So, these stress hormones can either directly dysregulate the functioning of the immune system or affect the hormones required in an immune response, indirectly, negatively influencing immune functioning, and thus health.

Not all stress is created equal, and the same is true of its impact on immune functioning. Short-term, acute stressors (lasting minutes), such as a fight with your partner or taking a major exam, are one thing. They may activate the immune system in potentially adaptive ways (Segerstrom & Miller, 2004). Chronic, long-term stressors, however, can be harmful to health. As Meghan experienced at the start of this chapter, long-term unemployment or chronic pain may oblige us to restructure key aspects of our lives, making things worse. Spouses of people with Alzheimer's disease or Parkinson's disease show higher rates of anxiety, depression, and illness (Frazier, Hooker, & Siegler, 1993; Hooker, Manoogian-O'Dell, Monahan, Frazier, & Shifren, 2000; Kiecolt-Glaser et al., 1996; Vedhara et al., 1999). They also do not benefit as much from the flu vaccine (Kiecolt-Glaser et al., 1996; Vedhara et al., 1999). Parents of children with cancer also show the effects of chronic stress (Miller, Cohen, & Ritchey, 2002). Their immune systems release lower levels of useful hormones than do parents of relatively healthy children, leaving them more vulnerable to infection and inflammation.

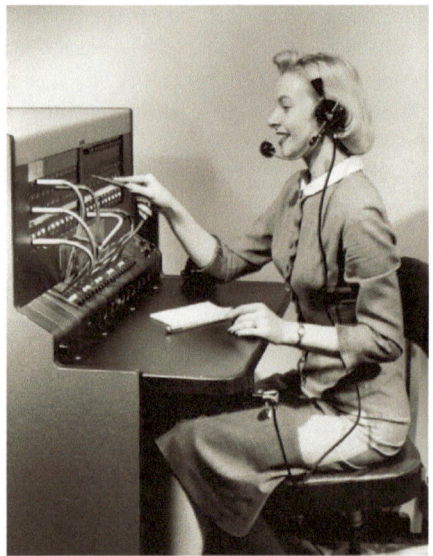

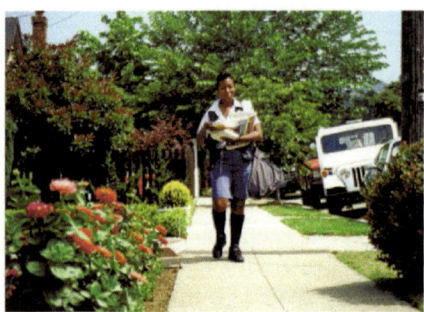

Photo 11.5   Just like telephone operators of the 1900s connected calls through a switchboard, the brain operates the CNS by sending messages along fixed pathways throughout the body. Meanwhile, the many parts of the immune system communicate directly with each other, much like how mail travels from its origin to its recipient.

Source: Superstock/Shutterstock (top) and Migdale Lawewnce/Getty Images (bottom)

Cutting-Edge Connections

Connections between the immune system and CNS continue to be explored. In the developmental line of research, for instance, a compromised immune system has been linked to age-related neurodegenerative diseases, such as dementia. Specifically, *microglia* (macro-phages that live in the brain and spinal cord) have been linked to maintenance of the CNS and the brain—so, when there is a dysfunction in these cells, disease may occur (Deczkowska et al., 2018). Microglia are able to detect deviations from homeostasis and send signals for repair. If researchers can identify the risk factors that cause changes in disease-associated microglia, they may be able to find ways to detect, offset, or reverse the course of disease (Deczkowska et al., 2018).

Another important new connection involves the interplay between the gut microbiome, the immune system, and the brain. Millions of neurons and nerves run along the *microbiota-gut-brain axis*—the brain influences the functioning of the gut through the autonomic nervous system, and the neurotransmitters and other chemicals produced in the gut influence the brain. Recent research has explored how bacteria in the gut help the immune system to develop, protecting us throughout our lives. In one study, laboratory mice bred to be born without any bacteria in their guts died quickly because they had no immunity to protect them (Hirayama et al., 1995; Sonnenberg & Artis, 2012). Other studies have shown that gut microbiota influence both innate and acquired immunity (Purchiaroni et al., 2013). Further research has shown that gut bacteria drive the development of harmful inflammation related to cardiovascular disease, cancers, Alzheimer's disease, and many other devastating diseases (Durack & Lynch, 2019).

Figure 11.2 shows the many ways in which gut microbiota influence the immune system. The bottom line is that a healthy gut means good health, and an unhealthy gut means illness. And there remain many other connections between the immune system and CNS that are yet to be investigated.

Thinking About Health

■ How do the immune system and CNS work together to promote health?

■ How does stress affect health, from a psychoneuroimmunological perspective?

■ What is the connection between the gut microbiome and the immune system?

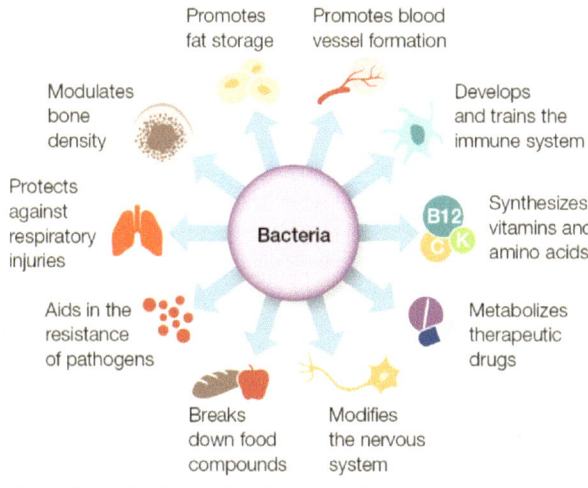

Figure 11.2   The Role of Gut Bacteria in the Immune System.

Information from Laukens, Brinkman, Raes, De Vos, and Vandenabeele (2015)

Autoimmune Diseases

We have seen how conditions, both physical and emotional, can compromise the immune system. Sometimes, however, the immune system is compromised by its own functioning. In an **autoimmune disease**, the immune system cannot distinguish between invading antigens and healthy tissues. In fact, the body's immune system begins to attack the body's own tissues and organs. The term *autoimmune disease* refers to a wide variety of illnesses that involve almost every human organ system—including the nervous, gastrointestinal, and endocrine systems; muscles, skin, and connective tissue; the blood and blood vessels; and the eyes and mouth. **Figure 11.3** shows the different parts of the body that can be affected by autoimmune disorders.

Types of Disease

Autoimmune disease was discovered more than 50 years ago by medical researchers baffled by the implausible, even contradictory, finding that the immune response sometimes attacks the body of its host (Rose, 2016). We now know that there are as many as 100 different types of autoimmune disease, and the immune system plays a role in approximately 40 additional diseases as well. Some autoimmune diseases are fairly common, such as rheumatoid arthritis, type 1 diabetes, and celiac disease, while others are quite rare. The incidence of autoimmune diseases is also on the rise (Lerner, Jeremais, & Matthias, 2015).

The American Autoimmune Related Diseases Association (AARDA) estimates that as many as 50 million Americans suffer from an autoimmune disease, making it one of the most prevalent illnesses. Meghan, in our opening story, is one of them. Autoimmune diseases and other specific conditions run in families and are more common in Hispanic

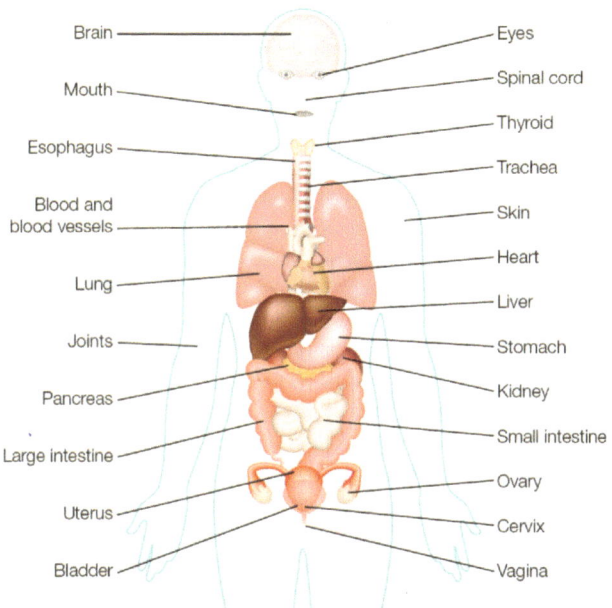

Figure 11.3   Body Parts Affected by Autoimmune Diseases.

Americans, as well as African American and Native American women. Of the 50 million Americans who have an autoimmune disease, 75% are women (AARDA, 2024). Moreover, having one autoimmune disease often leads to another. For example, a patient suffering from rheumatoid arthritis (RA) may be likely to also suffer from Hashimoto's thyroiditis.

What Causes Autoimmune Disease?

The causes of autoimmune disease are still not clear. Because women are at greater risk, hormones may play a role. A diagnosis of autoimmune disease is more likely in women in their twenties, when estrogen levels are high. In turn, testosterone, a hormone that women produce in only small amounts, may protect against autoimmune diseases.

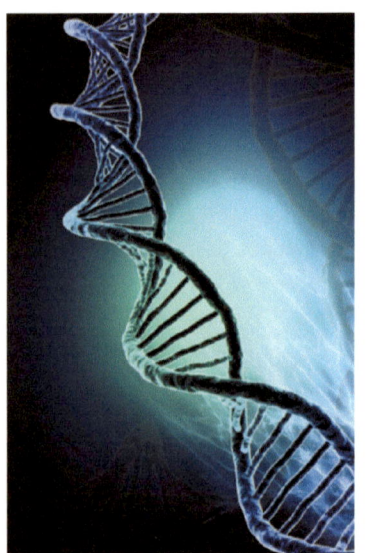

During pregnancy, women are also at risk. The cells developing in the fetus are not the mother's own cells; they have the DNA of the developing fetus. Nonself fetal cells introduced during pregnancy may have something to do with the higher rates of autoimmune disease in women. Higher rates of nonself fetal cells were found in the blood of women with scleroderma, a disease of the connective tissues, decades after pregnancy (Nelson et al., 1998). These findings may even complicate the picture of autoimmune disease as an attack on the body's own cells. Perhaps some autoimmune diseases actually arise when nonself cells mix with self cells—a condition known as *chimerism*. In *graft versus host disease*, sometimes seen after a bone-marrow transplant, the body mounts an immune attack on the grafted bone marrow cells. Could something similar be happening in autoimmune diseases as well?

Can genes promote disease or make its symptoms worse? Can environmental factors contribute to disease? Can viral infections, for example, trigger type 1 diabetes? We are still looking for the answers, all of which could lead to more effective treatment and prevention.

Photo 11.6   The effects of DNA on disease remain unclear. DNA likely plays a role in autoimmune diseases, which can be baffling to both patients and doctors in their causes and effects.

Diagnosis of Autoimmune Diseases

Living with an autoimmune disease is stressful, and simply trying to determine what is wrong can be frustrating. Many autoimmune diseases have symptoms, like aches and pains, similar to those of more familiar ailments. For example, some people who develop rheumatoid arthritis may first assume their achy joints are due to overexertion at the gym. They may experience flulike symptoms, such as fever, chills, aches and pains, and fatigue, and, as a consequence, may not seek treatment for symptoms of a more serious condition.

Many autoimmune diseases share symptoms with one another as well. Often the first symptoms of autoimmune disease are fatigue, muscle aches, and a low fever. Classic signs of an autoimmune disease—redness, swelling, heat, or pain—may be present, but only lab tests can confirm whether there are inflammatory markers in the blood. But then, winnowing down the possibilities becomes difficult.

For many patients, it takes a long time, multiple lab tests, and many doctor visits to arrive at a diagnosis. Recall Meghan's struggle at the start of our chapter. Adding to the difficulty is the fact that some autoimmune diseases are very rare. Although lupus, multiple sclerosis, type 1 diabetes, and rheumatoid arthritis are well known, patients may come to their doctors with an autoimmune disease yet to be named.

Treating Autoimmune Diseases

Autoimmune diseases are chronic and have no cure. They often have a trajectory of flare-ups, remission, and flare-ups yet again. Treatments thus focus on relieving discomfort, slowing the progression of the disease, if possible, and regaining quality of life. Patients with rheumatoid arthritis, for example, face the task of reconciling their threatened personal goals with their capabilities on a day-to-day basis (Arends, Bode, Taal, & van de Laar, 2016). A healthy rebalancing of a patient's life is required (de Ridder, Geenen, Kuijer, & van Middendorp, 2008). Having social support to help with these goals is especially important because the patient's psychological health becomes vulnerable, too (Arends et al., 2016; Sörensen, Rzeszutek, & Gasik, 2019).

Thinking About Health

■ How could a doctor mistake an autoimmune disease for another, more common illness?

■ What factors do you think might influence the development of an autoimmune disease? What future areas of study would you recommend for psychoneuroimmunological researchers?

HIV and AIDS

How can we apply what we have learned to specific diseases? Let's start with when the immune system fails, as in HIV/AIDS. **Acquired immune deficiency syndrome (AIDS)** is a disease marked by a compromised immune system. Its cause is **human immunodeficiency virus (HIV)**, a virus that targets the immune system and, over time, breaks down the body's surveillance and defense systems. Someone carrying the virus is *HIV positive*.

HIV spreads through the exchange of bodily fluids, such as blood and semen, in sexual activity, in shared contaminated needles, or in the birth of a baby to an infected mother. The exchange of bodily fluids may also occur in anal-receptive sex without a condom, which puts anyone who engages in this practice at risk—especially those involved in the sex trade. Child and adolescent runaways are also at greater risk, as are homeless youth (Slesnick, Kang, Bonomi, & Prestopnik, 2008).

Diagnosing HIV

As the virus progresses, it destroys or impairs the immune cells. This *immunodeficiency* is measured by cell counts in the blood. *CD4 cells*, also called *T-helper cells*, are a type of white blood cell designed to fight infection. They are produced in the spleen, the lymph nodes, and the thymus gland—all organs involved in the immune response. These cells move through the body in the bloodstream, looking to identify and destroy bacteria and viruses. The higher your CD4 count is, the stronger your immune system is.

Doctors use the CD4 count to determine the stage of HIV infection and to guide treatment. When someone is HIV positive, the virus binds to the surface of the CD4 cells and enters them. As these cells replicate, they reproduce the HIV infection. HIV also destroys CD4 cells, weakening the immune system and allowing the infected cells to take over. That is when other infections, called *opportunistic infections*, take advantage. They begin to develop, and HIV progresses to AIDS.

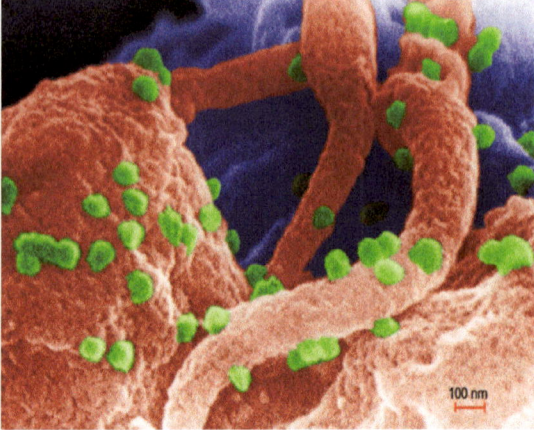

100 nm

Photo 11.7   The HIV virus binds to the surface of CD4 cells and destroys them, weakening the immune system, and eventually leading to AIDS.

Source: Centers for Disease Control and Prevention

How HIV Progresses

The time between exposure to the virus and the development of symptoms varies. Most people infected with HIV begin to see symptoms within 2 to 4 weeks, but some people do not see symptoms for years, possibly spreading the virus to others without knowing it. Once the HIV virus begins to proliferate, however, it moves through the body rapidly (this process is shown in **Figure 11.4**).

1. Acute Infection:	2. Clinical Latency:	3. AIDS:
During this time, large amounts of the virus are produced in the body.	During this stage of the disease, HIV reproduces at very low levels, although it is still active.	As CD4 cells fall below 200 cells/mm³, patients are considered to have progressed to AIDS.
Many, but not all, people develop flulike symptoms, often described as the "worst flu ever."	During this period, there may not be symptoms. With proper HIV treatment, people may live with clinical latency for several decades. Without treatment, this period lasts an average of 10 years, but some people may progress through this stage faster.	Without treatment, people typically survive 3 years.

Figure 11.4   Stages of HIV Infection.

Source: Information from AIDS.gov (2016)

First, a person will begin to experience flulike symptoms—such as swollen glands, sore throat, rash, muscle and joint aches, pains, fatigue, and headache. This acute infection stage is called **acute retroviral syndrome** (ARS, or *primary HIV infection*), and it is the body's natural response to the virus. During this phase, the CD4 count can drop drastically. The proportion of activated T lymphocytes circulating in the bloodstream is highly predictive of the time it takes for opportunistic infections to set in, and of survival time in general (Rodríguez-Alba et al., 2019).

Because of the mild early symptoms, people may not seek treatment. Even if they do seek treatment, neither they nor their doctor may suspect HIV. Yet early diagnosis is the key to successful treatment. The longer the virus goes undetected, the more strongly it will take hold.

Eventually, the immune system brings the viral level down, gradually reaching a level called *the viral set point*. At this point in the acute stage, the CD4 levels may rise, but they will never return to levels before the infection. The level of HIV in the blood is still very high, too, so patients are still highly contagious.

Clinical latency follows the acute stage. In this stage, the virus is living and reproducing within the body, but still not producing further symptoms. The virus is *latent*, or hidden, but it can still be spread to others. For a patient undergoing treatment, this stage can last for decades. Even in someone not undergoing treatment, clinical latency lasts, on average, for 10 years, although some people progress through this stage more quickly.

The final stage in the disease is AIDS. In this stage, the immune system cannot fight off opportunistic infections, such as pneumonia or Kaposi's sarcoma, a rare form of cancer. By this point, the viral load has increased, and the CD4 count has fallen again—to below 200 cells per cubic millimeter of blood (<200 cells/mm^3). By comparison, CD4 cell counts in someone with a healthy immune system will be between 500 and 1600 cells/mm^3. Without treatment, patients who progress to AIDS typically survive for about three years. Once dangerous opportunistic infections have taken hold, life expectancy falls to about one year (AIDS.gov, 2016).

Treatment for HIV/AIDS

HIV-positive patients who receive treatment can now expect to live a normal lifespan. Early diagnosis and treatment are thus crucial to reducing the burden of disease, increasing quality of life, and extending life.

Treatments aim at fortifying the immune system against the virus and slowing its progression. *Antiretroviral therapy*, also called *highly active retroviral therapy*, involves a combination of at least three drugs. The combination helps keep HIV levels low and reduces the likelihood that the virus will develop a resistance to the treatment. If the virus does develop a resistance to the first combination of drugs, or *first-line therapy*, or if the side effects are particularly bad, doctors may shift to another combination, or *second-line therapy*. There are now more than 20 FDA-approved antiretroviral drugs. Antiretroviral therapy is not a cure, but it can prevent the progression of the disease and stop people from becoming ill for many years.

Although there are many people throughout the world who do not have access to antiretroviral therapy, there are many who do, but who do not adhere to their treatment programs. This is especially a concern for HIV-positive illicit drug users. In a longitudinal study, both personal and contextual factors interfered with HIV-positive illicit drug users' ability to adhere to their treatment regimens. Specifically, those who were older when they began treatment were better at adhering to the regimen, whereas those who were homeless, used drugs daily, or had experienced violence or childhood abuse were less able to adhere to their treatment protocols (Lee, Milloy, Nosova, Walsh, & Kerr, 2019). Antiretroviral therapy is critical for disease management and life expectancy. Thus, it is important to find ways to increase self-efficacy and adherence to treatment among all patients.

Factors That Influence HIV Progression

People with access to treatment for HIV can live long, healthy lives. However, many factors influence the progression of the disease, including genetic makeup, how healthy the patient was when infected, how long before diagnosis and the start of treatment, how often the patient sees a health care provider, how well the patient adheres to treatment, and health-related lifestyle choices such as a healthy diet, exercise, and not smoking.

Other factors that influence the development of AIDS are age, gender, HIV subtype, the presence of other viruses, poor nutrition, and severe stress. Genetic factors, too, play a role. In the United States, the rate of death due to AIDS is higher in males than in females—and much higher in African Americans and Hispanics than in whites and Native Americans (Centers for Disease Control and Prevention, 2018b. Poverty and low income are associated with faster disease progression. This may be because poorer people tend to suffer from poorer health overall, less access to health care, more stress, a greater incidence of drug use, and discrimination (Bogart et al., 2010).

Psychosocial factors are part of the picture, too. Depression is linked to the progression of HIV symptoms, although not to CD4 cell counts (Cruess et al., 2003; Zorrilla, McKay, Luborsky, & Schmidt, 1996). Stress is also linked to a poorer prognosis even when socioeconomic factors are taken into account, but most important is how people cope with stress (Chapter 7). The influence of stress on the immune system may depend on the duration of the stress, gender, and the stage of the disease. Research shows no relationship between social support and HIV progression (Antoni, 2003). However, social support and positive states of mind are related to better adherence to medical treatment (Gonzalez et al., 2004).

Positive psychological factors, in turn, appear to slow the development of AIDS, much as with other diseases. Extraversion, conscientiousness, assertiveness, positive emotions, sociability, openness to ideas, and striving for achievement are all linked to higher CD4 counts and slowed progression of disease (Ironson et al., 2005). In a yearlong prospective study, researchers discovered that, whereas negative affect narrows HIV-positive patients' cognitive-behavioral

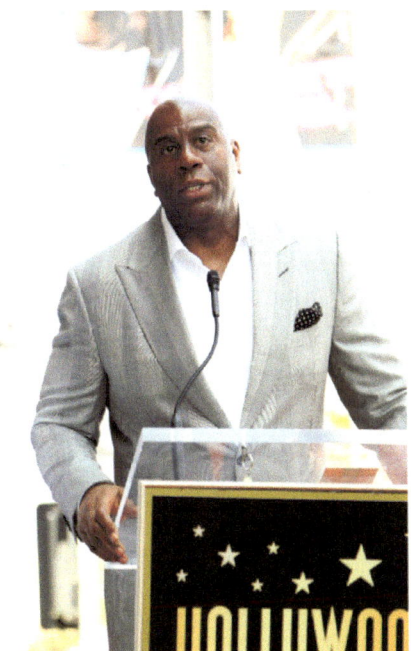

Photo 11.8 In 1991, star basketball player Magic Johnson announced his retirement, citing a recent diagnosis of HIV. Over the past three decades, Johnson has become an advocate for people with HIV/AIDS, partnering with the U.S. government and the United Nations in an effort to spread awareness and to reduce stigma. "The strides that we've made in 22 years—I've been all over the world talking about it," says Johnson. "But also a lot of people have died since then. So we're still in a big fight" (Jaslow, 2013).

responses to stress, positive affect broadens their responses, building their resources for coping. Additional resources may, in turn, increase quality of life (Rzeszutek & Gruszczyńska, 2019).

A Global Epidemic

HIV is a global issue: More than 39 million people worldwide are living with HIV (UNAIDS, 2024). In 2022 there were between 1 and 1.7 million new HIV infections. Although around the world up to 30 million people are on antiretroviral therapy for HIV, still approximately 630,000 people died of AIDS-related illness in 2022 (UNAIDS, 2024).

Sub-Saharan Africa is the most affected region, representing 77% of the worldwide total, although education and prevention have helped to slow the rate of new infections. Countries in East Africa have the second-highest rates of HIV/AIDS. In contrast, the incidence of AIDS has declined in more prosperous regions, such as the United States and Europe (WHO, 2015b).

One explanation for the spread of HIV in southern Africa has to do with *polygynous* relationships, in which a man has more than one wife or lover (Ragnarsson, Townsend, Thorson, Chopra, & Ekström, 2009; Reniers & Watkins, 2010). Unemployment and displacement as a result of poverty, famine, and war also contribute (Hanson & Hanson, 2008; Levinsohn, McLaren, Shisana, & Zuma, 2011). In West Africa, the main driver of disease is probably the sex trade (UNAIDS, 2012). In Niger, for example, the HIV rate was 36% among sex workers in 2011 (UNAIDS, 2012). The **Around the World** feature explores additional aspects of the HIV/AIDS epidemic in Africa.

Although more and more people have access to HIV treatment, the pandemic continues to outpace efforts to control it (Steinbrook, 2006). According to the Bill and Melinda Gates Foundation, the number of newly infected people outnumbers those who can get treatment by 2 to 1. There is still work to do to bring this global public health problem under control.

Thinking About Health

■ What is HIV/AIDS, how is it contracted, and how is it diagnosed?

■ What factors influence the progression of HIV/AIDS?

■ Why can some people live with HIV and never develop AIDS, while others die from the disease?

■ Why do you think that HIV/AIDS is still a global health problem?

Around *the* World

The HIV/AIDS Epidemic in Africa

Sub-Saharan Africa faces many barriers to an effective response to the HIV/AIDS epidemic. These countries lack the funding to support education, AIDS prevention, and medical treatment. However, the barriers are social and cultural as well. HIV brings with it shaming and discrimination, which discourage people from being tested, seeking treatment, and, most damaging of all, disclosing their HIV status. Cultural and religious beliefs all play a part (Mbonu, van den Borne, & De Vries, 2009), even among health care workers (Ahsan Ullah, 2011).

So does the status of women. As in much of the world, the HIV epidemic disproportionally affects women, who are twice as likely to be living with HIV/AIDS as are men in sub-Saharan Africa (UNAIDS, 2018 b). Women and girls there have less access to education, employment, and health care. They are often in relationships in which men are dominant and women are submissive, meaning that they cannot practice safer sex even when they know the risks. Violence against women is also a factor (Ellsberg & Betron, 2010; UNAIDS, 2018a). In response, the sixteenth International Conference on AIDS and STIs in Africa launched a task force on women, girls, gender equality, and HIV.

Legal barriers to prevention and treatment exist, too. Laws in several countries criminalize those who transmit the virus, whether through sexual activity or childbirth. While supporters justify this on public health or moral grounds, these laws discourage people from getting tested and disclosing their HIV status. Although some laws guarantee counseling and bar discrimination in employment and insurance, they nonetheless make people with HIV solely responsible for not spreading the disease.

Finally, one of the greatest barriers is ignorance. In South Africa, former president Thabo Mbeki wrote a letter to world leaders that appeared in the *Washington Post* in 2000. In it, he questioned the relationship between HIV and AIDS, suggesting that the actual cause of the disease is poverty. He suggested a diet of vegetables and opposed subsidies for drug treatment.

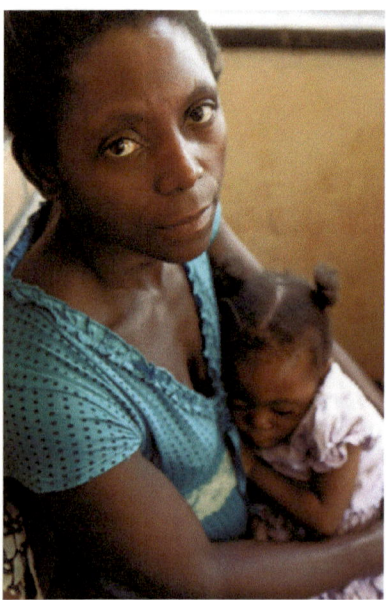

Photo 11.9   A woman waits to see a doctor at an AIDS relief clinic supported by Catholic Relief Services in Kitwe, Zambia.

Source: Jake Lyell/Alamy

Question:

What solutions can you offer to address each of the social and cultural barriers to an effective response to HIV/AIDS?

Cancer

Cancer is the name for more than 100 related diseases. Characteristic of all types of cancer, the orderly process of cellular division goes awry. Let's see why—and why the immune system fails to stop it.

What Is Cancer?

Cancer is a group of related diseases caused by the uncontrolled growth and spread of abnormal cells (American Cancer Society, 2024). Normally, the trillions of cells in the human body grow and divide to make new cells when and where the body needs them. When cells grow old or become damaged, they die and are removed from the body, and new cells grow in their place. In cancers, however, cells begin to divide without stopping and proliferate into surrounding tissues. Cancer is a biopsychosocial disease. Although its causes are still not fully understood, factors that increase the risk of cancer are known, and many of them are modifiable.

Cancer can begin in any part of the body, and types of cancer are usually named for where the cancer began. For example, lung cancer originates in the cells in the lungs; brain cancer originates in the brain. Sometimes, too, cancers are named for the type of cell that formed them, such as *squamous cell carcinoma*, named for cells found in the layers of the skin.

When rapid cell reproduction begins, cellular abnormalities then reproduce unchecked as well. In some cases, old or damaged cells do not die and instead reproduce less-healthy cells. In other cases, the body begins producing cells that are not needed. In all these cases, the extra cells may form growths, masses of tissue called **tumors**; see **Table 10.2**. Not all tumors are cancerous; there are harmless, or **benign**, tumors, too. But when tumors are **malignant**, they can invade nearby tissue, with dangerous results. However, while malignant tumors are always cancer, some cancers do not form tumors, such as in **leukemia**, a cancer of the blood.

When malignant tumors develop, some of these cells can break off and travel through the blood or lymph system to other locations. There, they can take hold and cause new tumors to develop. When a cancer has spread from one part of the body to another, it is said to have *metastasized*. This is common in later stages of cancer and is very serious. Regardless of where the cancer began, the most common sites for tumors to metastasize are the lungs, the liver, the brain, and the bones.

Benign tumors	Malignant tumors
Not cancerous	Cancerous
Do not spread	Spread to nearby tissue/organs
Do not grow back	Sometimes regrow after removal
Rarely life threatening—except brain tumors, which can be fatal	Dangerous and often life threatening if not treated

Table 11.1 Types of Tumors

How Do Cancer Cells Differ from Normal Cells?

What causes cells to grow out of control? Cancer cells differ from healthy cells in several ways (Cancer.gov, 2016):

- Cancer cells are not as specialized as normal cells. Although normal cells develop into distinct cell types with specific functions, cancer cells do not.
- Cancer cells are somehow able to ignore the chemical signals that tell cells to stop dividing or that initiate cell death. In normal cells, the body uses programmed cell death, or *apoptosis*, to rid itself of unneeded old or abnormal cells.
- Cancer cells can "take control" of normal cells, molecules, and blood vessels to feed the tumor. By co-opting nearby blood vessels, cancer cells create a **microenvironment**—a site in which the tumor can grow, obtain oxygen, and remove waste.

Recall that the immune system is designed to recognize and destroy unhealthy cells. Cancer cells also differ from healthy cells in how they evade the immune system:

- Cancer cells somehow "hide" from the immune system and proliferate undetected.
- As cancer cells grow into tumors, they begin to use the immune system to stay alive. They essentially manipulate the immune system into supporting tumor growth.

How Is Cancer Diagnosed?

When tumors can be seen or felt, a person is likely to seek medical attention. But many cancers are largely asymptomatic. When medical professionals suspect cancer, they will perform tests using an array of diagnostic procedures, including imaging, blood and urine sampling, tumor biopsy, endoscopic examinations, genetic testing, and surgery. Tissue or cellular samples are examined to determine if the proteins and genetic profile indicate cancer. If cancer is detected, its *stage* will be assessed to evaluate the progression and severity of the disease. Cancer stage refers to the extent or spread of the cancer, usually at diagnosis.

Staging is critical for effective treatment and prognosis. For most cancers, staging is based upon the size of the tumor and whether the cancer has spread to nearby lymph nodes or other areas of the body. The *TNM staging system* is the globally recognized standard for classifying the spread and severity of cancers:

- T stands for the size of the primary tumor;
- N stands for the presence or absence of involvement of the lymph nodes;
- M stands for whether or not the cancer has metastasized (moved to other areas of the body).

The TNM stages range from Stage 0, which is *in situ* (cancer cells only present within their original location) to Stage I (early cancer with a good prognosis) to Stage IV (the most advanced form, where the cancer has spread into the lymph nodes and other tissues and organs). Some cancers, like testicular cancer, do not use this staging system.

Cancers are treated in many different ways, depending on their type and staging. Treatments involve surgery, chemotherapy, and radiation, all of which are designed to remove or destroy the cancer cells. Once no more cancer cells are present in a person, the cancer is said to be in remission.

What Causes Cancer?

Many types of cancer have a genetic component. It originates in changes in the genes that control cell growth and division, and these mutations can be passed down from parents to offspring. Some breast and ovarian cancers, for example, run in families. Women who have a mother, sister, or daughter with a history of breast cancer are about twice as likely to develop breast cancer themselves (Metcalfe et al., 2013). Men also get breast cancer, but it is rare. Less than 1% of all breast cancer cases are diagnosed in men (Susan G. Komen, 2019). We can now do a blood test to determine whether a woman is carrying the genes that put her at greater risk for these cancers, genes known as *BRCA1* and *BRCA2*.

Not all cancers, however, are inherited. Environmental factors can also damage genes. A **carcinogen** is a substance that can cause cancer in living tissue. Examples are the chemicals in tobacco smoke, ultraviolet rays from the sun, some infections, and even an unhealthy diet. It can take more than 10 years from the exposure to carcinogens to the detection of cancer.

Although many cancers run in families, a family shares more than just genes. Families also share their lifestyle and environment. All these factors may act together or in sequence to cause cancer, and it can be difficult to tease apart the risks.

Who Is at Risk for Cancer?

It is difficult to estimate how many people have cancer at any point in time because cancer can be treated and go into remission. However, we can determine that 2 million new cases of cancer will be diagnosed this year (not including skin cancers, which are not required to be reported to cancer registries) in the United States. This year, about 611, 720 people are expected to die of cancer, totaling around 1660 deaths per day (National Cancer Institute, 2024). Cancer is the second-most-common cause of death in the United States after heart disease, and it accounts for one out of every four deaths (American Cancer Society, 2019; see **Figure 11.5**). Globally, there are 20 million new cases of cancer diagnosed annually and nearly 10 million people die from cancer (International Agency for Research on Cancer, 2024). The most common forms of cancer worldwide are lung, breast, and colorectal cancer.

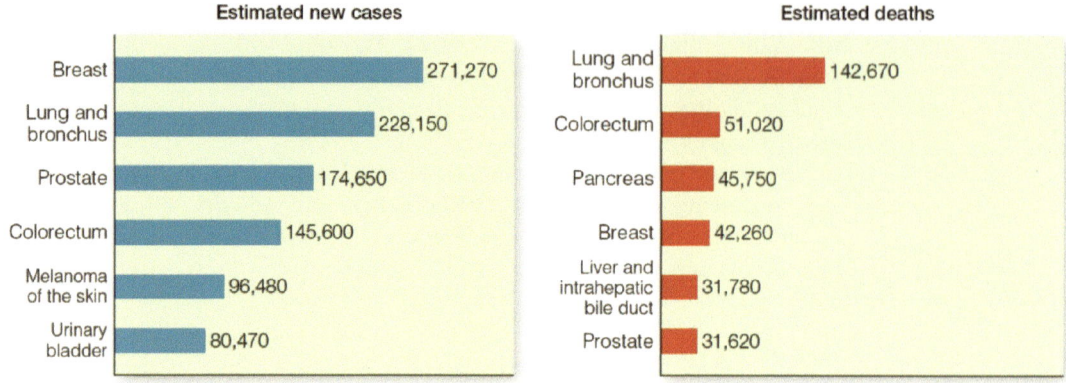

By cancer type, both sexes combined

Figure 11.5   Incidence and Mortality Rates Associated with Different Types of Cancer.

Source: Data from the American Cancer Society (2019)

What are some of the risk factors for cancer? Aging is the single biggest risk factor (Siegel, Miller, & Jemal, 2019), even if there is no family history of cancer. Adults aged 55 or older account for 80% of all cancer diagnoses (Siegel et al., 2019). The longer we live, the more everyday wear and tear our bodies sustain, resulting in cell damage.

Gender is also associated with cancer risk, as **Figure 11.6** shows. Thirty-nine percent of men and 38% of women will develop cancer at some point in their lifetimes (Siegel et al., 2019). Certain cancers are exclusive to men, such as testicular and prostate cancers, while others are exclusive to women, such as cervical and ovarian cancers.

We have already seen how genes affect the risk of cancer, but lifestyle is just as important. Excess weight and alcohol consumption are linked to cancer risk. People who smoke are 25 times more likely to develop lung cancer than are nonsmokers (Siegel et al., 2019). Only a few cancers are solely hereditary. Regardless of family history, a person may never develop breast cancer unless she or he engages in health-compromising behaviors.

Ethnicity, race, culture, and socioeconomic status (SES) may increase the risk of cancer as well. White women have the highest rates of cancer, while Black women have the highest death rates due to cancer (CDC, 2014a). In men, and especially Black men, have the highest rates of cancer and the highest death rates associated with cancer. Native Americans and Native Alaskans have the lowest incidence of cancers, while male Asians and Pacific Islanders have, overall, the lowest death rates (CDC, 2014a).

Ethnicity and SES often go together—and they often correspond to where you live. In their diversity, New York City neighborhoods are a good proxy for race and SES, and, sure enough, late-stage cancers are more prevalent in low-income and minority neighborhoods (Islami, Kahn, Bickell, Schymura, & Boffetta, 2013; Kanna, Narang, Atwal, Paul, & Azeez, 2009; Mandelblatt, Andrews, Kerner, Zauber, & Burnett, 1991; McCord & Freeman, 1990). In the

Trends in death rates for females, 1930–2016

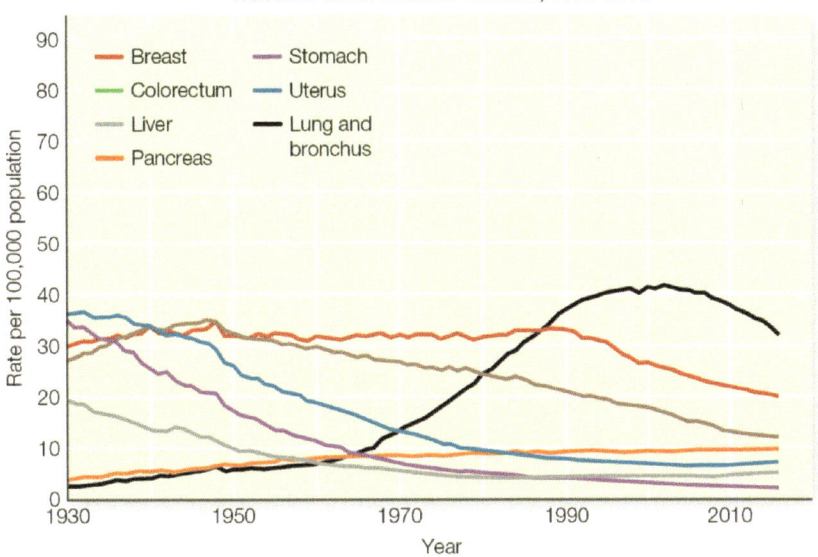

Trends in death rates for males, 1930–2016

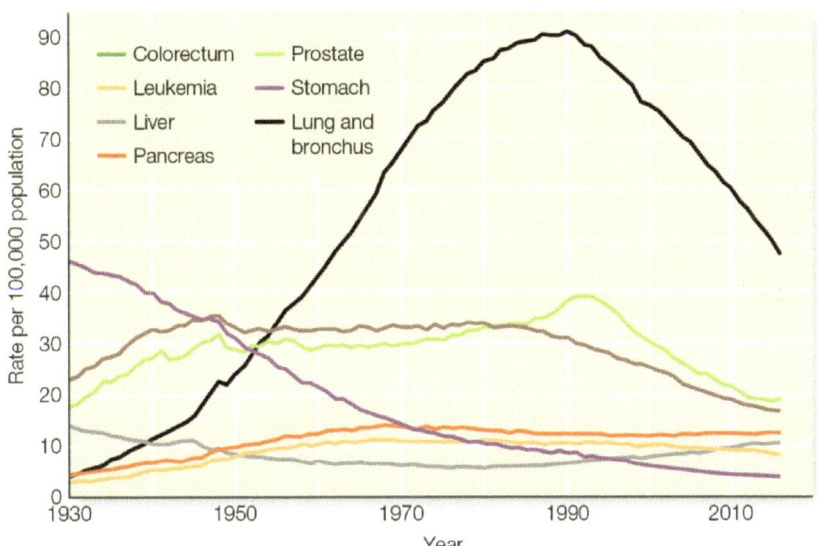

Figure 11.6   Death Rates * by Sex in the United States, All Cancers, 1930–2016.

Note: *Rates are per 100,000 and are age-adjusted to the 2000 U.S. standard population.

Source: Data from the American Cancer Society (2019)

United States as a whole, nonwhites and those of lower SES are at higher risk of late-stage cancers than are whites or those of higher SES (Islami et al., 2013). Around the world, the health disparities seen in cancer have to do with early detection and effective treatment. Countries where people have easy access to quality medical care have lower rates of cancer than those that do not.

Can we disentangle these factors? It is not easy, but one study did look at four geographically close but very different New York neighborhoods (Islami et al., 2013). It found 34,981 cancer cases, and all ethnic/racial groups were at higher risk than whites were for late-stage cancers (see **Table 10.3**). Was this because ethnic minorities had lower SES and, therefore, less access to health insurance, early detection, and treatment for cancer? Apparently, but not entirely: Race or ethnicity was a stronger predictor than was SES for late stage at diagnosis. Cultural beliefs, levels of education, language barriers, and immigrant status may also play a role.

Stress and Cancer

As with other immune-related diseases, stress can make a person more vulnerable to cancer by impairing the immune system. Major life events, such as the loss of a loved one or economic downturn, definitely increase the risk of breast cancer (Kruk, 2012). So do stressors going back as far as childhood (Bower et al., 2014). In turn, stress is a normal reaction to living with cancer, producing a vicious cycle (Costanzo, Stawski, Ryff, Coe, & Almeida, 2012; Diehl & Hay, 2013). As daily hassles bring down a patient's mood and ability to cope, physical symptoms such as exhaustion grow worse, and so does the cancer, although the precise mechanisms of this process are still unknown (Bower et al., 2014). Fatigue may persist for years, even after successful treatment (Bower et al., 2000).

It is not only the patient that has to live with cancer—the disease affects family members and loved ones, too (Lindberg & Wellisch, 2004). Posttraumatic stress disorder has been found in children who have had a parent die of cancer (Stoppelbein, Greening, & Elkin, 2006). Fortunately, there are ways to help. For example, mindfulness-based stress reduction can slow disease progression and enhance quality of life (Carlson, Speca, Patel, & Goodey, 2003; Huang, He, Wang, & Zhou, 2016).

Personality and Cancer Could there be a cancer-prone personality? As early as 1962, researchers were finding that some people were more prone to cancer than others of the same age (Kissen & Eysenck, 1962). The profile of the cancer-prone person includes a formidable list of negatives: emotional repression, anger, hostility, resentment, poor coping, taking on responsibilities even when stressed, pessimism, depression, hopelessness, excessive worry about others, and a need for approval (Kissen & Eysenck, 1962). It is not a pretty picture, but could it be true?

Although research support has been inconsistent, depression, anger, and hostility do seem to predispose people to illness. One meta-analysis showed a small but marginally significant link between depression and overall cancer risk (Oerlemans, van den Akker, Schuurman, Kellen, & Buntinx, 2007). A study using data from the NHANES program (see Chapter 9) found a much higher risk of death when a cancer patient was depressed as well (Onitilo, Nietert, & Egede, 2006). The links run the other way, too: Between 15% and 25% of cancer patients may experience depression (Agarwal, Hamilton, Moore, & Crandell, 2010). Depression may be a reaction to living with cancer, or it may be related to the changes in the brain due to cancer (Agarwal et al., 2010), but, in either case, it reduces a patient's quality of life (Ferreira et al., 2008) and influences mortality (Gallo et al., 2007; Lloyd-Williams, Shiels, Taylor, & Dennis, 2009).

Researchers are still exploring the links between personality and cancer. They hope to tease apart the roles of hormones, lifestyle, and psychological factors. For hormonal risk factors, they have singled out early age of menarche (menstruation), later age for first pregnancy, older age at menopause, and hormone replacement therapy after menopause. For lifestyle factors, they point to obesity, smoking, alcohol consumption, poor diet, and lack of physical activity.

The supposed cancer-prone personality has taken on the name type C. One hallmark of the **type C personality** is repressed expression of emotion. Another suggested personality trait that might make a person prone to cancer is *commitment*, or deferring one's own needs to the needs of others, such as spouses and children (Temoshok, 1987).

Breast cancer patients do rate significantly higher on commitment than healthy people, in part due to its effects on hormones and the immune system (Eskelinen & Ollonen, 2011). Yet, that alone is not evidence for a cancer-prone personality, and other studies have been just as skeptical (Lillberg, Verkasalo, Kaprio, Helenius, & Koskenvuo, 2002; Nakaya et al., 2003; Shapiro et al., 2001). In one study, type C personality actually related to a *decreased* risk of breast cancer (Grossarth-Maticek & Eysenck, 1990). Hostility does seem to increase the risk of smoking-related cancers (Lemogne et al., 2013). But does hostility directly change the course of disease, or does it only change smoking habits? The jury is still out.

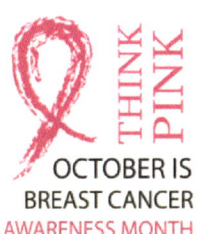

OCTOBER IS
BREAST CANCER
AWARENESS MONTH

Surviving Cancer

The good news is that the survival rates for cancers are increasing (see **Figure 11.6**). Seventy percent of whites and 63% of Blacks reach the 5-year relative survival rate (for all cancers). While survival rates vary by the type of cancer, they are also impacted by early diagnosis and treatment, age at diagnosis, and stage of cancer at diagnosis.

Public health campaigns regarding the dangers of tobacco are also surely helping. Cancer screenings and early detection may be helping as well. Together with better treatment, these measures are creating a huge population of survivors. The number of cancer survivors in the United States alone is expected to reach nearly 19 million by 2024. These survivors are changing the way we think about cancer. They also have special needs—in both health care and quality of life—that we are only beginning to understand.

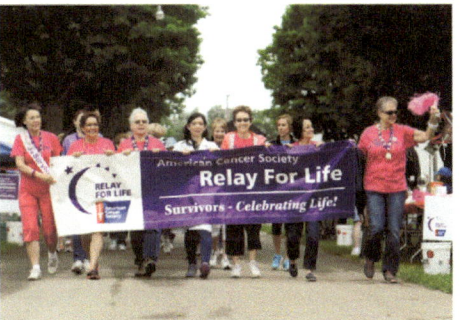

Photo 11.10 Annual events such as Breast Cancer Awareness Month and Relay for Life bring attention and funding to fighting cancer across the United States.

Source: AP Images/DON CAMPBELL

Thinking About Health

- How is cancer a psychoneuroimmunological disease?
- What are the biopsychosocial factors that influence the development and treatment of cancer?
- Why are health disparities involved in cancer, and what can be done to address them?
- What are the most important factors for living with cancer?

Arthritis

Like cancer, arthritis encompasses as many as 100 different conditions. **Arthritis** attacks the joints, bones, muscles, cartilage, or other connective tissues. The word *a rthritis* literally means joint inflammation—from the Greek *artho* (joint) and *itis* (inflammation). Arthritis is not just aches and pains, but a debilitating illness. It is the leading cause of disability in the United States.

Nearly 55 million Americans (or one in four adults) are suffering from arthritis today; however, this may be an underestimate, because many people do not seek medical treatment or are not diagnosed appropriately (Barbour, Helmick, Boring, & Brady, 2017). Revised estimates suggest that the number may be closer to 91.2 million adults who have either a clinical diagnosis of arthritis or joint pain consistent with a diagnosis of arthritis (Jafarzadeh & Felson, 2017).

Arthritis is correlated with age. In those over age 65, more than half of men and two-thirds of women have arthritis (Jafarzadeh & Felson, 2017). In addition, as the obesity epidemic increases, rates of arthritis increase as well—extra weight puts more stress on joints. Research shows, too, that women who are obese are 32% more likely to have severe joint pain (Barbour et al., 2017). And arthritis affects all races and ethnicities: Around 4 million Hispanic adults and 6 million blacks have doctor-diagnosed arthritis (Jafarzadeh & Felson, 2017).

In general, arthritis significantly impairs the lives of those who have it. Forty-four percent of patients report limitations in their activities (Barbour et al., 2017). Severe joint pain is also associated with higher rates of diabetes and significant psychological distress (Barbour et al., 2017). Although arthritis is not solely an autoimmune disease, it is one of the most common examples of the immune system gone rogue.

Types of Arthritis

Arthritis is not exclusively a disease of aging. Two thirds of those living with arthritis are younger than 65. In particular, **juvenile arthritis** is a set of autoimmune and inflammatory conditions that can develop at age 16 or younger. Although there are several subtypes of juvenile arthritis, affecting children worldwide of all races and ethnicities, it tends to affect girls more than boys, and has a prevalence of one to two children in every 1000 (Arthritis Foundation, 2018). Juvenile arthritis has a significant impact on children's mental health, well-being, and quality of life, and can lead to other comorbid health problems across the lifespan.

The most common type of arthritis, however, does become more common as we grow older. **Osteoarthritis** develops when the lining of the joints begins to wear away and the bones begin to grind on each other, causing pain, inflammation, and sometimes, joint disfigurement. It affects the fingers, knees, and hips, and may sometimes result from a previous injury, such as a childhood sports injury or a car accident in adulthood. Roughly 31 million Americans live with osteoarthritis (Arthritis Foundation, 2018). One third of military veterans of all ages have arthritis, as do athletes and others who have suffered injuries (Arthritis Foundation, 2018).

As with many chronic illnesses, depression is common in individuals who suffer from osteoarthritis. Depression can exacerbate the pain and distress

(Zautra & Smith, 2001). For example, a classically trained violinist who has practiced many hours per day for 40 years may have to give up playing and performing after osteoarthritis develops. The disease may rob her of her passion, her livelihood, and her sense of self.

Rheumatoid arthritis is an autoimmune disease in which the body's immune system mistakenly attacks the joints. What causes this to happen is still unknown, though scientists have begun to explore the origins of the disease (see the **In the News** feature). The abnormal immune response causes inflammation, primarily in the lining of the joints. The main symptoms are pain, swollen or reddish joints, and fatigue. Onset can sometimes be sudden and unexpected. One patient might wake up in the morning with severe pain and weakness, so much so that it is impossible to lift oneself out of bed. Another patient may experience soreness after a vigorous workout that just will not go away. RA is a progressive disease, and, over time, the inflammation can damage organs, such as the heart. It can lead to disability, deformity, a lower quality of life, and higher mortality (Brooks, 2006).

In the News

An Unlikely Culprit in Autoimmune Disease

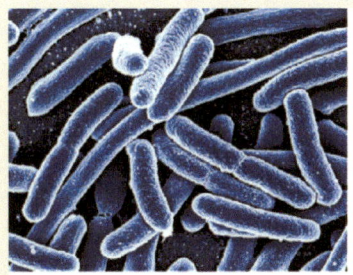

Could bacteria affect your chance of developing rheumatoid arthritis? What role does the microbiota-gut-brain axis play in the development of autoimmune diseases?

Although the cause of rheumatoid arthritis remains unknown, science has uncovered a surprising culprit: the bacteria that live in our intestines (Wells, Williams, Matey-Hernandez, Menni, & Steves, 2019). The intestines contain nearly 1000 different bacteria, and the evidence is growing that these microbiota may trigger chronic, noninfectious ailments such as RA. As Veena Taneja, an immunologist at the Mayo Clinic, wrote, "It's become more and more clear that these microbes can affect the immune system, even diseases that are not in your gut" (Kohn, 2015).

Could the increase in autoimmune diseases over the last few decades correspond to changes in our bacterial ecosystem? Meghan, the subject of our chapter-opening story who adopted a radical diet in order to

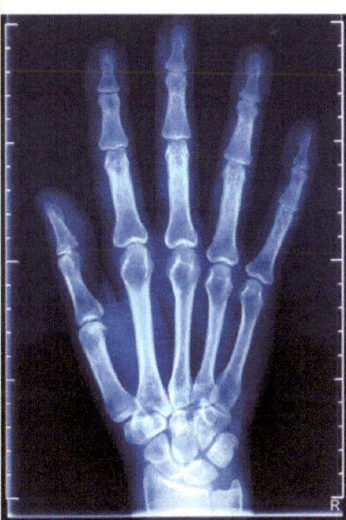

Photo 11.11

Source: PASIEKA/Getty Images (top) and BSIP/Science Source (bottom)

combat the symptoms of an autoimmune disease, might think so. These changes have come from alterations in diet and the overuse of antibiotics. Humans and the microbiota of the natural world are also simply less exposed to one another, as our daily activities have less to do with animals and plants.

How do these bacteria affect autoimmune diseases? Perhaps their very presence in our gut helps modulate the immune system. After all, two thirds of the body's immune cells exist in the gut. As the bacteria begin to disappear, immune cells may then begin to assault not only the microbiota, but also the body itself (Wells et al., 2019). Although scientists have not yet identified the microbiota that may trigger an autoimmune reaction, they are

getting closer, and soon it may be possible to use bacteria as medicine.

Do not go back to the grocery store for the "probiotic" yogurt you saw the other day, though. Most scientists say that products containing probiotics are mostly harmless, but completely untested. But a vegan diet may improve arthritis symptoms (McDougall, Bruce, Spiller, Westerdahl, & McDougall, 2002). In 10 or 15 years, the microbiome may be a key therapeutic option, suggesting that, in the future, we may well see our ailments treated by our diet.

Question: Why do you think immune cells are so common in the gut? What might they be protecting us against?

The severity of RA varies from person to person, and symptoms can vary from day to day. Flare-ups can last from days to months. Many RA sufferers report long periods of joint stiffness in the morning that wears off during the day. As the disease progresses, the flare-ups become more disabling.

About 1.5 million Americans have RA, with three times as many women afflicted as men. For women, RA usually begins to show symptoms between the ages of 30 and 60. For men, it emerges later in life. RA is more prevalent in older adults and is often comorbid with other conditions, such as age-related cognitive declines (Zwahr, Park, & Shifren, 1999). It is also associated with depression, and stress has been found to exacerbate its symptoms as well.

Treatment for Arthritis

Treatment for osteoarthritis involves maintaining a healthy weight, using anti-inflammatory pain relievers, and exercise. These changes allow for better coping and a higher quality of life (Zautra & Smith, 2001). Social support, especially understanding from spouse and family, is the key to adjustment. When diagnosed early and effectively treated, RA can be managed as well. Treatments include anti-inflammatory medications, pain relievers, rest, modification of daily activities, and regular exercise.

Thinking About Health

- What role does the immune system play in each of the different types of arthritis?
- How might these differences influence a patient's perception of their illness and their treatment?

Diabetes

There are two types of diabetes. **Type 1 diabetes**, or *early-onset diabetes*, appears when an autoimmune disease impairs the production of insulin, a hormone needed to convert sugar, starches, and other food into the energy we need. Although type 1 diabetes can appear at any age, it is most often diagnosed in childhood or adolescence. Type 1 was once called *juvenile diabetes* for just that reason. *Type 2 diabetes* usually develops later in life as a result of lifestyle and diet, as discussed in Chapter 9.

Type 1 Diabetes

In Chapter 10 we learned about the links among CVD and diabetes. So you might be wondering why diabetes is also covered in this chapter. The reason is because Type 1 diabetes develops when the immune system attacks and destroys the insulin-producing cells, called *beta cells*, in the pancreas. In a healthy person, insulin causes the cells in the liver, muscle, and fat tissue to absorb glucose and convert it to glycogen to be used as energy, and it keeps the amount of sugar in the bloodstream from getting too high. A dysfunction in insulin production can be life threatening.

The early symptoms of type 1 diabetes are excessive thirst and frequent urination, extreme hunger, sudden weight loss, extreme fatigue, irritability, blurred vision, nausea, and vomiting. These symptoms may appear abruptly and may be severe. Children with type 1 diabetes may also appear restless or apathetic, and they may have trouble in school. In some severe cases, a coma is the first sign of diabetes.

Hypoglycemia, or *low blood sugar*, occurs when there is too much insulin in the blood. Just how much is *too* much depends on the amount of food consumed and the level of physical activity, but the danger is real. Symptoms of hypoglycemia are sweating, trembling, hunger, rapid heartbeat, and confusion. When blood sugar drops sharply, the result is **diabetic shock**. If not treated quickly, it can lead to fainting, seizure, coma, and death.

People with diabetes are also at greater risk of kidney disease, heart disease, stroke, high blood pressure, neuropathy, foot ulcers that may require amputation, blindness, skin infections, and gum disease (see Chapter 9). These diseases can be reduced significantly by proper diabetes management.

Risk Factors for Diabetes

As many as 30 million adults in the United States (9.3% of the population) suffer from diabetes, and roughly 15,000 children and 15,000 adults are diagnosed with the disease each year in the United States alone (CDC, 2017d). New cases of diabetes have been rising over the past few decades, especially in white youth. Boys and girls are equally at risk.

Both genes and the environment may put someone at risk. Some 18 genetic locations have been implicated in the development of type 1 diabetes. If one identical twin has the disease, the other has a 33% chance of developing it. A child is more likely to inherit the disease from a father than from a mother. Yet many sufferers do not have a family history of the disease. Even if a close relative has diabetes, one has only a 10% chance of developing the disease.

Environmental triggers for the disease include the *enteric* viruses that attack the intestinal track. One family of enteric viruses, the *coxsackie* viruses, is a particular concern. Epidemics of mumps and congenital rubella have also led to cases of type 1 diabetes, another reminder of the importance of vaccination.

Other potential risk factors for type 1 diabetes include illness in early infancy, children born to older mothers, a mother who had preeclampsia during pregnancy, and several other autoimmune diseases—Grave's disease, Hashimoto's thyroiditis, Addison's disease, multiple sclerosis, and pernicious anemia.

Treatment for Diabetes

Hypoglycemia can be managed effectively through carefully monitored treatment, diet, and exercise. When the body fails to make insulin or cannot regulate it effectively, patients must take insulin in the form of a shot each day. The daily regimen for children with diabetes involves giving them a shot upon waking and monitoring their blood sugar with finger sticks throughout the day. When symptoms occur, they can quickly raise their blood sugar by sucking on a hard candy or drinking fruit juice. People with diabetes usually carry some form of sugar with them, just in case.

This regimen is complex and demanding, but it works (McGrady, Peugh, & Hood, 2014). Yet more than two thirds of adolescents and young adults with type 1 diabetes fail to comply fully (Hilliard, Wu, Rausch, Dolan, & Hood, 2013; McGrady et al., 2014; Petitti et al., 2009). Diabetes control is poorest around age 18 or 19, perhaps because of the transition to university and adulthood in general (Bryden et al., 2001). Faced with emotional, social, and academic challenges, these patients may forget or forgo treatment (McGrady et al., 2014; Peters & Laffel, 2011). Changes in hormone levels at puberty may also affect insulin levels and dosing.

In early childhood, treatment naturally falls to the parent, and the transition to self-management can be difficult (King, Berg, Butner, Butler, & Wiebe, 2014). The key is for parents to remain involved, but to also help the child assume responsibility and face many psychosocial and interpersonal challenges (King et al., 2014). With positive coping strategies and family support, people with diabetes can look forward to a high quality of life.

Understanding psychoneuroimmunology is essential to disease management—whether of autoimmune disease, HIV/AIDS, cancer, arthritis, or diabetes.

Thinking About Health

■ Compare and contrast what you learned about type 2 diabetes in Chapter 9 with what you have learned about type 1 diabetes in this chapter.

■ If you know someone who has grown up managing diabetes, how has the illness influenced that person's life?

■ What are some of the challenges in managing diabetes?

Chapter Summary

Psychoneuroimmunology is the study of the biological processes of the immune, endocrine, and nervous systems and how they interact with psychological processes to promote good health or to put individuals at risk for poor health. The immune system is the body's defense against illness. It works by recognizing antigens on the surfaces of cells and destroying foreign or unhealthy cells, and its defenses include inflammation and a complex network of cells, organs, hormones, and bacteria. We are all born with innate immunity, and we develop acquired immunity through exposure to our environment.

Immune-related disorders may occur when the immune system is compromised. Personality, stress, and environmental factors all play roles, as do genetics and heredity. In cancer, unhealthy cells evade or even co-opt the immune system, while in autoimmune diseases, the body attacks its own healthy cells. Certain forms of arthritis and type 1 diabetes are common examples of autoimmune diseases. From a mosquito bite to HIV/AIDS, the ever-evolving immune system is the perfect example of the biopsychosocial nature of health.

KEY TERMS ▶ psychoneuroimmunology p. 328, danger-associated molecular patterns p. 329, antigens p. 329, innate immunity (or *nonspecific immunity*) p. 330, acquired immunity (or *specific immunity*) p. 331, herd immunity p. 331, macrophages p. 332, lymphocytes p. 332, autoimmune disease p. 337, acquired immune deficiency syndrome (AIDS) p. 339, human immunodeficiency virus (HIV) p. 339, acute retroviral syndrome (ARS; or *primary HIV infection*) p. 341, clinical latency p. 341, cancer p. 345, tumors p. 345, benign p. 345, malignant p. 345, leukemia p. 345, microenvironment p. 346, carcinogen p. 347, type C personality p. 351, arthritis p. 352, juvenile arthritis p. 352, osteoarthritis p. 352, rheumatoid arthritis p. 353, type 1 diabetes (or *early-onset diabetes*) p. 355, hypoglycemia (or *low blood sugar*) p. 355, diabetic shock p. 355

CHAPTER 12

Chronic and Terminal Illnesses

Learning Outcomes

After reading this chapter, you should be able to:

- **Define** *chronic illness*, and describe the physical and emotional symptoms that chronically ill patients often experience.
- **Identify** the factors that influence coping with chronic illness.
- **Explain** the importance of quality of life.
- **Define** terminal illness and explain the stages of dying.
- **Identify** how causes of death vary across the lifespan.
- **Describe** what can be done to prepare for death and what factors lead to a "good" death.
- **Define** the death-with-dignity and right-to-die movements.
- **Explain** how culture influences death and bereavement.

After years of debilitating headaches, at the age of 29, Brittany Maynard was diagnosed with terminal brain cancer and told that she had 6 months to live. Brittany had glioblastoma multiforme, the most aggressive and lethal form of brain cancer. It spreads quickly to other parts of the body, and few patients survive (**Photo 12.1**).

After a long and careful assessment, she and her family chose to move to Oregon, the first state of the United States of America to pass death-with-dignity laws. These laws give terminally ill patients the option to take life-ending medication if dying becomes unbearably painful. Brittany met the legal and medical criteria for assisted death and was prescribed medication that would allow her to end her life peacefully and painlessly when and if she chose to do so.

Brittany was keenly aware that most people with terminal illness cannot choose to die on their own terms—what advocates of that option call "death with dignity." The laws in most states and countries do not permit it, and most families do not have the means to move. Brittany chose to use her terminal illness as an opportunity to begin a global

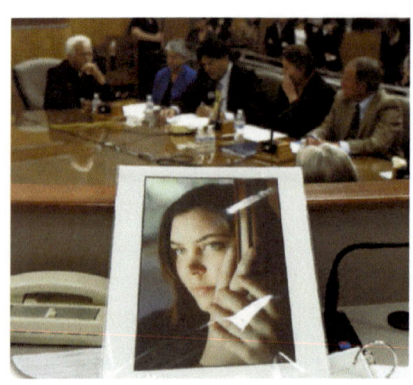

Photo 12.1

AP Images/Rich Pedroncelli

DOI: 10.4324/9781032643090-12

conversation. In a video that went viral, Brittany shared her controversial decision. For her, she explained, her decision was part of living each moment to the fullest in the face of imminent death. On November 1, 2014, two days after her husband's birthday, Brittany ended her life peacefully in her home, surrounded by her loved ones.

Would you have made the same decision as Brittany? Do you agree that all terminally ill patients should have the same choices? Millions of people around the world have been inspired by Brittany's strength and bravery, and her story has created a movement to expand access to assisted death so that no one in the terminal phase of chronic illness has to endure prolonged pain and suffering. Yet, many people condemn her decision to die and oppose making this option legal.

Patients, their caregivers, and their loved ones cope with chronic and terminal illness, dying, and death in many different ways. We will explore these issues in depth in this chapter, and we will also touch upon some of the attributes that lead to better coping and adaptation (see Chapter 13 for more on emotional health and well-being). But first, we must understand the trajectory of chronic illness, what it is like to be diagnosed with a chronic illness, what we mean by quality of life, and the biopsychosocial factors that influence decisions throughout life. We will also discuss the terminal phase of chronic illness, the stages of death and dying, end-of-life decisions, and grief and bereavement.

Chronic Illness

When you have a cold, an upset stomach, or body aches, you may feel dreadful, but you also know that you will feel better soon. As we saw in Chapter 1, *acute disorders* may be intense and serious, and they may cause pain and disability, but they are often curable and of limited duration—in other words, they go away. **Chronic illnesses** are diseases that, once you have them, are not curable and may last the rest of your life, creating significant life changes, stress, and discomfort.

The Impact of Chronic Illness

Chronic conditions range from mild, such as hearing impairment, to severe and life-threatening, such as cancer. There are many types of chronic illnesses, including cardiovascular disease, diabetes, arthritis, Alzheimer's and Parkinson's diseases, amyotrophic lateral sclerosis (called ALS or Lou Gehrig's disease), multiple sclerosis, asthma, cystic fibrosis, and osteoporosis. Although there is great variability in what is considered a chronic condition (specifically, in the amount of time that someone must live with a condition for it to be considered "chronic"), here we will adopt the Centers for Disease Control and Prevention definition that chronic conditions are conditions that last one year or longer and often require ongoing medical attention (CDC, 2019a).

Chronic illnesses are a global health challenge—perhaps the greatest health challenge we face today. The most recent global data from 2019 shows the top 10 leading causes of death (see **Figure 12.2**). In terms of lives lost, the top three disease categories—CVD, respiratory diseases, and neonatal conditions—account for 55% of all deaths worldwide (WHO, 2020). These data do not include deaths due to the COVID-19 pandemic. Although the COVID-19 pandemic was an acute and global catastrophe, for people who have long-COVID or continue to live with debilitating conditions brought on by exposure to the COVID-19 virus, COVID is a chronic condition.

Sixty percent of all Americans have at least one chronic condition, and 40% have multiple chronic conditions—and this proportion increases with age (CDC, 2019b). After age 65, nearly 85% of American adults have at least one chronic condition, and 60% have multiple chronic conditions (National Institute on Aging, 2017). This is due, as we saw in Chapter 1, to an increasing population of older adults, who are living longer than ever before. Although some chronic health problems, such as hearing deficits, type 1 diabetes, and asthma, are present from birth or early childhood, most chronic health problems emerge in midlife. Chronic illness is the main source of poor health, disability, and death in the United States, where it also accounts for the largest health care expenditure.

Chronic conditions are largely caused by lifestyle factors, such as tobacco use, secondhand smoke, excessive alcohol consumption, uncontrolled high blood pressure, poor diet, and a sedentary lifestyle. Adverse childhood experiences, poverty, and stress all play roles as well (Bauer, Briss, Goodman, & Bowman, 2014; Borja, Nurius, Song, & Lengua, 2019). Thus, the good news is that these conditions are often preventable. It is important for health psychologists to help people make lifestyle choices that will reduce their risk of long-term chronic illness. **Figure 12.1**, for example, shows which modifiable risk factors may lead to preventable cancers.

Physiological, psychological, and sociocultural factors all influence the risks and course of illness and affect how people cope with their condition. These factors include sex, age, economic stability, ethnicity, and religion. In turn, a biopsychosocial perspective helps in understanding the impact of chronic illness on a person's life.

The pain and discomfort associated with being ill can vary by disease. Some chronic conditions, for example, are noticeable and felt every day, such as chronic back pain. Others are less obvious, but still dangerous, such as high blood pressure or high cholesterol. Many chronic conditions have long periods of stability, interrupted

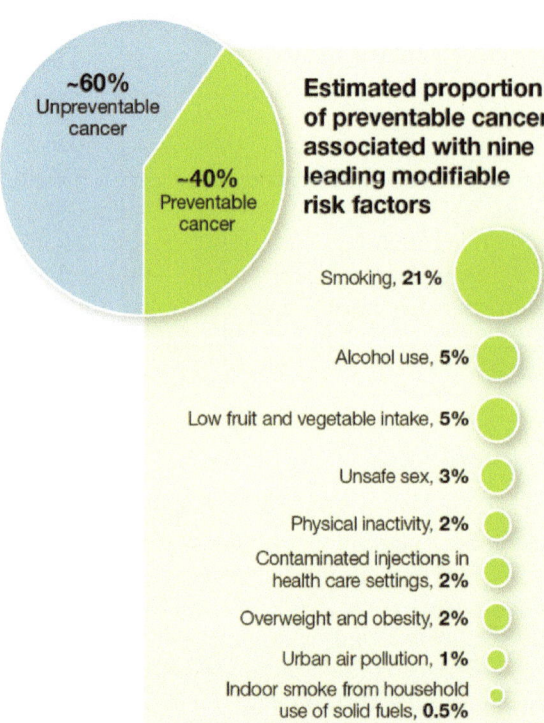

Figure 12.1   Modifiable risk factors associated with preventable cancer.

Source: Data from Danaei et al. (2005).

by acute episodes or flare-ups. Others are progressive, and each new stage poses different challenges. Some diseases require self-management through medication or lifestyle changes, while others require repeated treatments, surgery, or hospitalization. There may also be differences in the intensity and invasiveness of treatments, and these treatments may themselves create discomfort. Even the same disease may not be experienced in the same way by two different patients.

Health Disparities in Chronic Illness

Due to modern medical advances, life expectancy has increased overall. Fatalities due to acute and infectious diseases have become less common, thanks to vaccinations and antibiotics. Thus, most older adults in developed countries will die of chronic conditions. Worldwide, the leading causes of death today are cardiovascular diseases, as shown in **Figure 12.2** (see Chapter 9 for more on cardiovascular disorders).

However, the leading causes of death by sex and ethnicity vary. Chronic kidney disease, for instance, is found at significantly higher rates among African Americans than other groups in the United States (Lissanu et al., 2019). Although blacks and whites have a similar prevalence of early-stage kidney disease, blacks reach the threshold of life-threatening kidney failure more rapidly than whites do (Lissanu et al., 2019). Why? The answer is that African American kidney patients are more likely to have comorbid chronic conditions, such as obesity,

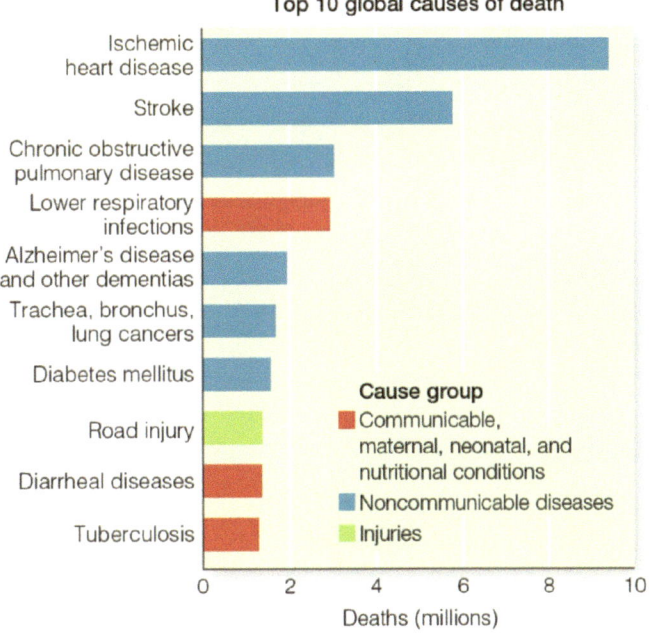

Figure 12.2   Leading causes of death worldwide.

Source: Data from World Health Organization (2018d).

diabetes, and hypertension, which put them at greater risk for severe kidney disease. They are also more likely to encounter socioeconomic stumbling blocks in receiving medical care and social support, making self-care and disease management more problematic (Lissanu et al., 2019). These biopsychosocial factors all come together to create a significant health disparity.

Elsewhere in the United States, health disparities also adversely affect the Latinx population, which suffers from rates of childhood obesity, adult diabetes, advanced and terminal cancers, and suicide attempts higher than in the general population (Ramírez García, 2019). These disparities can be attributed to social determinants of health such as economic and social resources, living conditions, social context, and cultural beliefs (Ramírez García, 2019). Among all minority populations, health inequities increase vulnerability to acute and chronic illnesses.

An underlying biopsychosocial factor of health disparities is economic disadvantage. In spite of the Affordable Care Act (ACA), low-income levels and poverty are still linked to a lack of health insurance in the United States. Although people without the financial resources for medical care can use free clinics that provide medical services for little or no expense, not everyone in need of this care can access it. For example, for patients residing in rural communities, where lower incomes are combined with distance from resources, visiting a clinic may be impossible (Theeke, Carpenter, Mallow, & Theeke, 2019). In addition, low socioeconomic status and financial insecurity are associated with higher levels of stressful experiences, such as divorce, death of a child, and violent assault (Cohen, Murphy, & Prather, 2019). Like dominos, the experience of one stressor can lead to another (Cohen et al., 2019), and the more stressors a person experiences, the more vulnerable that person becomes to chronic illness.

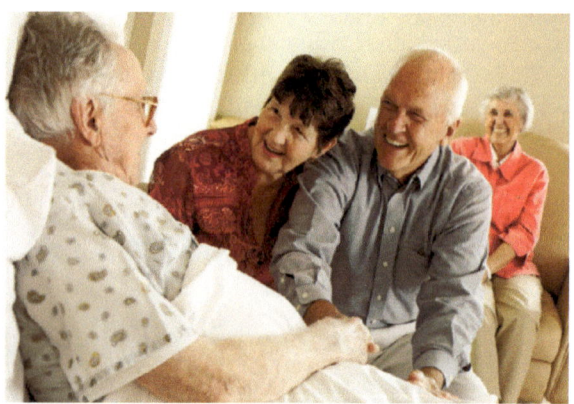

Photo 12.2   Social support can help alleviate the stress of chronic illness

Source: Design Pics Inc/Alamy

At the forefront of health psychology is the need to understand how social determinants and health disparities impact the experience of chronic illness. Biopsychosocial factors also influence the development, progression, and mortality associated with chronic and terminal conditions. The first step in addressing these disparities is to understand them (**Photo 12.2**).

Thinking About Health

■ If you have a chronic health condition, how does it affect your daily life? If you have multiple conditions, how do they interact with one another?

■ How is chronic illness largely preventable?

■ Why is chronic illness a global concern?

Emotional Responses to Chronic Illness

Chronic illness sets off a cascade of both physical and emotional changes. Finding a way to manage emotions is essential to living with a chronic condition. While many conditions cannot be cured, the stress, depression, and anxiety related to illness can be addressed.

Stress: An Emotional Roller Coaster

As we know from previous chapters, dealing with ambiguous symptoms and waiting for a diagnosis can be extremely stressful. For most people, a diagnosis comes after the experience of symptoms, doctors' visits, medical tests, and not knowing what is wrong. And once a patient has been given a diagnosis, new and different kinds of stressors emerge. A diagnosis is likely to release a flood of emotions: grief, shame, guilt, emptiness, loneliness, and sadness (Stanton & Revenson, 2011). A common first reaction is shock. There may be a sense of disbelief and disconnection from the situation. If feelings of shock do not give way to reality, the patient cannot begin to cope with the situation.

The unfolding of a chronic condition is different for everyone. Besides the physical pain and symptoms of illness, a patient may face relationship strains, possible loss of employment, and serious financial burdens. Most people report feeling distressed. People who have already experienced a number of stressful life events or have a history of depression can be at risk for greater distress upon diagnosis (American Psychological Association, Bourdeau, & Walters, 2013; Cohen et al., 2019). And this risk runs the other way as well: over 70 years of research demonstrates the association between stressful life events, perceived stress, and subsequent chronic illness (Cohen et al., 2019).

Stress can have both direct and indirect impacts on health and chronic illness (see Chapter 6). Specifically, the experience of stress increases the likelihood of developing a chronic condition, the progression and severity of symptoms, and, ultimately, mortality associated with the condition. Factors such as poor emotional regulation, anxiety, fear, and depression contribute to stress and chronic illness, just as poor physical health behaviors do. Stress does not cause disease—but it may weaken the immune system, create inflammation, and disrupt the balance of gut microbiota, all of which make the development of a chronic condition more likely. And living with chronic illness is stressful in itself. Stressful experiences that are a threat to a person's sense of self, competence, and social status—such as being diagnosed with or living with chronic illness—are especially "costly" in terms of negative health outcomes (Cohen, Gianaros, & Manuck, 2016).

Depression and Anxiety

Depression and anxiety are common emotional responses to chronic illness, especially for those with more than one condition (Liew, 2012). In a recent study of patients with rare chronic conditions, 42% reported moderate to severe depression, and 23% reported regularly experiencing anxiety (Uhlenbusch et al., 2019). High rates of depression and anxiety are found alongside the most common chronic conditions as well.

There are two pathways through which chronic illness can lead to depression. First, illness can involve neurochemical and structural changes in the brain; deficiencies in the immune system can also trigger depression (Liew, 2012; Shimoda & Robinson, 1999; Zautra, Burleson, Matt, Roth, & Burrows, 1994). Second, the pain, physical limitations, loss of independence and sense of self, feelings of helplessness, and interpersonal difficulties in living with illness can lead to depression (Friedman, Lyness, Delavan, Li, & Barker, 2008; Liew, 2012).

It is hard to know how many chronically ill patients are also depressed because depression is often not diagnosed. It may be mistaken for a normal reaction to illness, and symptoms such as fatigue may mimic the illness itself. Patients themselves may not realize they are depressed because they are more concerned for their physical health.

Sometimes negative emotions are a reaction to the illness, but sometimes they are **comorbid symptoms**: They exist alongside the illness and interact with it. In other words, chronic illness may cause depression, and depression may exacerbate chronic illness (Clarke & Currie, 2009). Each can worsen the other. For example, depression can lead to higher cholesterol levels and increase the risk of heart attack and the development of type 2 diabetes (Clarke & Currie, 2009). What accounts for these links? It may be that depression brings about lifestyle changes, or it may be that the neurobiological underpinnings of depression and certain chronic illnesses may interact. In general, behaviors fueled by depression and anxiety—such as avoidance, rumination, problematic social interactions, and perceived social constraints—lead to poorer adjustment to chronic illness (Uhlenbusch et al., 2019).

Depression may abate as the patient learns to cope with the illness. Or it may appear intermittently in response to changes in symptoms, prognosis, or treatments. For instance, someone with Parkinson's disease may experience bouts of depression with each new loss of motor function (Frazier, 2002).

Feelings of Loss

Chronic illness is often associated with feelings of loss—loss of identity, self-esteem, goals, activities, social connections, sleep, independence, and more (Carel, 2017; Frazier, 2000, 2002; Frazier & Hooker, 2006; Frazier, Cotrell, & Hooker, 2003; Frazier, Hooker, Johnson, & Kaus, 2000; Frazier, Johnson, Gonzalez, & Kafka, 2002; Turvey & Klein, 2008). These feelings tend to fluctuate from day to day, depending on levels of pain and discomfort, visits to the doctor, changes in medications and treatments and perceived competence at managing the illness. People living with HIV, for example, often report a loss of their very sense of self (Golub, Rendina, & Gamarel, 2013), which has a significant impact on perceptions of illness and health. This loss can deepen depression and lower quality of life. Although these emotions are a normal reaction to living with chronic illness, managing them is challenging all the same. People respond to

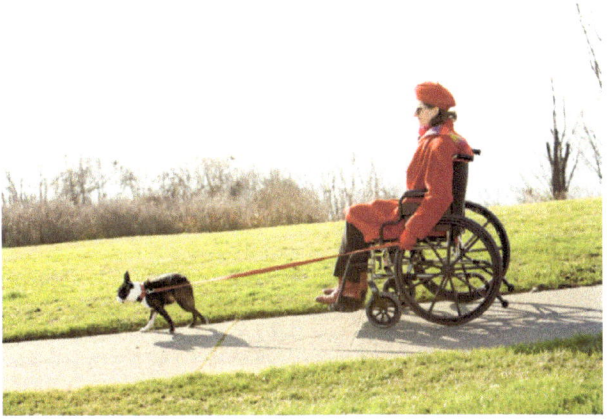

Photo 12.3   Adjusting to changes brought on by chronic illness can be akin to riding an emotional roller coaster of stress, depression, and anxiety. Fortunately, adaptation is possible

Source: Big Cheese Photo/Getty Images

these challenges in many different ways, depending on their personal, social, and economic resources (**Photo 12.3**).

Chronic illness has the potential to create dramatic changes in the lives of patients and their families (de Ridder, Geenen, Kuijer, & van Middendorp, 2008), affecting the self, work, productivity, economic stability, and social networks. The sense of loss affiliated with chronic illness can take two forms. **Clear loss** is the expected and obvious loss associated with tangible changes, such as the loss of mobility, eyesight, or motor abilities. **Ambiguous loss** is the sense of uncertainty that chronic illness causes, such as a lack of clarity about the course of the illness or fluctuating pain levels and capabilities (Boss & Couden, 2002).

The Trajectory of Chronic Illness

Some patients will shift from the initial shock of diagnosis to denial. Some may become paralyzed at the prospect of a lifelong illness and refuse to accept the diagnosis: "This can't be true." Others may simply withdraw. These emotional reactions may provide a protective buffer while the person is still not ready to accept the situation. Yet they can also stand in the way of coping with inevitable stress, depression, anxiety, and feelings of loss, or of getting needed medical treatment (Frazier, 2002; Golub, Gamarel, & Rendina, 2014; Stanton & Revenson, 2011).

For some, adjusting to life with a chronic illness can be similar to living with posttraumatic stress (Hefferon, Grealy, & Mutrie, 2009). For others, the stress, depression, and anxiety will abate. Patients may even come to see the experience of illness as a positive influence on their lives—an effect sometimes called *posttraumatic growth* (Carver, 1998; Golub, Gamarel, Rendina, Surace, & Lelutiu-Weinberger, 2013; Golub, Rendina, et al., 2013; Nolen-Hoeksema & Davis, 2002). In one study of arthritis patients, those who had social support and a sense of spirituality were more likely to transition from feelings of trauma to posttraumatic growth (Sörensen, Rzeszutek, & Gasik, 2019). It may seem surprising that resilience and other positive outcomes can result from negative health situations, as we will explore in Chapter 13.

> ## Thinking About Health
>
> - Describe the possible emotional reactions to living with chronic illness. What causes these reactions?
> - What are the two types of loss affiliated with chronic illness, and how do they differ?
> - How might emotional reactions change across the trajectory of chronic illness?

Coping with Chronic Illness

We know from Chapter 7 that effective coping strategies are crucial for good health. What we will see is how these strategies become even more important when learning to live with a chronic condition. Chronic illnesses force patients and their families to make significant emotional, behavioral, and social adjustments. If you recall the social readjustment rating scale (see Chapter 6; Holmes & Rahe, 1967), you will remember that the greater the change associated with a life event, the greater the stress. And having a chronic illness is high on the list of life-changing events.

Ambiguity, or not knowing what to expect, causes the greatest distress (Dunkel-Schetter, Feinstein, Taylor, & Falke, 1992; Frazier, 2002). After that comes the fear of future physical limitations and loss of functioning (Dunkel-Schetter et al., 1992; Frazier, 2002), fear of pain, fear of lifestyle changes, and fear of other forms of clear loss. Fortunately, active, problem-focused strategies can help patients cope more effectively, develop a sense of self-efficacy, and live a fuller life.

Coping Strategies

As we know, some coping strategies are more effective than others. Despite individual differences in the experience of disease, problem-focused coping strategies are the most beneficial overall (Frazier, 2002; Frazier et al., 2003). When people feel that something can be done to change a situation, they are more likely to feel competent enough to make those changes.

The chronically ill are less likely than others to adopt active, problem-focused coping strategies. That is because there is much less that they can control. The best approach is, then, to focus on managing emotions (Frazier, 2002). Patients who rely on avoidance, distractions, or withdrawal tend to experience greater distress, more problematic symptoms, poorer adjustment, and a poorer prognosis. In turn, patients who have a strong sense of control over their lives despite their illness are more likely to cope better. Consider how Brittany Maynard, from our chapter-opening story, did everything she could to address her illness. She researched her options and moved from one state to another so that she could have control over the end of her illness, have her loved ones around her, and become an activist for others struggling with terminal illnesses.

For physical stressors, a problem-focused strategy is especially beneficial. For an 80-year-old man with balance issues after a stroke, for example, a cane might help. For emotional stressors, a weekly support group can help by inviting patients to share their experiences of the disease. Some patients can avoid feeling like victims by making their illness part of their sense of self (Frazier, 2002). They may not be able to change the prognosis, but they can still find a way to accept and even master it. Sometimes just remembering that each day brings a new morning can provide a sense of optimism.

The key is being flexible (Cheng, Lau, & Chan, 2014). When patients tailor their coping to the situation, they can face it better. Take the case of patients with Parkinson's disease (Frazier, 2002). The symptoms of Parkinson's disease include physical impairments (shaking, tremors, and difficulty writing, walking, brushing teeth, or chewing food), emotional impairments (loneliness, anxiety, depression, or fear of the future), and social impairments (less social engagement, smaller social networks, or fewer opportunities to socialize). When patients with Parkinson's match their coping strategies to the type of stressor, they have a greater sense of well-being.

A Parkinson's patient who had been a dancer and dance instructor, for example, felt distress in simply walking. She was able to rise to a standing position, but that first step was torture: She felt paralyzed. One day, as she rose from the chair, her husband took her arms, placed one on his shoulder and the other on his waist, and asked her to dance. Much to their amazement, they waltzed right across the room. Obviously, she couldn't waltz everywhere. Still, whenever she wanted to walk, if her first few steps were fluid and dance-like, she was able to get where she needed to go without freezing or tremors. She had found a creative way of coping.

Adaptation

The trajectory of a chronic illness depends on the condition and the person. Some patients may actually improve with proper medical treatment and changes in lifestyle. However, some illnesses, like Parkinson's disease, become progressively worse—with greater loss of functioning and daily activities. Many chronic illnesses, too, end in death.

Nevertheless, human beings are resourceful, and most find a way to adapt to their illness. **Adaptation** is the process of coming to terms with and adjusting to illness. Clearly, adaptation depends on effective coping strategies, good medical care and self-care, and a supportive and understanding family and social network. Adaptation can help the patient maintain their lifestyle and functional abilities in the face of progressing disease and changing symptoms. It also helps to preserve a positive mind-set and to avoid distress (Stanton, Revenson, & Tennen, 2007). How can we measure adaptation? One way is to think about quality of life.

Quality of Life

Until recently, assessing quality of life was left to physicians. You were assumed to have a high quality of life if you were free of disease and a low quality of life if you had a disease, with no gray area in between. A biopsychosocial approach considers how living with a chronic condition affects the entirety of a patient's life—not just the illness and how to treat it, but overall well-being and life satisfaction as well. This approach can be used to understand which aspects of a patient's life are most at risk. It is useful in monitoring the trajectory of a disease and a life—and how changes in one influence changes in the other.

Quality of life is the degree of excellence and satisfaction that people report in their lives. It includes intimacy and relationships, work, school, leisure activities, hobbies, intellectual growth, how our bodies feel, what we are capable of doing, and our goals for the future. Finding the right balance among all of these aspects gives rise to our overall quality of life. More technically, the World Health Organization defines quality of life as individuals' perception of their lives within the context of the culture and value systems in which they live, and in relation to societal expectations, standards, concerns, and goals (Saxena & Orley, 1997). The different components of quality of life are presented in **Table 12.1**. The **Around the World** feature explores quality of life through the lens of culture.

Of course, you can feel differently about different aspects of your life. You might think, "My relationship with my partner makes my life rich and satisfying"—and, at the same time, be thinking, "I hate my dead-end job." These factors also affect one another. Illness, for instance, influences not just our physical self, but our emotional, social, and spiritual selves as well.

Physical health	Energy and fatigue
	Pain and discomfort
	Sleep and rest
Psychological	Body image and appearance
	Negative feelings
	Positive feelings
	Self-esteem
	Thinking, learning, memory, and concentration
Level of independence	Mobility
	Activities of daily living
	Dependence on medical substances and medical aids
	Work capacity
Social relationships	Personal relationships
	Social support
	Sexual activity
Environment	Financial resources
	Freedom, physical safety, and security
	Health and social care: accessibility and quality
	Home environment
	Opportunities for acquiring new information and skills
	Participation in and opportunities for recreation and leisure physical environment (pollution, noise, traffic, climate) transport
Spirituality	Religion
	Spirituality
	Personal beliefs

Source: Information from WHO (1997).

Table 12.1   Facets of quality of life

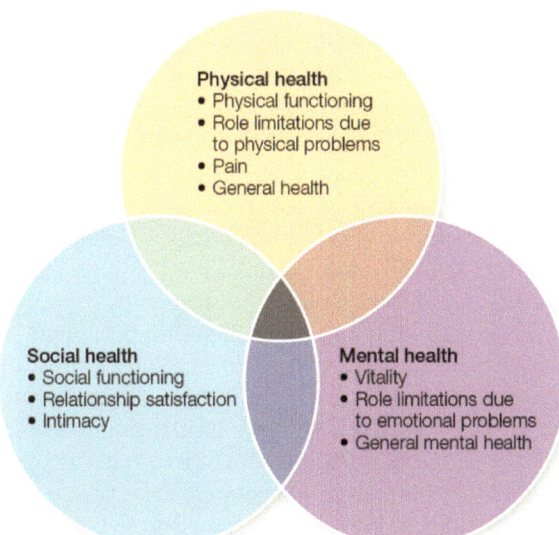

Figure 12.3   Dimensions of health-related quality of life: a biopsychosocial model.

Faced with acute illness, medical professionals focus on minimizing impairment and finding a cure. In chronic conditions that cannot be cured, however, the goal is to preserve health-related quality of life. **Health-related quality of life** involves physical functioning, emotional well-being, fatigue, social functioning, pain, any limitations due to health-related problems, and overall health (Ahlström & Sjöden, 1996; Koplas et al., 1999; Lawton, 1991; Stewart, Hays, & Ware, 1988). Like quality of life in general, it relies on the patient's self-report.

Medical professionals are now taking a "big picture" approach to treating the chronically ill (Landro, 2013). Quality of life is no longer just about adding years to life, but about adding life to years. Improving sleep, physical functioning, emotional health, satisfaction in relationships, and the ability to engage in leisure activities and work— all of these are important goals for medical care (see **Figure 12.3**).

Around *the* World

Is Quality of Life an American Concept?

Quality of life is influenced by age, sex, socioeconomic status, and cultural values (Eckermann, 2000; Mercier, Peladeau, & Tempier, 1998; Tov & Diener, 2009). Younger adults report higher quality of life, since they are less likely to have painful or limiting medical conditions. Compared to women of the same age, men are found to have higher quality of life as well, with less pain (Cherepanov et al., 2011). Socioeconomic status influences the quality of life in the expected way: the greater the financial advantage, the greater the quality of life (Cherepanov et al., 2011).

Interestingly, research on quality of life has been criticized for applying a Western standard for living well to other cultures (Shrestha & Zarit, 2012; Torres, Arroyo, Araya, & Pablo, 1999). The most widely used quality-of-life scales were created for and based on middle-class Americans and designed by researchers whose native language is English. And these measures do not always translate well (Guyatt, Feeny, & Patrick, 1993).

In cultures that value collectivism or interdependence, for example, quality of life looks different from those that value independence and individualism (Keith & Schalock, 1994). Respect for the elderly and family influences the quality of life for the Inuit elders of Canada (Collings, 2001) and Latinx people (Beyene, Becker, & Mayen, 2002). Indian cultures similarly place a high value on social networks and kinship (van Willigen & Chadha, 1999). Immigrants to the United States bring their cultural values with them—and how they adapt to a new culture ultimately influences their quality of life (Chappell, 2005).

Question:

How might the facets of health-related quality of life differ depending on the cultural background of the patient?

Many factors can influence a chronically ill patient's quality of life, including their perceptions of the illness, sense of control, and amount of disability (Helgeson & Zajdel, 2017). Maintaining healthy behaviors in the face of chronic illness is still very important. If you ask older people who have lost family and friends to illness—and who may be ill themselves—about the importance of health, they will tell you, "If you don't have your health, you don't have anything." They may talk about how a diagnosis of heart disease or diabetes was a "wake-up call"—a call to eat healthier and get more exercise. They know the importance of how they feel each and every day.

Because anxiety and depression are three times more common in patients with chronic illness, cultivating good mental health is especially important to the quality of life (National Collaborating Centre for Mental Health [UK], 2010). So is proper physical treatment. Often, medications or invasive procedures are as painful or debilitating as the illness itself. Think of the challenging rounds of chemotherapy and radiation experienced by someone with cancer. You may know someone who was diagnosed with cancer and chose to decline these options and simply let the disease take its course. These decisions are highly personal, and they typically come down to the impact of treatment on quality of life. Medical professionals thus work carefully with patients to find the right treatment plan for them.

At the more advanced stages of illness, preserving patients' independence is paramount. Many patients' greatest fears for the future are that they will become dependent on others (Frazier, 2002). From driving to feeding and dressing, most patients want to be able to perform daily tasks on their own.

Living with a chronic illness is a long-term process in which effective coping strategies, adaptation, and maintaining quality of life are crucial. At worst, ineffective coping strategies, resistance to adaptation, and declining quality of life can hasten the onset of disability and death from chronic illness. At best, living with chronic illness can present opportunities for growth, and the passage of time can influence the possibility of successful adaptation to and coping with life's new circumstances.

Thinking About Health

■ How do people typically cope with chronic illness? Which ways are beneficial, and which ways are detrimental?

■ What is an adaptation to long-term illness?

■ What factors affect the quality of life of people who have chronic illnesses?

Terminal Illness

Many chronic illnesses, especially those that develop in middle to late life, have a terminal phase ending in death. A **terminal illness** is a disease that cannot be cured or adequately treated and is expected to soon end in death. In this section, we explore the experiences of patients who are dying, the emotional responses to dying, the impact of terminal illness on loved ones and caregivers, and the process of healing, through grief and bereavement. We also discuss palliative and hospice care as well as the controversial decisions that patients face regarding their end-of-life care.

Death Across the Lifespan

In 2022, there were slightly more than three million deaths in the United States (Kochanek et al., 2024). The leading cause of death was heart disease, followed by cancer, accidents or unintentional injuries, chronic respiratory diseases, stroke, Alzheimer's disease, diabetes, influenza and pneumonia, kidney-related diseases, and suicide (Kochanek et al., 2024). The average life expectancy for someone born in the United States in 2022 is 77.5 years, up a year from 2021.

The causes of death differ across the lifespan (see **Tables 12.2** and **12.3**). For infants, congenital anomalies, low birth weight, complications during pregnancy, sudden infant death syndrome (SIDS), and unintentional injury are the primary causes of death (Murphy et al., 2018). In childhood, the most common cause of death is unintentional injury, with car crashes and death by firearms being the main culprits (Cunningham, Walton, & Carter, 2018). Unintentional injury remains the most common cause of death until age 44. For teens, suicide

	Age groups				
RANK	**<1**	**1–4**	**5–9**	**10–14**	**15–24**
1	Congenital anomalies	Unintentional injury	Unintentional injury	Unintentional injury	Unintentional injury
2	Short gestation	Congenital anomalies	Cancer	**Suicide**	**Suicide**
3	Maternal pregnancy comp.	Cancer	Congenital anomalies	Cancer	Homicide
4	SIDS	**Homicide**	**Homicide**	Congenital anomalies	Cancer
5	**Unintentional injury**	Heart disease	Heart disease	**Homicide**	Heart disease
6	Placenta cord. membranes	Influenza & pneumonia	Influenza & pneumonia	Heart disease	Congenital anomalies
7	Bacterial sepsis	Stroke	Chronic low respiratory disease	Chronic low r espiratory disease	Diabetes mellitus
8	Circulatory system disease	Sepsis	Stroke	Stroke	Influenza & pneumonia
9	Respiratory distress	Benign tumors	Sepsis	Influenza & pneumonia	Chronic low respiratory disease
10	Neonatal hemorrhage	Perinatal period	Benign tumors	Benign tumors	Complicated pregnancy

Source: Information from CDC (2019e).

Table 12.2 Top 10 causes of death in the United States, ages 0 to 24

RANK	Age groups				
	25–34	35–44	45–54	55–64	65+
1	**Unintentional injury**	**Unintentional injury**	Cancer	Cancer	Heart disease
2	**Suicide**	Cancer	Heart disease	Heart disease	Cancer
3	**Homicide**	Heart disease	**Unintentional injury**	**Unintentional injury**	Chronic low respiratory disease
4	Heart disease	**Suicide**	**Suicide**	Chronic low respiratory disease	Stroke
5	Cancer	**Homicide**	Liver disease	Diabetes mellitus	Alzheimer's disease
6	Liver disease	Liver disease	Diabetes mellitus	Liver disease	Diabetes mellitus
7	Diabetes mellitus	Diabetes mellitus	Stroke	Stroke	**Unintentional injury**
8	Stroke	Stroke	Chronic low respiratory disease	**Suicide**	Influenza & pneumonia
9	HIV	Sepsis	Sepsis	Sepsis	Nephritis
10	Complicated pregnancy	HIV	**Homicide**	Nephritis	Parkinson's disease

Source: Information from CDC (2019e).

Table 12.3   Top 10 causes of death in the United States, ages 25 to 65+

emerges as the second-most common cause of death. And as you can see in, chronic conditions begin to take hold in the middle years. In midlife to later life, the two leading causes of death are heart disease and cancer—deaths due to chronic illness.

Death and dying are difficult whenever they happen. However, our expectations about *who* dies and *when* influence the impact of death. Most of us expect, for example, that by later life (say, age 80 or later), older people will have chronic conditions that may end their lives. And, unless we know someone who is living with a rare, life-threatening illness, we do not typically expect death in children, teens, or young adults. When death is unexpected and "off time," such as when a young person dies, the impact on loved ones is more pronounced. Shock, shattered expectations, and unfinished business makes coping and grieving more difficult. In contrast, when an older person dies after a chronic or protracted illness, loved ones may cope better, having had time to anticipate and prepare for the devastation of death.

Theories About Death and Dying

Consciously or unconsciously, most people fear death (Becker, 1973). It is part of the human condition, and it influences almost everything we do (Greenberg & Arndt, 2012). **Death anxiety**, or fear of death and dying, can be an appropriate response to thinking about one's own death. It is a common theme in philosophy, anthropology, poetry, art, literature, music, film, and culture.

One theory devised to explain death anxiety has its roots in an ancient Sumerian text from 3000 B.C.E. called the *Epic of Gilgamesh* (Greenberg & Arndt, 2012). Gilgamesh's deep concerns about death propel him on an epic search for immortality. More recently, **terror management theory (TMT)** (Becker, 1973) explains death anxiety in relation to two simple observations. First, humans are animals driven to preserve and protect their own existence. The fight-or-flight response is one of the systems that has evolved to help us stay alive. Second, our uniquely human cognitive capacities provide us with the awareness that death is inevitable and can come at any time (Greenberg & Arndt, 2012). The ever-present fear, anxiety, or terror of death must be continuously managed, and it lies at the heart of all human motivation (Geller & Yagil, 2019). We also have the fundamental tendency to see ourselves and our world in ways that deny the precarious and transient nature of our own existence (Greenberg & Arndt, 2012), not unlike the beliefs that drive Gilgamesh in search of life everlasting.

TMT highlights our vulnerability to the deep-seated anxiety and dread we feel when we think about our mortality (Solomon & Greenberg, 2019; Van Tongeren, Green, Davis, Worthington, & Reid, 2013). Our culture, worldviews, and self-esteem, things that make us "uniquely human," help to buffer against this anxiety by providing a *symbolic immortality*—a belief that we will live on through our actions, legacy, or relationships with others after we die (Greenberg et al., 1990; Rosenblatt, Greenberg, Solomon, Pyszxzynski, & Lyon, 1989; Van Tongeren et al., 2013). The most obvious example of symbolic immortality is a religious belief in an afterlife. Symbolic immortality is also embodied in our national identity, the belief that humans are superior to animals, and our belief in heroes. They might be fictional heroes, such as T'Challa from *The Black Panther*, Luke Skywalker from *Star Wars*, or Daenerys Targaryen from *Game of Thrones*, or real-life heroes such as Nelson Mandela, Martin Luther King, Jr., and Marie Curie. Their stories give meaning to life, help us aspire to live well, and can vanquish the fear caused by the inevitability of death (**Photo 12.4**) (Allison & Goethals, 2014; Solomon & Greenberg, 2019; Van Tongeren et al., 2013).

TMT can also motivate people to adopt healthier behaviors in order to live longer. In one study, researchers experimentally manipulated *mortality salience*, the awareness that death is inevitable. Participants who were primed with mortality salience used an exercise bike more than those who were not

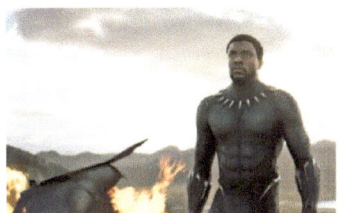 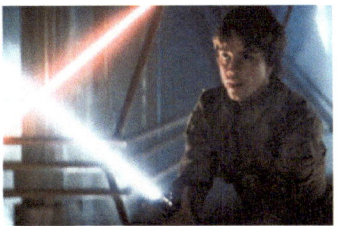 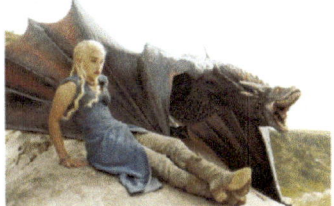

Photo 12.4 According to terror management theory, symbolic immortality acts as a buffer against death anxiety. Heroic characters who overcome death—such as T'Challa, Luke Skywalker, and Daenerys Targaryen—affirm the belief that our legacies will live on after we die

primed. As part of the same study, smokers primed with mortality salience were more likely to try to quit smoking than those who were not primed (Morris, Goldenberg, Arndt, & McCabe, 2018). These findings show that death anxiety can motivate behavior, whether or not a patient is at risk for a fatal disease (Greenberg & Arndt, 2012). When death is salient, people strive to bolster their self-esteem and minimize feelings of regret as well (Rudert, Reutner, Walker, & Greifeneder, 2015).

Some fascinating research on people's hopes and fears concerning their deaths shows that most people, both young and old, fear the pain associated with death more than death itself (Dark-Freudeman, 2022). Other fears include suffering and being a burden to others, and some people also expressed religious and spiritual concerns. Most also report that their hopes for a good death involve achieving a sense of closure. Most people would prefer to die in their sleep without pain, fear, or conscious awareness (Maxfield, Pyszczynski, & Solomon, 2013). But for those in the terminal phase of a protracted illness, death is no longer an abstract problem of the distant future, but rather an ever-present concern. Typical psychological defenses against death anxiety have been stripped away. For dying patients, finding meaning and reaffirming relationships with loved ones are often greater concerns than even physical symptoms and pain (Edmondson, Park, Chaudoir, & Wortmann, 2008). Consistent with TMT, those who take comfort in their religious beliefs experience less depression as they face death (Edmondson et al., 2008).

Time Left to Live

Someone with a terminal illness is expected to die soon, and yet the length of time until death can be hard to determine. Physicians can generally tell when the body has begun to break down by monitoring the functioning of critical organs, such as the heart and lungs. Unless the patient is within days or weeks of death, however, further prediction is difficult.

Doctors often overestimate remaining life expectancy, whether out of fear, ignorance, or concern for the patient's emotional well-being (Brody, 2007; Christakis, Smith, Parkes, & Lamont, 2000; Heyse-Moore & Johnson-Bell, 1987; Maltoni et al., 1994; Mayo Clinic, 2005). Unfortunately, overestimation can cause harm. As one physician said, "When we prognosticate and it turns out that the patient lives a longer life, then we can be joyous with them, but when we prognosticate and the patient ends up living a far shorter time, that's when we really do harm" (Brody, 2007). In one study of patients in end-of-life care, only 20% of the physicians' predictions were accurate, and 63% overestimated their patient's time left to live (Mayo Clinic, 2005). In another study, the median estimate was 90 days left to live, but the actual median survival time was 24 days. Overestimates tend to worsen when the physician has a long-standing relationship with the patient (Qualls & Kasl-Godley, 2011).

Although physicians are sometimes concerned about the negative impact of end-of-life discussions on their patients, research shows that, in fact, these

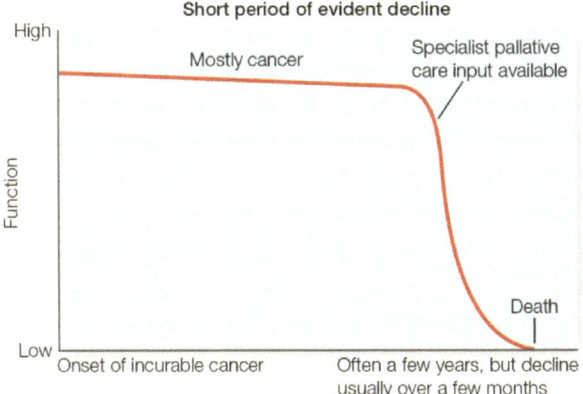

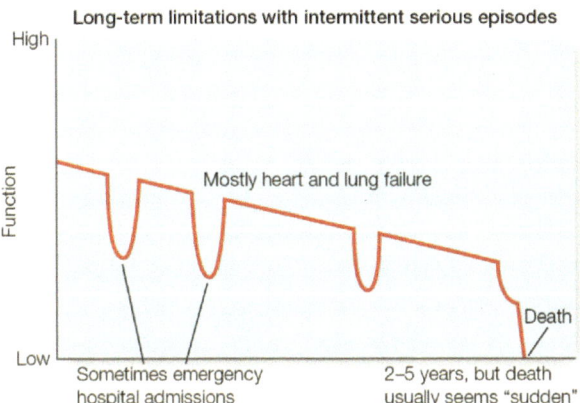

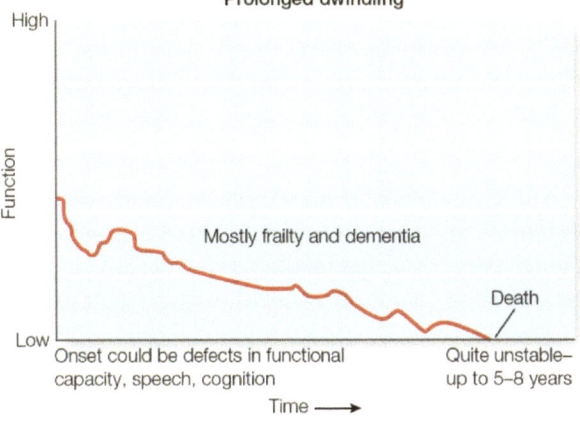

Figure 12.4   Three trajectories of dying.

Source: Data from Lynn and Adamson (2003).

discussions are beneficial for both terminal patients and their loved ones (Wright et al., 2008). Having these difficult discussions led to less aggressive end-of-life care and more referrals for hospice care, which, in turn, led to better quality of life in dying patients and better adjustment for bereaved loved ones (Wright et al., 2008). This is important because, at the end of life, the patient's decisions should matter most. Physicians, and loved ones, should ask patients how much they want to know about their condition and abide by the patient's wishes.

Ideally, dying patients and their loved ones know how long they have left together. This knowledge can help inform what treatments to pursue and what support systems to put in place. It allows patients to put their affairs in order, to fulfill remaining goals, and to say goodbye. Most importantly, a prognosis of impending death can open up conversations that will allow patients to die in the manner of their choosing. Like Brittany Maynard, they may choose to die with dignity.

Trajectories of Death

Many patients with life-threatening illnesses want to know something else, too: "What will happen to me?" Terminal illness has three common trajectories, and the prognosis depends on the trajectory.

The first trajectory (depicted in the top box of **Figure 12.4**) is marked by a period of decline followed by a short terminal phase, as is common in cancer. The decline is often gradual, and the patient may remain stable for weeks, months, or even years, barring unforeseen complications. This trajectory gives the patient and loved ones time to prepare. The last few months have brought noticeable changes in the patient's weight, activities, daily living, and ability to provide self-care (Lunney, Lynn, Foley, Lipson, & Guralnik, 2003).

The second trajectory (depicted in the middle box of **Figure 12.4**) is marked by a slow decline with periodic crises, followed by death. Chronic conditions such as heart failure and chronic obstructive pulmonary disease often have this trajectory. Crises and deteriorations in physical health often require hospitalization and intensive treatment. For example, a man in his seventies with congestive heart failure may be hospitalized for an acute downturn. He may recover after intensive care, but not to his previous level of functioning, and his health will become progressively worse. "He's always pulled through," his family may say, but any one acute episode can result in death. The timing of this trajectory and the number of episodes of recovery combine to make it difficult to know when death will happen. In one large study of patients with advanced heart failure, death occurred roughly six months before the date predicted (Levenson, McCarthy, Lynn, Davis, & Phillips, 2000).

The third trajectory (depicted in the bottom box of **Figure 12.4**) is marked by prolonged decline and a long, lingering, anticipated death. For people who escape cancer and acute organ system failure, most live to later ages and die of neurological conditions (such as Alzheimer's disease or other dementias), or generalized frailty and eventual organ failure. For dementia patients and their families, this trajectory can be devastating. It can take years or even decades, with levels of disability and dysfunction increasing slowly over time. There may or may not be acute episodes (a stroke, for example), but eventually, an infection, illness, or other event combined with degraded bodily functioning will prove fatal. Heart attacks, blood clots, strokes, kidney failure, lung infections, and multiple organ failure are the most frequent causes of death for Alzheimer's disease patients (Beard et al., 1996).

Dying

There is no such thing as a typical death. However, some symptoms are common to many who are dying. During the last six months of life, terminally ill patients may experience chronic fatigue and weakness and become less physically active. They may spend a lot of time sleeping. Weight loss and diminished appetite are common as well. Depending on the disease and the type of care they are receiving, pain may increase—whether diffuse pain or pain in specific areas of the body. A patient in hospice care will be given pain relief to lessen this symptom. As death approaches, the skin may become thin and irritated, and bed sores may develop. Eventually, bladder and bowel control is lost, which is a distressing time for both the dying patient and loved ones.

Some emotional changes have been common in the last six months as well. Many dying patients experience stress, anger, anxiety, or depression. They fear becoming a burden on loved ones, or feel guilty or resentful. Some may lose interest in the world around them because of sadness and a sense of impending loss—withdrawal may be a healthy way of coping with the end of life. Yet, many patients experience feelings of acceptance and contentment, which can be confusing to loved ones. Some may experience dying as a time of revelation, with a greater feeling of meaning or purpose in life. Some experience a heightened sense of spirituality, or seek a greater meaning to help alleviate fear and suffering.

Health care practitioners refer to a patient for whom death is imminent (within minutes to hours) as "transitioning" (Qualls & Kasl-Godley, 2011) or "actively dying" (Hospice Patients Alliance, 2019). Physically, this transition is usually orderly and undramatic. The progressive changes during this period are not medical emergencies and do not require emergency care, although hospice care will be provided to alleviate any pain associated with the process. There may be no pain at all (Qualls & Kasl-Godley, 2011). The body begins to shut down, starting with nonvital organs and functions (for example, the kidneys or gastrointestinal tract); this conserves energy to preserve the functioning of the heart and lungs for as long as possible. Eventually, however, there is not enough energy left, and physical systems cease to function.

People who are dying will begin to speak and move less. They may not respond to questions or to those around them. As the energy to support life fades, it becomes more difficult to talk, eat, or drink. The patient's hands may feel cold to the touch, as blood pressure and blood flow to the extremities gradually decrease. When a person is just hours from death, a new pattern of breathing occurs. Sometimes breathing is halted for a time before resuming—a condition called Cheyne–Stokes respiration, named by the physicians who first noticed it. Coughing may occur as fluids build up in the pharynx. This fluid can also cause "death rattles," a distressing sound to loved ones. As death approaches, skin color may change to a darker, duller hue, and fingernails may become bluish as well. Depending on changes to the central nervous system, the dying patient may be conscious and responsive, or unconscious and unresponsive.

Some patients will lapse into a *coma*—a deep state of unconsciousness from which they cannot be roused. They may still be able to hear what is said around them, but will not be able to respond. Hearing, in fact, is one of the last senses to go. If unconscious, dying patients may also be able to experience pain, but be unable to indicate that they are in pain. It is common for patients who are conscious at the end to experience hallucinations and delusions, which may be frightening for the patient or caregiver. It is important for everyone around to interact with the patient as if they can hear and understand what is going on until the very end. Friends and family should provide as much support and care as possible.

Are There Stages in Dying?

Elisabeth Kübler-Ross developed one of the first theoretical and empirical models of dying. Kübler-Ross, a Swiss American psychiatrist, observed a common psychological pattern in her patients that she summarized in a groundbreaking book, *On Death and Dying* (Kübler-Ross, 1969). Her model postulates five stages of dying. The model has been applied to other traumatic events as well, such as divorce, loss of employment, or the onset of chronic illness.

According to Kübler-Ross's model, the first stage, usually associated with learning that death is imminent, is *denial*, or refusing to believe a diagnosis. In the next stage, denial is replaced with *anger*. "Why me?" a patient might ask. "This is not fair," they might say. "Why would God let this happen?" In the third stage, *bargaining*, the sufferer pleads for more time. *Depression* follows, as the certainty and inevitability of impending death sink in. Finally, *acceptance* arrives, as the dying person comes to terms with impending death, assesses their life, and embraces mortality.

The model remains controversial. After decades of study, it lacks solid empirical support. Many dying patients do not experience any of these responses. Others experience some stages, but not others, and still others do not experience them in the prescribed order. Nevertheless, Kübler-Ross has helped medical practitioners anticipate the emotions of dying patients and better provide support for them.

As noted earlier, positive feelings may emerge in the process of dying, as in this quote from a 70-year-old woman battling metastatic breast cancer. She spoke of hope, just two months before she died:

> When I was first diagnosed, I was hoping for a cure. I just wanted the cancer to go away. I just wanted the cancer to go away. I know I am almost 70, but I just wanted to get rid of it and go on with my life. And I did all the chemo, and I was really hoping it would kill all the cancer. But the cancer came back and now it's all over my body. And now I am still hoping for different things. I hope for a day without pain, I hope for a good bowel movement. Now I hope for things in the very, very near future, typically the same day. I feel that hope is closer to me now; it's always very close. But hope does not go away. I will continue to hope for something until I die.
>
> (Qualls & Kasl-Godley, 2011, 50)

Spirituality is also important near the end of life. Spirituality is hard to define—it can refer not just to going to a church, a synagogue, or a mosque, but also to something more private and personal. Some people may turn to prayer, meditation, yoga, quiet reflection, or being in nature—whatever puts them in touch with something greater than themselves. It may allow them to let go of material or physical concerns and focus on self-awareness and finding meaning in the experience of dying. Spiritual feelings may also correspond with what Kübler–Ross considered the final stage in advanced illness: acceptance. As a patient dying of advanced lung cancer put it,

> These days I like to remember the past, but I also think about the meaning of life, about the meaning of my life, as a human being, you know? I mean, what is this all about? And I look at the stars at night and wonder about life on other planets and God. And I feel perfectly content just sitting there contemplating …. I am just happy being. I enjoy being alive, and contemplating my thoughts. And now that I know I am dying, being with myself is even more important.
>
> (Qualls & Kasl-Godley, 2011, 53)

It is important to recognize that the emotional responses of each dying patient are unique. These responses can be important for coping and for experiencing death with dignity.

Thinking About Health

■ What are the primary causes of death at different points in the lifespan?

■ How do theories of dying address death anxiety and explain the process of death?

■ What physical and emotional changes occur as one dies?

■ What do you think are the stages of dying?

The End of Life

It may be hard to imagine a good death, but the concept is simple: The dying patient's wishes for the end of life are observed. This allows patients to die with dignity in a way that is meaningful to them. They may wish to be at home with loved ones around, as Brittany Maynard was, or to be free of pain.

Medical professionals worldwide are trained to do everything possible to save and prolong lives. Having a patient die is contrary to their training. Many doctors seek to promote survival no matter how great the costs or how slim the chances (Qualls & Kasl-Godley, 2011). Unfortunately, there are some cases in which end-of-life care actually *decreases* quality of life and is counter to a patient's wishes. It is important to know what can be done to promote comfort for the dying patient and their loved ones.

Open communication is essential to ensuring a good death. It includes communication between patients, family, doctors, nurses, clergy, therapists, and social workers so that each knows what to expect. It also entails listening. When death is imminent, patients may want to cease treatments that are unpleasant and debilitating, letting the illness take its course. Or they may decide to avoid a painful death by taking life-ending medicines. Allowing the patient to articulate their wishes is important, even if it is not what the doctors or the family want to hear. Most of all, it enables the patient and family to prepare.

Advanced Care Planning

Advanced care planning may be initiated long before the end of life. The Patient Self-Determination Act of 1990 requires that all medical service providers—hospitals, nursing homes, home health agencies, hospice providers, and health maintenance organizations—provide patients with written notice of their decision-making rights. That includes the right of patients to make their own health care decisions and the right to accept or refuse medical treatment.

If a patient has given advanced care directives, the health care facility must abide by them. One kind of advanced care directive is a **do not resuscitate (DNR) order**. Written by a doctor and signed by the patient, it instructs health care providers not to perform cardiopulmonary resuscitation (CPR) if breathing stops or the heart stops beating.

In a **living will**, a patient specifies in detail which medical actions can (or cannot) be taken. It comes into play when patients are no longer able to make or articulate these decisions themselves. "If I suffer an incurable or irreversible, illness, disease, or condition," it might say, "and my attending physician determines that my condition is terminal, I direct that life-sustaining measures that would serve only to prolong my dying be withheld or discontinued." Here is an example of a living will.

ADVANCE HEALTH CARE DIRECTIVE

Living Will

I, _____, willfully and voluntarily make this declaration, in a sound mind, and after careful consideration, that:

(1) COMFORT CARE DIRECTIVE: I direct that my attending or primary care physician(s) provide treatment and care to alleviate pain or discomfort at all times even if it would accelerate my death.

(2) END-OF-LIFE DIRECTIVE: Health care providers and others involved in my care shall provide, withhold, or stop treatment in accordance with my choices indicated below: [CHECK ONE]

[___] (a) Directive NOT to Prolong Life. I choose not to prolong my life if (a) I have an incurable and irreversible disease, illness, or injury that will result in my death within a short time period, (b) I am in a comatose state and at least two doctors assert that I will not regain consciousness, or (c) high risks or encumbrances of treating me would offset any potential benefits, OR

[___] (b) Directive To Prolong Life. I declare that I want my life prolonged as long as possible within reasonable limits of health care standards and medical science.

(3) ADDITIONAL DIRECTIVES: (Here you can expand upon your instructions or add additional directions.)

I direct and declare that:

a) I do not want my life to be prolonged by the following measures: 1) cardiopulmonary resuscitation (CPR) or 2) ventilation (breathing machine). _____ _____

(4) PRIMARY PHYSICIAN:

I name and assign the following physician as my primary doctor:

_____

(name of physician)

_____

(address) (city) (state) (zip code)

(OPTIONAL) If the doctor that I have named in this document is not able or reasonably available to act as my primary physician, I name and assign the following physician as my primary care doctor:

_____

(name of physician)

_____

(address) (city) (state) (zip code)

(5) DONATION OF ORGANS AT DEATH (OPTIONAL):

Upon my death: (Mark applicable box)

[___] (a) I permit the removal and give any needed organs, tissues, or parts, OR

[___] (b) I permit the removal and give the following organs, tissues, or parts only.

_____

I direct that my instructions in this document be honored by my family and physician as my final directives should I become unable to give further instructions.

I am emotionally and mentally competent to make these decisions and fully understand their significance.

I execute this declaration, as my free and voluntary act, on this _____ day of _____, 20 _____.

_____

(Signature)

Address _____

SIGNATURES OF WITNESSES:

Executed on this _____ day of the month of _____, 20 _____, in the State of _____.

First Witness:

_____, residing at _____

(Signature Above)

_____

Second Witness:

_____, residing at _____

Hand in hand with a living will is a **durable power of attorney**. This document states who will act on the patient's behalf with regard to health decisions, private affairs, and business or legal issues. The person giving power of attorney must be of sound mind and able to articulate their wishes. The open dialogue that persons with power of attorney should have with dying patients should include their wishes with regard to burial, cremation, religious services, and personal assets or belongings. These wishes may be articulated verbally or in writing in a **last will and testament**.

Palliative and Hospice Care

Another role of advanced care planning is to ensure proper care. Knowing a patient's trajectory allows care providers and loved ones to "do everything possible." Within the context of both chronic and terminal illnesses, providing comfort care is extremely important. **Palliative care** is a type of specialized medical care designed to provide relief from the symptoms and pain of chronic illness and to improve the quality of life for the patient and family. **Hospice care** refers to another kind of specialized care, designed to provide support, comfort, and pain relief to patients with terminal illness. It ensures that the dying process is as pain-free and comfortable as possible.

Palliative care is given to patients with chronic illnesses, while hospice care is given to those at the end of life or in the dying phase of a terminal illness. Palliative care can be part of hospice care, and both types of care are designed to provide compassionate treatment and comfort, regardless of the stage of life. To be eligible for hospice care, a patient must have a prognosis of six months or fewer (sometimes a year or less) to live, although care continues if the patient lives longer. A certification from an attending physician is required.

Hospice care begins when cure-oriented treatments are no longer desirable (Qualls & Kasl-Godley, 2011). It is based on the fundamental belief that "each of us has the right to die pain-free and with dignity and that our families will receive the necessary support to allow us to do so" (National Hospice & Palliative Care Organization, 2019). Hospice care may take place in a hospital, a nursing home, or the patient's home, and usually involves a team of providers to address all aspects of the patient's life and medical care. Physicians, nurses, home health aides, social workers, and clergy may provide services. Often, hospice nurses and support staff are available around the clock. In the United States, Medicare, a national insurance program, covers the expenses.

Not everyone accepts hospice care. In societies that value prolonging life, it can seem like giving up hope (Qualls & Kasl-Godley, 2011). Still, patients should know that they will receive the full range of palliative care available, and their families will have bereavement support for a full year following death (**Photo 12.5**).

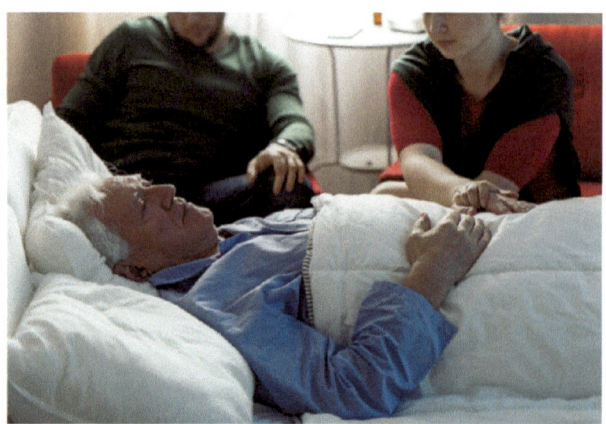

Photo 12.5 Having loved ones surround a dying patient offers comfort to both the patient and their family and friends, promoting acceptance of impending death.

Source: Photohraphee.eu/Shutterstock

Assisted Death and Euthanasia

Death with dignity is defined as an end-of-life decision that allows certain people who are eligible to legally request and receive medications from their physicians that will allow them to end their lives in a peaceful, humane, and dignified way. **Assisted death** (also called medical aid in dying, or physician-assisted dying), is a self-chosen, self-administered death with the help of another person, often a physician. As with Brittany Maynard, the physician may provide counseling about lethal doses of drugs or prescribe them. As of March 2023, 10 of the states in the United States have legalized physician-assisted death: California, Colorado, Hawaii, Maine, Montana, New Jersey, New Mexico, Oregon, Vermont, and Washington, D.C. Worldwide, assisted death is legal in Switzerland, Germany, Australia, Belgium, the Netherlands, Luxembourg, and Canada (Emanuel,

Onwuteaka-Philipsen, Urwin, & Cohen, 2016). A survey of practicing physicians showed that 20% received a request for physician-assisted death at some point in their medical careers (Back, Wallace, Starks, & Pearlman, 1996; Meier et al., 1998). The most common reason that patients request assistance in dying from physicians is to end or avoid suffering (Seller, Bouthillier, & Fraser, 2019).

Physician-assisted death is not to be confused with **euthanasia**, Greek for "good death." Euthanasia is the intentional termination of the life of a patient with an intractable terminal illness in an effort to end the patient's suffering. Here, the physician, rather than the patient, ends the life. As of 2019, *voluntary euthanasia*—euthanasia performed by the physician at the request of the patient— is legal in the Netherlands, Belgium, Colombia, Canada, and Luxembourg. *Involuntary euthanasia*—euthanasia performed without the patient's consent—is illegal in the United States.

In **active euthanasia**, medical personnel administer lethal drugs, often by injection, deliberately to cause death. In 1998, Dr. Jack Kevorkian gained national attention for videotaping himself administering a lethal medication to a 52-year-old man suffering from ALS. Network television broadcast the video one week later. Kevorkian was found guilty of committing second-degree murder and sent to prison. He served eight years of his sentence, but that did not stop him from advocating for euthanasia until his death in 2011.

In **passive euthanasia**, medical personnel simply withhold or end treatment, allowing nature to take its course. Examples include not putting a patient on life support, turning off respirators, ending medications, withholding food and water, and not resuscitating. When physicians provide high doses of morphine to control pain, despite the side effect of suppressing respiration and hastening death, it is also considered passive euthanasia (Batten, 2010). Administering these drugs is legal in most political jurisdictions, and most medical societies view it as ethical. Passive euthanasia is most commonly performed on patients in a persistent vegetative state from which they will never recover.

For any of us who have had a pet suffer from a painful illness, we know how hard it is to have the animal "put down." In essence, we are practicing euthanasia, but we know it is the humane thing to do. However, human euthanasia is highly controversial, as is assisted death. Advocates, many of whom are part of the right-to-die movement (like Brittany), see it as death with dignity and a basic human right. Opponents, many of them with strong religious convictions, may see the taking of a life for any reason as comparable to murder, a violation of religious doctrines that hold life sacred and dictate that one must not kill. Conversely, many religious people believe that drugs that end suffering are God-given, too.

Thinking About Health

■ What important legal documents and issues characterize the end of life?

■ What are the differences between palliative care and hospice care?

■ What is your position on assisted death and the right-to-die movement?

Coping with Loss

The loss of a loved one is always stressful, even when death results from a long battle with a painful illness and the family has had time to prepare. It means facing difficult end-of-life care issues—and then dealing with wakes, funerals, visitors, and often divisive legal and family issues. It also means facing a future without a loved one, a reality that people across different cultures come to terms with in a variety of ways.

Grieving

Grief is the mental suffering that results from loss, and it has physical, cognitive, behavioral, emotional, and social dimensions. **Mourning**, a conscious response to loss, involves deep sorrow, and often also includes symbolic gestures such as wearing black. Whenever people have lost a loved one, we say that they are in a period of **bereavement** as they work through their emotions.

We have already looked at one perspective on how we grieve. Elisabeth Kübler-Ross observed five stages of coping in her dying patients, and these stages may apply to the patients' family and friends as well. While her model is controversial in this context, too, patterns do emerge in how we experience grief. In the "first wave" after death, some people may experience feelings of disbelief, even when the death was expected (Zucker, 2009). They may not feel the emotions of loss at all—and may wonder what is wrong with them. This period may serve as a buffer, allowing time to prepare to cope with reality. The "second storm" is an intense period of grief, including denial, depression, anger, and hurt. In time, the acute emotions subside, and the griever is again able to engage in life. For most people, it takes about six months for these intense emotions to fade (Bonanno, 2004). Of course, while the symptoms of grief may dissipate, sadness remains. As one researcher said, "People continue to think about and miss their loved ones for decades. Loss is forever, but acute grief is not" (Konigsberg, 2011).

How we experience grief is determined by our personalities and how we cope with life (Konigsberg, 2011). So long as grievers are not harming themselves or others, any efforts at coping will be beneficial (Zucker, 2009). What is effective is what is right for you. Thinking back to how you have handled past challenges can help, too. "I am surprised I am so strong on my own," some might say. "I am just thankful we had time together before she died."

No one should have to grieve alone, if they don't choose to. Self-awareness, identifying thoughts and feelings, expressing emotions, and sharing grief with trusted friends and family are all important (Bonanno, 2009). Just being with others is often a source of comfort. Counselors and therapists who are trained to work with survivors can help, too.

Death Around the World

Although all humans share the experience of death, culture shapes *how* we experience it. In the United States, the end of life is often commemorated with services in a church, synagogue, or mosque, where prayers and memories of the deceased are shared. Some people follow the hearse to the cemetery, where flowers may be laid on a casket that is lowered into the ground. Mourners arrive at the family home carrying condolences and food to share. In the Jewish tradition, family and friends "sit shiva," a weeklong period of mourning. Some people choose to be cremated rather than buried, and their survivors may preserve or scatter their ashes.

In other cultures, the end of life is commemorated differently. Among the Tana Toraja in eastern Indonesia, death is a celebration—a lively affair that involves the whole village and can last for weeks (Swazey, 2015). Families save their finances for weeks, months, or years in order to send off their loved ones properly. Then, a sacrificial water buffalo "carries" the deceased's soul to the afterlife. Until then, the dead are spoken of as if they are merely sick or asleep. They are symbolically fed and cared for as if they were still alive (Swazey, 2015).

In the northwestern Philippines, the custom of the Benguet people is to blindfold the dead body and place it near the entrance to the home, while their Tinguian neighbors dress up their dead loved ones in their finest clothes and place them in a chair with a cigarette in their mouths (Swazey, 2015). Hollowed-out tree trunks are used to bury the dead by the Caviteño peoples, who also live in the Philippines, near Manila. In the northern Philippines, the people of Apayao bury dead relatives in the kitchen (Swazey, 2015). In Australia, Aboriginal people celebrate the dead by recovering their bones after decomposition, painting them, and wearing them to keep their dead loved ones near them. Eventually, the bones are placed in a cave or hollowed-out log. Although these practices greatly differ from Western ways of mourning, they are all forms of coping with loss, and they demonstrate the universal endurance of human relationships after death (**Photo 12.6**).

In Mongolia and Tibet, the Vajrayana Buddhists believe that the soul is released after death, leaving the body an empty vessel. To help the spirit and to allow the body to return to earth, the body is cut into pieces and taken to a high mountain

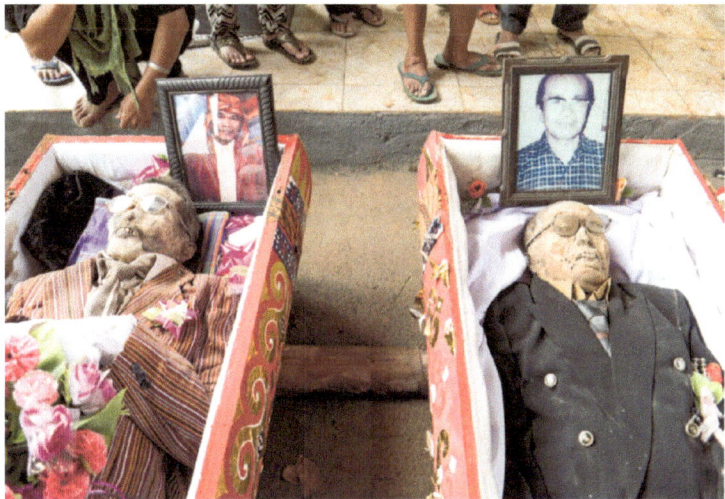

Photo 12.6   Until the funeral rites can be paid for, the Tana Toraja of Indonesia continue to care for their deceased loved ones as though they were merely sick or sleeping.

Source: Muslianshah Masrie/Alamy

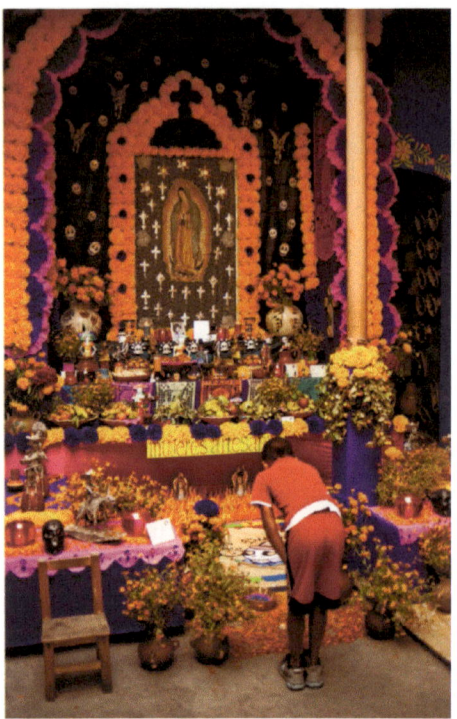

Photo 12.7 In preparation for El Día de los Muertos, altars are erected in private homes and public spaces to honor the dead.

peak, where it is left exposed to vultures and the elements—this is called a sky burial. After thousands of years, 80% of Tibetans still practice these unique forms of coping and closure today (Gouin, 2010).

El Día de los Muertos, the Day of the Dead, is a public holiday in Mexico, most often celebrated from November 1 to November 2. Families and friends use the time to remember loved ones who have died and to help them in their spiritual journey. Many families build private altars decorated with colorful skulls, marigolds (to call the dead to the altar with their vibrant color and sweet smell and to symbolize the fragility of life), and the favorite foods and drinks of the deceased. They will also visit the cemetery where the loved one is buried and leave special gifts on the grave. These practices are a healthy, communal form of coping, acknowledging the enduring influence of the deceased while accepting the finality of death.

Times are changing. As people become more environmentally conscious, funeral options worldwide are changing, too. A 2017 study from the National Funeral Directors Association (NFDA) found that 54% of Americans are looking into eco-friendly burial options (NFDA, 2017). In the United States, an environmentally friendly burial skips embalming and avoids the use of concrete vaults. Instead, biodegradable, woven-willow caskets are available. There are now many environmentally friendly cemeteries certified by the Green Burial Council. Another option is an artificial reef. Created by mixing the ashes of the dead with concrete, these creative structures are placed on the ocean floor and become a home and habitat for sea life (**Photos 12.7** and **12.8**).

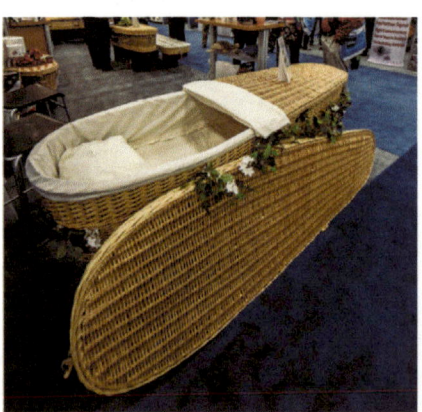

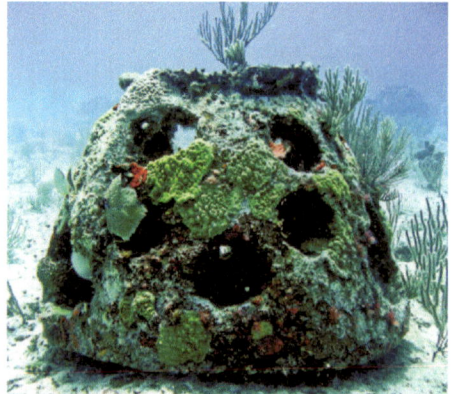

Photo 12.8 Environmentally friendly burial options, such as biodegradable woven-willow caskets and marine life-promoting reef remains, are becoming more popular.

As Kelli Swazey (2015), a cultural anthropologist, said, "I think it is safe to say that all humans will be intimate with death at least once in their lives." Still, she added, "Life doesn't end with death." Rather, as we have seen, the death of a loved one can be an opportunity to celebrate life and the transformative nature of relationships. Our relationships with our loved ones don't end when their lives do. When they die, we still have the opportunity for fond remembrance—and the chance to think about our own mortality as well. (See the **In the News** feature.)

In the News

What's on Your Bucket List?

Imagine that you are told that you have six months left to live. How would you want to spend your remaining time? What things would you want to do the most? What's on your bucket list? (**Photo 12.9**).

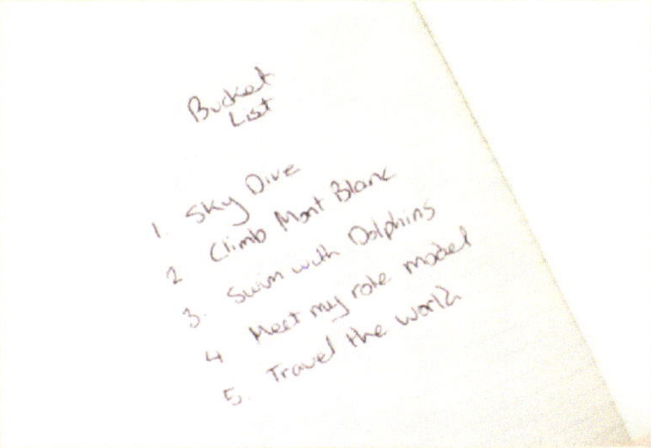

Photo 12.9

Source: Phil/Tinker/Shutterstock

A *bucket list* is a list of meaningful goals that someone wants to do or accomplish before they die (i.e., before they "kick the bucket"). Examples of items that might be on a bucket list include meeting your hero; learning a new language, sport, or skill; undertaking an extreme adventure (e.g., going on a safari, skydiving); or visiting a dreamed-of place. Bucket list goals differ from everyday goals in that they are often created with mortality in mind after awareness of the fragility and finitude of life becomes salient (Chu,

Grühn, & Holland, 2018). However, you don't have to be faced with death to develop a bucket list. Many people have them.

One interesting question is, How does the perception of time influence one's bucket list? Researchers wondered whether or not there would be differences between younger and older adults in the influence of differing time horizons on bucket list goals (Chu et al., 2018). They hypothesized that older adults and people who have a more constrained time horizon would report more bucket list goals related to intimacy, generativity (helping future generations), and ego-integrity (acceptance and awareness of self, including strengths, weaknesses, successes, and failures) than younger adults. Participants were randomly assigned to the limited time horizon group ("imagine you have six months to live") or the control group (with no time limitation at all), and asked to list five to twenty things they wanted to do or accomplish "before you die." Indeed, the researchers found that time horizon and age both influenced the types of bucket list goals, with goals related to intimacy, meaningfulness, and ego-integrity more prevalent in older people and those with only "six months to live." When the researchers conducted the exact same experiment, but with "one week to live" instead, they found that bucket list priorities shifted even further toward the intimate and meaningful.

Taken together, these findings highlight the influence of age and time horizon on our dreams and goals. With limited time, emotional connections and meaningful interactions became even more important.

Question: How might creating a bucket list cause you to rethink what is personally meaningful to you? What items would be on your bucket list?

Thinking About Health

■ How do survivors cope with death?

■ What cultural differences characterize societies' and people's reactions to death?

Chapter Summary

Lifestyle factors may lead to chronic conditions such as cardiovascular disease, diabetes, and cancer. Other chronic conditions, such as Alzheimer's disease and Parkinson's disease, emerge in later life and progressively worsen over time. Chronic illnesses can be treated, but not cured, so they must be managed for the rest of the patient's life. For patients with chronic illness and their families, learning to live with illness is imperative to preserving quality of life. Patients experience many different physical symptoms and emotional responses to chronic illness, and outcomes are better when coping efforts are tailored to specific stressors.

Many chronic conditions end with a terminal phase. A terminal illness is a life-ending illness or the dying phase of a chronic illness. There are different trajectories of death, corresponding to patterns of decline, which can help in understanding what a dying patient experiences. There may also be stages of dying and bereavement, marked by distinct emotional responses to death and dying. Important end-of-life considerations include hospice care, living wills, and what it means to die with dignity. Culture influences the experience of mourning and the emotional responses of survivors around the world.

KEY TERMS ▶   chronic illnesses p. 359, comorbid symptom p. 364, clear loss p. 365, ambiguous loss p. 365, adaptation p. 367, quality of life p. 368, health-related quality of life p. 369, terminal illness p. 370, death anxiety p. 372, terror management theory (TMT) p. 373, do not resuscitate (DNR) order p. 379, living will p. 379, durable power of attorney p. 381, last will and testament p. 381, palliative care p. 381, hospice care p. 382, assisted death p. 382, euthanasia p. 383, active euthanasia p. 383, passive euthanasia p. 383, grief p. 384, mourning p. 384, bereavement p. 384

CHAPTER 13

Healthcare Systems and Alternatives

Learning Outcomes

After reading this chapter, you should be able to:

- **Outline** the biopsychosocial factors that influence treatment seeking.
- **Explain** why some people misuse health care services.
- **Describe** the patient–practitioner relationship.
- **Compare** and contrast types of complementary and alternative medicines (CAMs).
- **Outline** the importance of the placebo effect.

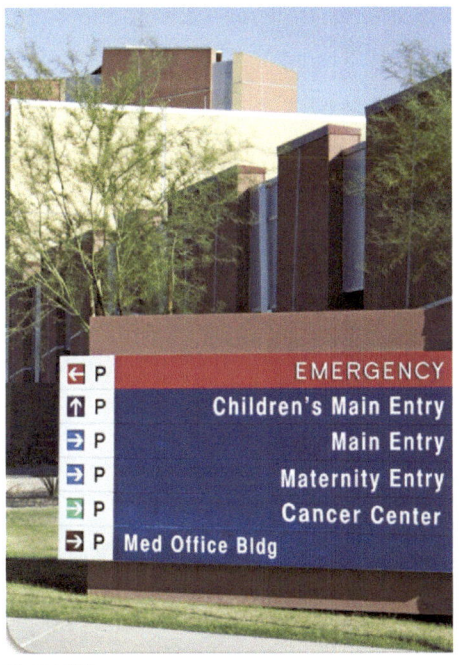

Photo 13.1

Paul Matthew Photography/Shutterstock

Mary Zupanc treats children with epilepsy. As a pediatric neurologist, she must often recommend brain surgery. You can imagine the fear and anxiety that parents feel when they hear this recommendation. Doctors are often the bearers of bad news, and they must help patients and their loved ones make difficult decisions. Dr. Zupanc always knew to come armed with all the right facts, but it wasn't until she became a patient herself that she learned how hard it is to be on the other side of the examining table (**Photo 13.1**).

A lifelong runner, Dr. Zupanc first suspected that something was wrong when she noticed her running times slowing (Zupanc, 2015). She also began to have visual problems and memory difficulties. After having a seizure, she underwent magnetic resonance imaging (MRI), which revealed a brain tumor that had caused the seizure and her visual problems. The tumor could have been growing for up to 20 years (Zupanc, 2015). Luckily, it was not cancerous, but still it had to be removed, and that meant brain surgery. She'd had to tell parents of children with epilepsy that same news many times. But now she was the patient, and now she, too, was afraid. "The possibility that I could die in surgery loomed large"—and so did the possibility that she would survive, but that she would not be the same person afterward (Zupanc, 2015).

It took four hours for surgeons to remove the two-inch tumor pressing on Dr. Zupanc's optic nerve and pituitary gland. Since then, she has had no seizures or visual problems, but surgery did have one lasting effect: It changed how she interacts with her patients. She knows now that statistics alone cannot calm a patient's fears (Zupanc, 2015). She understands the need for a sense of control over what is happening. Today, she often tells her patients her story—not just as their physician, but as their advocate and ally. Dr. Zupanc wants them to know that they are not alone.

What does Dr. Zupanc's story say about how physicians should be trained to interact with their patients? What can they do differently? Do you feel satisfied with the communication you have with your physician? In this chapter, we explore the experiences of patients as they seek treatment for health problems.

We'll examine the characteristics of health care in the United States and around the world, including the biopsychosocial and developmental influences on treatment seeking, patient–practitioner relationships, and quality of care. We'll discuss the health disparities in treatment-seeking and the differing perceptions of health care services. We'll also explore CMA and the power of the placebo effect to consider which options lead to the healthiest outcomes for the largest number of people.

Health Care Around the World

The quality of a nation's health care is tied to its economy. Citizens of prosperous countries are generally happier with their health care, while developing countries generally provide little or no health care coverage to their citizens. Developing countries may also have delayed technological advances, and shortages of physicians, clinics, and medicines. International disparities in health care may even compel people to seek care abroad (see **Figure 13.1;**.see the **Around the World** feature).

Many countries have **universal health care** (see **Table 13.1**)—health coverage for all citizens, regardless of income or employment. All citizens receive the health care they need at no personal expense. Doctor visits, specialized treatments, surgeries, and prescriptions are all covered. Many countries with economies comparable to the United States, such as Canada, Germany, Italy, Sweden, the Netherlands, and the United Kingdom, have universal health care. In the United Kingdom and Italy, physicians are employed by the government. In other countries with universal health care, doctors are privately employed, but the government sets their fees. Universal health care is far less expensive for the same quality of care (WHO, 2009a), although costs are rising. In some countries with universal health care, the health care is recognized as excellent; however, citizens complain of long waits, especially for diagnostic testing and elective surgeries. Still, the benefits often outweigh the hassles of waiting.

Many countries offer paid *parental leave* from work for families with newborn children. Apart from the United States, the only other country that does not provide paid maternity leave is Papua New Guinea, a country where 85% of the population derives their livelihood from agriculture (Addati, Cassirer, & Gilchrist, 2014). Many forward-thinking countries now also provide paid

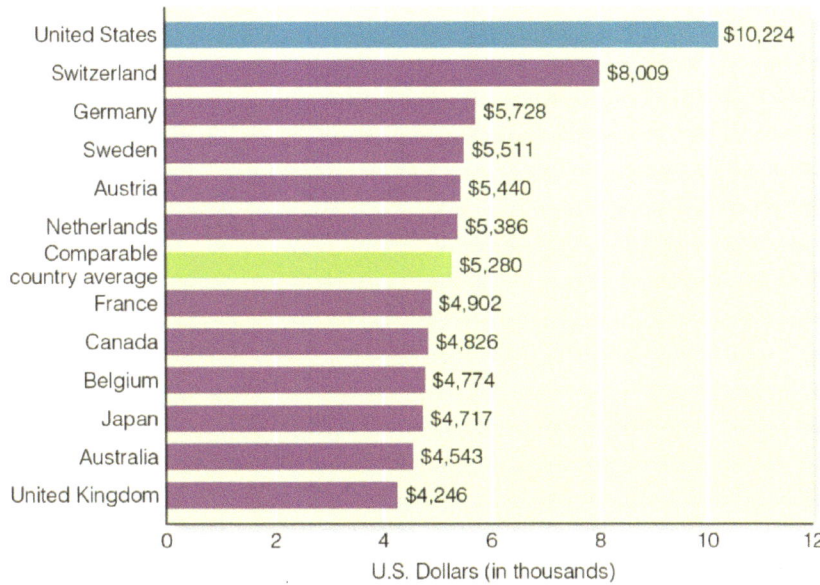

Figure 13.1   Healthcare expenditures worldwide.

Note: Health consumption expenditures per capita, U.S. dollars. Health consumption does not include investments in structures, equipment, or research.

Source: Data from Sawyer and Cox (2018).

Australia	Italy
Austria	Japan
Bahrain	Kuwait
Belgium	Luxembourg
Brunei	Netherlands
Canada	New Zealand
Cyprus	Norway
Denmark	Portugal
Finland	Singapore
France	Slovenia
Germany	South Korea
Greece	Spain
Hong Kong	Sweden
Iceland	Switzerland
Ireland	United Arab Emirates
Israel	United Kingdom

Table 13.1   A sample of countries with universal health care

paternity leave or allow parents to share paid leave. In the United States, the Family Medical Leave Act of 1993 allows most new parents to take up to 12 weeks off and still have their jobs when they return. However, they do lose their paychecks, and many must turn to public assistance or take on massive debt. Overall, only 17% of employers in the United States provide paid leave (Bureau of Labor Statistics, 2019). Small companies do not even have to guarantee that the parents' jobs will be held. Sweden, in contrast, provides 480 days fully paid for each child, for both parents—and parents can use those days any time before the child's eighth birthday. This practice saves companies money in the end, because talented employees are more likely to return to work (Wojcicki, 2014). When Google extended its paid maternity leave from three to five months, more than 50% of new mothers stayed on (Wojcicki, 2014).

Thinking About Health

- What are the differences between **Medicaid** and **Medicare**? Between single-payer and multipayer healthcare systems?
- What is the controversy surrounding the **Affordable Care Act**?
- How does the U.S. healthcare system differ from the systems in other countries?

Around *the* World

Medical Tourism

Approximately 15 million people (including over 1.4 million Americans) traveled to other countries for medical care (Crist et al., 2024). The most common destinations included Argentina, Thailand, Mexico, Singapore, India, Malaysia, Costa Rica, South Korea, Turkey, and Taiwan. Of all the destinations, Prince Court Medical Centre in Kuala Lumpur, Malaysia, was named the hospital that provides the very best care—not just for Malaysians, but also for a rising number of medical tourists (**Photo 13.2**) (International Medical Travel Journal, 2019).

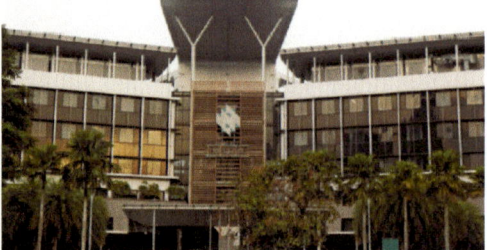

Photo 13.2   Malaysia's Prince Court Medical Centre in Kuala Lumpur is one of the most popular hospitals in the world for medical tourists.

Source: REUTERS/Alamy

A *medical tourist* is someone who travels to another country to seek medical care. Reasons for travel may include lower costs, a more familiar or hospitable culture, or therapies not available in one's own country (Gaines & Nguyen, 2014). Many Americans who go abroad lack health insurance or travel in pursuit of medical care not covered by their insurance. The most frequent types of care sought from abroad are dentistry, dermatology, cosmetic surgery, cardiac surgery, in vitro fertilization, gastric bypass surgery, liver and kidney transplants, and spine surgery (Crist et al., 2024). Although there are many risks associated with medical tourism, clearly these travelers think that the benefits outweigh the risks. Medical tourism is a multibillion-dollar industry, and it is growing every year.

One of the more controversial forms of medical tourism is transplant tourism—traveling for the purpose of receiving an organ. Transplant tourism is particularly risky, as some countries may have lax rules regarding the documentation of donors and organs, and patients may not receive important immunosuppressive drugs that prevent donor–host complications. Moreover, transplant tourism and organ trafficking go hand in hand, especially in less developed countries. In 2009, the WHO revised its guidelines to ensure that organ donations are made freely and ethically, not because of financial incentives.

Other medical tourists may be in search of a "fountain of youth": Antiaging is a big business. In many Asian countries, for example, researchers grow stem cells in the lab to target heart, muscle, blood, skin, and nerve cells. These specialized cells can then be implanted into a patient to replicate. The theory is that as old cells die, they are then replaced with new and youthful cells, essentially reversing aging. The richest and most energetic stem cells are said to be harvested from umbilical cord tissue in newborns. In the United States, the Food and Drug Administration has not approved many forms of stem cell therapies and heavily regulates their use—and no wonder: There is little empirical evidence to support the safety and long-term success of antiaging stem cell therapies. Still, people travel to Malaysia, Thailand, and other Asian countries to have these and other procedures. They may come back needing a vacation.

Question:

Under what circumstances would you consider traveling for medical care? What concerns might you have?

Who Seeks Treatment and Why?

Just as people vary greatly in the experience of illness, they also differ in their use of health care services. Not surprisingly, they also differ in their satisfaction with the care they receive.

In the United States, there were more than 9 million visits to a doctor's office in 2016 (Ashman, Rui, & Okeyode, 2019). Of those, 53% were to primary care physicians, and the most common complaint was coughing. A typical American adult sees a doctor an average of four times a year (CDC, 2016a). In the European Union, where many countries have universal health care, the average number of visits per year and per person is four to seven (Eurostat, 2017). In Europe, the most common reasons for seeking health care services are ear and respiratory infections, prenatal and pregnancy care, and chronic conditions such as obesity, cardiovascular disease, and cancer (Eurostat, 2017). But these are just the raw numbers. Who seeks healthcare services and why?

Age and Gender

Our use of health care services waxes and wanes across the lifespan (see **Figure 13.2**). It is high in infancy and childhood, because young children who begin to have more contact with other children become more prone to infections as they are still developing immunity (Cherry, Lucas, & Decker, 2010). The need for health services begins to decline in adolescence and continues to

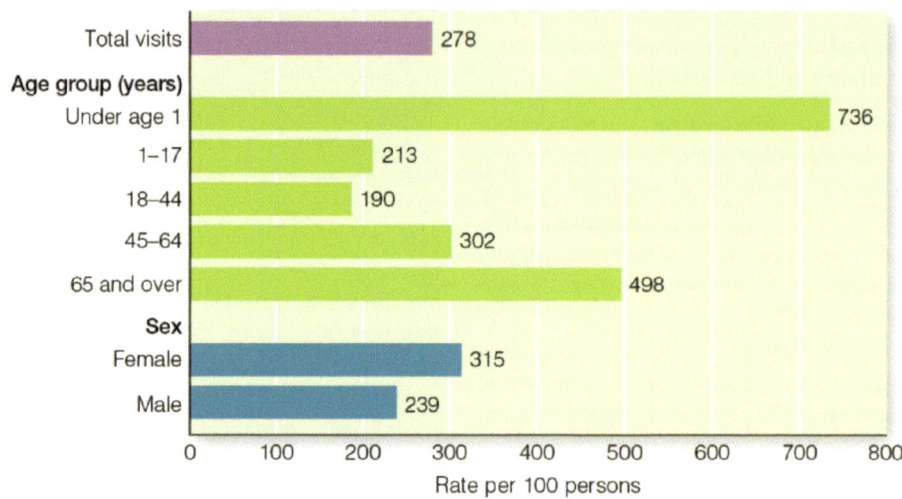

Figure 13.2   Rates of visits to the doctor in the United States, across the lifespan.

Source: Data from Ashman, Rui, and Okeyode (2019).

decline in young adulthood. During this period, many people visit their doctor only for annual exams. Health service utilization doesn't change again until late middle age and later life, as chronic conditions begin to emerge, and the use of health care services begins to rise again.

In general, women seek medical care at a higher frequency than men do (Bertakis, Azari, Helms, Callahan, & Robbins, 2000), and the gender difference begins to emerge in adolescence (Eiser, Havermans, Craft, & Kernahan, 1995; Klonoff & Landrine, 1992). Why? For one thing, women require specialized care for pregnancy and childbirth, and many seek annual health care from a specialist in obstetrics and gynecology or OB/GYN. Once they reach middle age, most women have annual mammograms to monitor for breast cancer. However, even when controlling for these gender-specific needs, women's use of healthcare services is still higher than men's. Women tend to have lower thresholds for pain and higher activation in brain regions when subjected to painful stimuli compared with men (Fillingim, 2000, 2003). As we saw in Chapter 8, women may report pain and be aware earlier of such symptoms as changes in body temperature and blood pressure (Kroenke & Spitzer, 1998; Leventhal, Diefenbach, & Leventhal, 1992). There are sociocultural explanations for differences in treatment-seeking as well. Because men are encouraged to endure pain and discomfort, they may persevere rather than seek treatment (Klonoff & Landrine, 1992).

There are some exceptions, though. Women tend to delay longer before going to an emergency department. Between 20% and 30% of women also put off seeking medical help for at least three months after noticing symptoms of breast cancer (Burgess et al., 2008).

Sociocultural Factors

In the United States, people who have low incomes use health services less frequently than wealthier people simply because they cannot afford to do so (Adler & Stewart, 2010). As we have already seen, the unequal availability of health care led to the Affordable Care Act. Along with Medicaid and Medicare, it may diminish the differences in who seeks care.

On average, low-income Americans are able to visit doctors less often and fill fewer prescriptions annually. They are also less likely to have a regular physician. When there *is* a health problem, low-income African Americans are more likely to visit an emergency department or outpatient clinic for care (Flack, Apelqvist, Keith, Trueman, & Williams, 2008). In addition, many physicians do not have offices in low-income neighborhoods, so economically disadvantaged people may have to travel farther for routine medical care. Preventive care is essential for offsetting the kinds of problems that lead to hospital visits.

Recent immigrants to the United States may be hesitant to seek medical care for another reason: They may have difficulty speaking English. Depending on their country of origin, some immigrants may also not trust the health care system in their new country.

Sociocultural factors also affect how quickly people recognize their symptoms and seek treatment. African Americans experience more chronic pain, more sleep disturbances, and more symptoms indicative of post-traumatic stress disorder and depression (Green et al., 2003). Yet they are less likely to visit a doctor and get medical care when they may need it. The symptoms of heart attack also present atypically more often in women and African Americans than in males and white Americans, adding to delays in seeking treatment (Lee, Bahler, Chung, Alonzo, & Zeller, 2000).

Recall the four stages of delay in obtaining treatment: appraisal delay, illness delay, behavioral delay, and medical delay (Anderson, Broad, & Bonita, 1995; see Chapter 8). People delay seeking treatment for many reasons. Fear, anxiety, minimizing the risk, disliking or not trusting the medical system, or simply not having time are all reasons why someone might put off going to the doctor. People's beliefs about their health also influence when and why they seek treatment. It may take some time for a person to decide if a symptom is serious. And people may not only misinterpret their symptoms, but also be reluctant to discuss them (Oberoi, Jiwa, McManus, & Hodder, 2015).

As we saw in Chapter 8, early diagnosis and treatment are essential for patients with many conditions, from cancer to cardiovascular disease. Regardless of sociocultural context, avoiding diagnosis and treatment can be life-threatening.

Misusing Health Services

Some people do not shy away from health care at all. In fact, they misuse health care services.

In Chapter 12, we learned the importance of identifying and treating anxiety and depression. These mental health problems often go undiagnosed and untreated. They are assumed to be a rational reaction to living with chronic illness, or the symptoms of depression are mistaken for symptoms of the chronic illness itself. However, the opposite also occurs: People may wrongly attribute their mental health symptoms to something physical.

People may go to urgent care or the emergency room with heart palpitations, difficulty breathing, chest pains, or nausea only to learn that they are suffering from an anxiety attack. Nearly 23% of people who present with cardiac symptoms may actually have anxiety or depression (Howren & Suls, 2011; Srinivasan & Joseph, 2004). Often, the physician may not realize the psychological origin of the symptoms and may order further tests and treatment. The result may be many more visits to physicians, prolonged hospital stays, and unnecessary prescriptions (de Jonge, Latour, & Huyse, 2003; Mitchell, Vaze, & Rao, 2009; Rubin, Cleare, & Hotopf, 2004). These patients are not malingering, nor actively pretending to be ill—neither they nor their physicians may know if or how to address physical symptoms that have a psychological origin.

Why do people misuse health care? First, the symptoms of mood and anxiety disorders, such as fatigue and rapid heart rate, can be physical. Patients may not know that they have a mood disorder. Second, many people still perceive mental health problems as stigmatizing and physical health problems as "legitimate." Seeking medical care can make their symptoms feel more acceptable. Third, patients may seek **secondary gains** —the positive things that come with being sick. Being ill allows them to indulge in much-needed rest, take time off from work, have others attend to their needs, and avoid burdensome responsibilities.

Illness anxiety disorder (formerly known as *hypochondriasis*) is when someone has an excessive concern for their health. People with this disorder are extremely attuned to their bodies and may end up in doctor's offices with problems that are imaginary or disproportionate to reality. To them, a new freckle may seem indicative of skin cancer. Indigestion from spicy foods could be food poisoning, or a headache could be a sign of a brain tumor.

Physicians must be attuned to the emotional as well as the physical issues of their patients. They need to ask questions: "Have you been feeling depressed lately? Have you lost interest in things that used to bring you pleasure? Are you experiencing any stress in your life?" As part of a routine checkup, they can also administer questionnaires that screen for mood and anxiety-related disorders (see **Table 13.2** for an example of a commonly used questionnaire). When the answers to these questions are *yes*, the doctor should refer the patient to a psychotherapist for counseling or a psychiatrist for a more thorough assessment (Means-Christensen, Arnau, Tonidandel, Bramson, & Meagher, 2005).

Thinking About Health

- Why do some people delay seeking treatment, and why do some people misuse health care services?
- What demographic and sociocultural factors influence treatment-seeking?
- The last time you sought treatment, what kinds of questions did the physician ask about your physical and mental health? Were you satisfied with the results of the treatment?

Over the last 2 weeks, how often have you been bothered by any of the following problems? *(Use "✓" to indicate your answer)*	Not at all	Several days	More than half the days	Nearly every day
1. Little interest or pleasure in doing things	0	1	2	3
2. Feeling down, depressed, or hopeless	0	1	2	3
3. Trouble falling or staying asleep, or sleeping too much	0	1	2	3
4. Feeling tired or having little energy	0	1	2	3
5. Poor appetite or overeating	0	1	2	3
6. Feeling bad about yourself—or that you are a failure or have let yourself or your family down	0	1	2	3
7. Trouble concentrating on things, such as reading the newspaper or watching television	0	1	2	3
8. Moving or speaking so slowly that other people could have noticed? Or the opposite—being so fidgety or restless that you have been moving around a lot more than usual	0	1	2	3
9. Thoughts that you would be better off dead or of hurting yourself in some way	0	1	2	3

For office coding   0   + _____   + _____   + _____

= Total Score : _____

If you checked off any problems, how difficult have these problems made it for you to do your work, take care of things at home, or get along with other people?

Not difficult at all	Somewhat difficult	Very difficult	Extremely difficult
☐	☐	☐	☐

Source: Research from Drs. Robert L. Spitzer, Janet B. W. Williams, Kurt Kroenke, and colleagues.

Table 13.2   Patient Health Questionnaire-9 (PHQ-9)

Compliance

Even when patients seek medical care, they don't necessarily follow their doctor's advice (DiMatteo, 2004). Following treatment correctly is called **compliance** (or *adherence*), and poor compliance is a factor in more than 125,000 deaths per year (Osterberg & Blaschke, 2005). More than half of Americans who seek advice from a physician do not adhere to that advice (DiMatteo, Giordani, Lepper, & Croghan, 2002). Poor compliance costs the United States $528.4 billion each year

(Watanabe, McInnis, & Hirsch, 2018). As former U.S. Surgeon General C. Everett Koop once said, "Drugs don't work in people who don't take them!"

In the United States, some 3.8 billion prescriptions are written annually, and yet at least half of them are not taken correctly or at all (Osterberg & Blaschke, 2005). Lack of compliance with medical treatment may run as high as 93% in some cases (DiMatteo et al., 2002). Overall, the average nonadherance rate is around 26%.

Rates of Compliance and Types of Treatment

It is difficult to estimate adherence reliably. Physicians tend to overestimate their patients' compliance, and patients are not always accurate in their reporting.

Noncompliance encompasses many different behaviors, from not taking prescribed medicines to not sticking to lifestyle changes, from not getting required tests to not showing up for doctor's appointments, and more. It can be a matter of forgetting, or it may be a conscious decision. Sometimes patients make their own modifications to recommended treatment, a behavior known as **creative nonadherence**. Suppose a doctor prescribes you a daily antibiotic for strep throat. You may think that, since you are feeling poorly, you should take multiple doses per day at first. And then, when you begin feeling better and your symptoms subside, you may stop taking the drug. But any modifications to a prescription can be dangerous (Haynes, McKibbon, & Kanani, 1996; O'Connor, 2006).

The rates of nonadherence are particularly high when it comes to treatments for gastrointestinal illnesses and cancer. They are lowest for sleep problems, pulmonary disorders, HIV/AIDS, arthritis, and diabetes (DiMatteo & Haskard, 2006). Compliance for acute, short-term health problems such as pneumonia or a stomach bug is around 67%, and compliance for treatments for chronic illnesses is between 50% and 55%. Short-term antibiotic treatments have a noncompliance rate of about one-third (Rapoff & Christophersen, 1982; West & Cordina, 2019). When it comes to keeping appointments, only 50% make it to the doctor's office, especially when health care involves preventive medicine (DiMatteo & DiNicola, 1982; West & Cordina, 2019). Doctors' suggestions to modify diet, quit smoking, or get exercise are rarely followed (Stilley, Bender, Dunbar-Jacob, Sereika, & Ryan, 2010; West & Cordina, 2019). For patients with cardiovascular disease, whose lives may depend on making lifestyle changes, up to 75% do not comply.

One reason for these differences in compliance is the nature of the illness and its treatment (Ingersoll & Cohen, 2008; Turk & Meichenbaum, 1991). Patients with an acute illness feel it every day—and also feel a strong desire to get back on their feet. If you have a respiratory infection right before a big event in your life, you might go to the doctor, get a prescription, and take it as prescribed to get better as quickly as possible. Conversely, patients with a chronic illness that requires long-term lifestyle changes and medications may slack off now and again. It may be that they "burn out" from their numerous daily responsibilities. Patients with diabetes, for example, must monitor their blood glucose levels, take regular medications or shots, follow a healthy diet, eat at regular intervals, and get exercise. Similarly, people whose prescriptions come with specific requirements, such as taking the medication on an empty stomach, with food, or in conjunction with other drugs or behaviors, may also become overwhelmed with the behavioral changes required of them (Ingersoll & Cohen, 2008; Insel, Reminger, & Hsiao, 2006). Some days, they may just want a break.

Overall, the longer someone has to take a medication, the less adherence there will be (Insel et al., 2006; Parrish, 1986). This may again have to do with the type of illness, but it may also be that some medications take longer to begin working, and patients give up on them too early. This is often the case with antidepressants or antianxiety medications, which may not produce signs of improvement for more than three weeks.

Side effects, too, often diminish compliance. Some antibiotics cause an upset stomach and some pain relievers affect libido. Medications for Parkinson's disease and cancer may have side effects on par with the symptoms they are taken to treat. The expense of medications can also motivate patients to skip them. They may feel the need to make their prescriptions last.

Who Complies?

Although age, gender, and socioeconomic status may influence adherence to treatment, these factors are not always predictive (Epstein & Cluss, 1982). Adherence in childhood is primarily the responsibility of the parent, which may benefit compliance—but then children may not be as conscientious about taking their medication when not supervised (Johnson, 1992). Middle-aged people with busy lives are most likely to forget. In general, older adults are more compliant, but once vision, hearing, and memory difficulties arise, compliance again tapers off (Park, 1999).

Women may be better at adherence if they are taking a birth control pill on a daily basis. The regular pill-taking becomes a habit. In non-English-speaking patients, language barriers may stand in the way of adherence (Pignone, DeWalt, Sheridan, Berkman, & Lohr, 2005). Some religious or cultural groups may have beliefs that conflict with taking medications. Some may try to find alternative approaches to treat their ailments.

So, who is likely to stick to treatment? A full answer involves the diagnosis, the kind of treatment, and the goals and beliefs of the patient. In general, though, if someone perceives an immediate threat or high risk, they are more likely to heed recommendations of change (see Chapter 3; Dolecek et al., 1986; Pederson, 1982).

One last thing that strongly affects compliance is the patient–practitioner relationship. Proper communication between doctor and patient affects not just compliance, but every aspect of the quality of care.

Thinking About Health

■ Why is treatment compliance important?

■ How does compliance relate to the type of treatment?

■ Given the factors that influence who complies and who does not, how can compliance be improved?

The Patient–Practitioner Relationship

Many patients complain about their experiences when seeing a doctor. They may feel that they had just begun to discuss what had brought them there—and the doctor was already writing a prescription and moving on to the next patient. Doctors being rushed, not taking the time to listen, not focusing on what the patient wants to discuss, and treating the patient brusquely are all common complaints.

These complaints may be valid. On average, physicians spend 20 minutes with patients—and the longer the visit, the higher the quality of care (Chen, Farwell, & Jha, 2009). As the patient describes the problem, the doctor interrupts and begins asking questions after, on average, just 23 seconds (Li, Magrabi, & Coiera, 2012). Medical providers also like to give care to patients with illnesses that are easy to diagnose and treat, as with acute conditions (Pandya, McHugh, & Batalova, 2011).

All patients want to understand what is ailing them (Schillinger, Bindman, Wang, Stewart, & Piette, 2004), but here, too, sociocultural differences affect what patients get from their doctors. In general, educated, young, non-Hispanic white women of higher socioeconomic status ask for more information about their condition and are more involved in their treatment than others (Levinson, Kao, Kuby, & Thisted, 2005; Turk-Charles, Meyerowitz, & Gatz, 1997). Questioning and involvement both lead to better outcomes (Auerbach, Krimgold, & Lefkowitz, 2000; Schillinger et al., 2004).

Patient-Centered and Doctor-Centered Medicine

Some doctors welcome interaction and communication with the patient. They ask open-ended questions and allow patients to take a more active role. Other doctors seek to dictate the interaction with patients. They ask questions that require only a yes or no answer, and they may well prevent the patient from providing more information. They feel that they need to stick strictly to business.

The more open approach is sometimes called **patient-centered care**, while the more authoritative approach is called **doctor-centered care** (Byrne & Long, 1976; Levenstein, McCracken, McWhinney, Stewart, & Brown, 1986). Some patients like to think of doctors as the authority, while others prefer to have a more egalitarian relationship with their physicians. When there is a mismatch between the doctor's style and the patient's expectations, it can lead to dissatisfaction with one's medical care and, ultimately, poorer quality of care. It can increase the patient's stress level, decrease the credibility of the diagnosis and treatment, and lower compliance (Auerbach, Martelli, & Mercuri, 1983; Cvengros, Christensen, Cunningham, Hillis, & Kaboli, 2009; Haug & Lavin, 1981; Keating, Guadagnoli, Landrum, Borbas, & Weeks, 2002; Miller & Mangan, 1983). In general, female physicians are more patient-centered, and they spend at least 10% more time with their patients (Krupat, Hsu, Irish, Schmittdiel, & Selby, 2004).

Doctor–Patient Dynamics: From a psychological perspective, the doctor–patient relationship is inherently imbalanced. Due to their expertise, the doctor has superiority over the patient, and this dynamic can give rise to various communication patterns. For example, a mismatch in personality factors between physicians and patients—such as a desire for control, submissiveness, dominance, aggression, and assertiveness—can create strained interactions (Namazi, Aramesh, & Larijani, 2016). Shared or divergent goals, preexisting beliefs about medicine, and cultural beliefs and expectations may also influence the doctor–patient relationship, for better or for worse. The actual conversations that physicians and health care practitioners have with their patients can also lead to problems. Patients may not understand the tests needed for a diagnosis, a diagnosis itself, or a course of treatment. Because patients depend on their physicians to provide them with the information they need to make the best treatment decisions (Clarke et al., 2015), communication problems can lead to confusion and lack of satisfaction with health care.

One factor that has been found to critically influence interpersonal dynamics in patient–practitioner communications is reciprocity. *Reciprocity* refers to a mutual sharing of feelings, thoughts, and behaviors, or the "give-and-take" in a professional or personal relationship. The mutual openness and respect of a reciprocal patient–practitioner relationship can reduce adverse outcomes, improve health, and increase satisfaction with the care received (Kelly, Agne, Meara, & Pawlik, 2019).

Many patients now experience their doctor's office visit within the context of technology, with e-mail and text reminders of upcoming visits, and computers recording information and guiding discussions and diagnoses. Patients generally have a positive attitude toward the use of technology in the examination room, and its use does not seem to affect the quality of their communication with the doctor (Antoun, Hamadeh, & Romani, 2019). In fact, as long as they perceive a balance between the doctor's paying attention to them and recording their information, patients are satisfied with their care (Antoun et al., 2019). Telehealth is changing the medical field in many ways, and it appears that it can improve doctor–patient communications as well.

Health Literacy

Patients may complain that doctors talk down to them, or use medical jargon, vocabulary that they cannot understand. Medical jargon can stand in the way of effective communication. Physicians cannot assume that all patients will understand the terms they use. These problems are often worse when the physician and patient have different cultural backgrounds or when there are language barriers (Halim, Yoshikawa, & Amodio, 2013).

The greater the patient's health knowledge, or **health literacy**, the greater their quality of care. Health literacy is defined as "the degree to which individuals have the capacity to obtain, process, and understand basic health information and services to make appropriate health decisions" (Anderson et al., 2019). It can be as simple as being able to read the label on a prescription—or as complex as fully understanding the doctor's diagnosis. Health literacy has emerged as one of the most important factors predicting positive or negative health outcomes. Lower health literacy is linked to poorer preventive care and worse health status, as well as more frequent hospitalizations and higher mortality rates (Allenbaugh, Spagnoletti, Rack, Rubio, & Corbelli, 2019).

As few as 12% of Americans have sufficient health literacy (U.S. Department of Health and Human Services, 2015). And over 85% of patients consider their

The Short Test of Functional Health Literacy (Nurss, Parker, Williams, & Baker, 2003) was designed to measure patients' ability to comprehend health-related materials. It asks patients to read and complete passages that relate to their treatment. For example, the patient might be asked to select the correct word in a sentence similar to this one:

Your doctor wants you to get an X-ray of your
a. diet.
b. stroke.
c. virus.
d. leg.

Figure 13.3   Example of an item from a Health Literacy Scale.

own health literacy to be poor (Allenbaugh et al., 2019; Rudd, 2007). How is your health literacy? In research settings, health literacy is measured using the technique shown in **Figure 13.3**. People are given a written passage describing a medical procedure. In each sentence, one or more words are left out, and the participant has to choose which word (or words) correctly completes the sentence. In essence, it is a test of reading comprehension for medical terms. Other questions ask whether a patient can accurately identify the milligrams of a dose and the dosing schedule of a medication. Others might ask the meaning of such terms as *mucus, sutures, glucose,* and *hypertension.*

Generally, people from less-educated, lower-income backgrounds do worse on tests of health literacy (DiMatteo & DiNicola, 1982; Egbert & Nanna, 2009; Nielsen-Bolman, Panzer, & Kindig, 2004). Demographic factors such as race/ethnicity and age are important to consider as well. Typically, low-income patients from minority backgrounds who have less than a high school education are at risk of health illiteracy, and being over the age of 65 increases that risk. (Developmentally, older patients may not be as health literate because of changes in the medical field over their lifetimes.) In a large, multiethnic, U.S.-based sample, lower health literacy was seen in Chinese, Hispanic, and black participants when compared to their white counterparts (Anderson et al., 2019). Moreover, the degree of acculturation to the United States—including factors such as not having been born in the United States, fewer familial generations living in the United States, and speaking languages other than English within the home—was also associated with lower health literacy. Researchers conclude that, especially within diverse communities, patients should be provided with greater health education and support. Health disparities and differences in health outcomes may be due, in part, to lower health literacy.

Physicians are still becoming aware of patients' needs for understanding. Fortunately, in the United States, ongoing initiatives by the American Medical Association and the Institute of Medicine are driving the education of health-care professionals about health literacy, providing evidence-based techniques that can be used in healthcare settings to improve communication (Allenbaugh et al., 2019). Health literacy and good communication between patient and healthcare provider are essential to the quality of medical care, treatment, recovery, and patient satisfaction.

Hospitalization

A good relationship between patient and practitioner is even more important in the place where the patient has the least say: the hospital. There are 6210 hospitals in the United States, and more than 36 million people are hospitalized in a given year (AHA, 2019a). Hospitals today provide many services, from lab work and tests to major surgery. As outpatient services have increased, longer hospital stays have decreased. However, as noted earlier, the average stay is still 4.8 days.

Being admitted to a hospital can be daunting. You may enter because of an illness that already has you scared. Once inside, you may lose autonomy and individuality, and you may be anxious about the outcome. You may interact with a host of healthcare providers who are new to you. You may experience pain, fever, physical and emotional fatigue, and sedation. You may also be subject to new and unfamiliar risks (see the **In the News** feature). All of these aspects may make it difficult to understand what is going on around you. One study showed that a typical patient was visited by hospital staff an average of five times per hour, though some patients had as many as 28 separate visits an hour (Cohen, Hyman, Rosenberg, & Larson, 2012). These visits were often from different specialists, with nurses having the highest frequency of room visits (45%), followed by medical staff (17%), nonclinical staff (hospital volunteers, 7%), and clinical staff (4%). Personal visitors were also common (23%). The length of visits lasted from 1 minute to 124 minutes, with an average of 3 minutes per visit (Cohen et al., 2012). Looked at from another angle, this study also showed that medical staff members visit an average of three patients per hour (Cohen et al., 2012). The rapid pace of care, coupled with the patient's anxiety, can easily lead to miscommunication.

Many hospitalized patients have a limited understanding of what is happening to them. In one survey, 68% did not understand their plan of care, only 32% could name their attending physician, and only 40% correctly named their nurses (O'Leary et al., 2010). Only 38% understood the procedures planned for the day, and their estimate of the length of their hospital stay matched the physician's estimate only 39% of the time.

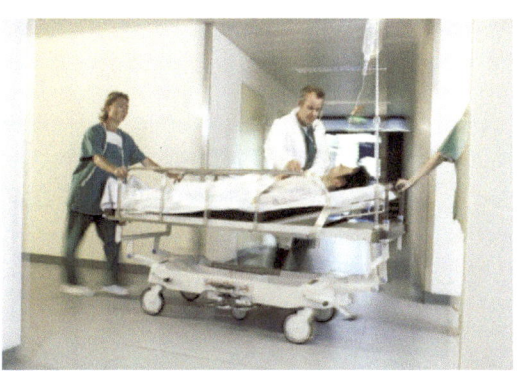

Photo 13.3   The many variables and unknowns associated with hospitalization can produce anxiety in patients and their loved ones. How can healthcare practitioners help relieve patients' worries and fears?

Source: Bikeriderlondon/Shutterstock

As we saw with Dr. Zupanc at the start of this chapter, even a physician with an intimate knowledge of how a hospital works can be afraid. For children, who may never have been in a hospital before, the fears are often compounded. They are away from their parents and sleeping in a strange place. Strangers are poking and prodding them. Parents feel stress and worry, too, and kids may pick up on their parents' fears. Caregivers should be especially concerned about communicating with younger patients and their parents to relieve their fears (**Photo 13.3**).

What Can Hospitals Do Better? As we have seen, when doctors show empathy and communicate well, treatment outcomes are better (Larson & Yao, 2005). Good communication leads to more positive perceptions of the physician and the quality of their care, decreases the length of hospitalization, lowers hospital costs, and lowers the risk of litigation (Swayden et al., 2012). Even simple things can make a big difference—such as making time to sit on the edge of a patient's bed to talk while making the daily rounds.

Patients' fears and anxieties can interfere with their understanding of medical procedures. Hospitals can act to reduce those fears. Providing patients with informative videos, for instance, can decrease their worry and better prepare them for surgery. Apps such as EASE and MyChart, through which doctors and nurses can provide text, photo, and video updates directly from the operating room, also help minimize anxiety by keeping patients' families informed (Jargon, 2019). In recent years, many hospitals have adopted the use of pre-operative videos and informative apps (Johnson, Lauver, & Nail, 1989; Mahler & Kulik, 1998).

Hospitals have highly focused operations designed to provide efficient, quality care (Brown & Fleisher, 2014). Staff work to create an environment that is comforting, relaxing, and appealing, especially for children. They are trained to be warm and accepting in their interactions with children and adults, and hospital rules are often flexible enough to allow parents to have as much contact with their children as they wish. These programs help overcome emotional distress and promote better postoperative adjustment (Gellert, 1958).

Think back to Dr. Zupanc. She learned that it is important for physicians to consider what is meaningful and comforting for the patient, as well as for their loved ones. Physicians should take time to help patients understand what is happening within them and around them. Both in and out of the hospital, the key is compassionate care and good communication.

Thinking About Health

■ What are the differences between patient-centered and doctor-centered care?

■ What is health literacy, and how does it affect the doctor–patient relationship?

■ What have experiences of hospitalization been like for you, your friends, or your family?

In the News

Hospital-Acquired Infections

If you find it frightening to enter a hospital, you might not be overreacting. The risk of hospital-acquired infections is real. These complications, also called *nosocomial infections*, can be life-threatening. In the words of physician and medical ethicist Atul

Gawande (2009), "This is the reality of intensive care: At any point, we are as apt to harm as we are to heal."

The lungs, wounds, urinary tract, or bloodstream can all become infected during a hospital stay. In some cases, an intravenous line is contaminated during insertion into the body. The infection can spread rapidly and may be fatal. Infections of intravenous lines are common enough that they are considered routine complications. Intensive care units alone place 5 million lines into patients each year, and after 10 days, 4% of those lines will become infected. That works out to 80,000 infected intensive care patients each year, and up to 28% of these infections will be fatal (Gawande, 2009). Recent research found that one out of every 25 hospital patients in the United States contracts a hospital-acquired infection (Agency for Healthcare Research and Quality [AHRQ], 2019). And surviving the infection means more time in the hospital. The good news is that the number of infections decreased between 2014 and 2017.

These are not the only risks of intensive care. According to one study, the average patient is subject to 178 actions per day, from the changing of bandages or bedding to the administering of drugs to the suctioning of the lungs—and every one of these actions poses a risk (Donchin et al., 1995; Gawande, 2009). Although doctors and nurses make errors only 1% of the time, this averages out to two errors a day per patient.

Evidence-based guidelines can reduce the risk of hospital-acquired infections. Protocols for uniforms, equipment sterilization, and regular hand washing are critical. In 2005, the World Health Organization (WHO) launched a Global Patient Safety Challenge to train hospital staff on how to minimize infections, and these efforts are ongoing (Sheikh et al., 2019; WHO, 2005). Slowly, the rates of hospital-acquired infections are coming down.

Question: Can you find the infection and error rates for hospitals in your area? How can hospital-acquired infections and medical errors be prevented?

Complementary and Alternative Medicine

People concerned about their health may seek treatment outside of conventional health services, providers, and medicines. They may look instead to CAM.

CAM is an overarching term for a wide array of approaches to prevent or treat disease, from ancient practices to New Age medicine, that exist outside of conventional Western medicine. Complementary approaches are used in conjunction with Western or conventional approaches and thus *complement* them. Alternative approaches are used *instead* of Western or conventional medicine.

Alternative medical practices emerged in the United States in the early- to mid-nineteenth century, as people sought to nourish what they considered the emotional and spiritual aspects of health (Ventola, 2010). These therapies were seen as "safe" and "natural." Even some conventional treatments have their roots in CAM. For example, the use of quinine, the most effective malaria treatment for more than 300 years, originates from therapy using Peruvian bark. Throughout history, plants have served as medicine, and as many as 70,000 plants have curing properties. Foxglove was used in ancient times to heal those who "have fallen from high places," or to combat swelling by dressing sores and ulcers. It led to the discovery of *digoxin*, an essential drug treatment for cardiovascular disease today. Morphine and codeine both derive from poppy plants.

CAM is not part of conventional medicine, because there is currently insufficient evidence that it is safe and effective (Barnes, Bloom, & Dhalhamer, 2008; Barnes, Bloom, & Nahin, 2008). That is, to date, there is not enough evidence-based science to merit these practices. Whereas Western drugs and medical treatments have to go through rigorous scientific study and approval by the FDA, many CAM therapies go untested. Products are also not regulated for dosage

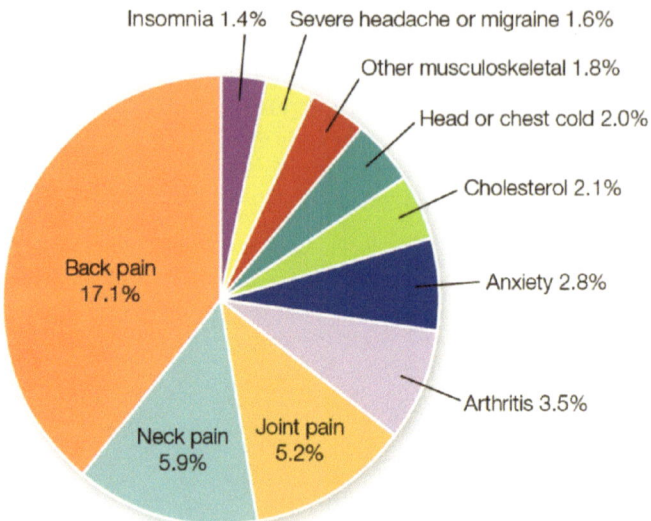

Figure 13.4   Most common conditions treated by CAM therapies.

Source: Data from Barnes, Bloom, and Dhalhamer (2008).

or composition. Formal training is not required for those who practice CAM, and many physicians do not have the knowledge to answer questions about it. Pharmacists, too, are generally unprepared to discuss a CAM therapy's mechanisms, dosage, efficacy, and side effects.

Nevertheless, up to 70% of Canadians and 60% of Americans use some kind of complementary therapies. For example, over 75% of American adults use dietary supplements, and 38% of Canadians use at least one natural health product (Vohra, Zorzela, Kemper, Vlieger, & Pintov, 2019). For preventing and treating diagnosed medical conditions, 36% of Americans and Canadians use CAM, and as many as 70% of parents use CAM for their children who have been diagnosed with chronic or life-threatening diseases (Shatnawi, Shafer, Ahmed, & Elbarbry, 2019; Vohra et al., 2019). In the United States, more than $33 billion is spent on nonconventional treatments annually—and rarely are these treatments covered by health insurance. When people have health problems, they may seek whatever they think will alleviate their pain (see **Figure 13.4**). The growing prevalence of CAM has driven medical scientists to conduct evidence-based research to determine which types of CAM really are safe and effective, and what their benefits are.

Kinds of Alternative Medicine

What, then, are people using? See **Figure 13.5**.

Surprise! Dietary supplements and natural products are the most popular alternative medicines, with fish oil and glucosamine being the most popular. Mind and body practices—such as yoga, meditation, and massage—are also rising in popularity.

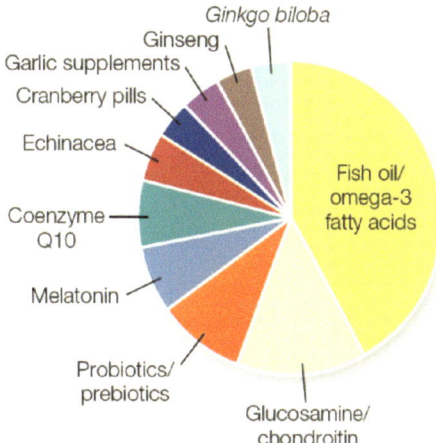

Most popular mind and body practices

Most popular natural products

Figure 13.5   Most common CAM approaches in the United States.

Source: Information from Clarke, Black, Stussman, Barnes, and Nahin (2015).

These are the top four dietary supplements:

■ *Fish oil*, which provides omega-3 fatty acids, is taken for cardiovascular health.

■ *Glucosamine*, an amino sugar, is used to reduce pain and inflammation of the joints, such as osteoarthritis. It is also taken in conjunction with chondroitin, a chemical found in cartilage around the joints.

■ *Probiotics*, live bacteria and yeasts, are thought to promote a balanced microbiome and digestive system.

■ *Melatonin*, a hormone, is taken as a sleep aid. Found in animals, plants, fungi, and bacteria, it may help the body mimic a response to the daily onset of darkness.

Again, not all of these supplements have been proven effective.

CAM falls into five categories (Ventola, 2010): whole medical systems, mind-body techniques, biologically based therapies, manipulative mind-body techniques, and energy therapies. Let's look at each of these and explore their cultural roots outside of Western medicine.

Whole Medical Systems Traditional Chinese medicine has its roots in the belief that illnesses and disorders are caused by improper flow of the life force *qi* (pronounced *chee*) through the body. For more than 2500 years, practitioners of Chinese medicine have been using diet, medicinal herbs, massage, meditation, and acupuncture (Harvard College, 2007; National Center for Complementary & Integrative Health, 2017). They believe that these practices restore the balance of opposing energy sources (*yin* and *yang*), heat and cold, external and internal, and deficiency and excess.

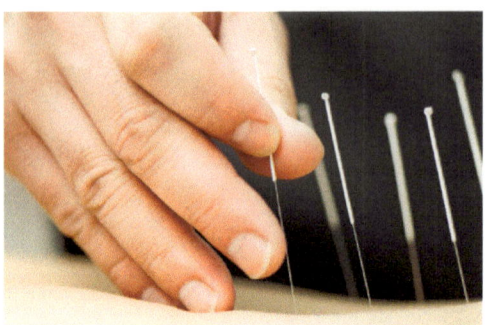

Photo 13.4 Some people believe acupuncture to be an effective treatment for pain, stress, nausea, and other symptoms of the disease.

Acupuncture involves inserting fine needles into the skin and the tissue beneath to release blocked *qi*. Pressure, heat, ultrasound, lasers, or a low-voltage electrical current can be applied to the needle as well. Acupuncture is not painful, but many people report a tingling sensation. An estimated 3 million American adults have acupuncture each year (Barnes, Bloom, & Nahin, 2008). (**Photo 13.4**).

Acupuncture has been shown to be effective in treating disorders from tennis elbow to posttraumatic stress disorder (Hollifield, Sinclair-Lian, Warner, & Hammerschlag, 2007; Tsui & Leung, 2002). It has been used to relieve nausea from chemotherapy and to treat addiction. However, the evidence suggests that acupuncture can treat only symptoms, such as pain, not an underlying disorder (Vickers et al., 2012). The technique releases neurotransmitters, possibly endorphins, in the brain that may act as painkillers. Given that pain is of great importance to those suffering from it, it is not surprising that acupuncture has become so popular.

Originating in India more than 4000 years ago, **Ayurveda** is another CAM technique based on theories of a proper balance in the body's life force. Practitioners evaluate the patient based on overall appearance, symptoms, behaviors, lifestyle, urine, and stool. From this, they design a treatment plan that may include diet, herbs, massage, meditation, and yoga. They may also inject fluid into the rectum to cause a bowel movement, or they may flush out the nose with a saline solution. There is very little evidence-based research to support Ayurvedic practices.

Homeopathy consists of a small dose of what in large doses causes the illness. The more diluted the substance, the more potent the cure is thought to be. The remedies, which originated in Germany in the late 1700s, include the use of plant and animal extracts as well as minerals. These substances are said to activate the body's innate capacity to heal itself. There is no scientific evidence to support this theory.

Mind-Body Techniques and Biologically Based Therapies: Meditation, relaxation techniques, guided imagery, hypnotherapy, and biofeedback are examples of **mind-body techniques**. They involve focusing attention on one's body to promote relaxation and mindfulness. There is little empirical evidence to show that these techniques are effective at treating illness. With their emphasis on mindfulness, they may, however, help people cope with the stress, pain, and ambiguity of illness.

Biologically based therapies, such as diet therapy, use naturally occurring substances to treat ailments. Although a healthy diet is good, and some diets are widely accepted as healthful, there is little empirical evidence that they promote healing. Any dietary changes should be discussed with your physician and monitored carefully.

Herbalism is the oldest biologically based therapy—and, indeed, the oldest known form of health care. Although herbs sound harmless enough, they may have side effects, contain impurities, or interact with other drugs. For example, patients who take warfarin, a blood thinner, could bleed to death if they also take the herb ginseng. St. John's wort can cause dangerously high blood pressure when combined with aged cheese, Chianti wine, or other foods that contain tyramine.

Orthomolecular therapy involves the use of combinations of vitamins, minerals, and amino acids. However, these supplements are not regulated, and the doses often far exceed what we normally consume. The doses in megavitamins, for example, are much higher than the FDA's recommended daily allowances. Orthomolecular therapies have no proven benefits and can be toxic.

Another biologically based therapy, chelation, involves injecting a synthetic solution (ethylenediaminetetraacetic acid, or EDTA) to bind with and remove toxins from the bloodstream. Chelation therapy is widely used to treat lead poisoning in Western medicine, but its effectiveness and safety are still under investigation.

Mind-Body Manipulative Techniques: In addition, **mind-body manipulative techniques** involve physically manipulating the body. They include chiropractic care, massage, Rolfing, reflexology, and postural reeducation.

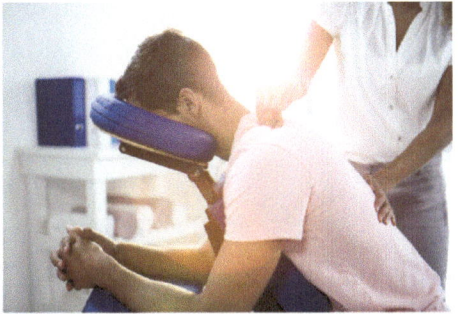

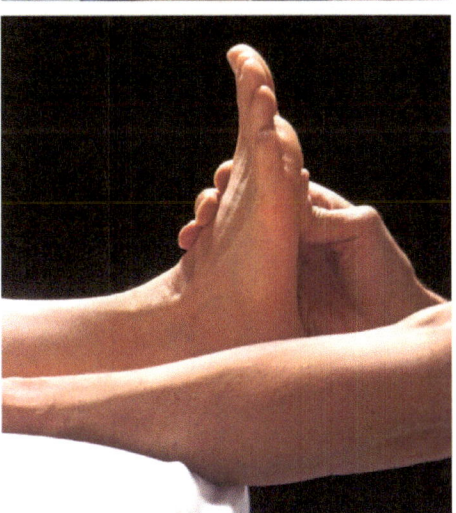

Photo 13.5   Both chiropractors (top) and Rolfers (bottom) seek to correct posture and bodily alignment in their patients. Chiropractors use massage, along with other spine manipulation methods, to treat pain and discomfort. Rolfers apply deep stimulation to the body's connective tissue in order to treat pain.

Source: Wavebreakmedia/Shutterstock (top) and Tomas del amo/Alamy (bottom)

Chiropractic care manipulates the spine, using massage, heat and ice, and exercises, and provides education about positive lifestyle changes. It is used to treat lower back pain, neck pain, joint immobility, and headaches. Between 1997 and 2006, the number of people seeking chiropractic treatment increased by 57% (Davis, Sirovich, & Weeks, 2010). The jury is still out on whether chiropractic care is effective at relieving acute pain. There is no consistent evidence that it is effective for patients with chronic pain (Ernst, 2004; Shaw et al., 2010) or in treating other issues, such as insomnia or the symptoms of menopause (Goto et al., 2014; Kingston, Raggio, Spencer, Stalaker, & Tuchin, 2010).

Rolfing is a form of deep-tissue massage, based on the belief that good health depends on correct body alignment. It was developed more than 50 years ago by Dr. Ida Rolf and involves manipulating connective tissue throughout the body, called fascia. There is no scientific evidence that Rolfing has any benefits.

Massage therapy can range from stroking to kneading. It has been shown to reduce nausea and vomiting in patients undergoing cancer treatment and to relieve stress, pain, muscle soreness, fatigue, and constipation. It may improve the development of infants with low birth weight and help in controlling asthma. In combination with exercise or traditional medicine, massage has also proven helpful for patients with fibromyalgia (Li, Wang, Feng, Yang, & Sun, 2014) and multiple sclerosis (Negahban, Rezaie, & Goharpey, 2013). It is not clear whether it is the actual tissue manipulation or simply the human touch that improves these conditions (**Photo 13.5**).

Energy Therapies: Another alternative therapy, **energy therapy**, claims to draw on a universal life force in and around the body. This includes the use of magnets, yoga, and Reiki. Magnet-based therapies apply magnetic fields or pulsed electrical fields to relieve pain. There is no evidence of any benefit from this treatment, although medically administered electromagnetic pulses can jump-start the healing of bone fractures. High-frequency magnetic stimulation of the brain has also been used to treat major depression and obsessive-compulsive disorder, but it is less effective than ordinary electroconvulsive therapy (Berlim, Van den Eynde, & Daskalakis, 2013).

Reiki is a Japanese practice that channels energy through the "laying on of hands" to promote healing. Reiki may help to relieve stress and has been shown to promote quality of life in terminally ill patients (Henneghan & Schnyer, 2013) and in women undergoing chemotherapy for breast cancer (Orsak, Stevens, Brufsky, Kajumba, & Dougall, 2015). However, this evidence should be interpreted with caution. (The cancer patients had reported improvements even before the Reiki was performed.)

People seek out alternative and complementary treatments for many reasons. They may feel dissatisfaction with their existing health care, they may be guided by cultural beliefs and practices, or they may just want to try everything possible to reduce pain. However, patients should choose carefully. Unproved therapies are unlikely to help, and they may have serious side effects. They could even be life-threatening.

Thinking About Health

■ Which CAM practices have scientific evidence to support them? Which do not?

■ How willing are you to rely on CAM therapies, and why?

The Placebo Effect

When it comes to our health, we want to feel better as quickly as possible—and sometimes we do, for just that reason. Some treatments work because we want them to. This is the **placebo effect**, and it is powerful. We introduced the placebo effect in Chapter 2, where we discussed its role in experimental research in health psychology. How and why, though, do placebos work?

Placebos as Treatment

A *placebo* (Latin for "I shall please") is basically a fake treatment. A typical example of one is when doctors prescribe an inactive substance such as sugar, distilled water, or saline solution; sham surgical procedures are also sometimes used in research. The patient thinks that the placebo will provide benefits, and so it does. The term originates from the fourteenth century, referring to hired mourners at funerals. These people would show up and begin wailing, crying *"Placebo Domino in regione vivorum"* (from Psalm 114, "I shall please the Lord"). The mourners were stand-ins for members of the family, brought in to give the funeral a credible feel (de Craen, Kaptchuk, Tijssen, & Kleijnen, 1999).

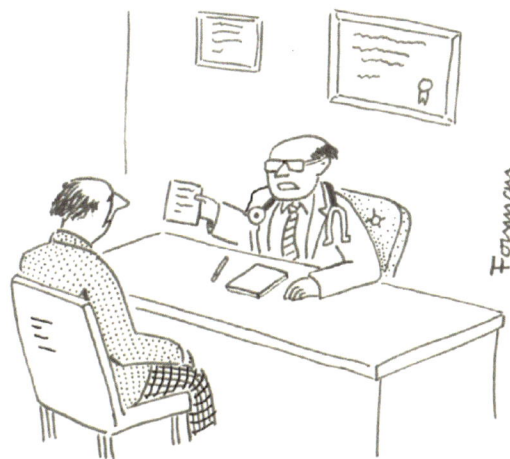

Photo 13.6   *"This is only a placebo, but trust me, it works!"*

Source: Kresten Forsman/www.CartoonStock.com

Placebos first appeared in medicine in the late eighteenth century, more to placate than to benefit the patient (Hooper & Quincy, 1811). In early medicine, treatments were largely hopeless, and the physician's role, according to sixteenth-century surgeon Ambroise Paré, was to "cure occasionally, relieve often, and console always." Yet placebos proved more powerful than those physicians knew.

Placebos help primarily because the patient expects that they will help. Sometimes, the doctor's orders are all it takes to feel better. Jan, a patient with an eating disorder, was going through physical and emotional distress. Her mother gave her a pill container with five small pink pills. If things "got really, really bad," Jan should take one or two, and she would feel better. Jan kept the vial of pills with her at all times for 10 years. She never used them, and yet her mood improved, and she made it through that dark period. She has since sought treatment and recovered fully from her eating disorder, but she still credits that little vial of pills (a placebo) for helping her (**Photo 13.6**).

Placebos in Clinical Trials

Before a drug is available for sale in the United States, it must undergo extensive clinical trials to prove that it is safe and effective. A safe drug is free of dangerous side effects, and an effective drug is more effective than a placebo. For that very reason, placebos play a critical role in drug testing.

To establish a drug's efficacy and safety, a rigorous scientific process is used. In a double-blind experiment, as we saw in Chapter 2, one group of patients receives drug treatment and another group receives placebo treatment. The experiment is "double-blind" because neither the researcher nor the patients themselves know which pill they have been given. Only after the study has ended do the researchers examine the code of the pills to determine which group of patients received the drug and which received the placebo. Patients often report improvements after taking the placebo; if there is significant improvement from the actual drug over and above any improvement from the placebo, the drug is considered beneficial.

Why Placebos Work

The placebo effect shows something that we have encountered often: the ability of the mind to influence the body. A placebo can alter the experience of pain, the quantity of white blood cells in the immune system, and the brain chemistry of a Parkinson's patient (LeBlanc, 2014). But why? There are several theories to explain how placebos work.

Meaning theory (or *meaning response theory*) points to the symbolism associated with treatment and the cultural factors behind it (Barrett et al., 2006; Moerman, 2002). It asks what we see when we look at treatment. For example, maybe we think that two pills work better than one, capsules work better than tablets, injections are better than pills, and branded pills work better than generic ones. The more expensive the pill, the more effective it is assumed to be. Pills that are pink, orange, or red (warm colors) are associated with stimulants, and pills that are green or blue (cool colors) are associated with sedatives or depressants (de Craen, Roos, De Vries, & Kleijnen, 1996; LeBlanc, 2014). Meaning theory also supports the importance of the doctor–patient relationship. A warm, enthusiastic bedside manner increases the effectiveness of treatment—and even of placebos (Di Blasi, Harkness, Ernst, Georgiou, & Kleijnen, 2001).

Expectancy theory points instead to what a patient is led to believe. In one classic study, undergraduates received a placebo cream, called Trivaricane, to lessen the pain of an electrical stimulation (Montgomery & Kirsch, 1996). The participants were greeted at the University Student Health Center and introduced to an experimenter wearing a white lab coat. The experimenter told them that they were part of a clinical trial, testing a new topical anesthetic. Trivaricane, they were told, had proved effective in preliminary studies at other universities. The participants completed a medical screening form, and the experimenter donned surgical gloves "to protect against overexposure." The cream was then applied from a tube to one of the subject's index fingers with a cotton swab. One finger was treated with the placebo Trivaricane, and the other finger was left untreated. The "medication" was allowed to "take effect," before a mildly painful electrical shock was administered to both fingers. After one minute, participants were asked to rate the intensity of the pain. The result was an overwhelming decrease in pain for fingers "treated" with the Trivaricane (Montgomery & Kirsch, 1996). Other tests of the expectancy theory have involved an alcohol placebo (Hull & Bond, 1986), placebo (decaffeinated) coffee (Flaten, Aasli, & Blumenthal, 2003; Kirsch, 1999; Kirsch & Sapirstein, 1998), and placebo antidepressants and sedatives (Jensen & Karoly, 1991; Kirsch & Sapirstein, 1998).

Could the medically charged context have made the difference? Think of the health center, the white lab coat, the surgical gloves, the appearance of a pharmaceutical company, and more. *Classical conditioning*, however, offers another explanation: The idea is that the placebo effect is learned. For example, placebo "aspirin" pills work because of our associations with actual aspirin (Ader, 1997; Benedetti et al., 2009; LeBlanc, 2014). We know from experience to associate pain relief with aspirin's shape, color, and taste. Thus, we feel the effects that we expect based on past experience.

Whatever the explanation, medically prescribed treatments make people feel better. And again, they work best when the patient understands the diagnosis and trusts the physician. When doctors and patients have a positive relationship and good communication, treatment will be more beneficial, and the patient's health is more likely to improve.

Thinking About Health

■ What is the placebo effect, and why does it work?

■ What personal experiences do you have with the placebo effect?

Chapter Summary

Healthcare services differ around the world and within the United States. They include office visits, urgent care, telemedicine, emergency departments, inpatient and outpatient care, and long-term care in an assisted living facility or nursing home. In countries without universal health care, health insurance options can limit the availability of health care, especially for lower-income people, but the Affordable Care Act has changed that for some U.S. citizens. Interpersonal and sociocultural factors determine who uses health care services—and who is likely to delay using them or misuse them. Many of the same factors explain why some people have a difficult time following their doctor's recommendations, the problem of noncompliance. The quality of the patient–practitioner relationship depends on effective communication, especially in the hospital setting. Physicians should avoid medical jargon and encourage reciprocity and health literacy. Alternative and complementary treatments are growing in popularity, but many do not stand up to empirical evidence. The placebo effect has an important role in the approval process for pharmaceutical and medical treatments in the United States.

KEY TERMS ▶ Medicaid p. 392, Medicare p. 392, Affordable Care Act (ACA) p. 392, universal health care p. 390, secondary gains p. 396, illness anxiety disorder p. 396, compliance (or *adherence*) p. 397, creative nonadherence p. 398, patient-centered care p. 400, doctor-centered care p. 400, health literacy p. 401, complementary and alternative medicine (CAM) p. 405, acupuncture p. 408, ayurveda p. 408, homeopathy p. 408, mind-body techniques p. 408, biologically based therapies p. 408, mind-body manipulative techniques p. 409, energy therapies p. 409, placebo effect p. 410

CHAPTER 14

Achieving Emotional Health and Well-Being and Future Directions in Health Psychology

Learning Outcomes

After reading this chapter, you should be able to:

- **Define** *positive psychology* and explain why we study it.
- **Outline** the developmental and sociocultural influences on well-being and resilience.
- **Identify** potential interventions for increasing well-being.
- **Describe** the future of health psychology.
- **Identify** the global and sociocultural challenges the health psychology field will face.
- **Name** some of the health psychology field's emerging areas.
- **Explain** how one would become a health psychologist and identify other careers in the field of health.

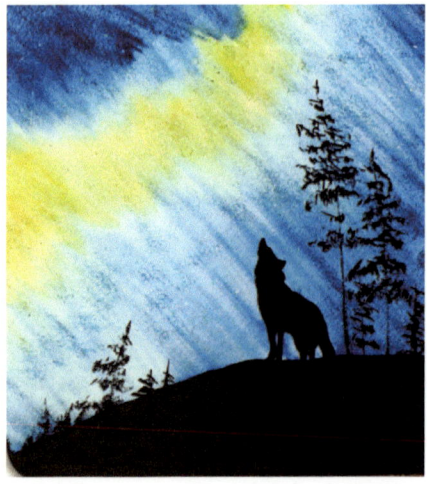

Photo 14.1

Nikolaj2/Getty Images

There is a Cherokee parable called Two Wolves that describes a conversation between a grandfather and his grandson:

An old Cherokee man is teaching his grandson about life. "A fight is going on inside me," he says to the boy.

"It is a terrible fight and it is between two wolves. One is evil," he continues. "He is anger, envy, sorrow, regret, greed, arrogance, self-pity, guilt, resentment, inferiority, lies, false pride, superiority, and ego. The other one is good. He is joy, peace, love, hope, serenity, humility, kindness, benevolence, empathy, generosity, truth, compassion, and faith. The same fight is going on inside you—and inside every other person, too."

The grandson thinks about this for a minute and then asks his grandfather, "Which wolf will win?"

His grandfather simply replies, "The one you feed."(Photo 14.1).

As a graduate student interviewing caregivers and their spouses who were living with Alzheimer's disease or

DOI: 10.4324/9781032643090-14

Parkinson's disease, my aim was to learn which coping strategies helped them adjust to these chronic, devastating, and life-altering conditions. In meeting hundreds of patients and caregivers, I learned that knowing which strategies are better in certain circumstances is important—but this knowledge didn't answer the bigger, more important questions. Why, I kept asking myself, do some people become the masters of their illness and others the victims? Why do some people see their health as a conquerable challenge, while others feel overwhelmed by it? Is personality the key? Is it values? Is it faith? Is it social support and valuable resources? Who chooses which wolf to feed, and why? I wondered if, perhaps, the biopsychosocial model could help tease apart these questions.

What is it about our culture, our personalities, our circumstances, and our experiences that influences who we become?

We all want to be happy and live satisfying lives. Good health contributes to a fulfilling life, and poor health impairs our quality of life. In turn, genetic predisposition, environmental factors, and risky behaviors may all have negative health outcomes. Throughout this book, we have explored health from a biopsychosocial approach. Although it is important to understand the role of biological, psychological, and social factors in poor health outcomes, it is equally important to explore these links in the context of positive health outcomes. How we adapt to life's challenges depends in large part on *which wolf we feed*, as the Cherokee parable says. Knowing which cognitive styles and personal resources lead to better outcomes can help us all make choices that contribute to emotional health and well-being.

In this chapter, we explore the positive psychology of health. And then we turn to the future of the field of health psychology. We look at how biopsychosocial factors influence our approach to and management of our health, and how we can achieve positive outcomes: high quality of life and well-being. We also examine the characteristics, types, and qualities of happiness, well-being, and resilience in the United States and around the world. As we have seen so often in previous chapters, personality, culture, spirituality, and humor intersect with genetics, health, and illness

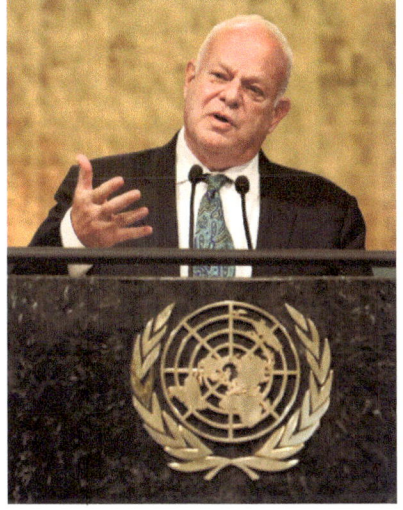

Photo 14.2   "If psychologists wish to improve the human condition, it is not enough to help those who suffer. The majority … also need examples and advice to reach a richer and more fulfilling existence," wrote Martin Seligman, the father of the positive psychology movement (Seligman & Csikszentmihalyi, 2000).

Source: J. Countless/Getty Images

Positive Psychology and Well-Being

The field of psychology has been changing. It is no longer just about understanding psychological dysfunction but also about how psychologically healthy people can live happier and more fulfilled lives. This new approach, called **positive psychology**, studies optimal human functioning (Seligman & Csikszentmihalyi, 2000) and what makes life most worth living (Peterson, Park, & Sweeney, 2008). The field seeks to discover what fosters the best and what remedies the worst in life, and it challenges scientists and practitioners alike to think about strengths as well as weaknesses. It considers what makes life good and explores adaptations to challenging health outcomes (**Photo 14.2**).

The Development of Positive Psychology

Positive psychology emerged in 1998 when Martin Seligman, then president of the American Psychological Association, made it the centerpiece of his presidency. In less than a decade, positive psychology had taken off, and its popularity is still growing among the general public, the academic community, and mental health providers. Already it has helped identify and promote positive approaches to living within the context of economic, sociocultural, developmental, mental, and physical health challenges.

Positive psychology goes hand in hand with the movement away from the biomedical model and toward the biopsychosocial model. Both are based on the idea that happiness, or a good life, is not just the absence of what is bad, problematic, or emotionally challenging. Rather, learning how to be happy is just as important as learning how to avoid feeling bad. Keep in mind, however, that we are discussing evidence-based, empirically sound psychological science—not untested self-help.

Since its inception the area of positive psychology has experienced several waves of theory and research. The first wave when the field began was focused simplistically on understanding well-being and flourishing (Lomas & Ivtzan, 2016; van Zyl et al., 2024). The second wave pursued the complexity of flourishing integrating the dynamic nature of both positive and negative experiences as influences on positive outcomes, such as post-traumatic growth. The third wave focused on broadening the concept of positive psychology to think about the interactional and intersectional nature of individuals within their social systems, cultures, and contexts (van Zyl et al., 2024). As with many new movements, positive psychology is still developing. But most would agree that research has helped to elucidate what makes us happy and what makes life worth living, even within the context of difficult health conditions. The true test of this approach is whether these findings hold up over time and lead to useful programs that help people to be happier.

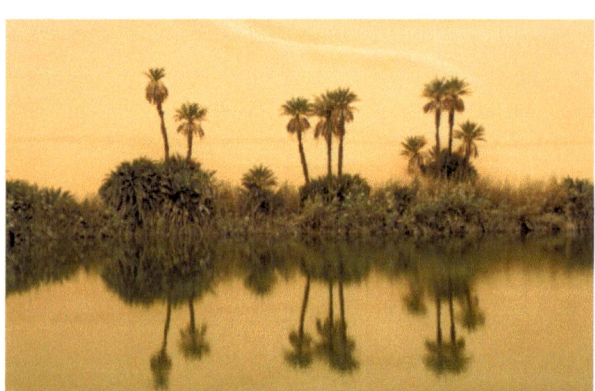

Photo 14.3   Understanding adaptation is like seeing a mirage. Although an optimal state of health and high quality of life may appear to be easily understood, researchers and clinicians find it difficult to define how we adapt to achieve each

Source: JK reortage/Alamy

Adaptation

Understanding how people adapt to the complex nature of health and illness has been likened to a desert mirage. From a distance, good health and adjustment to living with illness appear clear, and yet, just as researchers and clinicians try to define them, they can seem to disappear (Dubos, 1961; Walker, Jackson, & Littlejohn, 2004).

That is because *adaptation* is not just an achievement: It is a process. As we adapt to our changing lives, we adjust our thoughts and behaviors to make the situation more favorable or suitable for ourselves. In adapting, we use conscious awareness and personal choices to create greater consistency in our lives (**Photo 14.3**) (Roy & Andrews, 1999; Weinert, Cudney, & Spring, 2008).

In the context of health, adaptation happens all the time. People make lifestyle choices and behavioral changes to be healthier, to have more energy, and to improve their mood and self-esteem. They make changes in response to feeling sick, as with a cold, the flu, or a stomach virus. Adaptation is also necessary when one is diagnosed with a chronic condition, has to undergo surgery, develops physical disabilities, or becomes a caregiver for a loved one with a chronic illness (see Chapter 12). All of these are highly stressful situations, demanding significant adjustment to a new distressing reality (Kleftaras & Psarra, 2012; Psarra & Kleftaras, 2013). In each, too, depression is a common symptom. Although some people manage to adapt successfully, others fail to adjust to and accept their circumstances (Psarra & Kleftaras, 2013).

Many factors may assist in adaptation—from positive personality traits such as optimism and resilience to a sense of control or meaning in life. In one study, researchers examined factors that promoted positive adaptation during a major life transition that confronts millions of college freshmen every year—adapting to college. Students who had an optimistic thinking style were more likely to have a positive adjustment to college (Leary & DeRosier, 2012; Umuco et al., 2024).

We will examine the factors that help in adaptation more in depth later in the chapter. First, we need a clear understanding of the optimal state of health.

Thinking About Health

- Considering what you have learned about the biopsychosocial perspective, how might positive psychology influence health and behavior?

- How might understanding illness contribute to positive psychology and adaptation?

Health, Wellness, and Well-Being

It is tempting to say that health is simply the absence of disease—tempting, but also wrong. As we saw in Chapter 1, health, illness, and well-being intersect. Our health affects and is affected by many facets of our lives, from employment and income to our social activities, our moods, and our overall well-being (Binder & Coad, 2013).

Throughout this book, we have examined health-promoting behaviors, good coping strategies, and the positive impact they have on our health. We have seen the importance of getting enough sleep, eating well, exercising, fostering a sense of control, being connected to others, having financial stability, and not smoking. These and more all come together to create *wellness*. In addition, we have considered health-compromising behaviors, poor lifestyle choices, and their negative impact. We have explored stress and seen how living with chronic illness in its terminal phase can challenge one's sense of self and quality of life. Yet people facing health crises can adapt and grow in the face of these challenges, attaining *well-being*. To understand how and why, it helps to distinguish between *wellness* and *well-being*.

Wellness

Wellness is good physical and mental health. There are varying degrees of wellness, even for those who are ill: It is a continuum (as seen in **Figure 14.1** and Chapter 1). Good health is important for a high level of wellness; chronic disorders, poor health, and pain significantly reduce wellness. Our health, both mental and physical, often changes, so wellness is a dynamic concept. It involves integrating and balancing one's physical and mental states (Dunn, 1977), including body, mind, and spirit (Bezner, Adams, & Steinhardt, 1997).

The **wheel of wellness** (Kauppi et al., 2023; Sweeney & Witmer, 1991; Witmer & Sweeney, 1992; Witmer, Sweeney, & Myers, 1998) considers seven factors that contribute to an optimal state of health, encompassing every domain of our lives: spiritual, emotional, intellectual, physical, social, environmental, and financial. **Figure 14.2** shows how it might apply to college students. As you can see, there are simple ways that you can live better to achieve greater wellness. The ability to self-regulate, identify with one's work, and maintain valuable friendships are the strongest predictors of wellness (Hermon & Hazler, 1999).

Other approaches to wellness have identified as many as 12 different factors. A sense of self-worth and a sense of control over one's life are crucial, and illness can take its toll on both. Emotional awareness, coping effectively, and realistic beliefs are important, as are good stress management and creative problem-solving. Sound identity, including cultural identity, helps to shore up one's sense of self in the face of health challenges (see Chapter 7). In turn, these components of wellness vary by gender, culture, and point in the lifespan.

Finally, maintaining a sense of humor is essential in the face of crises of any sort (Proyer et al., 2018; Tandler & Proyer, 2022). Recognizing and appreciating funny things (Solomon, 1996) lead to beneficial physical changes: A hearty laugh causes the skeletal muscles to relax, boosts the immune system, and

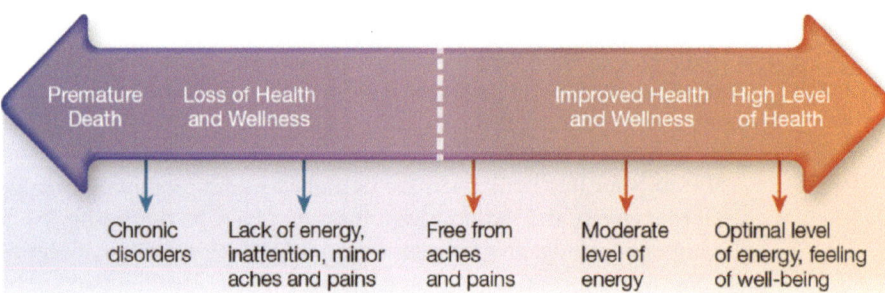

Figure 14.1   The illness–wellness continuum in the context of well-being.

Source: Information from Ryan and Travis (1981)

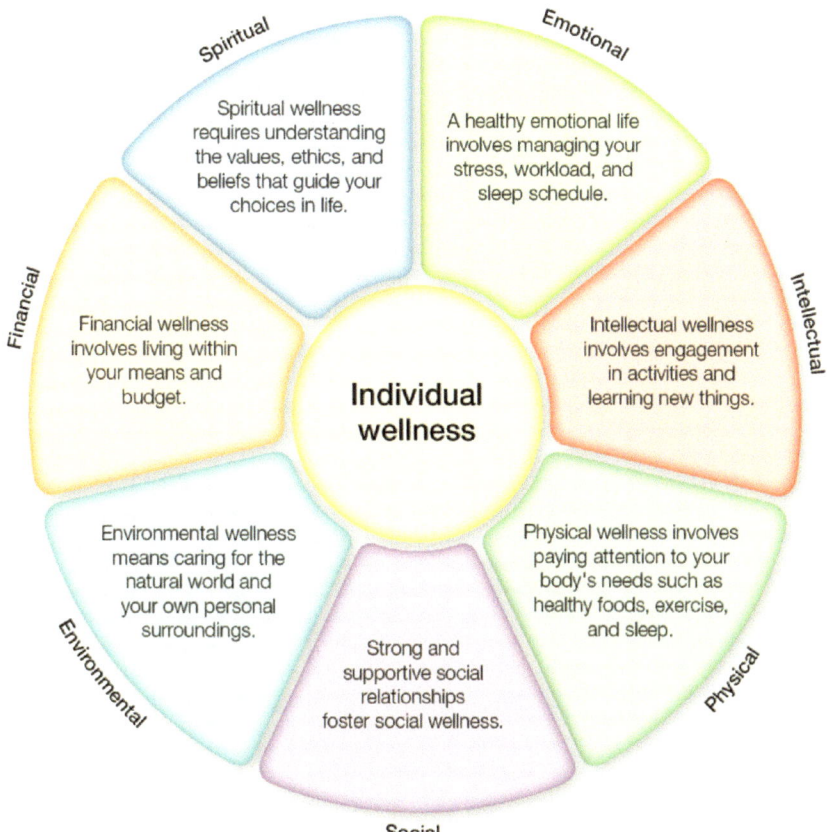

Figure 14.2   The wheel of wellness for college students.

Source: Information from Sweeney and Witmer (1991)

stimulates heart rate and circulation—bringing an influx of energy and nutrients to vital organs. A sense of humor also aids in digestion and, through the release of endorphins in the brain, enhances wellness and a sense of well-being (Erdman, 1991). In addition, it lessens symptoms of depression, provides pain relief (Carroll, 1990), boosts self-esteem, and lowers perceived stress (Kuiper, Martin, & Olinger, 1993). People with a good sense of humor tend to be more positive and respond better to both positive and negative life events (Martin, Kuiper, Olinger, & Dance, 1993; Solomon, 1996). Looking on the bright side helps promote self-awareness and social cohesion, diffusing conflicts and reducing feelings of hostility (Burns, 1989; Burns, Johnson, Mahoney, Devine, & Pawl, 1996; Morreall, 1991; Richman, 1995).

In addition to having a good sense of humor, playfulness across the life span and especially in adulthood is linked to many positive outcomes from better coping, increased life satisfaction and well-being, to better relationships with others, higher work-life balance and greater satisfaction at work (Clifford et al., 2024; Frazier et al., 2024; Lubbers et al., 2023; Shen, 2020; Tandler et al., 2024).

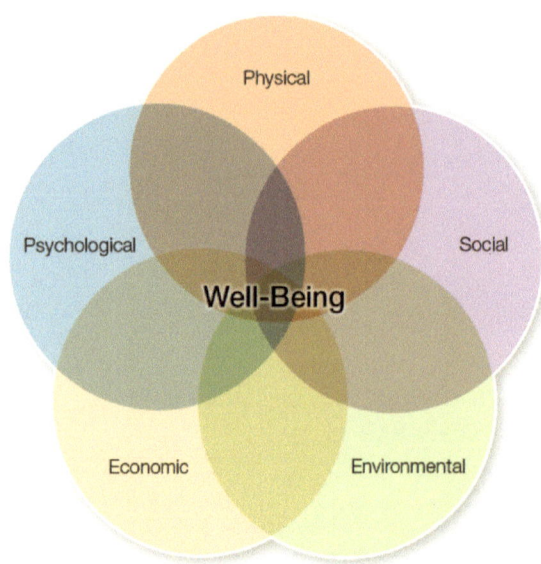

Figure 14.3   Factors that contribute to well-being.

Greater wellness may be part of what differentiates a patient who sees opportunities for growth even in the face of chronic illness from a patient who feels helpless and overwhelmed. As the old Cherokee story goes, where you fall on the illness—wellness continuum may be, in large part, due to which wolf you choose to feed.

Well-Being

Well-being is how we *feel* about ourselves and our lives, and it, too, has many components. People high in well-being are curious about what goes on around them and enjoy what they do. They have positive relationships and a sense of control in their lives. Well-being also encompasses a sense of fulfillment and purpose in life (Whitbourne & Ebmeyer, 2013).

Well-being is a biopsychosocial concept, and its physical, psychological, and social aspects engage and influence one another (as shown in **Figure 14.3**). So, too, do the influences of the environment and our socioeconomic status. *Physical well-being* is the knowledge that we can function typically in such activities as bathing, dressing, eating, and moving around (U.S. Department of Health & Human Services, 2000a). *Emotional well-being* comes from having intact cognitive capacities and minimal fear, anxiety, stress, depression, or other negative emotions. Finally, *social well-being* is the ability to derive fulfillment from social, familial, and intimate engagement with others.

Psychology began to focus on well-being in 1989 when Carol Ryff saw a gap in research on aging and health: No one focused on the positive outcomes. Like the wheel of wellness, Ryff's concept of well-being encompasses many different factors:

- *autonomy*: living in accord with one's personal convictions
- *environmental mastery*: the ability to manage one's own life
- *personal growth*: reaching full potential
- *positive relationships*: fulfilling relations with others
- *purpose in life*: a sense that life has meaning and direction
- *self-acceptance*: self-awareness and acceptance of oneself

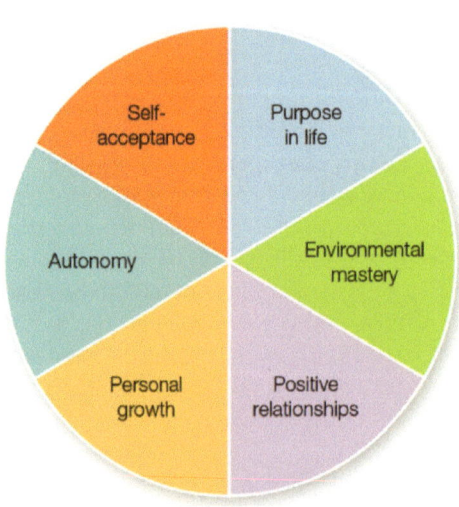

Figure 14.4   Dimensions of well-being.

Source: Information from Ryff (2014)

Autonomy

High scorer	Is self-determining and independent; able to resist social pressures to think and act in certain ways; regulates behavior from within; evaluates self by personal standards
Low scorer	Is concerned about the expectations and evaluations of others; relies on judgment of others to make important decisions; conforms to social pressures to think and act in certain ways

Environmental mastery

High scorer	Has a sense of mastery and competence in managing the environment; controls complex array of external activities; makes effective use of surrounding opportunities; able to choose or create contexts suitable to personal needs and values
Low scorer	Has difficulty managing everyday affairs; feels unable to change or improve surrounding context; is unaware of surrounding opportunities; lacks sense of control over external world

Personal growth

High scorer	Has a feeling of continued development; sees self as growing and expanding; is open to new experiences; has sense of realizing potential; sees improvement in self and behavior over time; is changing in ways that reflect more self-knowledge and effectiveness
Low scorer	Has a sense of personal stagnation; lacks sense of improvement or expansion over time; feels bored and uninterested in life; feels unable to develop new attitudes or behaviors

Positive relationships

High scorer	Has warm, satisfying, trusting relationships with others; is concerned about the welfare of others; capable of strong empathy, affection, and intimacy; understands give and take of human relationships
Low scorer	Has few close, trusting relationships with others; finds it difficult to be warm, open, concerned about others; is isolated and frustrated in interpersonal relationships; not willing to make compromises to sustain important ties with others

Purpose in life

High scorer	Has goals in life and a sense of direction; feels there is meaning to present and past life; holds beliefs that give life purpose; has aims and objectives for living
Low scorer	Lacks a sense of meaning in life; has few goals or aims; lacks sense of direction; does not see purpose in past life; has no outlooks or beliefs that give meaning

Self-acceptance

High scorer	Possesses a positive attitude toward the self; acknowledges and accepts multiple aspects of self, including good and bad qualities; feels positive about past life
Low scorer	Feels dissatisfied with self; is disappointed with what has occurred in past life; is troubled by certain personal qualities; wishes to be different

Source: Information from Ryff (2014).

Table 14.1 Dimensions of the psychological well-being scale

As Ryff's model suggests, as shown in **Figure 14.4** and more in-depth in **Table 14.1**, many factors can influence well-being—from gender, age, and education to income, employment status, social and intimate relationships, and personality (Binder & Coad, 2013). One of the strongest correlates of well-being, however, is health: The healthier you feel, the higher your well-being is likely to be (Dolan & Peasgood, 2008; Easterlin, 2003). Disabilities lower overall well-being (Brickman, Coates, & Janoff-Bullman, 1978; Oswald & Powdthavee, 2008; Uppal, 2006), as do rheumatoid arthritis, gastric distress, migraines, epilepsy, pain, and drug and alcohol abuse (Binder & Coad, 2013). Treatments for chronic and life-threatening illnesses also affect well-being.

Hedonic and Eudaimonic Well-Being

We can also distinguish between *hedonic* and *eudaimonic* well-being—or well-being as happiness and well-being as fulfillment. Many people believe that there is more to life than simple pleasures, and true well-being comes from doing something virtuous and worthwhile. For them, a meaningful life encompasses service to something higher than themselves.

Hedonic well-being is the experience of positive emotional states, such as joy, happiness, contentment, and satisfaction (Kashdan, Biswas-Diener, & King, 2008). The term derives from *hedonia*, or seeking pleasure and relaxation. It is the belief that you are getting the things you want and thus experiencing happiness (Kraut, 1979). A vast amount of research has demonstrated that **positive affect**—pleasurable emotions such as happiness, joy, enthusiasm, and contentment—is associated with many health benefits. These include better cardiovascular health, better outcomes in the context of chronic diseases (including cancer and HIV), and even a longer life (Pressman, Jenkins, & Moskowitz, 2019). More specifically, positive affect is associated with hedonic well-being, and both have been associated with longevity (Pressman & Cohen, 2005), slower progression of disease, and less pain (Pressman et al., 2019). To determine if you have an inclination toward positive affect, see **Table 14.2**.

Eudaimonic well-being is a sense of meaning and purpose in life. It goes beyond hedonic happiness to include personal growth, intrinsic motivation, vitality, wisdom, and maturity (Bauer & McAdams, 2010; Frazier, Barreto, & Newman, 2012; Frazier et al., 2024; Ryff, 2013). The term derives from the Latin word *daimon*, or one's true nature. It is the integration of our true self with our environment, which leads to authentic self-expression and the feeling of being alive (Ryan & Deci, 2001; Ryff, 2013; Sheldon, Corcoran, & Prentice, 2019). It is the pursuit of life activities that are most congruent with our values and sense of self (Vittersø, 2004). The ancient Greek philosopher Plato spoke of *eudemonia* as "the good composed of all goods, an ability that suffices for living well." His pupil Aristotle argued similarly for a life that actualizes human potential (as translated by Broadie & Rowe, 2002; Young, 1985). People who are high in eudemonia do things because the activities are worthwhile and because they benefit others (Huta, Park, Peterson, & Seligman, 2003).

Since eudaimonic well-being is now recognized as a critical ingredient for health, lessening physical and cognitive decline with aging is an important goal. Recently, researchers designed an 8-week program called "Lighten UP!" to promote eudaimonic well-being in older adults by training them to identify and nurture positive emotions (Friedman et al., 2019). The techniques were designed to increase meaningful life engagement and help people negotiate negative experiences across all aspects of their lives. The findings showed that,

This scale consists of a number of words that describe different feelings and emotions. Read each item and then list the number from the scale below next to each word. **Indicate to what extent you feel this way right now, that is, at the present moment,** *OR* **indicate the extent you have felt this way over the past week (circle the instructions you followed when taking this measure).**

1	2	3	4	5
Very Slightly or Not at All	A Little	Moderately	Quite a Bit	Extremely

_____ 1. Interested	_____ 11. Irritable
_____ 2. Distressed	_____ 12. Alert
_____ 3. Excited	_____ 13. Ashamed
_____ 4. Upset	_____ 14. Inspired
_____ 5. Strong	_____ 15. Nervous
_____ 6. Guilty	_____ 16. Determined
_____ 7. Scared	_____ 17. Attentive
_____ 8. Hostile	_____ 18. Jittery
_____ 9. Enthusiastic	_____ 19. Active
_____ 10. Proud	_____ 20. Afraid

Scoring instructions:

Positive Affect Score: Add the scores on items 1, 3, 5, 9, 10, 12, 14, 16, 17, and 19. Scores can range from 10 to 50, with higher scores representing higher levels of positive affect. Mean Scores: Momentary = 29.7 (SD = 7.9); Weekly = 33.3 (SD = 7.2)

Negative Affect Score: Add the scores on items 2, 4, 6, 7, 8, 11, 13, 15, 18, and 20. Scores can range from 10 to 50, with lower scores representing lower levels of negative affect. Mean Scores: Momentary = 14.8 (SD = 5.4); Weekly = 17.4 (SD = 6.2)

Table 14.2   The positive and negative affect schedule (panas) questionnaire

after the program, older adults reported significantly higher eudaimonic well-being, even six months later. Programs such as these demonstrate that our affect and attitudes can change across the lifespan and that these changes are good for our health, especially in later life, when there are many challenges to health and well-being.

Well-being across the lifespan

Well-being changes across the adult lifespan. Younger and middle-aged adults see themselves as improving over time in eudaimonic well-being, whereas older adults often anticipate declines (Frazier et al., 2012; Ryff, 2014). And personal growth and purpose in life do appear to decline with age. In adults older than 65, feeling younger leads to higher well-being, perhaps because feeling younger late in life is tied directly to health. Older adults who feel better also tend to feel younger (Ward, 2010).

At any age, however, higher well-being depends on a realistic perspective on ourselves and our health (Frazier et al., 2012; Lachman, Röcke, Rosnick, & Ryff, 2008). Whenever we face a challenge, from chronic illness to a change at work, our well-being is at stake. With each adverse outcome, whether a hearing or visual impairment or unemployment, the overall quality of life tends to decline, independent of age, sex, education, or frailty (Andrew, Fisk, & Rockwood, 2012). People who have higher environmental mastery, autonomy, and personal growth tend to navigate the changes better (Frazier et al., 2012). People with greater well-being have fewer chronic conditions, are more productive in life and work, and are less likely to need or use health care services (Keyes & Grzywacz, 2005). Lower levels of well-being are associated with greater mortality five years after a life challenge (Andrew et al., 2012).

Successful Aging: The renowned architect Frank Lloyd Wright once said, "The longer I live, the more beautiful life becomes." *Gerontologists*, psychologists who focus on studying the end of the lifespan, argue that now that people are living longer, maintaining well-being and quality of life for as long as possible, rather than just avoiding disease or disability, is the goal. The idea is to "add life to years," not merely to add years to a life. This is **successful aging**, defined as a low probability of disease and disability coupled with high cognitive and physical functioning and active engagement in life (Rowe & Kahn, 1997; Friedman et al., 2019).

Gerontologists speak of the *well-being paradox*, in which older adults who have significant health challenges (including disease and disability) still report high levels of subjective well-being. Those of us who are younger might wonder: How can you be happy with all those aches and pains? Research shows that younger and older adults do not hold the same expectations about what later life and the aging process are like (Castel, 2019). For instance, in one large-scale study of people aged 75 or older, 80% said they were "happy" or "very happy" (Castel, 2019; Taylor, 2009). The effect of older adults may skew more positively.

Many theories and models of successful aging have developed to capture and articulate what people can do to offset disease, prolong functioning, and remain actively engaged in life. From the perspective of developmental science and health psychology, we can make lifestyle choices at any age that will increase our chances of successful aging. In the words of jazz musician Eubie Blake, "If I knew I was going to live this long, I would have taken better care of myself" (Castel, 2019). This quote captures what we have tried to emphasize in this book—that we all can live a life that leads to lifelong good health. Our attitudes and beliefs, happiness and life satisfaction, engagement in mental enrichment and physical exercise, and positive social relationships are the keys to successful aging and adding life to years.

Spirituality and Well-Being

Religion and spirituality are important social and psychological resources, especially late in life (Daaleman, Perera, & Studenski, 2004; Forlenza & Vallada, 2018). *Religion* refers to an organized social system. It encompasses beliefs in the divine or supernatural power, and it often involves rituals such as prayer and attending church, temple, or mosque (Koenig, 2018; Koenig, Larson, & Larson, 2001). *Spirituality* is a feeling of being moved by things outside oneself. Both religion and spirituality have been found to relate to well-being (Rippentrop, 2005).

More than 3000 empirical studies and over 100 reviews of the literature have shown the powerful impact of religion and spirituality on health (Oman, 2018). Religion has been linked to perceived health, energy, vitality, and longevity, as well as better recovery from illness and reduced risk of disease and disability (George, Larson, Koenig, & McCullough, 2000; Koenig, 2018; Rippentrop, 2005). Religious involvement has been associated with better outcomes in patients with coronary heart disease, hypertension, stroke, immune-related disease, and functional impairment (Koenig, 2018; Koenig, McCullough, & Larson, 2001). Religion can be a way of coping with the stress of illness (Jozwiak, 2007). Religious involvement is also consistently associated with lower mortality (McCullough, Hoyt, Larson, Koenig, & Thoresen, 2000). One reason may be that people active in religion often have a healthier lifestyle, with less drinking or smoking (Krause, 2008), and consistent opportunities for social interaction, as we saw in Chapter 3 with the health behaviors associated with longevity in people of the Mormon faith.

In one study (Horton, 2015), researchers asked emerging adults (a phase of the life span that covers the transition from adolescence to full-fledged adulthood) a series of open-ended questions (based on Wallace, Forman, Caldwell, & Willis, 2003) about their perception of the impact of religion on their lives, especially in regard to health. The questions probed young adults' evolving definition of religion and the factors that influence their faith but also asked them to consider what negative effects religion might have upon their health as well as what positive health behaviors religion might promote. Compared with white young adults, young African Americans were more likely to say that religion has helped them cut down on risky behaviors, such as substance abuse and unsafe sex when they thought God would not approve (Horton, 2015). However, several white young adults also said that God makes them accountable for their behaviors. One participant said that inspiration from God helps her keep her weight at a healthy level (Horton, 2015).

Psychologists have tried to use people's religious beliefs to help them manage a health problem, such as in the context of the obesity epidemic (Horton, 2015; Hummer, Rogers, Nam, & Ellison, 1999; Koenig, 2018; Koenig, Larson, & Larson, 2001). Social support within religious contexts, such as Bible studies, can foster and encourage greater physical activity among congregants (Kanu, Baker, & Brownson, 2008; Kim & Sobal, 2004), and can be a channel to teach obesity prevention (Ayers et al., 2010). The value of religion and spirituality as a social and psychological resource has been found across different denominations and practices (Kim-Prieto, 2014).

Health and Well-Being

Good health is important to well-being—and well-being is important to good health. Exercise, a healthy diet, and optimal sleep are all correlated with higher well-being, while poor body image lowers well-being (Carr & Friedman, 2005;

McKinley, 1999). Moreover, body esteem and well-being can both change over time (McKinley, 2006).

When it comes to disease, well-being is also crucial. Those with a greater purpose in life are at lower risk for mild cognitive impairment and even Alzheimer's disease (Boyle, Buchman, Barnes, & Bennett, 2010). They show lower mortality as well (Boyle et al., 2012). Well-being, in turn, is compromised by hypertension and congestive heart failure. One study looked at women with fibromyalgia, a painful disorder characterized by musculoskeletal pain, fatigue, and memory and mood problems. Although these patients reported lower well-being than healthy women—and the greater the disability, the greater the impact on well-being—a positive sense of well-being aided adaptation to symptoms and lessened the uncertainties of the disease (Anema, Johnson, Zeller, Fogg, & Zetterlund, 2009). In patients with rheumatoid arthritis, those with a greater sense of environmental mastery are less likely to develop depression. Women with greater environmental mastery and positive relations with others, especially a spouse, are also at less risk for preterm labor (Facchinetti, Ottolini, Fazzio, Rigatelli, & Volpe, 2007). Cancer survivors, and their caregiving spouses, tend to be high in social well-being, spirituality, and personal growth (Ruini & Vescovelli, 2013; Weiss, 2004).

Enhancing Well-Being

Many approaches to therapy can enhance emotional, psychological, social, and physical well-being (Fava, 1999). For example, in one unique study, a video game designed to strengthen well-being worked well for the visually impaired young adults who played it (Di Cagno et al., 2013).

Other approaches focus on positive psychology. Patients with depression and anxiety disorders were taught to keep daily diaries in which they recorded positive experiences, such as positive relations with others. They then discussed these experiences in their therapy sessions. Over time, they learned how not to stand in the way of positive experiences and how to enrich and expand upon them instead (Fava & Sonino, 2005; Fava et al., 2004; Fava, Rafanelli, Tomba, Guidi, & Grandi, 2011; Ruini & Fava, 2009; Ryff, 2014). The technique was so successful that many were able to discontinue their drug therapy, and the benefits were still evident after six years. The success of well-being therapy suggests that it may help those coping with chronic illnesses or significant health problems as well. The benefits of interventions grounded in positive psychology are seen across all ages and stages of life (Peng et al., 2024; Söderlund et al., 2024).

Thinking About Health

■ What is wellness, and how does it differ from well-being?

■ What factors influence well-being? What are the different types of well-being?

■ What steps can you take to enhance your own well-being?

Resilience

Resilience is the ability to successfully adapt and recover in the face of acute stress, trauma, or chronic adversity (Charney, 2004; see Chapter 7). It is being able to sustain recovery and even grow from a long-term stressful experience. It includes how we recover or rebound from stressors, and how long it takes to regain equilibrium (Zautra, Hall, & Murray, 2010). It is our "ordinary magic" (Masten, 2001).

An emphasis on resilience is part of a major shift in thinking about health and wellness—from the *biomedical model*, focused on curing disease, to the *biopsychosocial model*, emphasizing the forces that create good health. The concept originates from the study of children who survive difficult or abusive home environments (for example, adverse childhood experiences; see Chapter 6). Resilience is not simply the absence of disease, but the process of cultivating healthy mental, emotional, and physical habits.

We can think of resilience as having three overlapping steps (Zautra, Arewasikporn, & Davis, 2010). The first step is recovery or a return to baseline functioning. The second step is moving forward with little disruption. Finally, there can be growth, or moving beyond former levels of adaptation. Each step is important to recovering health.

Sources of Resilience

What accounts for resilience? Like coping, which we studied in Chapter 7, resilience involves the interaction between internal capacities, such as optimism or a sense of control, and external resources, such as family and community. Some initial distress in the face of a stressful situation is normal and even beneficial for adaptation.

Although several of the "Big 5" personality traits relate to resilience, resilience itself is not a personality trait (see Chapter 7). While personality traits are internal and unchanging, resilience is dynamic, and resilient people can change how they cope with stress. Here are just some of the resources on which they can draw (Dunkel Schetter & Dolbier, 2011):

- *dispositional resources*, such as emotional stability and empathy
- *ego-related resources*, such as a sense of autonomy and a positive self-image
- *interpersonal resources*, such as family support and quality relationships
- *culturally based beliefs*, such as spirituality and concerns for benevolence and justice
- *behavioral and cognitive skills*, such as mindfulness, social skills, and creativity
- *other resources*, such as socioeconomic status, a healthy diet, and exercise

Resilience is not just important for those living at risk. In fact, it is the norm and may even be universal (Gallo, Bogart, Vranceanu, & Matthews, 2005; Zautra, Arewasikporn et al., 2010), and feats of resilience are common across the

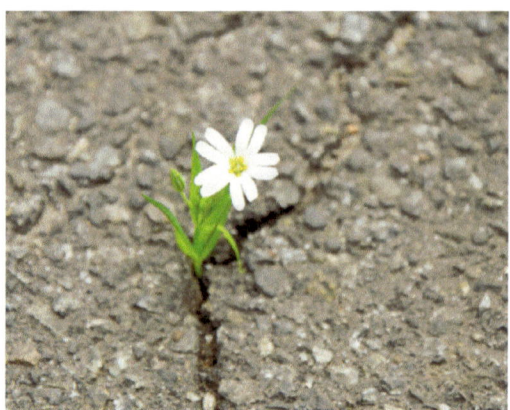

Photo 14.4   Resilience is a process, encapsulating recovery, forward movement, and positive growth after stressful or traumatic experiences.

Source: Kathriba/Shutterstock

lifespan (Bonanno, 2004; Garmezy, 1991; Greve & Staudinger, 2006). People who have faced poverty, childhood emotional abuse, war, natural disaster, or cancer do not always develop mental or physical health problems. Rather, they may develop a strong sense of growth in adversity, and that sense provides a buffer against future stressors and health challenges (**Photo 14.4**).

Although the concept of resilience arose from studies of children who were invincible in the face of traumatic, high-risk, or adverse situations, people of all ages can speak of "finding a silver lining," "discovering what really matters in life," "learning how much others cared," or "uncovering hidden strengths" (Zautra, 2003). Of course, many people are at risk for a life-threatening illness. Yet, today, most adults older than 65 can expect to live an average of 20 additional years, and only 20% of them will suffer from disability (Zautra, Arewasikporn et al., 2010). The golden years are much more golden now than they were 25 years ago. Now, people in the United States (and around the world) are better educated about health.

Sociocultural influences are also important to resilience. Communities matter: Think of the resilience of El Paso residents after the mass shooting of August 2019, or of Kyoto Animation staff after the arson attack in July 2019, where neighbors or even strangers helped one another in the face of trauma. In addition, how ethnic minorities adapt to illness and infirmity may relate to how they sustain themselves in the face of the trauma of racism (Becker & Newsom, 2005). For example, Hispanics with a strong attachment to their heritage have significantly better health outcomes (Fuentes-Afflick, Hessol, & Perez-Stable, 1999; Gould, Madan, Qin, & Chavez, 2003).

It might seem that the burdens of aging are greater for racial and ethnic minorities (Dowd & Bengtson, 1978), but all groups can overcome adversity through self-determination and community (Becker & Newsom, 2005; James, 1994). **Sojourner syndrome** is a concept developed by Arline T. Geronimus (1993) that highlights the unique and cumulative health disparities experienced by African American women that arise from the historical and ongoing effects of racism, sexism, and social oppression. It takes its name from Sojourner Truth, a formerly enslaved women who became an African American abolitionist and advocate for women's rights   (Becker & Newsom, 2005; Taylor & Chatters, 1991; Warren-Findlow, 2019; Wimberly, 2001). The story of Sojourner Truth's life draws attention to both the unimaginable pain and suffering that was inflicted upon her and how she used those life experiences to fight for the rights of others. Her story demonstrates what it means to be resilient.

Resilience and Health

Although life is filled with stress, chronic long-term stress is bad for health (see Chapter 6; Baum, Garofalo, & Yali, 1999; Dunkel Schetter & Dolbier, 2011;

Thoits, 2010). It can be devastating to live with a life-threatening medical condition, such as cancer, HIV, or Alzheimer's disease. Here, resilience can literally be a matter of life and death (Bower & Hayes, 1998; Dunkel Schetter & Dolbier, 2011; Pakenham & Cox, 2009; Park, Chmielewski, & Blank, 2010; Xu & Roberts, 2010). Empirical evidence shows that positive emotions, like those that give rise to resilience, are linked in many ways to longevity and survival (Xu & Roberts, 2010). Positive adaptation to breast cancer, for example, gives women a greater sense of control over their disease, bolsters their self-esteem, and increases their optimism for the future (Taylor, 1983).

Surprisingly, it may be easier to adapt to a serious health condition that is permanent rather than temporary (Smith, Loewenstein, Jankovic, & Ubel, 2009). In other words, people who are *objectively* better off might be *subjectively* worse off because they believe their health situation will improve. How can this be? It may be that hoping one's circumstances will improve can impede adaptation (Smith et al., 2009). This may relate to the *disability paradox* (Levine, 1987): Many people with serious and debilitating disabilities (such as disfigurement, chronic pain, and physical handicap) report a higher quality of life when by objective measures (to outside observers, or compared with people who do not have a disability) they should be worse off and suffering (Albrecht & Devlieger, 1999; Webb, 2019). Patients across a wide range of health conditions typically say that they have greater happiness and quality of life than do healthy people who imagine themselves with the same conditions (Ashby, O'Hanlon, & Buxton, 1994; Ubel, Loewenstein, Schwarz, & Smith, 2005). They are attempting to find the balance between the good and the bad in their lives—much like the Cherokee belief in "the one you feed." That balance in mind, body, and spirit is what leads to the overall experience of a high quality of life (Albrecht & Devlieger, 1999; Ubel et al., 2005; Ubel, Loewenstein, & Jepson, 2003). It is the ability to adapt, find meaning, and maintain emotional health in the face of disability, and it is crucial to resilience.

In the case of injury, rape, war, and natural disasters, we can observe trauma-related psychopathology, such as *posttraumatic stress disorder* (PTSD), but also positive outcomes, or *posttraumatic growth* (see Chapter 11). More than one-third of survivors of the attacks on the World Trade Center on 9/11 who were surveyed were resilient (Bonanno, Galea, Bucciarelli, & Vlahov, 2006). PTSD was twice as likely in people who were in the Twin Towers at the time of the attack than in those who merely witnessed the attacks from outside. Yet more than half the people in both these groups were resilient. Evidently, resilience can be learned in a variety of contexts (see the **In the News** feature).

Thinking About Health

■ What is resilience, and where does it come from?

■ Given its sources, how can resilience be improved?

■ If you know someone who has suffered from trauma or serious illness, how has resilience influenced that person's health?

Happiness and Hope

Is happiness good for your health? Are happy and hopeful people healthy people? There is certainly ample evidence that depression, anxiety, and stress can negatively affect health. Is the converse also true? The answers are all yes.

Happiness

Although we all think we know what happiness is, psychologists define **happiness** as the appreciation of life as a whole—or how much you like the life you lead (Veenhoven, 2008). It is essentially having lots of positive affect and little negative affect (Diener, 2000; Diener & Lucas, 1999). And that turns out to be important for good health.

Happiness is built on good relationships, fulfilling work, spirituality, and a passion for life. What doesn't matter, surprisingly, is money (Vohs & Baumeister, 2011), although spending money on others can make us happy (Dunn, Aknin, & Norton, 2008). Overall, that feeling of having "a good day" has three common features: autonomy, competence, and connection to others. In other words, happiness is the freedom to make our own decisions, to feel competent at whatever we are doing, and to share our lives with others. College students who took an online course in positive psychology that taught them how to maximize their happiness and wellbeing had less anxiety and depression and higher levels of happiness (Smith et al., 2023) showing that we can improve our lives by focusing on being happy. Dr. Laurie Santos at Yale University has taught what is perhaps the most popular college course ever! Yale University doesn't even have a room big enough for all the students who want to take this course each semester. Her course is "The Science of Well-being" and from the data that Dr. Santos has collected on over four million students who have taken her course the results are profound: students are, on average, 17% happier after taking her course than they were on the first day! (Yaden et al., 2021). Dr. Santos's class at Yale is available online for anyone who wants to take it for free. Additionally, you can also learn how to be happier through the "Pursuit-of-Happiness" programs online.

Even centenarians report high levels of happiness, including the positive feeling of having a good laugh (Jopp & Smith, 2006). These folks have not just beaten the odds, and they do not necessarily benefit from higher levels of education, income, or social status. Rather, both prospective and longitudinal studies show that mere happiness serves as a protective factor in relation to health and mortality (Steptoe, 2019). Some researchers theorize that we each have a set point of happiness, much like a set point of weight. They argue that we return to that set point as we adapt to changing circumstances. It may be a genetic predisposition, and it may account for as much as 50% of happiness, as opposed to only 10% that can be attributed to life circumstances. Yet that still leaves 40% that we can hope to control through the power of change (Lyubomirsky, Sheldon, & Schkade, 2005). In one novel study that used *ecological momentary assessment*, participants reported their levels of happiness at scheduled or random times during the day, week, and month to demonstrate day-to-day fluctuations in happiness. Results from these assessments show that happiness, even over the course of a single day, has an impact on survival (Steptoe & Wardle, 2011). Like weight loss, happiness is not just luck. It requires both daily, and lasting, commitments (Lyubomirsky, 2008).

Hope

If you are faced with an obstacle, what do you do? Do you actively look for ways around it? Do you persist or give up? If you are usually able to find another path to your goals, chances are you have a hopeful outlook on life.

There is no agreed-upon definition of hope. Some have called it a trait, a state, a personal attribute, an experience, an emotion, or even a life force (Southerland et al., 2016). Regardless, *hope* has affective, cognitive, and behavioral components. Unlike fear, which is an automatic emotional response, hope is an emotional and cognitive process.

Hope involves having goals for each day and for the future. It derives from a sense of success, along with the energy and the ability to find pathways to get there (Snyder, 2002; Snyder, Rand, & Sigmon, 2002). Hope consistently relates to better outcomes, whether in academics, athletics, psychological adjustment, or physical health. It is associated with greater adherence to medical regimens and higher levels of satisfaction with medical treatment (Makarem, Hunt, Mudambi, & Aaronson, 2010; Nekolaichuk, 2015). When a doctor tells a patient that he needs to lose weight to avoid a heart attack, hope assists with the challenges of sticking to a new diet and exercise.

Related to hope is **agency**—the sense that our behavior is under our control. It includes a belief that we can change the environment, as well as be changed by it. We do so not only through what we think and feel but also through what we choose to do or not do.

Happiness, Hope, and Health

There are many benefits of positive emotional states (Steptoe, 2019; Zautra, 2003). Happiness opens doors to other desirable outcomes, such as good performance at school, satisfaction at work, close and fulfilling intimate and social relationships, good health, and a long life. It is also an important buffer against the damaging effects of disappointments and setbacks, including health crises (Peterson, 2006).

There is plenty of evidence that the happier you are, the better your health (Steptoe, 2019; Veenhoven, 2008; Veenhoven & Hagerty, 2006) and the longer your life (Lyyra, Törmäkangas, Read, Rantanen, & Berg, 2006; Veenhoven, 2008). This association exists at the personal and global levels (see the **Around the World feature). For example, a longitudinal study of Catholic nuns found that happiness, love, and hope at an early age were predictive of longer life (Siahpush, Spittal, & Singh, 2008). Similarly, a 20-year longitudinal study of Finnish twins found that happiness was associated with lower mortality (Koivumaa-Honkanen et al., 2000). The correlation holds regardless of age, gender, socioeconomic status, and personality—and across nations (Helliwell, 2001; Helliwell, Layard, & Sachs, 2015; Pierewan & Tampubolon, 2015). The correlation is also higher in people with illness than those without, making the importance of happiness to health outcomes clearer still. Not that happiness cures disease and makes people well again—it does not (Veenhoven, 2008). Rather, it helps us maintain health and adapt to chronic illness.

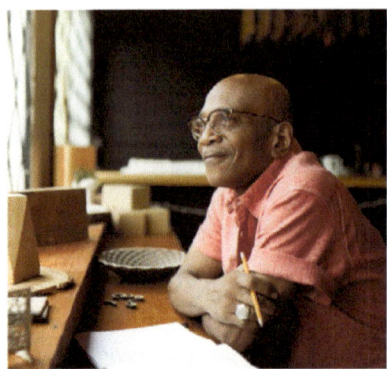

Photo 14.5 Happiness and hope are both crucial factors of a healthy lifestyle.

Source: Hero Images/Getty Images

How does happiness protect against poor health? First, as we saw in Chapter 6, chronic unhappiness triggers the fight-or-flight response, which can elevate blood pressure and lower immune functioning. Conversely, a positive mood may lead to better immune functioning (Pressman & Cohen, 2005). Second, happy people appear to be more health conscious and to take better care of their health, at least in part because they are more self-confident and open to new experiences (Zautra, 2003). They are more likely to have a well-balanced diet, watch their weight, engage in sports, and attend to symptoms of illness (Ormel, 1980; Schulz & Decker, 1985; Veenhoven, 2008). Happy people engage in fewer health-compromising behaviors, as well, with lower rates of drinking and smoking (Veenhoven, 2008). Finally, happy people have more friends and more satisfying close relationships (Photo 14.5).

Around *the* World

Global Happiness

Happiness is now considered a measure of social progress and a worthy goal for public policy worldwide. Global happiness is assessed by surveying people around the world on a scale from 0 (*the worst possible life*) to 10 (*the best possible life*). International differences are due to factors such as financial recession, war, natural disaster, quality of governance, and social support (Helliwell, Layard, & Sachs, 2019; Sachs, 2019). Women around the world report that their lives are slightly better than men's lives, regardless of where they live. Happiness around the world is highest in younger age groups.

Happiness also differs by country, in surprising ways. The top 10 happiest and 10 least happy countries are shown in the figure (The United States is number 19 in the global happiness list, and it is continually falling down the list.) (Photo 14.6).

Question:

According to the figure, what factors explain the perception of happiness around the world? Why do you think there are global differences in this magnitude?

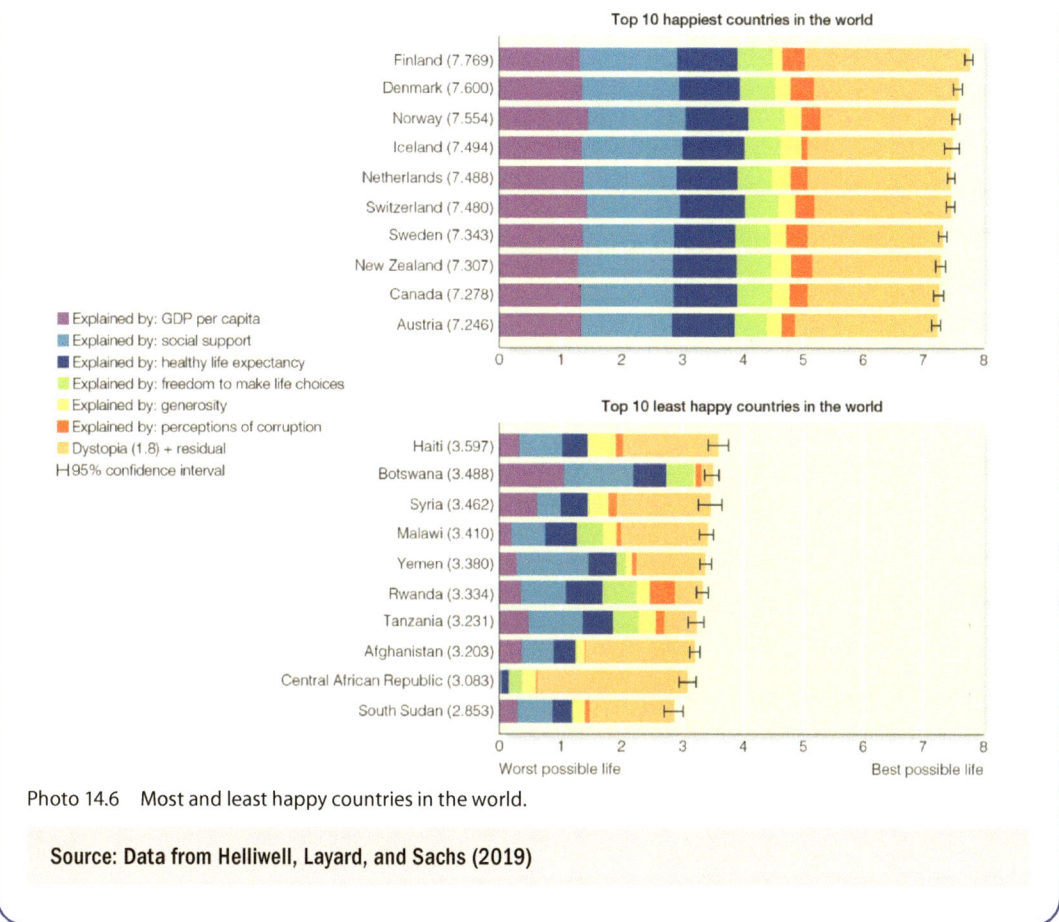

Photo 14.6   Most and least happy countries in the world.

Source: Data from Helliwell, Layard, and Sachs (2019)

What's love got to do with it? A 2010 paper with that name reported on the daily happiness, social functioning, and perceived health of married octogenarians. Although happiness may decline with age for both men and women, marital satisfaction buffers the day-to-day impact of poor health (Waldinger & Schulz, 2010). Recalling my experiences as a graduate student (in the chapter opening story), I certainly saw this firsthand in the spouse caregivers of patients with devastating illnesses. My conversations with hundreds of patients about their experiences taught me that, as the Cherokee saying goes, coping and adapting to stress depends on whichever wolf—positive or negative—you feed.

Thinking About Health

■ Do you think that there is a set point to happiness? Why or why not?

■ How does a sense of hope influence your life?

■ How does agency relate to happiness and hope?

The Future of Health Psychology

Like any science, the field of health psychology is always changing and always teaching us something new. Health psychology is a relatively young discipline, but it has grown by leaps and bounds. In 50+ years, it has become one of the most active and vibrant areas within the field of psychology.

Health psychologists are still focused on research and clinical practice in order to understand good mental and physical health, but changes in our society and the world have changed their work. Today, promoting health, education, and well-being are paramount goals, as we have seen throughout this book. Research, health advocacy, and disease prevention have led to many achievements and created new opportunities, but there is still so much to be done.

In this chapter, we will examine what lies ahead for the field of health psychology. First, we will examine the most important new directions in health psychology. We will see how health psychology must continue to develop in the context of the biopsychosocial model, within both basic and applied science and in areas of contemporary importance. Then we will look at career options for people, who want to contribute to this growing field.

Revisiting the Biopsychosocial Model

The field of health psychology has advanced tremendously due, in part, to the guiding principles of the *biopsychosocial model*. When George Engel (1977) introduced this model in 1977, he advocated for a move away from conceptualizing health purely in terms of pathology, disease, and disability. He believed that the existing biomedical model was short-sighted and did not consider the whole human being experiencing a health problem. Rather, Engel's goal was to motivate health care practitioners to consider the psychosocial aspects of health, treatment, and illness as well (Bolton & Gillett, 2019).

Since its inception, the biopsychosocial model has dominated the field of health psychology. It has significantly shaped science, health care, and health policy and has led to improvements in all areas of health (Bolton & Gillett, 2019). However, some scholars are critical of the model (Bolton & Gillett, 2019). Critics argue that it lacks predictive and explanatory power—that is, that the model provides a useful way to think about health, but that it is too difficult to actually measure what and how things happen within the context of individuals with disease. To this day, establishing causation among biological, psychological, and social factors is a challenge—a challenge that, hopefully, the next wave of health psychologists and medical scientists will tackle.

New approaches to clinical care, such as culturally competent and person-centered models of care, demonstrate the importance of considering how illness uniquely impacts each person's health and well-being. The biopsychosocial model is also integral to considering social determinants of health and how they lead to health disparities. So, while criticism of the biopsychosocial model exists, it is still the best way to conceptualize health.

Thinking About Health

■ What is the significance of the biopsychosocial model?

Lifespan and Development

One area of critical importance to the future of health psychology is a shift in demographics (Siegler, Bosworth, Davey, & Elias, 2012). The population is changing within the United States and around the world—and the most salient changes are in ethnic diversity and aging. More than ever, they oblige us to take a developmental perspective across the lifespan.

This *lifespan developmental perspective* is also necessary because health habits form early. Health psychologists must find ways to cultivate positive health values, healthy habits, and resilience throughout the lifespan. Developmental research that begins early in childhood and follows people into later life is critical to the success of health promotion. Throughout this book, we have seen the value of longitudinal studies for understanding health.

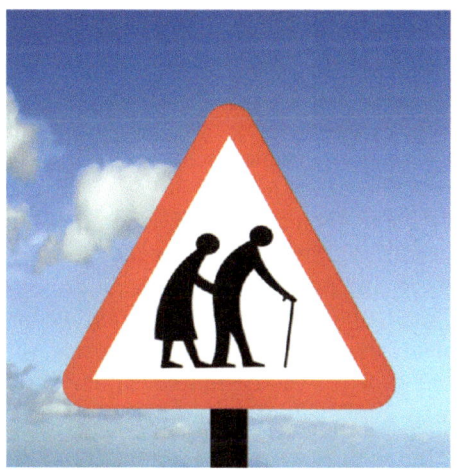

Photo 14.7   Around the world, populations are aging at rapid rates. At the same time, life expectancies are rising. Should we change traditional images of aging? How can the lifespan developmental perspective influence our answer to this question?

Source: Peter Etchells/Shutterstock

Prenatal Development and Childhood

Ongoing research on prenatal development points to several crucial issues. Educating pregnant women about the risks of smoking cigarettes and vaping is one worldwide health priority. Maternal smoking is associated with an increased risk of cardiovascular disease in future adults. During pregnancy, nicotine can cross the placenta and produce higher nicotine concentrations in the fetus's cardiovascular system, leading to hypertension and cardiovascular disorders later in life. Smoking during pregnancy can lead to other significant health complications for both the mother and the fetus as well, such as impaired fetal development, preterm birth, and lower birth weights (Xiao, Dasgupta, Li, Huang, & Zhang, 2014). Sudden infant death syndrome (SIDS) is also linked to smoking during pregnancy, and it doesn't take much: Just one cigarette a day doubles the risk that the child will die of SIDS. Recent research shows that 22% of instances of SIDS can be traced to the mother smoking while pregnant (**Photo 14.7**) (Anderson et al., 2019).

The **fetal origins of disease hypothesis** states that risk factors for many chronic conditions may be established before birth (Barker, Eriksson, Forsén, & Osmond, 2002; Xiao et al., 2014). However, helping pregnant women to quit smoking and vaping is challenging, and efforts so far have had only limited success. Some studies show a higher rate of abstinence in pregnant smokers who receive drug therapy (Myung et al., 2012), but other approaches are important as well. In Great Britain, 97 studies showed positive effects of smoking cessation interventions, with as many as 11 different components (Greaves et al., 2011):

- *Quit guides*: take-home, patient-focused guides to quitting
- *Counseling*: from a range of practitioners, from obstetricians to peers
- *Peer support*: social support while quitting, often involving a "buddy"
- *Groups*: support groups or group counseling
- *Partnering*: identifying the smoking patterns of friends and family
- *Information*: pamphlets, videos, and other educational materials
- *Nicotine replacement*: pharmacological therapies
- *Incentives*: both financial and symbolic rewards
- *Biological feedback*: ultrasound images and stress tests to show the effects of smoking on the fetus
- *Personal follow-up*: further encouragement, including postpartum
- *Assessment:* other follow-up, to assess the success of intervention

Given the limited success of these measures so far, health psychologists need to find better ways to educate and motivate women to avoid nicotine during pregnancy.

Good health habits established in childhood set the stage for a long and healthy life (Smith, Orleans, & Jenkins, 2004). Yet very little research has focused on the developmental factors that influence how health behaviors develop during childhood. How can we instill health promotion in both parents and children? A healthy diet, an active lifestyle, good oral hygiene, regular physical examinations, vaccinations, and the use of seat belts are all crucial. So is early education on the risks of unsafe sex, smoking, drugs, and alcohol.

Across the lifespan, but especially in prenatal and child development, the concept of *preemptive medicine* has taken hold. This medical approach advocates for prediction, prospective diagnosis, and preventive interventions to offset the development of later disease (Sata, 2019). It also involves using genetic and physiological information to evaluate the risk that potential diseases will become reality and to determine the effectiveness of certain treatments. Using what we know about risks that develop prenatally or early in development, we can use preemptive medicine to begin lifestyle changes and positive health interventions early in order to offset the possibility of negative health outcomes.

Adolescence and Emerging Adulthood

Adolescence and emerging adulthood present more opportunities and challenges. Here, too, health choices set the stage for the rest of one's life. As part of normal development, adolescents may experiment with diet, exercise, sexual activity, substance use, and risky behaviors that have the potential to affect health both in the short term and across the lifespan (see Chapter 5; Park, Scott, Adams, Brindis, & Irwin, 2014). For instance, precursors of cardiovascular disease (e.g., high blood pressure, excess body fat, and buildup of plaques in the arteries) can be seen in adolescence. Disturbingly, less than half of American teenagers have good cardiovascular health, suggesting that these teens may develop heart disease in midlife (Chiang et al., 2019).

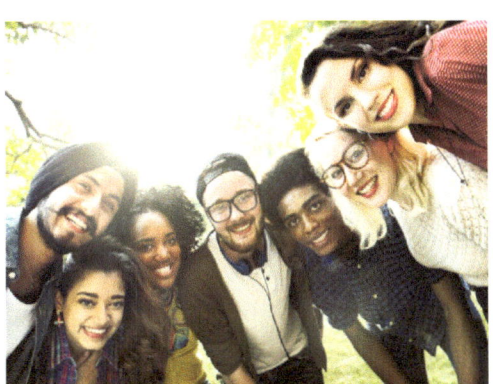

Photo 14.8 Emerging adults show positive trends toward better health in the areas of exercise, sexual activity, and tobacco use.

Source: Rawpixel.com/Stutterstock

One factor that causes inflammation and elevates the risk of later cardiovascular disease is stress. And the stress of adolescence is particularly powerful (Chiang et al., 2019). Yet, something as simple as having clear goals and hopes for the future can serve as a valuable stress-reduction tool in the teen years. Positive future expectations can offset the risk of disease and promote healthy development, especially in vulnerable racial and ethnic minority male teenagers (Prince, Epstein, Nurius, Gorman-Smith, & Henry, 2019).

The transition from adolescence to young adulthood is more challenging still. There are encouraging trends toward better sexual and reproductive health, decreased tobacco use, and more frequent exercise in this age group. Yet young adults have poorer self-reported health than adolescents, and they fare worse than other age groups in many health risks. For example, emerging adults are four times more likely to drink and drive than adolescents (Park et al., 2014). Young adult males (especially Native Americans) are more likely to die in car crashes than females (**Photo 14.8**) (CDC, 2017c; Park et al., 2014).

Health psychologists are investigating how choices made during adolescence and emerging adulthood are sensitive to culture and context. Other research is focusing on positive health interventions in college, especially in the context of alcohol use.

Adulthood

The major life tasks of adulthood include establishing a career, finding a partner, and becoming a parent (Havighurst, 1972; McCormick, Kuo, & Masten, 2011). Each of these life tasks relates to a change in lifestyle, and each presents a ripe opportunity for research.

Establishing one's career may require long hours spent commuting and sitting at a desk, with additional life stressors from pressure at work to managing finances, all of which can negatively affect health. Finding a partner can also be stressful, and whether dating websites and apps help or hinder the development of healthy relationships remains to be determined (Choi, Wong, & Fong, 2018; Hobbs, Owen, & Gerber, 2017). Becoming a parent may bring great joy and excitement, but it can also have a negative impact on health, leading to weight gain and decreased physical activity (Nasuti et al., 2014; Rhodes et al., 2014). Retrospective research shows that more than 50% of previously active women are no longer active five years into motherhood (McIntyre & Rhodes, 2009). Australian mothers were two times more likely to be inactive and sedentary than nonmothers four years after delivery. Compared to nonmothers, first- and second-time Canadian moms showed significantly lower perceived behavioral control, motivation, and confidence that they could be physically active only 12 months after delivery (Rhodes et al., 2014). Although most research thus far has focused on mothers, fathers also experience similar or even greater declines (Rhodes et al., 2014). These findings point to the need for health psychologists to develop more effective interventions for adults during the transition to parenthood.

Midlife to Later Life

Health behaviors continue to influence the risk of chronic illness throughout adulthood. Obesity, a sedentary lifestyle, smoking, sun exposure, unsafe sex, poor stress management, and a lack of emotionally fulfilling relationships can all lead to poor health outcomes. By midlife to later life, most health behaviors have been well established, and getting people to change their habits is hard, even in the face of life-threatening illness. Still, behavioral change is always possible. A challenge for health psychologists is to find more effective ways to motivate people with an entrenched lifestyle. It shouldn't take a brush with death to scare us into change.

As mentioned in Chapter 1, the aging of the population both within the United States and around the world presents many issues for health psychology (see **Around the World** feature). People are living longer, and longer lives mean greater opportunities for personal fulfillment and continued contributions to society (Friedman et al., 2019). But at the end of life, there is often disease, discomfort, disability, and a loss of independence as well. Health psychologists can play a role in understanding and optimizing the balance among these aspects of later life like Aidan wants to do.

Around *the* World

Population Aging and Careers in Gerontology

Population aging is taking place in nearly all countries (United Nations, 2017). In 2017, 962 million people around the world were older than 60 years, more than twice as many as in 1980. By 2050, the number of older adults will double again to reach over 2 billion people. That means that there will be more older adults than children. The fastest-growing segment of the older population worldwide is people over the age of 80 years old, who will represent 425 million people by 2050.

The aging of the population presents important challenges to medicine, health care, and health psychology. In developed countries, older adults are the main consumers of health care, and they have an increasing number of chronic conditions that need long-term medical and behavioral management. With the growing population of older adults, the focus on identifying and changing health behaviors becomes more important as well (Siegler et al., 2012). Health psychology must address the risk factors for chronic illness and identify and promote successful aging.

Professionals who focus on researching and providing care for older adults are called *g erontologists.* While many of the health problems faced by older adults are the same as those for other age groups, aging presents several unique challenges. First among these is Alzheimer's disease (AD), the sixth leading cause of death in the United States today. Currently, one out of nine older people has AD, and as the population grows, this number will reach an alarming 13.8 million by 2050. Providing appropriate care to AD patients and their caregivers is crucial to maintaining health, well-being, and quality of life for as long as possible.

Dementia is another age-related illness that gerontologists address. Because it impacts a person's memory, attention, and communication skills, dementia makes carrying out the activities of daily living difficult. Dementia is very common in later life and increases with age. According to the Health and Retirement Survey, 5% of people in their seventies have dementia, while nearly 38% of people in

their nineties suffer from it (Kuchibhatla et al., 2019). Dementia can be comorbid with a number of different diseases, such as type 2 diabetes. Older adults with diabetes are at greater risk for dementia and heart disease and can suffer from many other disease-related complications that negatively impact their quality of life.

Gerontologists include psychologists, physicians, social workers, nursing home administrators, and any other career that specializes in aging and later life. There are many training programs in gerontology that can lead to fulfilling and impactful careers in the health sector, and, as the world population ages, employment opportunities will continue to increase.

Question:

Why are gerontology careers growing in number and importance? Might improving the lives of older adults be of interest to you?

As populations age, health psychologists will focus on health situations in which there is *comorbidity*, or multiple coexisting conditions (see Chapter 5). For instance, because rates of cognitive impairment rise in later life, health psychologists will have to be trained in neuropsychology as well as health science. In addition, health psychologists are not only concerned with improving the quality of life and well-being of patients with chronic conditions but with improving the well-being of their loved ones and caregivers, too. The burden of care often takes a toll on the mental and physical health of caregivers (see Chapter 12; Hooker, Frazier, & Monahan, 1994), which means that health psychologists should also be trained in social and clinical psychology. Just as the characteristics of populations will change, so, too, will the knowledge required to further health psychology.

Thinking About Health

■ Why is it important to view health from a developmental perspective across the lifespan?

■ What steps can people take at any stage in the lifespan to improve their health outcomes?

Health Disparities

Health disparities, or health differences between groups, will be another growing focus for the field of health psychology, both globally and within the United States (see Chapter 1). Disparities arise from poor health, risk factors for disease, and limited access to health care—especially among those with social, economic, and environmental disadvantages. And these factors can combine with race, ethnicity, gender, sexual orientation, and disability to influence health, imposing a higher burden of illness, injury, disability, and mortality.

Increased research and applied efforts can help to identify and cultivate awareness of the differences in health outcomes. Yet, research on health disparities accounts for only 10% of the current research budget at the National Institutes of Health (NIH; Alvidrez & Stinson, 2019). To address this weakness, the NIH has developed a strategic plan for guiding research on minority health and health disparities over the next five years, with the goal of moving beyond merely identifying the factors that contribute to health disparities and implementing actual interventions (Pérez-Stable & Collins, 2019). These interventions have the greatest opportunity to make a difference and can help the communities at greatest risk.

Global Health Disparities

Although dramatic gains in life expectancy have occurred since 2000, significant health inequalities across countries persist (WHO, 2024j). There is a 33-year discrepancy in life expectancy among countries. A child born in Sierra Leone may live to age 50, while a child born in Japan could live to the ripe old age of 85 (WHO, 2016b). In Chad, every fifth child will not reach age five (~20%), while in Europe, mortality among children younger than five is only 1.3% (WHO, 2011). There is no biological or genetic reason for these differences.

Cancer disparities pose another global health challenge. Cancer incidence around the world is expected to exceed 21 million new cases by 2030, with about two-thirds of new diagnoses in low- and middle-income countries (Chawla et al., 2013). These diagnoses will be devastating, because these countries also have limited resources for treating cancer.

Addressing global health disparities will require an integrative biopsychosocial approach. Socioeconomic status is the biggest driver of these disparities—followed by limited access to preventive services and treatment, poor quality of care, lack of knowledge, and problems with the distribution of resources. Cultural beliefs, such as fatalism and reliance on traditional healers, are also potential barriers to treatment and services. Interventions can help establish new beliefs and behaviors. Education can improve patient awareness and encourage preventive medicine (Chawla et al., 2013).

Health Disparities Within the United States

There are significant gaps in health outcomes within the United States, too. As in most countries, these differences stem from inequities in social status, income, ethnicity, gender, disability, and sexual orientation. Infants born to African American

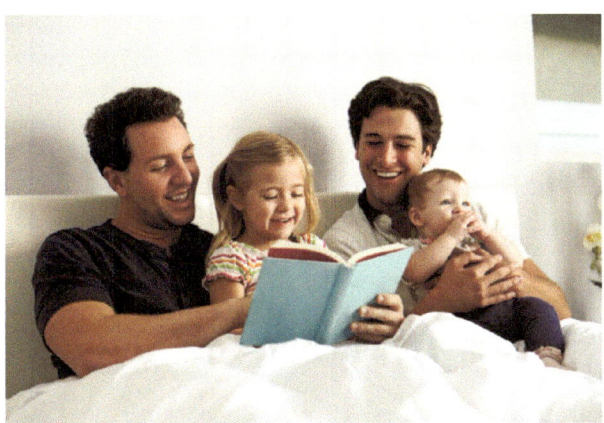

Photo 14.9   The increased empathy offered by cultural-sensitivity training and person-centered care has helped reduce healthcare disparities for LGBTQ families.

Source: Monkey Business Images/Stutterstock

mothers, for example, are nearly three times more likely to die than infants of other races and ethnicities (MacDorman & Mathews, 2011), and African American men are more likely to die of cancer than men from any other ethnic group (CDC, 2017a). Overall, Blacks and Hispanics have poorer health and health behaviors than whites.

While the population is aging, countries around the world are also becoming more culturally and ethnically diverse. In the United States, which is already a diverse country, people of color will account for more than half of the population by 2050. Thus, health psychologists must do more to understand the drivers of cultural and ethnic health disparities and to address them (**Photo 14.9**).

Another example of health disparities can be seen in access to care for lesbian, gay, bisexual, transgender, and queer/questioning (LGBTQ+) families (Telazzi & Colombo, 2024). In 2015, former U.S. president Barack Obama declared June to be Lesbian, Gay, Bisexual, and Transgender Pride Month. He called on all citizens of the United States to eliminate prejudice and to celebrate the diversity of the American people. In spite of these actions, LGBTQ people and students still experience microaggressions, bullying, and discrimination (Hood, Sherrell, Pfeffer, & Mann, 2019). In a recent study at a large public university, LGBTQ college students reported that their campus healthcare centers were uninformed, unaccepting, and discriminatory toward them, characteristics that were attributed to the ignorance of healthcare staff in regard to LGBTQ issues (Hood et al., 2019). This study is an example of how cultural sensitivity training and person-centered care approaches are still lacking in many areas and continue to contribute to health disparities. As we see next, however, health care is becoming increasingly available to diverse populations.

Thinking About Health

■ If you were a health psychologist addressing health disparities, what issues would you choose to tackle? What interventions would you choose to employ?

Becoming a Health Psychologist

Aidan's goal is to become a clinical health psychologist. He is drawn to this career by a deep appreciation of how mental, emotional, and social factors influence physical well-being. His goal is to help patients manage the cognitive and behavioral factors that alter how they cope with and adjust to chronic illness. Future health psychologists like Aidan generally begin their studies by enrolling in relevant courses, including biology, public health, economics, nutrition, and psychology. They obtain experience in a lab and become involved in research, often starting as undergraduates, and sometimes pursuing an advanced degree.

However, for many college students interested in health psychology, pursuing an advanced degree is out of the question because of time or financial constraints. Yet all is not lost. Students with a bachelor's degree in psychology and an interest in health can pursue other trajectories as well. Many jobs have arisen to meet the needs of an aging population and the obesity epidemic, including health coaching and health advocating, as we will see below.

Health psychologists typically hold a PhD or PsyD. Applicants to PhD programs often apply to work with a mentor who is conducting research in their area of interest. Their degree may be in health psychology, but doctoral programs in clinical, developmental, counseling, social, or experimental psychology also have specialized health psychology tracks. Graduate students can expect to acquire a broad repertoire of professional skills.

Applied health psychologists work directly with patients, and this track, too, requires further study. Students who pursue a PhD often choose between a general psychology program, focused on research and teaching, and a clinical health psychology program. Clinical programs help them master both science and clinical practice. Many also prepare students for licensure and board certification from the American Board of Professional Psychology (www.health-psych.org). Board certification generally requires students to complete a one-year internship or residency before obtaining their doctorate.

After graduate school, many students pursue a postdoctoral fellowship. It might be in a university medical center, a university laboratory, or a health center outside academia for further research or clinical training. The fellowship hones a research psychologist's skills, offers experience in pursuing funding, and builds one's program of research and professional accomplishments.

All of these steps take time. Health psychologists have generally completed four years of undergraduate education, an average of five years of graduate training, and up to three years of internship or postdoctoral training—even before taking their first professional position. As Aidan will surely find, though, those years are rewarding in themselves.

Careers for Health Psychologists

Careers for health psychologists usually intersect with the health care system. They do so directly when a psychologist works in a primary care or inpatient setting. They do so as well for those specializing in pain management, rehabilitation, women's health, oncology, smoking cessation, addiction, weight loss, or headache management. Other careers, such as psychotherapy, intersect with the health care system indirectly. Health psychologists also work at colleges and universities to conduct research, teach, and mentor students.

Still others work for corporations and government agencies, in communities, or in public policy.

Many clinical psychologists work in assessment, using surveys and interviews. Others work with patients, through individual or group therapy or through support groups. They help patients and caregivers adapt and cope with disease or teach them how to modify health behaviors. Health psychologists may also design or provide health and wellness workshops for healthy people, or they may work in hospitals, where they assist medical staff in providing the most effective health care. Health psychologists also serve as consultation liaisons in hospitals or primary care offices and may facilitate treatment and recovery by serving as the go-between for staff and patients.

Health psychologists conducted much of the research cited in this book. They are often the scientists at the forefront of research on HIV, cancer, psychosomatic illness, compliance with and relapse from medical regimens, health promotion, and the influences of psychological, social, and cultural factors on a wide range of health problems (health-psychology.org). They may study chronic pain, eating disorders, obesity, diabetes, cancer, cardiovascular disease, autoimmune disorders, sleep disorders, and terminal illnesses.

As we saw in Chapter 1, the goal of health psychology is to uncover the causes and development of disease—but that's not all. Research in health psychology also helps individuals develop a healthy lifestyle. Health psychologists study the effectiveness of treatments. They examine ways of coping with and adjusting to stress, pain, and serious health problems. Health psychologists also work as epidemiologists, who study disease patterns within larger populations (see Chapter 2). And health psychologists often work with neuroscientists to understand what causes disease, and to determine the best treatment, rehabilitation, and recovery strategies. New fields of research are developing all the time.

Health Coaches: Not everyone has the time or money to pursue the long and challenging path to a traditional healthcare career. Innovative careers, however, are opening the field of health psychology to others. One such career is health coaching.

A **health coach** (or *wellness coach*) helps clients attain a healthy and sustainable lifestyle. Health coaching challenges people to develop their inner strengths, wisdom, values, and motivation, and it helps them transform their goals into actions. Health coaches are authorities on wellness and serve as mentors, providing education and enabling behavioral modification. There are different types of health coaches. Some are skilled at identifying what is holding a person back and what will bring change. Many work in private practice or in conjunction with a doctor's office, spa, gym, physical and occupational rehabilitation center, or weight-loss center.

Health coaches are credentialed and have training in the science of behavioral change. They may also have training in psychology, behavior analysis, nutrition, physical therapy, medicine, or nursing. Many universities offer certificate programs, covering theoretical foundations, a patient-centered approach, motivational interviewing, behavioral change, disease-specific coaching, positive psychology and mindfulness, and the scope, practice, referrals, and ethics of health coaching. Certification may take up to a year.

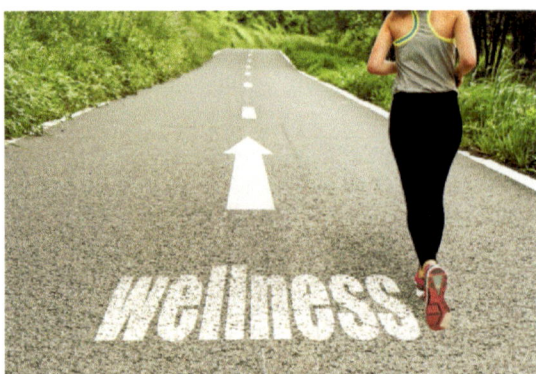

Photo 14.10   Need a health coach? They may provide new and affordable directions to a healthy lifestyle.

Health coaching arose from the intersection of positive psychology and health psychology. It has become popular as healthcare costs rise and more companies are turning to wellness programs for their employees. Health coaches have also become a viable alternative to help patients manage chronic illness. As the wellness revolution unfolds, their role will become even more important (**Photo 14.10**).

Health Advocates: Imagine that you are told you have a serious illness. What do you do next? It is easy to become overwhelmed by our complex medical and insurance systems. A whole new career has emerged as a result.

Health advocates are clinical consultants who guide patients and caregivers through the health care maze. They help patients understand their treatment options and make the right choices. They often coordinate services with specialists, hospitals, insurance companies, ancillary providers, and other health care professionals. They may also arrange end-of-life plans and

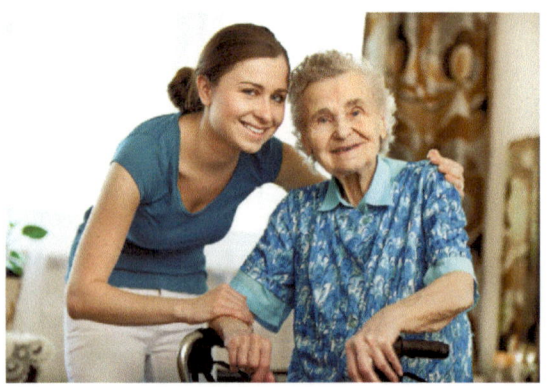

Photo 14.11   A health advocate guides patients through their health care options.

organize forms and medical records for insurance companies, nursing homes, and other services. Health advocates and other allied health professionals are also involved in preventive medicine and improving lifestyle choices. They aim to provide timely access to care, remove obstacles, promote adjustment, and improve quality of life. They are essentially project managers for health care (**Photo 14.11**).

Health advocates may also be called patient advocates, case managers, care coordinators, geriatric care managers, or elder care professionals. Training for future health advocates may require one course or a series of courses, and some programs offer certificates upon completion. Clinical health advocates are often nurses, doctors, physician assistants, nurse practitioners, or social workers who already have experience in health care. Some may have helped a loved one suffering from disease. Health advocacy offers new opportunities to contribute to the future of health psychology.

Thinking About Health

■ What are the training options for a career in health psychology?

■ Which professional path in health psychology interests you most?

Chapter Summary

Positive psychology has helped us recognize how individuals can live a healthy life, reduce the risk of negative health outcomes, and cope more effectively when dealing with health challenges. Many interpersonal factors influence well-being and wellness. They include personality factors, such as positive affect, extraversion, optimism, and an internal locus of control. They also include tailoring one's coping efforts to the specific situation and finding social support. We can contrast hedonic well-being, or feelings of happiness, with eudaimonic well-being, or a sense of fulfillment. Resilience is not just the avoidance of stress or the absence of poor health but also the "everyday magic" of recovery. It differentiates people who,

when faced with life-altering health challenges, see them as opportunities for growth. Together, these ideas can help us maintain happiness, hope, and good mental and physical health. The field of health psychology is changing because the world is changing. Our aging and diversifying population points to the need for a biopsychosocial and lifespan developmental approach to health care, while global and national health disparities point to the need to focus on the social and economic determinants of health. Access to health care, with the advent of telemedicine and climate change, is also changing health outcomes. Health psychologists can address these issues. For those who want to work in the field, innovative careers are available, including health coaching and health advocacy.

KEY TERMS ▶ fetal origins of disease hypothesis p. 435, health coach (or *wellness coach*) p. 443, health advocates p. 444, positive psychology p. 415, wellness p. 418, wheel of wellness p. 418, well-being p. 420, hedonic well-being p. 422, positive affect p. 422, eudaimonic well-being p. 422, successful aging p. 424, resilience p. 427, sojourner syndrome p. 428, happiness p. 430, agency p. 431

References

Abbey, A., Zawacki, T., Buck, P. O., Clinton, A. M., & McAuslan, P. (2004). Sexual assault and alcohol consumption: What do we know about their relationship and what types of research are still needed? *Aggression and Violent Behavior*, *9*(3), 271–303.

Abel, E. L., & Sokol, R. J. (1986). Fetal alcohol syndrome is now leading cause of mental retardation. *Lancet*, *328*(8517), 1222.

Abrahamsson, S. S., Bütikofer, A., & Karbownik, K. (2023). *Swallow this: Childhood and adolescent exposure to fast food restaurants, BMI, and cognitive ability (no. w31226)*. National Bureau of Economic Research.

Abu-Kaf, S., & Braun-Lewensohn, O. (2019). Coping resources and stress reactions among Bedouin Arab adolescents during three military operations. *Psychiatry Research*, *273*, 559–566.

Adamo, S. A. (2012). The effects of the stress response on immune function in invertebrates: An evolutionary perspective on an ancient connection. *Hormones and Behavior*, *62*(3), 324–330.

Adan, R. A. H., & Kaye, W. H. (Eds.). (2011). *Behavioral neurobiology of eating disorders*. Berlin: Springer.

Addati, L., Cassirer, N., & Gilchrist, K. (2014). *Maternity and paternity at work: Law and practice across the world*. Geneva: International Labor Office. Retrieved from http://www.ilo.org/wcmsp5/groups/public/—dgreports/—dcomm/—publ/documents/publication/wcms_242615.pdf

Ader, R. (1981). *A historical account of conditioned immunobiologic responses* (Vol. 321). New York, NY: Academic Press.

Ader, R. (1997). The role of conditioning in pharmacotherapy. In A. Harrington (Ed.), *The placebo effect: An interdisciplinary exploration* (pp. 138–165). Cambridge, MA: Harvard University Press.

Ader, R., & Cohen, N. (1981). Conditioned immuno pharmacologic responses. *Psychoneuroimmunology*, *281*, 319.

Adler, N. E., Boyce, T., Chesney, M. A., Cohen, S., Folkman, S., Kahn, R. L., & Syme, S. L. (1994). Socioeconomic status and health: The challenge of the gradient. *American Psychologist*, *49*(1), 15–24.

Adler, N. E., & Stewart, J. (2010). Preface to the biology of disadvantage: Socioeconomic status and health. *Annals of the New York Academy of Sciences*, *1186*(1), 1–4.

Agarwal, M., Hamilton, J. B., Moore, C. E., & Crandell, J. L. (2010). Predictors of depression among older African American cancer patients. *Cancer Nursing*, *33*(2), 156–163.

Agency for Healthcare Research and Quality. (2019, January). AHRQ national scorecard on hospital-acquired conditions updated baseline rates and preliminary results 2014–2017. Retrieved from https://www.ahrq.gov/sites/default/files/wysiwyg/professionals/quality-patient-safety/pfp/hacreport-2019.pdf

Agrawal, A., & Lynskey, M. T. (2008). Are there genetic influences on addiction: Evidence from family, adoption and twin studies. *Addiction*, *103*(7), 1069–1081.

Ahlström, G., & Sjödén, P. O. (1996). Coping with illness-related problems and quality of life in adult individuals with muscular dystrophy. *Journal of Psychosomatic Research*, *41*(4), 365–376.

Ahmad, F. B., Cisewski, J. A. (2023). *Quarterly provisional estimates for selected indicators of mortality, 2020-Quarter 3, 2022*. National Center for Health Statistics. National Vital Statistics System, Vital Statistics Rapid Release Program.

Ahsan Ullah, A. K. (2011). HIV/AIDS-related stigma and discrimination: A study of health care providers in Bangladesh. *Journal of the International Association of Physicians in AIDS Care*, *10*(2), 97–104.

AIDS.gov. (2016). *Stages of HIV infection*. Retrieved from https://www.aids.gov/hiv-aids-basics/just-diagnosed-with-hiv-aids/hiv-in-your-body/stages-of-hiv/

Aitken, V. (2015). Grieving Scot saw his weight drop to under four stone after struggling to cope with deaths of his mum and grandfather. *Daily Record*. Retrieved from http://www.dailyrecord.co.uk/news/health/grieving-scot-saw-weight-drop-7079197

Ajzen, I., & Fishbein, M. (1980). *Understanding attitudes and predicting social behavior*. Englewood Cliffs, NJ: Pearson.

Ajzen, I., & Madden, T. J. (1986). Prediction of goal-directed behavior: Attitudes, intentions, and perceived behavioral control. *Journal of Experimental Social Psychology, 22*(5), 453–474.

Akkermann, K., Kaasik, K., Kiive, E., Nordquist, N., Oreland, L., & Harro, J. (2012). The impact of adverse life events and the serotonin transporter gene promoter polymorphism on the development of eating disorder symptoms. *Journal of Psychiatric Research, 46*(1), 38–43.

Alabas, O. A., Tashani, O. A., & Johnson, M. I. (2013). Effects of ethnicity and gender role expectations of pain on experimental pain: A cross-cultural study. *European Journal of Pain, 17*(5), 776–786.

Albers, M. (2018). Achieving competitive neutrality step-by-step. *World Competition, 41*(4), 495–512.

Albrecht, G. L., & Devlieger, P. J. (1999). The disability paradox: High quality of life against all odds. *Social Science & Medicine, 48*(8), 977–988.

Aldwin, C. M. (1991). Does age affect the stress and coping process? Implications of age differences in perceived control. *Journal of Gerontology, 46*(4), P174–P180.

Aldwin, C., Folkman, S., Schaefer, C., Coyne, J. C., & Lazarus, R. S. (1980, September). *Ways of coping: A process measure*. Presented at 88th Annual Meeting of the American Psychological Association, Montreal, Quebec.

Algafly, A. A., & George, K. P. (2007). The effect of cryotherapy on nerve conduction velocity, pain threshold and pain tolerance. *British Journal of Sports Medicine, 41*(6), 365–369.

Alhalal, E. (2018). Obesity in women who have experienced intimate partner violence. *Journal of Advanced Nursing, 74*(12), 2785–2797.

Al-Hasani, R., & Bruchas, M. R. (2011). Molecular mechanisms of opioid receptor-dependent signaling and behavior. *Anesthesiology, 115*(6), 1363–1381.

Allen, J. P. (2005). *The art of medicine in ancient Egypt*. New York, NY: Metropolitan Museum of Art.

Allenbaugh, J., Spagnoletti, C. L., Rack, L., Rubio, D., & Corbelli, J. (2019). Health literacy and clear bedside communication: A curricular intervention for internal medicine physicians and medicine nurses. *MedEdPORTAL: The Journal of Teaching and Learning Resources, 15*.

Allison, S. T., & Goethals, G. R. (2014). "Now he belongs to the ages": The heroic leadership dynamic and deep narratives of greatness. In G. R. Goethals, S. T. Allison, R. M. Kramer, & D. M. Messick (Eds.), *Conceptions of leadership: Enduring ideas and emerging insights* (pp. 167–183). New York, NY: Palgrave Macmillan.

Almeida, D. M., Charles, S. T., & Neupert, S. D. (2008). Commentary: Assessing health behaviors across individuals, situations, and time. In K. W. Schaie & R. P. Abeles (Eds.), *Social structure and aging individuals* (pp. 97–111). New York, NY: Springer.

Almeida, D. M., Neupert, S. D., Banks, S. R., & Serido, J. (2005). Do daily stress processes account for socioeconomic health disparities? *Journals of Gerontology Series B: Psychological Sciences and Social Sciences, 60*(Special Issue 2), S34–S39.

Alt, D. (2018). Students' wellbeing, fear of missing out, and social media engagement for leisure in higher education learning environments. *Current Psychology, 37*(1), 128–138.

Alvidrez, J., & Stinson, N., Jr. (2019). Sideways progress in intervention research is not sufficient to eliminate health disparities. *American Journal of Public Health, 109*(S1), S102–S104. doi: 10.2105/AJPH.2019.304953

Alzahrani, S. G., Watt, R. G., Sheiham, A., Aresu, M., & Tsakos, G. (2014). Patterns of clustering of six health-compromising behaviours in Saudi adolescents. *BMC Public Health, 14*, 1215. doi: 10.1186/1471-2458-14-1215

Alzheimer's Association. (2023). *Alzheimer's disease facts and figures*. Retrieved from https://www.alz.org/alzheimers-dementia/facts-figures

American Academy of Dermatology. (2019). *Skin cancer*. Retrieved from https://www.aad.org/media/stats/conditions/skin-cancer

American Autoimmune Related Diseases Association. (2024). *Autoimmune disease statistics*. Retrieved from https://autoimmune.org/wp-content/uploads/2019/12/1-in-5-Brochure.pdf

American Cancer Society. (2019). *Cancer facts & figures 2019*. Retrieved from https://www.cancer.org/content/dam/cancer-org/research/cancer-facts-and-statistics/annual-cancer-facts-and-figures/2019/cancer-facts-and-figures-2019.pdf

American Cancer Society. (2024). *Cancer facts & figures 2024*. Retrieved from https://www.cancer.org/research/cancer-facts-statistics/all-cancer-facts-figures/2024-cancer-facts-figures.html

American Heart Association. (2017, November). *Understanding blood pressure readings*. Retrieved from https://www.heart.org/en/health-topics/high-blood-pressure/understanding-blood-pressure-readings

American Heart Association. (2024). *High blood pressure*. Retrieved from *https://www.heart.org/en/health-topics/high-blood-pressure*

American Hospital Association. (2019a, January). *Fast facts on U.S. hospitals, 2019*. Retrieved from https://www.aha.org/statistics/fast-facts-us-hospitals

American Institute of Stress. (2018). *How stress affects your body*. Retrieved from https://www.stress.org/stress-effects

American Pain Society. (2014, October 9). Adolescent chronic pain costs $19.5 billion a year in the United States. *Journal of Pain*. Retrieved from http://americanpainsociety.org/about-us/press-room/adolescent-chronic-pain-news-release

American Psychiatric Association. (2013). *Diagnostic and statistical manual of mental disorders* (5th ed.). Washington, DC: Author.

American Psychological Association. (2017). Stress in America: The state of our nation. *Stress in America Survey*.

American Psychological Association. (2019). *Managing your distress in the aftermath of a mass shooting*. Retrieved from https://www.apa.org/helpcenter/mass-shooting

American Psychological Association, Bourdeau, T. L., & Walters, A. (2013). *Coping with a diagnosis of chronic illness*. Retrieved from http://www.apa.org/helpcenter/chronic-illness

American Psychosomatic Society. (2001). *Mission statement*. Retrieved from http://www.psychosomatic.org/AnMeeting/PastEvents/archive/mission.html

Amra, B., et al. (2017). The association of sleep and late-night cell phone use among adolescents. *Jornal de Pediatria, 93*(6), 560–567.

Anderson, R. J., & Brice, S. (2011). The mood-enhancing benefits of exercise: Memory biases augment the effect. *Psychology of Sport and Exercise, 12*, 79–82.

Anderson, N. E., Broad, J. B., & Bonita, R. (1995). Delays in hospital admission and investigation in acute stroke. *BMJ, 311*(6998), 162.

Anderson, P. M., & Butcher, K. E. (2006). Childhood obesity: Trends and potential causes. *Future Child, 16*(1), 19–45.

Andersen, B. L., Cacioppo, J. T., & Roberts, D. C. (1995). Delay in seeking a cancer diagnosis: Delay stages and psychophysiological comparison processes. *British Journal of Social Psychology, 34*(Pt 1), 33–52.

Anderson, T. M., Ferres, J. M. L., Ren, S. Y., Moon, R. Y., Goldstein, R. D., Ramirez, J. M., & Mitchell, E. A. (2019). Maternal smoking before and during pregnancy and the risk of sudden unexpected infant death. *Pediatrics, 143*(4), e20183325.

Andersen, A. E., & Holman, J. E. (1997). Males with eating disorders: Challenges for treatment and research. *Psychopharmacology Bulletin, 33*(3), 391–397.

Anderson, J., & Rainie, L. (2023). *Themes: The best and most beneficial changes in digital life that are likely by 2035*. Pew Research Center. Retrieved from https://www.pewresearch.org/internet/2023/06/21/themes-the-best-and-most-beneficial-changes-in-digital-life-that-are-likely-by-2035/

Anderson, M., Stein Merkin, S., Everson Rose, S. A., Widome, R., Seeman, T., Rodriguez, C., & Lutsey, P. L. (2019). Abstract P394: Health literacy within a diverse community-based cohort: The multi-ethnic study of atherosclerosis. *Circulation, 139*(Suppl. 1), AP394.

Anderson, S. E., & Whitaker, R. C. (2010). Household routines and obesity in US preschool-aged children. *Pediatrics, 125*(3), 420–428.

Andoy-Galvan, J. A., Sriram, S., Kiat, T. J., Xin, L. Z., Shin, W. J., & Chinna, K. (2023). Obesogenic environment in the medical field: First year findings from a five-year cohort study. *F1000Research, 12*, 550.

Andreeva, V. A., Tavolacci, M. P., Galan, P., Ladner, J., Buscail, C., Péneau, S., … Julia, C. (2019). Sociodemographic correlates of eating disorder subtypes among men and women in France, with a focus on age. *Journal of Epidemiology and Community Health, 73*(1), 56–64.

Andrew, M. K., Fisk, J. D., & Rockwood, K. (2012). Psychological well-being in relation to frailty: A frailty identity crisis? *International Psychogeriatrics, 24*(8), 1347–1353.

Anema, C., Johnson, M., Zeller, J. M., Fogg, L., & Zetterlund, J. (2009). Spiritual well-being in individuals with fibromyalgia syndrome: Relationships with symptom pattern variability, uncertainty, and psychosocial adaptation. *Research and Theory for Nursing Practice*, *23*(1), 8–22.

Annan, K. A. (2000). *We the peoples: The role of the United Nations in the 21st century*. New York, NY: United Nations. Retrieved from http://www.un.org/en/events/pastevents/pdfs/We_The_Peoples.pdf

Annas, G. J., & Grodin, M. A. (Eds.). (1992). *The Nazi doctors and the Nuremberg Code: Human rights in human experimentation*. New York, NY: Oxford University Press.

Antoni, M. H. (2003). Stress management effects on psychological, endocrinological, and immune functioning in men with HIV infection: Empirical support for a psychoneuroimmunological model. *Stress*, *6*(3), 173–188.

Antonovsky, A. (1967). Social class, life expectancy and overall mortality. *Milbank Memorial Fund Quarterly*, *45*(2), 31–73.

Antoun, J., Hamadeh, G., & Romani, M. (2019). Effect of computer use on physician-patient communication using interviews: A patient perspective. *International Journal of Medical Informatics*, *125*, 91–95.

Anyiwe, K., Erman, A., Hassan, M., Feld, J. J., Pullenayegum, E., Wong, W. W., & Sander, B. (2024). Characterising the effectiveness of social determinants of health-focused hepatitis B interventions: A systematic review. *The Lancet Infectious Diseases*, *24*, e366–e385.

Araújo, J., Cai, J., & Stevens, J. (2018). Prevalence of optimal metabolic health in American adults: National Health and Nutrition Examination Survey 2009–2016. *Metabolic Syndrome and Related Disorders*, *17*(1), 46–52.

Arends, R. Y., Bode, C., Taal, E., & van de Laar, M. A. (2016). The longitudinal relation between patterns of goal management and psychological health in people with arthritis: The need for adaptive flexibility. *British Journal of Health Psychology*, *21*, 469–489. doi: 10.1111/bjhp.12182

Arleo, E. K., Dashevsky, B. Z., Reichman, M., Babagbemi, K., Drotman, M., & Rosenblatt, R. (2013). Screening mammography for women in their 40s: A retrospective study of the potential impact of the U. S. Preventive Service Task Force's 2009 breast cancer screening recommendations. *AJR American Journal of Roentgenology*, *201*(6), 1401–1406.

Armitage, C. J. (2009). Is there utility in the transtheoretical model? *British Journal of Health Psychology*, *14* (Pt 2), 195–210.

Armitage, C. J., & Arden, M. A. (2012). A volitional help sheet to reduce alcohol consumption in the general population: A field experiment. *Prevention Science*, *13*(6), 635–643.

Arslan, N., Aslan Ceylan, J., & Hatipoğlu, A. (2023). The relationship of fast food consumption with sociodemographic factors, body mass index and dietary habits among university students. *Nutrition & Food Science*, *53*(1), 112–123. https://doi.org/10.1108/NFS-01-2022-0003

Arthritis Foundation. (2018). *Arthritis by the numbers: Book of trusted facts & figures*. Retrieved from https://www.arthritis.org/Documents/Sections/About-Arthritis/arthritis-facts-stats-figures.pdf

Asendorpf, J. B. (1993). Beyond temperament: A two-factorial coping model of the development of inhibition during childhood. In K. Rubin & J. Asendorpf (Eds.), *Social withdrawal, inhibition, and shyness in childhood* (pp. 265–289). Hillsdale, NJ: Erlbaum.

Ashby, J., O'Hanlon, M., & Buxton, M. J. (1994). The time tradeoff technique: How do the valuations of breast cancer patients compare to those of other groups? *Quality of Life Research*, *3*(4), 257–265.

Ashman, J. J., Rui, P., & Okeyode, T. (2019, January). Characteristics of office-based physician visits, 2016. *Centers for Disease Control and Prevention*. Retrieved from https://www.cdc.gov/nchs/products/databriefs/db331.htm

Asthana, H. S. (2012). Psycho-social correlates of obesity: An empirical study. *Social Science International*, *28*(2), 233–251.

Auerbach, J. A., Krimgold, B. K., & Lefkowitz, B. (2000). *Improving health: It doesn't take a revolution* (Issue 298). Washington, DC: Academy for Health Services Research and Health Policy.

Auerbach, S. M., Martelli, M. F., & Mercuri, L. G. (1983). Anxiety, information, interpersonal impacts, and adjustment to a stressful health care situation. *Journal of Personality and Social Psychology*, *44*(6), 1284–1296.

Auter, Z. (2017). *U.S. uninsured rate rises to 12.3% in third quarter*. Retrieved from https://news.gallup.com/poll/220676/uninsured-rate-rises-third-quarter.aspx?g_source=HEALTH_INSURANCE&g_medium=topic&g_campaign=tiles

Averill, J. R., Ekman, P., Ellsworth, P. C., Frijda, N. H., Lazarus, R., Scherer, K. R., & Davidson, R. J. (1994). How is evidence of universals in antecedents of emotion explained? In P. Ekman & R. J. Davidson (Eds.), *The nature of emotion: Fundamental questions* (pp. 144–177). New York, NY: Oxford University Press.

Ayers, J. W., Hofstetter, C. R., Irvin, V. L., Song, Y., Park, H., Paik, H., & Hovell, M. F. (2010). Can religion help prevent obesity? Religious messages and the prevalence of being overweight or obese among Korean women in California. *Journal for the Scientific Study of Religion*, *49*(3), 536–549.

Back, S. E., Flanagan, J. C., Killeen, T., Saraiya, T. C., Brown, D. G., Jarnecke, A. M., … Brady, K. T. (2023). COPE and oxytocin for the treatment of co-occurring PTSD and alcohol use disorder: Design and methodology of a randomized controlled trial in US military veterans. *Contemporary Clinical Trials*, *126*, 107084.

Back, A. L., Wallace, J. I., Starks, H. E., & Pearlman, R. A. (1996). Physician-assisted suicide and euthanasia in Washington State: Patient requests and physician responses. *Journal of the American Medical Association*, *275*(12), 919–925.

Baer, P. E., Garmezy, L. B., McLaughlin, R. J., Pokorny, A. D., & Wernick, M. J. (1987). Stress, coping, family conflict, and adolescent alcohol use. *Journal of Behavioral Medicine*, *10*, 449–466.

Bagherian-Sararoudi, R., Sanei, H., Attari, A., & Afshar, H. (2012). Type D personality is associated with hyperlipidemia in patients with myocardial infarction. *Journal of Research in Medical Sciences*, *17*(6), 543–547.

Bailis, D. S., Chipperfield, J. G., & Perry, R. P. (2005). Optimistic social comparisons of older adults low in primary control: A prospective analysis of hospitalization and mortality. *Health Psychology*, *24*(4), 393–401.

Bair, M. J., Wu, J., Damush, T. M., Sutherland, J. M., & Kroenke, K. (2008). Association of depression and anxiety alone and in combination with chronic musculoskeletal pain in primary care patients. *Psychosomatic Medicine*, *70*(8), 890–897.

Baker, T. B., Piper, M. E., McCarthy, D. E., Majeskie, M. R., & Fiore, M. C. (2004). Addiction motivation reformulated: An affective processing model of negative reinforcement. *Psychological Review*, *111*(1), 33–51.

Bales, K. L., van Westerhuyzen, J. A., Lewis-Reese, A. D., Grotte, N. D., Lanter, J. A., & Carter, C. S. (2007). Oxytocin has dose-dependent developmental effects on pair-bonding and alloparental care in female prairie voles. *Hormones and Behavior*, *52*, 274–279.

Ballard, J. (2018, June 28). *One in five Americans has stuck to their 2018 New Year's Resolution*. Retrieved from https://today.yougov.com/topics/lifestyle/articles-reports/2018/06/28/2018-new-years-resolutions-update

Ball, K., & Kenardy, J. (2002). Body weight, body image, and eating behaviours: Relationships with ethnicity and acculturation in a community sample of young Australian women. *Eating Behaviors*, *3*(3), 205–216.

Ball, N. J., Miller, K. E., Quigley, B. M., & Eliseo-Arras, R. K. (2018). Alcohol mixed with energy drinks and sexually related causes of conflict in the barroom. *Journal of Interpersonal Violence*. Advance online publication. doi: 10.1177/0886260518774298

Bandura, A. (1989). Social cognitive theory. In R. Vasta (Ed.), *Annals of child development, vol. 6. Six theories of child development* (pp. 1–60). Greenwich, CT: JAI Press.

Bandura, A. (1991). Self-efficacy mechanism in physiological activation and health-promotion behavior. In J. Madden (Ed.), *Neurobiology of learning, emotion, and affect* (pp. 229–269). New York, NY: Raven.

Bandura, A. (1995). *Self-efficacy in changing societies*. Cambridge, UK: Cambridge University Press.

Bandura, A. (1998). Health promotion from the perspective of social cognitive theory. *Psychology & Health*, *13*, 623–649.

Banerjee, A. (2024). Disparities by social determinants of health: Links between long COVID and cardiovascular disease. *Canadian Journal of Cardiology*, *40*(6), 1123–1134.

Banfield, J., Wyland, C. L., Macrae, C. N., Münte, T. F., & Heatherton, T. F. (2005). The cognitive neuroscience of self-regulation. In R. F. Baumeister & K. D. Vohs (Eds.), *The handbook of self-regulation* (pp. 63–83). New York, NY: Guilford.

Barańczuk, U. (2019). The five factor model of personality and emotion regulation: A meta-analysis. *Personality and Individual Differences*, *139*, 217–227.

Barbour, K., Helmick, C., Boring, M., Brady, T. (2017). Vital signs: Prevalence of doctor-diagnosed arthritis and arthritis-attributable activity limitation—United States 2013–2015. *Morbidity and Mortality Weekly Report*, *66*(9), 246–253.

Barbour, K. E., Helmick, C. G., Theis, K. A., Murphy, L. B., Hootman, J. M., Brady, T. J., & Cheng, Y. J. (2013). Prevalence of doctor-diagnosed arthritis and arthritis-attributable activity limitation—United States, 2010–2012. *Morbidity and Mortality Weekly Report*, *62*(44), 869–873.

Barefoot, K. N., Warren, J. C., & Smalley, K. B. (2017). Women's health care: The experiences and behaviors of rural and urban lesbians in the USA. *Rural and Remote Health*, *17*, 3875.

Barker, D. J., Eriksson, J. G., Forsén, T., & Osmond, C. (2002). Fetal origins of adult disease: Strength of effects and biological basis. *International Journal of Epidemiology*, 31(6), 1235–1239.

Barnes, P., Bloom, B., & Dhalhamer, J. (2008). *CAM use in 2007: Data from the national health interview survey*. Hyattsville, MD: National Centers for Health Statistics.

Barnes, P. M., Bloom, B., & Nahin, R. L. (2008). Complementary and alternative medicine use among adults and children: United States, 2007. In *CDC national health statistics report* (Vol. 12, pp. 1–24). Bethesda, MD: National Center for Complementary and Integrative Health. Retrieved from https://nccih.nih.gov/news/camstats/2007

Baron, K. G., Reid, K. J., Kern, A. S., & Zee, P. C. (2011). Role of sleep timing in caloric intake and BMI. *Obesity (Silver Spring)*, 19(7), 1374–1381.

Barrett, B., Muller, D., Rakel, D., Rabago, D., Marchand, L., & Scheder, J. C. (2006). Placebo, meaning, and health. *Perspectives in Biology and Medicine*, 49(2), 178–198.

Batten, D. (Ed.) (2010). Euthanasia. In *Gale Encyclopedia of American Law* (3rd ed., Vol. 4, pp. 257–263). Detroit: Gale, Cengage Learning.

Bauer, U. E., Briss, P. A., Goodman, R. A., & Bowman, B. A. (2014). Prevention of chronic disease in the 21st century: Elimination of the leading preventable causes of premature death and disability in the USA. *Lancet*, 384(9937), 45–52.

Bauer, J. J., & McAdams, D. P. (2010). Eudaimonic growth: Narrative growth goals predict increases in ego development and subjective well-being 3 years later. *Developmental Psychology*, 46(4), 761–772.

Bauer, U. E., & Plescia, M. (2014). Addressing disparities in the health of American Indian and Alaska Native people: The importance of improved public health data. *American Journal of Public Health*, 104(Suppl. 3), S255–S257. doi: 10.2105/AJPH.2013.301602

Bauer, I., & Wrosch, C. (2011). Making up for lost opportunities: The protective role of downward social comparisons for coping with regrets across adulthood. *Personality and Social Psychology Bulletin*, 37(2), 215–228.

Baum, A. (1990). Stress, intrusive imagery, and chronic distress. *Health Psychology*, 9, 653–675.

Baum, A., Garofalo, J. P., & Yali, A. (1999). Socioeconomic status and chronic stress: Does stress account for SES effects on health? *Annals of the New York Academy of Sciences*, 896(1), 131–144.

Baumeister, R., & Tierney, J. (2012). *Willpower: Rediscovering the greatest human strength*. London, UK: Penguin.

Baumeister, R. (2018). *Self-regulation and self-control: Selected works of Roy F. Baumeister*. Routledge.

Bayer, V., Robert-McComb, J. J., Clopton, J. R., & Reich, D. A. (2017). Investigating the influence of shame, depression, and distress tolerance on the relationship between internalized homophobia and binge eating in lesbian and bisexual women. *Eating Behaviors*, 24, 39–44.

Bazo Perez, M., & Frazier, L. D. (2024). Risk and resilience in eating disorders: Differentiating pathways among psychosocial predictors. *Journal of Eating Disorders*, 12(1), 62.

Bazo Perez, M., Hayes, T. B., & Frazier, L. D. (2023). Beyond generalized anxiety: The association of anxiety sensitivity with disordered eating. *Journal of Eating Disorders*, 11(1), 173.

Beard, C. M., Kokmen, E., Sigler, C., Smith, G. E., Petterson, T., & O'Brien, P. C. (1996). Cause of death in Alzheimer's disease. *Annals of Epidemiology*, 6(3), 195–200.

Beauchamp, G. K., & Mennella, J. A. (2009). Early flavor learning and its impact on later feeding behavior. *Journal of Pediatric Gastroenterology and Nutrition*, 48(Suppl. 1), S25–30. doi: 10.1097/MPG.0b013e31819774a5

Beaudoin, C. E. (2011). Hurricane Katrina: Addictive behavior trends and predictors. *Public Health Reports*, 126(3), 400–409.

Beck, J., Garcia, R., Heiss, G., Vokonas, P. S., & Offenbacher, S. (1996). Periodontal disease and cardiovascular disease. *Journal of Periodontology*, 67(10 Suppl.), 1123–1137.

Beck, J., Loretz, E., & Rasch, B. (2023). Stress dynamically reduces sleep depth: Temporal proximity to the stressor is crucial. *Cerebral Cortex*, 33(1), 96–113.

Becker, E. (1973). *The denial of death*. New York, NY: Free Press.

Becker, M. H. (1979). Understanding patient compliance: The contributions of attitudes and other psychosocial factors. In S. J. Cohen (Ed.), *New directions in patient compliance* (pp. 1–31). Lexington, MA: Lexington Books.

Becker, G., & Newsom, E. (2005). Resilience in the face of serious illness among chronically ill African Americans in later life. *Journals of Gerontology Series B: Psychological Sciences and Social Sciences*, 60(4), S214–S223.

Becker, M. H., & Rosenstock, I. M. (1984). Compliance with medical advice. In A. Steptoe & A. Mathews (Eds.), *Health care and human behavior* (pp. 175–208). London, UK: Academic Press.

Beecher, H. K. (1946). Pain in men wounded in battle. *Annals of Surgery, 123*(1), 96–105.

Beecher, H. K. (1956). Relationship of significance of wound to pain experienced. *Journal of the American Medical Association, 161*(17), 1609–1613.

Beecher, H. K. (1959). *Measurement of subjective responses: Quantitative effects of drugs*. New York, NY: Oxford University Press.

Bégin, C., Turcotte, O., & Rodrigue, C. (2019). Psychosocial factors underlying symptoms of muscle dysmorphia in a non-clinical sample of men. *Psychiatry Research, 272*, 319–325.

Belloc, N. B., & Breslow, L. (1972). Relationship of physical health status and family practices. *Preventive Medicine, 1*, 409–421.

Belsky, J., Houts, R. M., & Fearon, R. M. (2010). Infant attachment security and timing of puberty: Testing an evolutionary hypothesis. *Psychological Science, 21*, 1195–1201.

Benedetti, F., Lanotte, M., Colloca, L., Ducati, A., Zibetti, M., & Lopiano, L. (2009). Electrophysiological properties of thalamic, subthalamic and nigral neurons during the antiparkinsonian placebo response. *Journal of Physiology, 587*(Pt 15), 3869–3883.

Benjamin, E. J., Virani, S. S., Callaway, C. W., Chang, A. R., Cheng, S., Chiuve, S. E., ... Ferguson, J. F. (2018). Heart disease and stroke statistics—2018 update: A report from the American Heart Association. *Circulation, 137*(12), e67–e492.

Bennett, C. (2010). Early/ancient history. In J. Holland (Ed.), *The pot book: A complete guide to cannabis*. Rochester, VT: Park Street Press.

Bennett, M. P., & Lengacher, C. A. (2006). Humor and laughter may influence health. I. History and background. *Evidence Based Complementary and Alternative Medicine, 3*(1), 61–63.

Benotsch, E. G., Snipes, D. J., Martin, A. M., & Bull, S. S. (2013). Sexting, substance use, and sexual risk behavior in young adults. *Journal of Adolescent Health, 52*(3), 307–313.

Berenson, G. S., Srinivasan, S. R., Bao, W., Newman, W. P., Tracy, R. E., & Wattigney, W. A. (1998). Association between multiple cardiovascular risk factors and atherosclerosis in children and young adults. *New England Journal of Medicine, 338*(23), 1650–1656.

Berenson, G. S., Wattigney, W. A., Tracy, R. E., Newman, W. P., Srinivasan, S. R., Webber, L. S., ... Strong, J. P. (1992). Atherosclerosis of the aorta and coronary arteries and cardiovascular risk factors in persons aged 6 to 30 years and studied at necropsy (The Bogalusa Heart Study). *American Journal of Cardiology, 70*(9), 851–858.

Berkman, L. F., & Breslow, L. (1983). *Health and ways of living: The Alameda County Study*. New York, NY: Oxford University Press.

Berlim, M. T., Van den Eynde, F., & Daskalakis, Z. J. (2013). Clinical utility of transcranial direct current stimulation (tDCS) for treating major depression: A systematic review and meta-analysis of randomized, double-blind and sham-controlled trials. *Journal of Psychiatric Research, 47*(1), 1–7.

Bermudez, V. N., Fearon-Drake, D., Wheelis, M., Cohenour, M., Suntai, Z., & Scullin, M. K. (2022). Sleep disparities in the first month of college: Implications for academic achievement. *Sleep Advances, 3(1)*, zpac041.

Berry, J. W. (1992). Acculturation and adaptation in a new society. *International Migration, 30*(s1), 69–85.

Berry, J. W., Kim, U., Minde, T., & Mok, D. (1987). Comparative studies of acculturative stress. *International Migration Review, 21*(3), 491–511.

Bertakis, K. D., Azari, R., Helms, L. J., Callahan, E. J., & Robbins, J. A. (2000). Gender differences in the utilization of health care services. *Journal of Family Practice, 49*(2), 147–152.

Beyene, Y., Becker, G., & Mayen, N. (2002). Perception of aging and sense of well-being among Latino elderly. *Journal of Cross-Cultural Gerontology, 17*(2), 155–172.

Bezner, J., Adams, T. B., & Steinhardt, M. A. (1997). Relationship of body dissatisfaction to physical health and wellness. *American Journal of Health Behavior, 21*(2), 147–155.

Bill & Melinda Gates Foundation. (2024). *The Bill & Melinda gates foundation commits $922 million to advance global nutrition to help women and children*. Retrieved from https://www.gatesfoundation.org/ideas/media-center/press-releases/2021/09/922m-commitment-to-global-nutrition-and-food-systems

Billings, A. G., & Moos, R. H. (1984). Coping, stress, and social resources among adults with unipolar depression. *Journal of Personality and Social Psychology, 46*, 877–891.

Binder, M., & Coad, A. (2013). "I'm afraid I have bad news for you ...": Estimating the impact of different health impairments on subjective well-being. *Social Science & Medicine, 87*, 155–167.

Blackmore, D. G., Golmohammadi, M. G., Large, B., Waters, M. J., & Rietze, R. L. (2009). Exercise increases neural stem cell number in a growth hormone-dependent manner, augmenting the regenerative response in aged mice. *Stem Cells, 27*, 2044–2052.

Blake, H. M. (2019). Botanical treatments in cancer pain management. In A. Gulati, V. Puttanniah, B. M. Bruel, W. Rosenberg, & J. C. Hung, (Eds.), *Essentials of interventional cancer pain management* (pp. 503–506). New York, NY: Springer.

Blanchflower, D. G., & Oswald, A. J. (2017). Unhappiness and pain in modern America: A review essay, and further evidence, on Carol Graham's Happiness for All?. IZA Discussion Papers, No. 11184. Bonn, Germany: Institute of Labor Economics (IZA).

Bleuler, M. (1963). Conception of schizophrenia within the last fifty years and today [abridged]. *Proceedings of the Royal Society of Medicine, 56*(10), 945–952.

Bloomgarden, Z. T. (2004). Type 2 diabetes in the young: The evolving epidemic. *Diabetes Care, 27*(4), 998–1010.

Blumenthal, J. A., Babyak, M. A., Doraiswamy, P. M., Watkins, L., Hoffman, B. M., Barbour, K. A., ... Sherwood, A. (2007). Exercise and pharmacotherapy in the treatment of major depressive disorder. *Psychosomatic Medicine, 69*(7), 587–596. doi: 10.1097/PSY.0b013e318148c19a

Blumenthal, J. A., Babyak, M. A., Hinderliter, A., Watkins, L. L., Craighead, L., Lin, P.-H., ... Sherwood, A. (2010). Effects of the DASH diet alone and in combination with exercise and weight loss on blood pressure and cardiovascular biomarkers in men and women with high blood pressure: The ENCORE Study. *Archives of Internal Medicine, 170*(2), 126–135. doi: 10.1001/archinternmed.2009.470

Bodell, L. P., Hames, J. L., Holm-Denoma, J. M., Smith, A. R., Gordon, K. H., & Joiner, T. E. (2012). Does the stress generation hypothesis apply to eating disorders? An examination of stress generation in eating, depressive, and anxiety symptoms. *Journal of Affective Disorders, 142*(1–3), 139–142.

Boehm, J. K., & Kubzansky, L. D. (2012). The heart's content: The association between positive psychological well-being and cardiovascular health. *Psychological Bulletin, 138*, 655–691. doi: 10.1037/a0027448

Bogart, L. M., Howerton, D., Lange, J., Setodji, C. M., Becker, K., Klein, D. J., & Asch, S. M. (2010). Provider-related barriers to rapid HIV testing in U.S. urban non-profit community clinics, community-based organizations (CBOs) and hospitals. *AIDS and Behavior, 14*(3), 697–707.

Bogel-Burroughs, N., & Peters, J. W. (2020, April 20). 'You have todisobey': Protesters gather to defy stay-at-home orders. *The New York Times.* Retrieved from https://www.nytimes.com/2020/04/16/us/coronavirus-rulesprotests.html

Bolger, N., & Amarel, D. (2007). Effects of social support visibility on adjustment to stress: Experimental evidence. *Journal of Personality and Social Psychology, 92*(3), 458–475.

Bolger, N., DeLongis, A., Kessler, R. C., & Schilling, E. A. (1989). Effects of daily stress on negative mood. *Journal of Personality and Social Psychology, 57*, 808–818.

Bolton, D., & Gillett, G. (2019). Biopsychosocial conditions of health and disease. In *The biopsychosocial model of health and disease* (pp. 109–145). New York, NY: Palgrave.

Bo, S., Musso, G., Beccuti, G., Fadda, M., Fedele, D., Gambino, R., ... Cassader, M. (2014). Consuming more of daily caloric intake at dinner predisposes to obesity: A 6-year population-based prospective cohort study. *PLoS One, 9*(9), e108467. doi: 10.1371/journal.pone.0108467

Bonanno, G. A. (2004). Loss, trauma, and human resilience: Have we underestimated the human capacity to thrive after extremely aversive events? *American Psychologist, 59*(1), 20–28.

Bonanno, G. A. (2009). *The other side of sadness: What the new science of bereavement tells us about life after loss.* New York, NY: Basic Books.

Bonanno, G. A., Galea, S., Bucciarelli, A., & Vlahov, D. (2006). Psychological resilience after disaster: New York City in the aftermath of the September 11th terrorist attack. *Psychological Science, 17*(3), 181–186.

Bongers, P., de Graaff, A., & Jansen, A. (2016). "Emotional" does not even start to cover it: Generalization of overeating in emotional eaters. *Appetite, 96*, 611–616.

Borja, S., Nurius, P. S., Song, C., & Lengua, L. J. (2019). ACEs to adult adversity trends among parents: Socioeconomic, health, and developmental implications. *Children and Youth Services Review, 100*. doi: 10.1016/j.childyouth.2019.03.007

Borland, R., Partos, T. R., Yong, H.-H., Cummings, K. M., & Hyland, A. (2012). How much unsuccessful quitting activity is going on among adult smokers? Data from the International Tobacco Control Four Country cohort survey. *Addiction, 107*(3), 673–682. doi: 10.1111/j.1360-0443.2011.03685.x

Borup, G., Mikkelsen, K. L., Tønnesen, P., & Christrup, L. L. (2015). Exploratory survey study of long-term users of nicotine replacement therapy in Danish consumers. *Harm Reduction Journal, 12*, 2.

Boschi, V., Iorio, D., Margiotta, N., D'Orsi, P., & Falconi, C. (2001). The three-factor eating questionnaire in the evaluation of eating behaviour in subjects seeking participation in a dietotherapy programme. *Annals of Nutrition and Metabolism, 45*(2), 72–77.

Boss, P., & Couden, B. A. (2002). Ambiguous loss from chronic physical illness: Clinical interventions with individuals, couples, and families. *Journal of Clinical Psychology, 58*(11), 1351–1360.

Bosworth, H. B., Oddone, E. Z., & Weinberger, M. (Eds.). (2006). *Patient treatment adherence: Concepts, interventions, and measurement.* Mahwah, NJ: Erlbaum.

Bower, J. E., Ganz, P. A., Desmond, K. A., Rowland, J. H., Meyerowitz, B. E., & Belin, T. R. (2000). Fatigue in breast cancer survivors: Occurrence, correlates, and impact on quality of life. *Journal of Clinical Oncology, 18*(4), 743–753.

Bower, J. E., Greendale, G., Crosswell, A. D., Garet, D., Sternlieb, B., Ganz, P. A., ... Cole, S. W. (2014). Yoga reduces inflammatory signaling in fatigued breast cancer survivors: A randomized controlled trial. *Psychoneuroendocrinology, 43*, 20–29.

Bower, A. M., & Hayes, A. (1998). Mothering in families with and without a child with disability. *International Journal of Disability, Development and Education, 45*(3), 313–322.

Boyle, P. A., Buchman, A. S., Barnes, L. L., & Bennett, D. A. (2010). Effect of a purpose in life on risk of incident Alzheimer disease and mild cognitive impairment in community-dwelling older persons. *Archives of General Psychiatry, 67*(3), 304–310.

Boyle, P. A., Buchman, A. S., Wilson, R. S., Yu, L., Schneider, J. A., & Bennett, D. A. (2012). Effect of purpose in life on the relation between Alzheimer disease pathologic changes on cognitive function in advanced age. *Archives of General Psychiatry, 69*(5), 499–505.

Brailovskaia, J., Ozimek, P., Rohmann, E., & Bierhoff, H. W. (2023). Vulnerable narcissism, fear of missing out (FoMO) and addictive social media use: A gender comparison from Germany. *Computers in Human Behavior, 144*, 107725.

Brandow, B. (2015, November 23). *Locus of control.* Retrieved from http://www.debtdiscipline.com/locus-of-control/

Brantley, P. J., Dutton, G. R., Grothe, K. B., Bodenlos, J. S., Howe, J., & Jones, G. N. (2005). Minor life events as predictors of medical utilization in low income African American family practice patients. *Journal of Behavioral Medicine, 28*, 395–401.

Breasted, J. H. (Trans. and Ed.). (1991). *The Edwin Smith Surgical Papyrus: Published in facsimile and hieroglyphic transliteration with translation and commentary in two volumes.* Chicago, IL: University of Chicago Press. (Original work published 1930.)

Breen, F. M., Plomin, R., & Wardle, J. (2006). Heritability of food preferences in young children. *Physiology & Behavior, 88*(4–5), 443–447.

Breslau, N., Roth, T., Rosenthal, L., & Andreski, P. (1996). Sleep disturbance and psychiatric disorders: A longitudinal epidemiological study of young adults. *Biological Psychiatry, 39*(6), 411–418.

Breslow, L., & Enstrom, J. E. (1980). Persistence of health habits and their relationship to mortality. *Preventive Medicine, 9*, 469–483.

Breton, É., Côté, S. M., Dubois, L., et al. (2023). Childhood overeating and disordered eating from early adolescence to young adulthood: A longitudinal study on the mediating role of BMI, victimization and desire for thinness. *Journal of Youth and Adolescence, 52*, 1582–1594. doi: 10.1007/s10964-023-01796-5

Brewerton, T. D., & George, M. S. (1993). Is migraine related to the eating disorders? *International Journal of Eating Disorders, 14*(1), 75–79.

Brickman, P., Coates, D., & Janoff-Bulman, R. (1978). Lottery winners and accident victims: Is happiness relative? *Journal of Personality and Social Psychology, 36*(8), 917–927.

Broadbent, E. Petrie, K. J., Main, J., & Weinman, J. (2006). The brief illness perception questionnaire (BIPQ). *Journal of Psychosomatic Research, 60*, 631–637.

Broadie, S., & Rowe, C. (Eds.), (trans. 2002). *Aristotle Nichomachean ethics: Translation, introduction, and commentary.* New York, NY: Oxford University Press.

Brody, H. (2014). Stories and the biopsychosocial model. *Philosophy, Psychiatry, & Psychology, 21*(3), 191–193.

Brody, J. E. (2007, March 6). Tough question to answer, tough answer to hear. *New York Times.* Retrieved from http://www.nytimes.com/2007/03/06/health/06mbrody.html?_r=0

Brooks, P. M. (2006). Rheumatoid arthritis: Aetiology and clinical features. *Medicine, 34*(10), 379–382.

Brooks, S., Rowley, S., Broadbent, E., & Petrie, K. J. (2012). Illness perception ratings of high-risk newborns by mothers and clinicians: Relationship to illness severity and maternal stress. *Health Psychology, 31*(5), 632–639.

Brosschot, J., Godaert, G., Benschop, R., Olff, M., Ballieux, R., & Heijnen, C. (1998). Experimental stress and immunological reactivity: A closer look at perceived uncontrollability. *Psychosomatic Medicine, 60*, 359–361.

Brown, C. R., & Fleisher, D. S. (2014). The bi-cycle concept— Relating continuing education directly to patient care. *Journal of Continuing Education in the Health Professions*, *34*(2), 141–148.

Brown, S. A., McGue, M., Maggs, J., Schulenberg, J., Hingson, R., Swartzwelder, S., … Murphy, S. (2008). A developmental perspective on alcohol and youths 16 to 20 years of age. *Pediatrics*, *121*(Suppl. 4), S290–S310.

Brown, T. L., Phillips, C. M., Abdullah, T., Vinson, E., & Robertson, J. (2011). Dispositional versus situational coping: Are the coping strategies African Americans use different for general versus racism-related stressors? *Journal of Black Psychology*, *37*(3), 311–335.

Brownell, K. D. (1982). Obesity: Understanding and treating a serious, prevalent, and refractory disorder. *Journal of Consulting and Clinical Psychology*, *50*, 820–840.

Brownell, K. D., Marlatt, G. A., Lichtenstein, E., & Wilson, G. T. (1986). Understanding and preventing relapse. *American Psychologist*, *41*(7), 765–782.

Brummett, B. H., Babyak, M. A., Williams, R. B., Barefoot, J. C., Costa, P. T., & Siegler, I. C. (2006). NEO personality domains and gender predict levels and trends in body mass index over 14 years during midlife. *Journal of Research in Personality*, *40*, 222–236.

Bryce, R., Guajardo, C., Ilarraza, D., Milgrom, N., Pike, D., Savoie, K., et al. (2017). Participation in a farmers' market fruit and vegetable prescription program at a federally qualified health center improves hemoglobin A1C in low income uncontrolled diabetics. *Preventive Medicine Reports*, *7*, 176–179. doi: 10.1016/j.pmedr.2017.06.006

Bryden, K. S., Peveler, R. C., Stein, A., Neil, A., Mayou, R. A., & Dunger, D. B. (2001). Clinical and psychological course of diabetes from adolescence to young adulthood: A longitudinal cohort study. *Diabetes Care*, *24*(9), 1536–1540.

Buettner, D. (2005, November). Longevity, the secrets of a long life. *National Geographic*.

Buettner, D. (2015). *The Blue Zones solution: Eating and living like the world's healthiest people*. Washington, DC: National Geographic Society.

Burgard, S. A., & Ailshire, J. A. (2013). Gender and time for sleep among U.S. adults. *American Sociological Review*, *78*(1), 51–69. doi: 10.1177/0003122412472048

Burgess, C. C., Bish, A. M., Hunter, H. S., Salkovskis, P., Michell, M., Whelehan, P., & Ramirez, A. J. (2008). Promoting early presentation of breast cancer: Development of a psycho-educational intervention. *Chronic Illness*, *4*(1), 13–27.

Burkhauser, R. V., & Cawley, J. (2008). Beyond BMI: The value of more accurate measures of fatness and obesity in social science research. *Journal of Health Economics*, *27*(2), 519–529. doi: 10.1016/j.jhealeco.2007.05.005

Burns, D. D. (1989). *The feeling good handbook*. New York, NY: Penguin Group.

Burns, J. W., Johnson, B. J., Mahoney, N., Devine, J., & Pawl, R. (1996). Anger management style, hostility and spouse responses: Gender differences in predictors of adjustment among chronic pain patients. *Pain*, *64*(3), 445–453.

Burns, J. W., Quartana, P., Gilliam, W., Gray, E., Matsuura, J., Nappi, C., … Lofland, K. (2008). Effects of anger suppression on pain severity and pain behaviors among chronic pain patients: Evaluation of an ironic process model. *Health Psychology*, *27*(5), 645–652.

Burston, J. J., Wiley, J. L., Craig, A. A., Selley, D. E., & Sim-Selley, L. J. (2010). Regional enhancement of cannabinoid CB_1 receptor desensitization in female adolescent rats following repeated Delta-tetrahydrocannabinol exposure. *British Journal of Pharmacology*, *161*(1), 103–112. doi: 10.1111/j.1476-5381.2010.00870.x

Bynum, M. S., Burton, E. T., & Best, C. (2007). Racism experiences and psychological functioning in African American college freshmen: Is racial socialization a buffer? *Cultural Diversity and Ethnic Minority Psychology*, *13*(1), 64–71.

Byrne, P. S., & Long, B. E. (1976). *Doctors talking to patients: A study of the verbal behaviours of general practitioners consulting in their surgeries*. London, UK: Her Majesty's Stationery Office.

Caceres, B. A., Brody, A. A., Halkitis, P. N., Dorsen, C., Yu, G., & Chyun, D. A. (2018). Sexual orientation differences in modifiable risk factors for cardiovascular disease and cardiovascular disease diagnoses in men. *LGBT Health*, *5*(5), 284–294. doi: 10.1089/lgbt.2017.0220

Cahn, B. R., & Polich, J. (2006). Meditation states and traits: EEG, ERP, and neuroimaging studies. *Psychological Bulletin*, *132*(2), 180–211.

Calhoun, K. S., & Burnette, M. M. (1983). Etiology and treatment of menstrual disorders. *Behavioral Medicine Update*, *5*(4), 21–26.

Cancer.gov. (2016). *What is cancer?* Retrieved from https://www.cancer.gov/about-cancer/understanding/what-is-cancer

Cannon, W. B. (1932). *The wisdom of the body*. New York, NY: Norton.

Cappell, H., & Greeley, J. (1987). Alcohol and tension reduction: An update on research and theory. In H. T. Blane & K. E. Leonard (Eds.), *Psychological theories of drinking and alcoholism* (pp. 15–54). New York, NY: Guilford.

Cardona Cano, S., Tiemeier, H., Van Hoeken, D., Tharner, A., Jaddoe, V. W., Hofman, A., … Hoek, H. W. (2015). Trajectories of picky eating during childhood: A general population study. *International Journal of Eating Disorders, 48*(6), 570–579.

Cardoso, C., Ellenbogen, M. A., Serravalle, L., & Linnen, A. M. (2013). Stress-induced negative mood moderates the relation between oxytocin administration and trust: Evidence for the tend-and-befriend response to stress? *Psychoneuroendocrinology, 38*(11), 2800–2804.

Cardoso, C., Linnen, A. M., Joober, R., & Ellenbogen, M. A. (2012). Coping style moderates the effect of intranasal oxytocin on the mood response to interpersonal stress. *Experimental and Clinical Psychopharmacology, 20*(2), 84–91.

Cardoso-Moreno, M. J., & Tomás-Aragones, L. (2017). The influence of perceived family support on post surgery recovery. *Psychology, Health and Medicine, 22*(1), 121–128.

Carel, H. (2017). Illness and its experience: The patient perspective. In T. Schramme & S. Edwards (Eds.), *Handbook of the philosophy of medicine* (pp. 1–13). Dordrecht, the Netherlands: Springer Science+Business Media.

Carey, M. P., Kalra, D. L., Carey, K. B., Halperin, S., & Richard, C. S. (1993). Stress and unaided smoking cessation: A prospective investigation. *Journal of Consulting and Clinical Psychology, 61*, 831–838.

Carlson, L. E., Speca, M., Patel, K. D., & Goodey, E. (2003). Mindfulness-based stress reduction in relation to quality of life, mood, symptoms of stress, and immune parameters in breast and prostate cancer outpatients. *Psychosomatic Medicine, 65*(4), 571–581.

Carnell, S., Haworth, C. M., Plomin, R., & Wardle, J. (2008). Genetic influence on appetite in children. *International Journal of Obesity (London), 32*(10), 1468–1473.

Carney, R. M., Freedland, K. E., Miller, G. E., & Jaffe, A. S. (2002). Depression as a risk factor for cardiac mortality and morbidity: A review of potential mechanisms. *Journal of Psychosomatic Research, 53*(4), 897–902.

Carpenter, S., Rigaud, M., Barile, M., Priest, T. J., Perez, L., & Ferguson, J. B. (1998). *An interlinear transliteration and English translation of portions of the Ebers Papyrus possibly having to do with diabetes mellitus.* Annandale-on-Hudson, NY: Bard College. Retrieved from http://bxscience.edu/ourpages/ auto/2008/11/10/43216077/egypt%20medicine.pdf

Carretero, O. A., & Oparil, S. (2000). Essential hypertension part I: Definition and etiology. *Circulation, 101*(3), 329–335.

Carr, D., & Friedman, M. A. (2005). Is obesity stigmatizing? Body weight, perceived discrimination, and psychological well-being in the United States. *Journal of Health and Social Behavior, 46*(3), 244–259.

Carr, D., & Jaffe, K. (2012). The psychological consequences of weight change trajectories: Evidence from quantitative and qualitative data. *Economics & Human Biology, 10*(4), 419–430. doi: 10.1016/j.ehb.2012.04.007

Carroll, J. L. (1990). The relationship between humor appreciation and perceived physical health. *Psychology: A Journal of Human Behavior, 27*(2), 34–37.

Carter, J. C., Van Wijk, M., & Rowsell, M. (2019). Symptoms of "food addiction" in binge eating disorder using the Yale Food Addiction Scale version 2.0. *Appetite, 133*, 362–369.

Cartwright, M., Wardle, J., Steggles, N., Simon, A. E., Croker, H., & Jarvis, M. J. (2003). Stress and dietary practices in adolescents. *Health Psychology, 22*, 362–369.

Carver, C. S. (1997). You want to measure coping but your protocol's too long: Consider the brief COPE. *International Journal of Behavioral Medicine, 4*(1), 92–100.

Carver, C. S. (1998). Resilience and thriving: Issues, models, and linkages. *Journal of Social Issues, 54*(2), 245–266.

Carver, C. S. (2004). Self-regulation of attention and affect. In R. F. Baumeister & K. D. Vohs (Eds.), *Handbook of self-regulation: Research, theory, and applications* (pp. 13–29). New York, NY: Guilford.

Carver, C. S., & Connor-Smith, J. (2010). Personality and coping. *Annual Review of Psychology, 61*, 679–704. doi: 10.1146/annurev.psych.093008.100352

Carver, C. S., Scheier, M. F., & Segerstrom, S. C. (2010). Optimism. *Clinical Psychology Review, 30*(7), 879–889.

Carver, C. S., Scheier, M. F., & Weintraub, J. K. (1989). Assessing coping strategies: A theoretically based approach. *Journal of Personality and Social Psychology, 56*(2), 267–283.

Casey, B. J., Kosofsky, B. E., & Bhide, P. G. (Eds.). (2014). Teenage brains: Think different? [Special issue]. *Developmental Neuroscience, 36*(3–4).

Cash, T. F., & Smolak, L. (2011). *Body image: A handbook of science, practice, and prevention.* (2nd ed.). New York, NY: Guilford.

Cassells, E. L., Magarey, A. M., Daniels, L. A., & Mallan, K. M. (2014). The influence of maternal infant feeding practices and beliefs on the expression of food neophobia in toddlers. *Appetite, 82,* 36–42.

Castel, A. (2019). *Better with age: The psychology of successful aging.* New York, NY: Oxford University Press.

Castellini, G., Caini, S., Cassioli, E., Rossi, E., Marchesoni, G., Rotella, F., … Ricca, V. (2023). Mortality and care of eating disorders. *Acta Psychiatrica Scandinavica, 147*(2), 122–133.

Cavanaugh, K. V., Kruja, B., & Forestell, C. A. (2014). The effect of brand and caloric information on flavor perception and food consumption in retrained and unrestrained eaters. *Appetite, 82,* 1–7.

CBS News. (2023). *Stanford student says social media led to near fatal eating disorder.* Retrieved from https://www.cbsnews.com/sanfrancisco/news/stanford-student-says-social-media-led-to-near-fatal-eating-disorder/

CDC. (2022). COMMIT. Retrieved from https://www.cdc.gov/obesity/initiatives/commit/index.html#:~:text=Childhood%20Obesity%20is%20a%20Serious,year%2Dolds%20(13%25).

Center for Behavioral Health Statistics and Quality. (2015). *Behavioral health trends in the United States: Results from the 2014 National Survey on Drug Use and Health* (HHS Publication No. SMA 15-4927, NSDUH Series H-50). Retrieved from http://www.samhsa.gov/data/

Center for Countering Digital Hate. (2023). *TikTok's toxic trade.* Retrieved from https://counterhate.com/wp-content/uploads/2023/09/TikToks-Toxic-Trade-Steroids-and-Steroid-Like-Drugs.pdf

Centers for Disease Control and Prevention. Get the facts: Added sugars. Retrieved from https://www.cdc.gov/nutrition/data-statistics/added-sugars.html

Centers for Disease Control and Prevention. (2011c). *The obesity epidemic* [Online video]. Retrieved from https://www.cdc.gov/cdctv/diseaseandconditions/lifestyle/obesity-epidemic.html

Centers for Disease Control and Prevention. (2011d). Quitting smoking among adults—United States, 2001–2010. *Morbidity and Mortality Weekly Report, 60*(44), 1513–1519. Retrieved from https://www.cdc.gov/mmwr/preview/mmwrhtml/mm6044a2.htm?s_cid=%20mm6044a2.htm_w

Centers for Disease Control and Prevention. (2014a). *Breast cancer rates by race and ethnicity.* Retrieved from https://www.cdc.gov/breast-cancer/statistics/?CDC_AAref_Val=https://www.cdc.gov/cancer/breast/statistics/

Centers for Disease Control and Prevention. (2015a). *About underlying cause of death, 1999–2015.* Retrieved from http://wonder/cdc.gov/ucd-icd10.html

Centers for Disease Control and Prevention. (2016a). *Ambulatory care use and physician office visits.* Retrieved from https://www.cdc.gov/nchs/fastats/physician-visits.htm

Centers for Disease Control and Prevention. (2016b). *Smoking & tobacco use: Fast facts.* Retrieved from https://www.cdc.gov/tobacco/data_statistics/fact_sheets/fast_facts/

Centers for Disease Control and Prevention. (2017a). *Cancer rates by race/ethnicity and sex.*

Centers for Disease Control and Prevention. (2017c). *Injury prevention and control: Motor vehicle safety.*

Centers for Disease Control and Prevention. (2017d). *National diabetes statistics report, 2017.*

Centers for Disease Control and Prevention. (2018b, November). *HIV surveillance report, 2017.* Retrieved from https://www.cdc.gov/hiv/pdf/library/reports/surveillance/cdc-hiv-surveillance-report-2017-vol-29.pdf

Centers for Disease Control and Prevention. (2018e). *Smoking is down, but almost 38 million American adults still smoke.*

Centers for Disease Control and Prevention. (2019a, March). *About chronic diseases.*

Centers for Disease Control and Prevention. (2019b, April). *Chronic diseases in America.*

Centers for Disease Control and Prevention. (2019c, May). *Measles (rubeola).*

Centers for Disease Control and Prevention. (2019e, April). *Ten leading causes of death and injury.* Retrieved from https://www.cdc.gov/injury/wisqars/LeadingCauses.html

Cervero, F. (2012). *Understanding pain: Exploring the perception of pain.* Cambridge, MA: MIT Press.

Chambless, D. L., & Hollon, S. D. (1998). Defining empirically supported therapies. *Journal of Consulting and Clinical Psychology, 66*(1), 7–18.

Chang, L. H., Couvy-Duchesne, B., Liu, M., Medland, S. E., Verhulst, B., Benotsch, E. G., … GSCAN Consortium. (2019). Association between polygenic risk for tobacco or alcohol consumption and liability to licit and illicit substance use in young Australian adults. *Drug and Alcohol Dependence, 197,* 271–279.

Chappell, N. L. (2005). Perceived change in quality of life among Chinese Canadian seniors: The role of involvement in Chinese culture. *Journal of Happiness Studies, 6*(1), 69–91.

Charney, D. S. (2004). Psychobiological mechanisms of resilience and vulnerability: Implications for successful adaptation to extreme stress. *American Journal of Psychiatry, 161*(2), 195–216.

Chawla, N., Butler, E. N., Lund, J., Warren, J. L., Harlan, L. C., & Yabroff, K. R. (2013). Patterns of colorectal cancer care in Europe, Australia, and New Zealand. *Journal of the National Cancer Institute. Monographs, 46*, 36–61.

Chekroud, S. R., Gueorguieva, R., Zheutlin, A. B., Paulus, M., Krumholz, H. M., Krystal, J. H., & Chekroud, A. M. (2018). Association between physical exercise and mental health in 1–2 million individuals in the USA between 2011 and 2015: A cross-sectional study. *The Lancet Psychiatry, 5*(9), 739–746.

Chen, L. M., Farwell, W. R., & Jha, A. K. (2009). Primary care visit duration and quality: Does good care take longer? *Archives of Internal Medicine, 169*(20), 1866–1872.

Cheng, Y., & Grühn, D. (2014). Age differences in reactions to social rejection: The role of cognitive resources and appraisals. *Journals of Gerontology Series B: Psychological Sciences and Social Sciences, 70*(6), 830–839. doi: 10.1093/geronb/gbu054

Cheng, C., Lau, H. P., & Chan, M. P. (2014). Coping flexibility and psychological adjustment to stressful life changes: A meta-analytic review. *Psychological Bulletin, 140*(6), 1582–1607.

Chenlu G., & Scullin, M. K. (2020). Sleep health early in the coronavirus disease 2019 (COVID-19) outbreak in the United States: Integrating longitudinal, cross-sectional, and retrospective recall data. *Sleep Medicine, 73*, 1–10,

Chen, E., Strunk, R., Bacharier, L., Chan, M., & Miller, G. E. (2010). Socioeconomic status associated with exhaled nitric oxide responses to acute stress in children with asthma. *Brain, Behavior, and Immunity, 24*, 444–450.

Chen, L., Zhernakova, D. V., Kurilshikov, A., Andreu-Sánchez, S., Wang, D., Augustijn, H. E., Vich Vila, A., Weersma, R. K., Medema, M. H., Netea, M. G., et al. (2022). Influence of the microbiome, diet and genetics on inter-individual variation in the human plasma metabolome. *Nature Medicine, 28*, 2333–2343.

Cherepanov, D., Palta, M., Fryback, D. G., Robert, S. A., Hays, R. D., & Kaplan, R. M. (2011). Gender differences in multiple underlying dimensions of health-related quality of life are associated with sociodemographic and socioeconomic status. *Medical Care, 49*(11), 1021–1030.

Cherny, N. I., & Foley, K. M. (1996). Nonopioid and opioid analgesic pharmacotherapy of cancer pain. *Hematology/Oncology Clinics of North America, 10*(1), 79–102.

Cherry, D., Lucas, C., & Decker, S. L. (2010). *Population aging and the use of office-based physician services* (NCHS data brief no. 41). Retrieved from http://www.cdc.gov/nchs/data/databriefs/db41.pdf

Cheung, B. M., & Li, C. (2012). Diabetes and hypertension: Is there a common metabolic pathway? *Current Atherosclerosis Reports, 14*(2), 160–166.

Chiang, J. J., Park, H., Almeida, D. M., Bower, J. E., Cole, S. W., Irwin, M. R., … Fuligni, A. J. (2019). Psychosocial stress and C-reactive protein from mid-adolescence to young adulthood. *Health Psychology, 38*(3), 259.

Choi, N. G., DiNitto, D. M., & Marti, C. N. (2016). Older-adult marijuana users and ex-users: Comparisons of sociodemographic characteristics and mental and substance use disorders. *Drug and Alcohol Dependency, 165*, 94–102.

Choi, E. P. H., Wong, J. Y. H., & Fong, D. Y. T. (2018). An emerging risk factor of sexual abuse: The use of smartphone dating applications. *Sexual Abuse, 30*(4), 343–366.

Chow, D. S.-K., Au, E. W. M., & Chin C.-Y. (2008). Predicting the psychological health of older adults: Interaction of age based rejection sensitivity and discriminative facility. *Journal of Research in Personality, 42*, 169–182.

Christakis, N. A., & Fowler, J. H. (2007). The spread of obesity in a large social network over 32 years. *New England Journal of Medicine, 357*, 370–379.

Christakis, N. A., Smith, J. L., Parkes, C. M., & Lamont, E. B. (2000). Extent and determinants of error in doctors' prognoses in terminally ill patients: Prospective cohort study. Commentary: Why do doctors overestimate? Commentary: Prognoses should be based on proved indices not intuition. *BMJ, 320*(7233), 469–472.

Christensen, A. J., Benotsch, E. G., Wiebe, J. S., & Lawton, W. (1995). Coping with treatment-related stress: Effects on patient adherence in hemodialysis. *Journal of Consulting and Clinical Psychology, 63*(3), 454–459.

Chu, Q., Grühn, D., & Holland, A. M. (2018). Before I die: The impact of time horizon and age on bucket-list goals. *GeroPsych: The Journal of Gerontopsychology and Geriatric Psychiatry, 31*(3), 151.

Chu, M. D., Karnati, A., He, Z., & Lerman, K. (2024). Characterizing online eating disorder communities with large language models. arXiv preprint arXiv:2401.09647.

Chun, C. A., Enomoto, K., & Sue, S. (1996). Health care issues among Asian Americans. In P. M. Kato & T. Mann (Eds.), *Handbook of diversity issues in health psychology* (pp. 347–365). New York, NY: Plenum.

Chun, C.-A., Moos, R. H., & Cronkite, R. C. (2006). Culture: A fundamental context for the stress and coping paradigm. In P. T. P. Wong and L. C. J. Wong (Eds.), *Handbook of multicultural perspectives on stress and coping* (pp. 29–53). New York, NY: Springer.

Citron, M. L., Johnston-Early, A., Boyer, M., Krasnow, S. H., Hood, M., & Cohen, M. H. (1986). Patient-controlled analgesia for severe cancer pain. *Archives of Internal Medicine, 146*(4), 734–736.

Clark, M. M., Abrams, D. B., Niaura, R. S., Eaton, C. A., & Rossi, J. S. (1991). Self-efficacy in weight management. *Journal of Consulting and Clinical Psychology, 59*(5), 739–744. doi: 10.1037/0022-006X.59.5.739

Clarke, T. C., Black, L. I., Stussman, B. J., Barnes, P. M., & Nahin, R. L. (2015). Trends in the use of complementary health approaches among adults: United States, 2002–2012. *National Health Statistics Reports, 79*, 1.

Clarke, D. M., & Currie, K. C. (2009). Depression, anxiety and their relationship with chronic diseases: A review of the epidemiology, risk and treatment evidence. *Medical Journal of Australia, 190*(7 Suppl.), S54–S60.

Clarke, M. A., Moore, J. L., Steege, L. M., Koopman, R. J., Belden, J. L., Canfield, S. M., … Kim, M. S. (2015). Health information needs, sources, and barriers of primary care patients to achieve patient-centered care: A literature review. *Health Informatics Journal, 22*, 992–1016. doi: 10.1177/1460458215602939

Clifford, C., Paulk, E., Lin, Q., Cadwallader, J., Lubbers, K., & Frazier, L. D. (2024). Relationships among adult playfulness, stress, and coping during the COVID-19 pandemic. *Current Psychology, 43*(9), 8403–8412.

Coelho, G. V., Hamburg, D. A., & Adams, J. E. (1974). *Coping and adaptation.* Oxford, UK: Basic Books.

Cohen, R. Y., Brownell, K. D., & Felix, M. R. (1990). Age and sex differences in health habits and beliefs of schoolchildren. *Health Psychology, 9*, 208–224.

Cohen, S., Doyle, W. J., Alper, C. M., Janicki-Deverts, D., & Turner, R. B. (2009). Sleep habits and susceptibility to the common cold. *Archives of Internal Medicine, 169*, 62–67.

Cohen, S., Doyle, W. J., Turner, R. B., Alper, C. M., & Skoner, D. P. (2003). Emotional style and susceptibility to the common cold. *Psychosomatic Medicine, 65*(4), 652–657.

Cohen, S., Frank, E., Doyle, W. J., Skoner, D. P., Rabin, B. S., & Gwaltney, J. M. (1998). Types of stressors that increase susceptibility to the common cold in healthy adults. *Health Psychology, 17*, 214–223.

Cohen, S., Gianaros, P. J., & Manuck, S. B. (2016). A stage model of stress and disease. *Perspectives on Psychological Science, 11*(4), 456–463.

Cohen, S., Glass, D. C., & Phillips, S. (1979). Environment and health. In H. E. Freeman, S. Levine, & L. G. Reeder (Eds.), *Handbook of medical sociology* (3rd ed., pp. 134–149). Englewood Cliffs, NJ: Prentice Hall.

Cohen, B., Hyman, S., Rosenberg, L., & Larson, E. (2012). Frequency of patient contact with health care personnel and visitors: Implications for infection prevention. *Joint Commission Journal on Quality and Patient Safety, 38*(12), 560–565.

Cohen, S., Kamarck, T., & Mermelstein, R. (1983). A global measure of perceived stress. *Journal of Health and Social Behavior, 24*, 385–396.

Cohen, S., & McKay, G. (1984). Social support, stress and the buffering hypothesis: A theoretical analysis. In A. Baum, J. E. Singer, & S. E. Taylor (Eds.), *Handbook of psychology and health, Vol. 4. Social psychological aspects of health* (pp. 253–267). Hillsdale, NJ: Erlbaum.

Cohen, S., Murphy, M. L., & Prather, A. A. (2019). Ten surprising facts about stressful life events and disease risk. *Annual Review of Psychology, 70*, 577–597.

Cohen, R., Newton-John, T., & Slater, A. (2021). The case for body positivity on social media: Perspectives on current advances and future directions. *Journal of Health Psychology, 26*(13), 2365–2373.

Cohen, S., Tyrrell, D. A., & Smith, A. P. (1991). Psychological stress and susceptibility to the common cold. *New England Journal of Medicine, 325*, 606–612.

Cohen, S., & Wills, T. A. (1985). Stress, social support, and the buffering hypothesis. *Psychological Bulletin, 98*(2), 310–357.

Cohn, S. K., Jr. (2008). 4 Epidemiology of the Black Death and successive waves of plague. *Medical History Supplement, (27)*, 74–100.

Cohn, M. A., Mehl, M. R., & Pennebaker, J. W. (2004). Linguistic markers of psychological change surrounding September 11, 2001. *Psychological Science, 15*(10), 687–693.

Colcombe, S. U., Erickson, K. I., Scalf, P. E., Kim, J. S., Prakash, R., McAuley, E., … Kramer, A. F. (2006).

Aerobic exercise training increases brain volume in aging humans. *Journals of Gerontology. Series A, Biological Sciences and Medical Sciences, 61*(11), 1166–1170.

Cole, S. W., Hawkley, L. C., Arevalo, J. M., & Cacioppo, J. T. (2011). Transcript origin analysis identifies antigen presenting cells as primary targets of socially regulated gene expression in leukocytes. *Proceedings of the National Academy of Sciences of the USA, 108*(7), 3080–3085.

Cole, S. W., Hawkley, L. C., Arevalo, J. M., Sung, C. Y., & Cacioppo, J. T. (2007). Social regulation of gene expression in human leukocytes. *Genome Biology, 8*(9), R189.

Collings, P. (2001). "If you got everything, it's good enough": Perspectives on successful aging in a Canadian Inuit community. *Journal of Cross-Cultural Gerontology, 16*(2), 127–155.

Collins, S. R., Gunja, M. Z., Doty, M. M., & Bhupal, H. K. (2018, May 1). First look at health insurance coverage in 2018 finds ACA gains beginning to reverse: Findings from the Commonwealth Fund Affordable Care Act Tracking Survey, Feb.–Mar. 2018. *To the Point* (blog). Commonwealth Fund.

Collins, F. S., Morgan, M., & Patrinos, A. (2003). The Human Genome Project: Lessons from large-scale biology. *Science, 300*, 286–290.

Collins, R. L., Taylor, S. E., & Skokan, L. A. (1990). A better world or a shattered vision? Changes in life perspectives following victimization. *Social Cognition, 8*(3), 263–285.

Colzato, L. S., Kramer, A. F., & Bherer, L. (2018). Editorial special topic: Enhancing brain and cognition via physical exercise. *Journal of Cognitive Enhancement, 2*(2), 135–136.

Compas, B. E., Connor-Smith, J. K., Saltzman, H., Thomsen, A. H., & Wadsworth, M. E. (2001). Coping with stress during childhood and adolescence: Problems, progress, and potential in theory and research. *Psychological Bulletin, 127*(1), 87–127.

Compas, B. E., Jaser, S. S., Bettis, A. H., Watson, K. H., Gruhn, M. A., Dunbar, J. P., … Thigpen, J. C. (2017). Coping, emotion regulation, and psychopathology in childhood and adolescence: A meta-analysis and narrative review. *Psychological Bulletin, 143*(9), 939.

Condén, E., Rosenblad, A., Wagner, P., Leppert, J., Ekselius, L., & Åslund, C. (2017, January 1). Is type D personality an independent risk factor for recurrent myocardial infarction or all-cause mortality in post-acute myocardial infarction patients? *European Journal of Preventive Cardiology.* doi: 10.1177/2047487316687427

Constantine, M. G., Alleyne, V. L., Caldwell, L. D., McRae, M. B., & Suzuki, L. A. (2005). Coping responses of Asian, Black, and Latino/Latina New York City residents following the September 11, 2001 terrorist attacks against the United States. *Cultural Diversity and Ethnic Minority Psychology, 11*(4), 293–308.

Conversano, C., Rotondo, A., Lensi, E., Della Vista, O., Arpone, F., & Reda, M. A. (2010). Optimism and its impact on mental and physical well-being. *Clinical Practice and Epidemiology in Mental Health, 6,* 25–29.

Cooke, L. J. (2004). The development and modification of children's eating habits. *Nutrition Bulletin, 29*(1), 31–35. doi: 10.1111/j.1467-3010.2003.00388.x

Cooke, L. J., Haworth, C. M., & Wardle, J. (2007). Genetic and environmental influences on children's food neophobia. *American Journal of Clinical Nutrition, 86*(2), 428–433.

Cooper, M. L. (2002). Alcohol use and risky sexual behavior among college students and youth: Evaluating the evidence. *Journal of Studies on Alcohol and Drugs, 14,* 101–117.

Corte, C., Lee, C. K., Stein, K. F., & Raszewski, R. (2022). Possible selves and health behavior in adolescents: A systematic review. *Self and Identity, 21*(1), 15–41.

Cosme, D., Ludwig, R. M., & Berkman, E. T. (2019). Comparing two neurocognitive models of self-control during dietary decisions. *Social Cognitive and Affective Neuroscience, 14*(9), 957–966.

Costa, A., Carrión, S., Puig-Pey, M., Juárez, F., & Clavé, P. (2019). Triple adaptation of the mediterranean diet: Design of a meal plan for older people with oropharyngeal dysphagia based on home cooking. *Nutrients, 11*(2), 425.

Costa, P. T., & McCrae, R. R. (1984). Personality as a lifelong determinant of well-being. In C. Malatesta & C. Izard (Eds.), *Affective processes in adult development and aging* (pp. 141–157). Beverly Hills, CA: Sage.

Costa, P. T., Jr., & McCrae, R. R. (1987). Neuroticism, somatic complaints, and disease: Is the bark worse than the bite? *Journal of Personality, 55*(2), 299–316.

Costanzo, P. R., Reichmann, S. K., Friedman, K. E., & Musante, G. J. (2001). The mediating effect of eating self-efficacy on the relationship between emotional arousal and overeating in the treatment-seeking obese. *Eating Behaviors*, *2*, 363–368.

Costanzo, E. S., Stawski, R. S., Ryff, C. D., Coe, C. L., & Almeida, D. M. (2012). Cancer survivors' responses to daily stressors: Implications for quality of life. *Health Psychology*, *31*(3), 360–370.

Coughlin, S. S. (2019a). Social determinants of breast cancer risk, stage, and survival. *Breast Cancer Research and Treatment*, *177*, 537–548.

Coughlin, S. S. (2019b). Epidemiology of breast cancer in women. *Advances in Experimental Medicine and Biology*, *1152*, 9–29.

Courtenay, W. H. (2000). Constructions of masculinity and their influence on men's well-being: A theory of gender and health. *Social Science & Medicine*, *50*(10), 1385–1401.

Coyne, J. C., & Gottlieb, B. H. (1996). The mismeasure of coping by checklist. *Journal of Personality*, *64*(4), 959–991.

Creamer, M., Burgess, P., & Pattison, P. (1992). Reaction to trauma: A cognitive processing model. *Journal of Abnormal Psychology*, *101*, 452–459.

Crean, R. D., Crane, N. A., & Mason, B. J. (2011). An evidence-based review of acute and long-term effects of cannabis use on executive cognitive functions. *Journal of Addiction Medicine*, *5*(1), 1–8. doi: 10.1097/ADM.0b013e31820c23fa

Crescioni, A. W., Ehrlinger, J., Alquist, J. L., Conlon, K. E., Baumeister, R. F., Schatschneider, C., & Dutton, G. R. (2011). High trait self-control predicts positive health behaviors and success in weight loss. *Journal of Health Psychology*, *16*(5), 750–759.

Crist, M., et al. (2024). Medical Tourism: CDC Yellow Book 2024. Retrieved from https://wwwnc.cdc.gov/travel/yellowbook/2024/health-care-abroad/medical-tourism

Critchley, H. D., & Garfinkel, S. N. (2017). Interoception and emotion. *Current Opinion in Psychology*, *17*, 7–14.

Cruess, D. G., Antoni, M. H., Gonzalez, J., Fletcher, M. A., Klimas, N., Duran, R., … Schneiderman, N. (2003). Sleep disturbance mediates the association between psychological distress and immune status among HIV-positive men and women on combination antiretroviral therapy. *Journal of Psychosomatic Research*, *54*(3), 185–189.

Cullen, K. W., Baranowski, T., Owens, E., Marsh, T., Rittenberry, L., & de Moor, C. (2003). Availability, accessibility, and preferences for fruit, 100% fruit juice, and vegetables influence children's dietary behavior. *Health Education and Behavior*, *30*, 615–626.

Cunningham, R. M., Walton, M. A., & Carter, P. M. (2018). The major causes of death in children and adolescents in the United States. *New England Journal of Medicine*, *379*(25), 2468–2475.

Curry, C. W., Felt, D., Kan, K., Ruprecht, M., Wang, X., Phillips II, G., & Beach, L. B. (2021). Asthma remission disparities among US youth by sexual identity and race/ethnicity, 2009–2017. *The Journal of Allergy and Clinical Immunology: In Practice*, *9*(9), 3396–3406.

Curry, S. G., & Marlatt, G. A. (1985). Unaided quitters' strategies for coping with temptations to smoke. In S. Shiffman & T. A. Wills (Eds.), *Coping and substance use* (pp. 243–265). New York, NY: Academic.

Cvengros, J. A., Christensen, A. J., Cunningham, C., Hillis, S. L., & Kaboli, P. J. (2009). Patient preference for and reports of provider behavior: Impact of symmetry on patient outcomes. *Health Psychology*, *28*(6), 660–667.

d'Abreu, A., Castro-Olivo, S., & Ura, S. K. (2019). Understanding the role of acculturative stress on refugee youth mental health: A systematic review and ecological approach to assessment and intervention. *School Psychology International*, *40*(2), 107–127.

Daaleman, T. P., Perera, S., & Studenski, S. A. (2004). Religion, spirituality, and health status in geriatric outpatients. *Annals of Family Medicine*, *2*(1), 49–53.

Dabelea, D., Mayer-Davis, E. J., Saydah, S., Imperatore, G., Linder, B., Divers, J., … Hamman, R. F. (2014). Prevalence of type 1 and type 2 diabetes among children and adolescents from 2001 to 2009. *JAMA*, *311*(17), 1778–1786.

Dai, W., Zhou, J., Li, G., Zhang, B., Ma, N. (2021). Maintaining normal sleep patterns, lifestyles and emotion during the COVID-19 pandemic: The stabilizing effect of daytime napping. *Journal of Sleep Research*, *30*, e13259.

Dalal, H. M., Doherty, P., & Taylor, R. S. (2015). Cardiac rehabilitation. *BMJ*, *351*, h5000.

Dalessio, D. J. (1994). Diagnosing the severe headache. *Neurology*, *44*(5 Suppl. 3), S6–S12.

Daley, S. E., Hammen, C., Burge, D., Davila, J., Paley, B., Lindberg, N., & Herzberg, D. S. (1997). Predictors of the generation of episodic stress: A longitudinal study of late adolescent women. *Journal of Abnormal Psychology*, *106*(2), 251–259.

Danaei, G., Vander Hoorn, S., Lopez, A. D., Murray, C. J., Ezzati, M., & Comparative Risk Assessment collaborating group (Cancers). (2005). Causes of cancer in the world: Comparative risk assessment of nine behavioural and environmental risk factors. *Lancet, 366*(9499), 1784–1793.

Danialan, R., Gopinath, A., Phelps, A., Murphy, M., & Grant-Kels, J. M. (2012). Accurate identification of melanoma tumor margins: A review of the literature. *Expert Review of Dermatology, 7*(4), 343–358.

Dankel, S. J., Loenneke, J. P., & Loprinzi, P. D. (2016). Mild depressive symptoms among Americans in relation to physical activity, current overweight/obesity, and self-reported history of overweight/obesity. *International Journal of Behavioral Medicine, 23*(5), 553–560.

Danner, D. D., Darnell, K. R., & McGuire, C. (2011). African American participation in Alzheimer's disease research that includes brain donation. *American Journal of Alzheimer's Disease and Other Dementias, 26*(6), 469–476. doi: 10.1177/1533317511423020

Dark-Freudeman, A., & Bensadon, B. A. (2022). Advance care planning: End-of-life hopes and fears among community dwelling adults. *Journal of Health Psychology, 27*(14), 3177–3189.

Dark-Freudeman, A., & West, R. L. (2016). Possible selves and self-regulatory beliefs: Exploring the relationship between health selves, health efficacy, and psychological well-being. *The International Journal of Aging and Human Development, 82*(2–3), 139–165.

Davidson, K. W., Trudeau, K. J., & Smith, T. W. (2006). Introducing the new *Health Psychology* series "Evidence-based treatment reviews": Progress not perfection. *Health Psychology, 25*(1), 1–2.

David, J. P., & Suls, J. (1999). Coping efforts in daily life: Role of Big Five traits and problem appraisals. *Journal of Personality, 67*(2), 265–294.

Davies, A., Burnette, C. B., & Mazzeo, S. E. (2020). Real women have (just the right) curves: investigating anti-thin bias in college women. Eating and Weight Disorders-Studies on Anorexia, Bulimia and Obesity, 25, 1711–1718.

Davila, J. (2001). Refining the association between excessive reassurance seeking and depressive symptoms: The role of related interpersonal constructs. *Journal of Social and Clinical Psychology, 20*(4), 538–559.

Davis, M. A., Sirovich, B. E., & Weeks, W. B. (2010). Utilization and expenditures on chiropractic care in the United States from 1997 to 2006. *Health Services Research, 45*(3), 748–761.

Davis, K. D., Taylor, S. J., Crawley, A. P., Wood, M. L., & Mikulis, D. J. (1997). Functional MRI of pain- and attention-related activation in the human cingulate cortex. *Journal of Neurophysiology, 77*(6), 3370–3380.

Davis, M. C., Twamley, E. W., Hamilton, N. A., & Swan, P. D. (1999). Body fat distribution and hemodynamic stress response in premenopausal obese women: A preliminary study. *Health Psychology, 18*(6), 625–633.

de Bruijn, G.-J. (2011). Exercise habit strength, planning and the theory of planned behavior: An action control approach. *Psychology of Sport and Exercise, 12*(2), 106–114.

de Castro, J. M. (2009).When, how much and what foods are eaten are related to total daily food intake. *British Journal of Nutrition, 102*(8), 1228–1237.

de Craen, A. J., Kaptchuk, T. J., Tijssen, J. G., & Kleijnen, J. (1999). Placebos and placebo effects in medicine: Historical overview. *Journal of the Royal Society of Medicine, 92*(10), 511–515.

de Craen, A. J., Roos, P. J., De Vries, A. L., & Kleijnen, J. (1996). Effect of colour of drugs: Systematic review of perceived effect of drugs and of their effectiveness. *BMJ, 313*(7072), 1624–1626.

de Ferranti, S. D., Gauvreau, K., Ludwig, D. S., Neufeld, E. J., Newburger, J. W., & Rifai, N. (2004). Prevalence of the metabolic syndrome in American adolescents: Findings from the Third National Health and Nutrition Examination Survey. *Circulation, 110*(16), 2494–2497.

de Jonge, P., Latour, C. H., & Huyse, F. J. (2003). Implementing psychiatric interventions on a medical ward: Effects on patients' quality of life and length of hospital stay. *Psychosomatic Medicine, 65*(6), 997–1002.

de Ridder, D., Geenen, R., Kuijer, R., & van Middendorp, H. (2008). Psychological adjustment to chronic disease. *Lancet, 372*(9634), 246–255.

de Vos, C. C., Meier, K., Zaalberg, P. B., Nijhuis, H. J., Duyvendak, W., Vesper, J., … Lenders, M. W. (2014). Spinal cord stimulation in patients with painful diabetic neuropathy: A multicentre randomized clinical trial. *Pain, 155*(11), 2426–2431.

Deczkowska, A., Keren-Shaul, H., Weiner, A., Colonna, M., Schwartz, M., & Amit, I. (2018). Disease-associated microglia: A universal immune sensor of neurodegeneration. *Cell, 173*(5), 1073–1081.

Deloitte Access Economics. (2020). *The social and economic cost of eating disorders in the United States of America: A report for the strategic training initiative for the prevention of eating disorders and the academy for eating disorders*. Retrieved from https://www.hsph.harvard.edu/striped/report-economic-costs-of-eating-disorders/

DeLongis, A., Coyne, J. C., Dakof, G., Folkman, S., & Lazarus, R. S. (1982). Relationship of daily hassles, uplifts, and major life events to health status. *Health Psychology, 1*(2), 119–136.

DeLongis, A., Folkman, S., & Lazarus, R. (1988). The impact of daily stress on health and mood: Psychological social resources as mediators. *Journal of Personality and Social Psychology, 54*, 486–495.

Dennis, A., Cuthbertson, D. J., Wootton, D., Crooks, M., Gabbay, M., Eichert, N., ... Banerjee, A. (2023). Multi-organ impairment and long COVID: A 1-year prospective, longitudinal cohort study. *Journal of the Royal Society of Medicine, 116*(3), 97–112.

Denny, K. N., Loth, K., Eisenberg, M. E., & Neumark-Sztainer, D. (2013). Intuitive eating in young adults: Who is doing it, and how is it related to disordered eating behaviors? *Appetite, 60*(1), 13–19. doi: 10.1016/j.appet.2012.09.029

Denollet, J. (1993). Biobehavioral research on coronary heart disease: Where is the person? *Journal of Behavioral Medicine, 16*(2), 115–142. doi: 10.1007/BF00844889

Denollet, J., Sys, S. U., & Brutsaert, D. L. (1995). Personality and mortality after myocardial infarction. *Psychosomatic Medicine, 57*(6), 582–591.

DePue, J. D., Clark, M. M., Ruggiero, L., Medeiros, M. L., & Pera, V. (1995). Maintenance of weight loss: A needs assessment. *Obesity Research, 3*, 241–248.

Desharnais, R., Jobin, J., Côté, C., Lévesque, L., & Godin, G. (1993). Aerobic exercise and the placebo effect: A controlled study. *Psychosomatic Medicine, 55*, 149–154.

Dew, M. A., Hoch, C. C., Buysse, D. J., Monk, T. H., Begley, A. E., Houck, P. R., ... Reynolds, C. F. III. (2003). Healthy older adults' sleep predicts all-cause mortality at 4 to 19 years of follow-up. *Psychosomatic Medicine, 65*, 63–73.

Dhabhar, F. S. (2009). A hassle a day may keep the pathogens away: The fight-or-flight stress response and the augmentation of immune function. *Integrative and Comparative Biology, 49*(3), 215–236.

Di Blasi, Z., Harkness, E., Ernst, E., Georgiou, A., & Kleijnen, J. (2001). Influence of context effects on health outcomes: A systematic review. *Lancet, 357*(9258), 757–762.

Di Cagno, A., Iuliano, E., Aquino, G., Fiorilli, G., Battaglia, C., Giombini, A., & Calcagno, G. (2013). Psychological well-being and social participation assessment in visually impaired subjects playing Torball: A controlled study. *Research in Developmental Disabilities, 34*(4), 1204–1209.

Di Cesare, M., Perel, P., Taylor, S., Kabudula, C., Bixby, H., Gaziano, T. A., ... Pinto, F. J. (2024). The heart of the world. *Global Heart, 19*(1), 11.

Díaz-Marsá, M., Carrasco, J. L., López-Ibor, M., Moratti, A., Montes, A., Ortiz, T., & López-Ibor, J. J. (2011). Orbitofrontal dysfunction related to depressive symptomatology in subjects with borderline personality disorder. *Journal of Affective Disorders, 134*(1–3), 410–415.

Dickerson, D. L., Brown, R. A., Klein, D. J., Agniel, D., Johnson, C., & D'Amico, E. J. (2019). Overt perceived discrimination and racial microaggressions and their association with health risk behaviors among a sample of urban American Indian/Alaska Native adolescents. *Journal of Racial and Ethnic Health Disparities, 6*(4), 733–742. doi: 10.1007/s40615-019-00572-1

DiClemente, C. C., & Hughes, S. O. (1990). Stages of change profiles in outpatient alcoholism treatment. *Journal of Substance Abuse, 2*(2), 217–235.

Didžiokaite, G., Saukko, P., & Greiffenhagen, C. (2018). The mundane experience of everyday calorie trackers: Beyond the metaphor of Quantified Self. *New Media and Society, 20*(4), 1470–1487. doi: 10.1177/1461444817698478

Diehl, M., & Hay, E. L. (2013). Personality-related risk and resilience factors in coping with daily stress among adult cancer patients. *Research in Human Development, 10*(1), 47–69.

Diener, E. (2000). Subjective well-being: The science of happiness and a proposal for a national index. *American Psychologist, 55*(1), 34–43.

Diener, E., & Lucas, R. E. (1999). Personality and subjective well-being. In D. Kahneman, E. Diener, & N. Schwarz (Eds.), *Well-being: Foundations of hedonic psychology* (pp. 213–229). New York, NY: Russell Sage Foundation.

DiMatteo, M. R. (2004). Variations in patients' adherence to medical recommendations: A quantitative review of 50 years of research. *Medical Care, 42*(3), 200–209.

DiMatteo, M. R., & DiNicola, D. D. (1982). *Achieving patient compliance: The psychology of the medical practitioner's role.* New York, NY: Pergamon Press.

DiMatteo, M. R., Giordani, P. J., Lepper, H. S., & Croghan, T. W. (2002). Patient adherence and medical treatment outcomes: A meta-analysis. *Medical Care, 40*(9), 794–811.

DiMatteo, M. R., & Haskard, K. B. (2006). Further challenges in adherence research: Measurements, methodologies, and mental health care. *Medical Care, 44*(4), 297–299.

DiMatteo, M. R., Haskard, K. B., & Williams, S. L. (2007). Health beliefs, disease severity, and patient adherence: A meta-analysis. *Medical Care, 45*(6), 521–528.

Dinarello, C. A. (2000). Proinflammatory cytokines. *Chest, 118*(2) 503–508.

Dolan, P., & Peasgood, T. (2008). Measuring well-being for public policy: Preferences or experiences? *Journal of Legal Studies, 37*(S2), S5–S31.

Dolecek, T. A., Milas, N. C., Van Horn, L. V., Farrand, M. E., Gorder, D. D., Duchene, A. G., … Randall, B. L. (1986). A long-term nutrition intervention experience: Lipid responses and dietary adherence patterns in the Multiple Risk Factor Intervention Trial. *Journal of the American Dietetic Association, 86*(6), 752–758.

Dollard, J., Kearney, P., Clarke, G., Moloney, G., Cryan, J. F., & Dinan, T. G. (2015). A prospective study of C-reactive protein as a state marker in Cardiac Syndrome X. *Brain, Behavior, and Immunity, 43*, 27–32.

Doll, J., & Orth, B. (1993). The Fishbein and Ajzen Theory of Reasoned Action applied to contraceptive behavior: Model variants and meaningfulness. *Journal of Applied Social Psychology, 23*(5), 395–415.

Domínguez-Álvarez, B., López-Romero, L., Isdahl-Troye, A., Gómez-Fraguela, J. A., & Romero, E. (2020). Children coping, contextual risk and their interplay during the COVID-19 pandemic: A Spanish case. *Frontiers in Psychology, 11*, 577763.

Domínguez, F., Fuster, V., Fernández-Alvira, J. M., Fernández-Friera, L., López-Melgar, B., Blanco-Rojo, R., … Ordovás, J. M. (2019). Association of sleep duration and quality with subclinical atherosclerosis. *Journal of the American College of Cardiology, 73*, 2.

Donchin, Y., Gopher, D., Olin, M., Badihi, Y., Biesky, M., Sprung, C. L., … Cotev, S. (1995). A look into the nature and causes of human errors in the intensive care unit. *Critical Care Medicine, 23*(2), 294–300.

Donoho, C. J., Seeman, T. E., Sloan, R. P., & Crimmins, E. M. (2015). Marital status, marital quality, and heart rate variability in the MIDUS cohort. *Journal of Family Psychology, 29*(2), 290–295.

Doremus-Fitzwater, T. L., & Spear, L. P. (2016). Reward-centricity and attenuated aversions: An adolescent phenotype emerging from studies in laboratory animals. *Neuroscience & Biobehavioral Reviews, 70*, 121–134.

Dosh, S. A. (2002). The treatment of adults with essential hypertension. *Journal of Family Practice, 51*(1), 74–80.

Doufas, A. G., Panagiotou, O. A., & Ioannidis, J. P. A. (2012). Concordance of sleep and pain outcomes of diverse interventions: An umbrella review. *PLoS One, 7*(7), e40891.

Dovey, T. M., Staples, P. A., Gibson, E. L., Halford, J. C. (2008). Food neophobia and 'picky/fussy'eating in children: A review. *Appetite, 50*, 181–193.

Dowd, J. J., & Bengtson, V. L. (1978). Aging in minority populations. An examination of the double jeopardy hypothesis. *Journal of Gerontology, 33*(3), 427–436.

Draper, P., & Harpending, H. (1982). Father absence and reproductive strategy: An evolutionary perspective. *Journal of Anthropological Research, 38*(3), 255–273.

Dryhurst, S., Schneider, C. R., Kerr, J., Freeman, A. L. J., Recchia, G., van der Bles, A. M., Spiegelhalter, D., & Van Der Linden, S. (2020). Risk perceptions of COVID-19 around the world. *Journal of Risk Research, 23*(7–8), 994–1006. doi: 10.1080/13669877.2020.1758193

Dubbert, P. M., Rappaport, N. B., & Martin, J. E. (1987). Exercise in cardiovascular disease. *Behavior Modification, 11*(3), 329–347.

Dubos, R. (1961). *Mirage of health: Utopias, progress and biological change* (pp. 235–236). Garden City, NY: Doubleday.

Dubow, E. F., Pargament, K. I., Boxer, P., & Tarakeshwar, N. (2000). Initial investigation of Jewish early adolescents' ethnic identity, stress, and coping. *Journal of Early Adolescence, 20*(4), 418–441.

Duckworth, A. L., Tsukayama, E., & Geier, A. B. (2010). Self-controlled children stay leaner in the transition to adolescence. *Appetite, 54*(2), 304–308.

Dunkel Schetter, C., & Dolbier, C. (2011). Resilience in the context of chronic stress and health in adults. *Social and Personality Psychology Compass, 5*(9), 634–652.

Dunkel-Schetter, C., Feinstein, L. G., Taylor, S. E., & Falke, R. L. (1992). Patterns of coping with cancer. *Health Psychology, 11*(2), 79–87.

Dunn, H. L. (1977). *High level wellness: A collection of twenty-nine short talks on different aspects of the theme "high-level wellness for man and society."* Thorofare, NJ: Charles B. Slack.

Dunn, E. W., Aknin, L. B., & Norton, M. I. (2008). Spending money on others promotes happiness. *Science, 319*(5870), 1687–1688.

Durack, J., & Lynch, S. V. (2019). The gut microbiome: Relationships with disease and opportunities for therapy. *Journal of Experimental Medicine, 216*(1), 20–40.

Dziurowicz-Kozłowska, A. H. (2010). Health-related quality of life in obesity. *Acta Neuropsychologica, 8*(3), 284–296.

Easterlin, R. A. (2003). Building a better theory of well-being. *IZA discussion paper no. 742.* Retrieved from https://ssrn.com/abstract=392043

Eaton, D. K., Kann, L., Kinchen, S., Shanklin, S., Flint, K. H., Hawkins, J., … Wechsler, H. (2012, June 8). Youth risk behavior surveillance—United States, 2011. *Surveillance Summaries* (Vol. 61(SS04), pp. 1–162). U.S. Department of Health and Human Services, Centers for Disease Control and Prevention. Retrieved from https://www.cdc.gov/mmwr/preview/mmwrhtml/ss6104a1.htm

Echavez, C. (2015). U.S. government finally banning chimp research. *Science Times*. Retrieved from http://www.sciencetimes.com/articles/7769/20151123/government-finally-banning-chimp-research.htm

Eckermann, L. (2000). Gendering indicators of health and well-being: Is quality of life gender neutral? *Social Indicators Research*, *52*(1), 29–54.

Eddy, K. T., Thomas, J. J., Hastings, E., Edkins, K., Lamont, E., Nevins, C. M., … Becker, A. E. (2015). Prevalence of DSM-5 avoidant/restrictive food intake disorder in a pediatric gastroenterology healthcare network. *International Journal of Eating Disorders*, *48*(5), 464–470.

Edmondson, D., Park, C. L., Chaudoir, S. R., & Wortmann, J. H. (2008). Death without God: Religious struggle, death concerns, and depression in the terminally ill. *Psychological Science*, *19*(8), 754–758.

Edwards, J. R. (1988). The determinants and consequences of coping with stress. In C. L. Cooper & R. Payne (Eds.), *Causes, coping, and consequences of stress at work* (pp. 233–263). Chichester, UK: Wiley.

Egbert, N., & Nanna, K. M. (2009). Health literacy: Challenges and strategies. *OJIN: The Online Journal of Issues in Nursing*, *14*(3). Retrieved from http://www.nursingworld.org/MainMenuCategories/ANAMarketplace/ANAPeriodicals/OJIN/TableofContents/Vol142009/No3Sept09/Health-Literacy-Challenges.html

Eiser, C., Havermans, T., Craft, A., & Kernahan, J. (1995). Development of a measure to assess the perceived illness experience after treatment for cancer. *Archives of Disease in Childhood*, *72*(4), 302–307.

Eitan, T., & Gazit, T. (2023). No social media for six hours? The emotional experience of Meta's global outage according to FoMO, JoMO and internet intensity. *Computers in Human Behavior*, *138*, 107474.

Ekkekakis, P., & Petruzzello, S. J. (2000). Analysis of the affect measurement conundrum in exercise psychology: I. Fundamental issues. *Psychology of Sport and Exercise*, *1*(2), 71–88.

Ekman, P. E., & Davidson, R. J. (Eds.). (1994). *The nature of emotion: Fundamental questions*. New York, NY: Oxford University Press.

Elfhag, K., & Linné, Y. (2005). Gender differences in association of eating pathology between mothers and their adolescent offspring. *Obesity Research*, *13*(6), 1070–1076.

Elfhag, K., & Morey, L. C. (2008). Personality traits and eating behavior in the obese: Poor self-control in emotional and external eating but personality assets in restrained eating. *Eating Behavior*, *9*(3), 285–293.

Elfhag, K., & Rössner, S. (2005). Who succeeds in maintaining weight loss? A conceptual review of factors associated with weight loss maintenance and weight regain. *Obesity Review*, *6*(1), 67–85.

Elfhag, K., Tholin, S., & Rasmussen, F. (2008). Consumption of fruit, vegetables, sweets and soft drinks are associated with psychological dimensions of eating behaviour in patients and their 12-year-old children. *Public Health Nutrition*, *11*(9), 914–923.

Ellsberg, M., & Betron, M. (2010). *Spotlight on gender: Preventing gender-based violence and HIV: Lessons from the field* (pp. 1–4). USAID. Retrieved from https://www.k4health.org/sites/default/files/AIDSTAR-One_Gender_Spolight_Gender-based_violence.pdf

Elwy, A. R., Yeh, J., Worcester, J., & Eisen, S. V. (2011). An illness perception model of primary care patients' help seeking for depression. *Qualitative Health Research*, *21*(11), 1495–1507.

Emanuel, E. J., Onwuteaka-Philipsen, B. D., Urwin, J. W., & Cohen, J. (2016). Attitudes and practices of euthanasia and physician-assisted suicide in the United States, Canada, and Europe. *JAMA*, *316*(1), 79–90.

Emch, M., Feldacker, C., Islam, M. S., & Ali, M. (2008). Seasonality of cholera from 1974 to 2005: A review of global patterns. *International Journal of Health Geographics*, *7*, 31. doi: 10.1186/1476-072X-7-31

Eng, T. R., & Butler, W. T. (Eds.). (1997). *Summary: The hidden epidemic: Confronting sexually transmitted diseases* (p. 43). Washington (DC): National Academy Press.

Engel, G. L. (1977). The need for a new medical model: A challenge for biomedicine. *Science*, *196*, 129–136.

Engel, G. L. (1980). The clinical application of the biopsychosocial model. *American Journal of Psychiatry*, *137*(5), 535–544.

Enstrom, J. E., & Breslow, L. (2008). Lifestyle and reduced mortality among active California Mormons, 1980–2004. *Preventive Medicine*, *46*(2), 133–136.

Epel, E. S., McEwen, B., Seeman, T., Matthews, K., Castellazzo, G., Brownell, K. D., … Ickovics, J. R. (2000). Stress and body shape: Stress-induced cortisol secretion is consistently greater among women with central fat. *Psychosomatic Medicine*, *62*(5), 623–632.

Epstein, L. H., & Cluss, P. A. (1982). A behavioral medicine perspective on adherence to long-term medical regimens. *Journal of Consulting and Clinical Psychology, 50*(6), 950–971.

Epstein, L. H., Raja, S., Daniel, T. O., Paluch, R. A., Wilfley, D. E., Saelens, B. E., & Roemmich, J. N. (2012). The built environment moderates effects of family-based childhood obesity treatment over 2 years. *Annals of Behavioral Medicine, 44*(2), 248–258.

Erdman, L. (1991). Laughter therapy for patients with cancer. *Oncology Nursing Forum, 18*(8), 1359–1363.

Erikson, E. H. (1968). *Identity, youth, and crisis.* New York, NY: Norton.

Ernst, E. (2004). Manual therapies for pain control: Chiropractic and massage. *Clinical Journal of Pain, 20*(1), 8–12.

ERR-256, U.S. (2024). Department of Agriculture, Economic Research Service. Retrieved from https://www.ers.usda.gov/webdocs/publications/90023/err256_summary.pdf?v=0

Eskelinen, M., & Ollonen, P. (2011). Assessment of general anxiety in patients with breast disease and breast cancer using the Spielberger STAI self evaluation test: A prospective case-control study in Finland. *Anticancer Research, 31*(5), 1801–1806.

Estabrooks, P. A., Bradshaw, M., Dzewaltoski, D. A., & Smith-Ray, R. L. (2008). Determining the impact of Walk Kansas: Applying a team-building approach to community physical activity promotion. *Annals of Behavioral Medicine, 36*, 1–12.

Etter, J.-F., & Bullen, C. (2011). Electronic cigarette: Users profile, utilization, satisfaction and perceived efficacy. *Addiction, 106*, 2017–2028.

Eurostat. (2017). *Healthcare activities statistics—consultations.* Retrieved from http://ec.europa.eu/eurostat/statistics-explained/index.php/Healthcare_activities_statistics_-_consultations

Everson, S. A., Lynch, J. W., Kaplan, G. A., Lakka, T. A., Sivenius, J., & Salonen, J. T. (2001). Stress-induced blood pressure reactivity and incident stroke in middle-aged men. *Stroke, 32*, 1263–1270.

Facchinetti, F., Ottolini, F., Fazzio, M., Rigatelli, M., & Volpe, A. (2007). Psychosocial factors associated with preterm uterine contractions. *Psychotherapy and Psychosomatics, 76*(6), 391–394.

Faith, M. S., Heo, M., Keller, K., & Pietrobelli, A. (2013). Child food neophobia is heritable, associated with less compliant eating, and moderates familial resemblance for BMI. *Obesity (Silver Spring), 21*, 1650–1655. doi: 10.1002/oby.20369

Fan, M., Sun, D., Zhou, T., Heianza, Y., Lv, J., Li, L., Qi, L. (2020). Sleep patterns, genetic susceptibility, and incident cardiovascular disease: A prospective study of 385 292 UK biobank participants. *European Heart Journal, 41*(11), 1182–1189.

FAO, IFAD, UNICEF, WFP and WHO. (2023). *The State of Food Security and Nutrition in the World 2023. Urbanization, agrifood systems transformation and healthy diets across the rural–urban continuum.* Rome: FAO. https://doi.org/10.4060/cc3017en

Farooqi, I. S., & O'Rahilly, S. (2005). Monogenic obesity in humans. *Annual Review of Medicine, 56*, 443–458.

Farr, R., & Marková, I. (1995). Professional and lay representations of health, illness and handicap: A theoretical overview. In I. Marková & R. Farr (Eds.), *Representations of health, illness and handicap* (pp. 93–110). Chur, Switzerland: Harwood Academic.

Fassino, S., Leombruni, P., Pierò, A., Daga, G. A., Amianto, F., Rovera, G., & Rovera, G. G. (2002). Temperament and character in obese women with and without binge eating disorder. *Comprehensive Psychiatry, 43*, 431–437.

Fava, G. A. (1999). Well-being therapy: Conceptual and technical issues. *Psychotherapy and Psychosomatics, 68*(4), 171–179.

Fava, G. A., Rafanelli, C., Tomba, E., Guidi, J., & Grandi, S. (2011). The sequential combination of cognitive behavioral treatment and well-being therapy in cyclothymic disorder. *Psychotherapy and Psychosomatics, 80*(3), 136–143.

Fava, G. A., Ruini, C., Rafanelli, C., Finos, L., Conti, S., & Grandi, S. (2004). Six-year outcome of cognitive behavior therapy for prevention of recurrent depression. *American Journal of Psychiatry, 161*(10), 1872–1876.

Fava, G. A., & Sonino, N. (2005). The clinical domains of psychosomatic medicine. *Journal of Clinical Psychiatry, 66*(7), 849–858.

Favieri, F., Marini, A., & Casagrande, M. (2021). Emotional regulation and overeating behaviors in children and adolescents: A systematic review. *Behavioral Sciences, 11*(1), 11F.

Feinstein, R. E., & deGruy, F. V., III. (2011). Difficult patients: Personality disorders and somatoform complaints. In R. E. Rakel & D. P. Rakel (Eds.), *Textbook of family medicine* (8th ed., pp. 1037–1059). Philadelphia, PA: Elsevier Saunders.

Feldman, P. J., Cohen, S., Doyle, W. J., Skoner, D. P., & Gwaltney, J. M., Jr. (1999). The impact of personality on the reporting of unfounded symptoms and illness. *Journal of Personality and Social Psychology, 77*(2), 370–378.

Feldman, M. B., & Meyer, I. H. (2007). Eating disorders in diverse lesbian, gay, and bisexual populations. *International Journal of Eating Disorders, 40*(3), 218–226. doi: 10.1002/eat.20360

Feldman, D. I., Theodore Robison, W., Pacor, J. M., Caddell, L. C., Feldman, E. B., Deitz, R. L., … Blaha, M. J. (2018). Harnessing mHealth technologies to increase physical activity and prevent cardiovascular disease. *Clinical Cardiology, 41*(7), 985–991.

Feldman, R., Weller, A., Zagoory-Sharon, O., & Levine, A. (2007). Evidence for a neuroendocrinological foundation of human affiliation: Plasma oxytocin levels across pregnancy and the postpartum period predict mother-infant bonding. *Psychological Science, 18*, 965–970.

Feldman, H. H., & Woodward, M. (2005). The staging and assessment of moderate to severe Alzheimer disease. *Neurology, 65*(6, Suppl. 3), S10–S17.

Feldt, K. S. (2000). The checklist of nonverbal pain indicators (CNPI). *Pain Management Nursing, 1*(1), 13–21.

Feng, S., Mäntymäki, M., Dhir, A., Salmela, H. (2021). How self-tracking and the quantified self promote health and well-being: Systematic review. *Journal of Medical Internet Research, 23*(9), e25171. doi: 10.2196/25171.

Ferguson, E., Williams, L., O'Connor, R. C., Howard, S., Hughes, B. M., Johnston, D. W., … O'Carroll, R. E. (2009). A taxometric analysis of type-D personality. *Psychosomatic Medicine, 71*(9), 981–986.

Ferreira, K. A., Kimura, M., Teixeira, M. J., Mendoza, T. R., da Nóbrega, J. C., Graziani, S. R., & Takagaki, T. Y. (2008). Impact of cancer-related symptom synergisms on health-related quality of life and performance status. *Journal of Pain and Symptom Management, 35*(6), 604–616.

Festinger, L. (1954). A theory of social comparison processes. *Human Relations, 7*(2), 117–140.

Field, T. (2012). Prenatal exercise research. *Infant Behavior and Development, 35*(3), 397–407.

Fields, L. C., Brown, C., Skelton, J. A., Cain, K. S., & Cohen, G. M. (2021). Internalized weight bias, teasing, and self-esteem in children with overweight or obesity. *Childhood Obesity, 17*(1), 43–50.

Fillingim, R. B. (2000). Sex, gender, and pain: Women and men really are different. *Current Review of Pain, 4*(1), 24–30.

Fillingim, R. B. (2003). Sex-related influences on pain: A review of mechanisms and clinical implications. *Rehabilitation Psychology, 48*(3), 165–174.

Finch, B. K., Frank, R., & Vega, W. A. (2004). Acculturation and acculturation stress: A social-epidemiological approach to Mexican migrant farmworkers' health. *International Migration Review, 38*(1), 236–262.

Fischer, P., Ai, A. L., Aydin, N., Frey, D., & Haslam, S. A. (2010). The relationship between religious identity and preferred coping strategies: An examination of the relative importance of interpersonal and intrapersonal coping in Muslim and Christian faiths. *Review of General Psychology, 14*(4), 365–381.

Fishbein, M., & Ajzen, I. (1975). *Belief, attitude, intention, and behavior: An introduction to theory and research*. Reading, MA: Addison-Wesley.

Fishman, S. M. (2007). Recognizing pain management as a human right: A first step. *Anesthesia and Analgesia, 105*(1), 8–9.

Flack, S., Apelqvist, J., Keith, M., Trueman, P., & Williams, D. (2008). An economic evaluation of VAC therapy compared with wound dressings in the treatment of diabetic foot ulcers. *Journal of Wound Care, 17*(2), 71–78.

Flanagan, J. C., Allan, N. P., Calhoun, C. D., Badour, C. L., Maria, M. S., Brady, K. T., & Back, S. E. (2019). Effects of oxytocin on stress reactivity and craving in veterans with co-occurring PTSD and alcohol use disorder. *Experimental and Clinical Psychopharmacology, 27*(1), 45.

Flaten, M. A., Aasli, O., & Blumenthal, T. D. (2003). Expectations and placebo responses to caffeine-associated stimuli. *Psychopharmacology, 169*(2), 198–204.

Flay, B. (2005, September 8). *Integrating theories of adolescent behavior: The theory of triadic influence*. Presented at NAS/IOM, Washington, DC. Retrieved from http://www.powershow.com/view/3d782e-YjA5N/Integrating_Theories_of_Adolescent_Behavior_The_Theory_of_Triadic_Influence_powerpoint_ppt_presentation

Flay, B. R., & Petraitis, J. (1994). The theory of triadic influence: A new theory of health behavior with implications for preventive interventions. *Advances in Medical Sociology, 4*, 19–44.

Flay, B. R., Snyder, F. J., & Petraitis, J. (2009). The theory of triadic influence. In R. J. DiClemente, R. A. Crosby, & M. C. Kegler (Eds.), *Emerging theories in health promotion practice and research* (2nd ed., pp. 451–510). San Francisco, CA: Jossey-Bass.

Fleetwood, S. (2021). A definition of habit for socio-economics. *Review of Social Economy, 79*(2), 131–165.

Fleming, M. (2010, November). *Playboy Interview: Robert Downey Jr.* Retrieved from http://www.dandychick.com/rdjfilmguide/institute/rlpby.php

Fleming, C. M., Eisenberg, N., Catalano, R. F., Kosterman, R., Cambron, C., Hawkins, J. D., … Watrous, J. (2019). Optimizing assessment of risk and protection for diverse adolescent outcomes: Do risk and protective factors for delinquency and substance use also predict risky sexual behavior? *Prevention Science, 20*(5), 788–799. doi: 10.1007/s11121-019-0987-9

Flor, H. (2012). New developments in the understanding and management of persistent pain. *Current Opinion in Psychiatry, 25*(2), 109–113.

Folkman, S. (2008). The case for positive emotions in the stress process. *Anxiety, Stress, & Coping, 21*(1), 3–14.

Folkman, S., & Lazarus, R. S. (1980). An analysis of coping in a middle-aged community sample. *Journal of Health and Social Behavior, 21*(3), 219–239.

Food and Agriculture Organization of the United Nations. (2024a). *Dietary guidelines*. Retrieved from https://www.fao.org/nutrition/education/food-dietary-guidelines/home/en/

Ford, E. S, Bergmann, M. M., Boeing, H., Li, C., & Capewell, S. (2012). Healthy lifestyle behaviors and all-cause mortality among adults in the United States. *Preventive Medicine, 55*(1), 23–27. PMID:22564893.

Forlenza, O. V., & Vallada, H. (2018). Spirituality, health and well-being in the elderly. *International Psychogeriatrics, 30*(12), 1741–1742.

Francis, L. A., & Susman, E. J. (2009). Self-regulation and rapid weight gain in children from age 3 to 12 years. *Archives of Pediatrics and Adolescent Medicine, 163*(4), 297–302.

Franco, O. H., Massaro, J. M., Civil, J., Cobain, M. R., O'Malley, B., & D'Agostino, R. B. (2009). Trajectories of entering the metabolic syndrome: The Framingham Heart Study. *Circulation, 120*(20), 1943–1950.

Frank, G. K. (2015). Advances from neuroimaging studies in eating disorders. *CNS Spectrums, 20*(4), 391–400.

Frank, G. K., Reynolds, J. R., Shott, M. E., Jappe, L., Yang, T. T., Tregellas, J. R., & O'Reilly, R. C. (2012). Anorexia nervosa and obesity are associated with opposite brain reward response. *Neuropsychopharmacology, 37*(9), 2031–2046.

Frank, D., Swedmark, J., & Grubbs, L. (2004). Colon cancer screening in African American women. *ABNF Journal, 15*, 67–70.

Franko, D. L., Striegel-Moore, R. H., Thompson, D., Schreiber, G. B., & Daniels, S. R. (2005). Does adolescent depression predict obesity in black and white young adult women? *Psychological Medicine, 35*(10), 1505–1513.

Fraser, E. D. G., & Rimas, A. (2010). *Empires of food: Feast, famine, and the rise and fall of civilizations*. New York, NY: Simon & Schuster.

Frazier, L. D. (2000). Coping with disease-related stressors in Parkinson's disease. *Gerontologist, 40*(1), 53–63.

Frazier, L. D. (2002). Stability and change in patterns of coping with Parkinson's disease. *International Journal of Aging and Human Development, 55*(3), 207–231.

Frazier, L. D., et al. (2024). The role of adult playfulness in eudaimonic well-being.

Frazier, L. D., Barreto, M. L., & Newman, F. L. (2012). Self-regulation and eudaimonic well-being across adulthood. *Experimental Aging Research, 38*(4), 394–410.

Frazier, L. D., Cotrell, V., & Hooker, K. (2003). Possible selves and illness: A comparison of individuals with Parkinson's disease, early-stage Alzheimer's disease, and healthy older adults. *International Journal of Behavioral Development, 27*(1), 1–11.

Frazier, L. D., & Hooker, K. (2006). Possible selves in adult development: Linking theory and research. In C. Dunkel & J. Kerpelman (Eds.), *Possible selves: Research and application* (pp. 41–59). Hauppauge, NY: Nova Science Publishers.

Frazier, L. D., Hooker, K., Johnson, P. M., & Kaus, C. R. (2000). Continuity and change in possible selves in later life: A 5-year longitudinal study. *Basic and Applied Social Psychology, 22*(3), 237–243.

Frazier, L. D., Hooker, K., & Siegler, I. C. (1993). Longitudinal studies of aging in social and psychological gerontology. *Reviews in Clinical Gerontology, 3*(4), 415–426.

Frazier, L. D., Johnson, P. M., Gonzalez, G. K., & Kafka, C. L. (2002). Psychosocial influences on possible selves: A comparison of three cohorts of older adults. *International Journal of Behavioral Development, 26*(4), 308–317.

Frazier, L. D., Newman, F. L., & Jaccard, J. (2007). Psychosocial outcomes in later life: A multivariate model. *Psychology and Aging, 22*(4), 676–689.

Frazier, P., & Schauben, L. (1994). Causal attributions and recovery from rape and other stressful life events. *Journal of Social and Clinical Psychology, 13*(1), 1–14.

Frazier, L. D., Vaccaro, J. A., Garcia, S., Fallahazad, N., Rathi, K., Shrestha, A., & Perez, N. (2015). Diet self-efficacy and physical self-concept of college students at risk for eating disorders. *Journal of Behavioral Health, 4*(4), 97–100.

Fredriksen-Goldsen, K. I., Cook-Daniels, L., Kim, H. J., Erosheva, E. A., Emlet, C. A., Hoy-Ellis, C. P., … Muraco, A. (2014). Physical and mental health of transgender older adults: An at-risk and underserved population. *Gerontologist, 54*(3), 488–500.

Freedman, D. S., Khan, L. K., Dietz, W. H., Srinivasan, S. R., & Berenson, G. S. (2001). Relationship of childhood obesity to coronary heart disease risk factors in adulthood: The Bogalusa Heart Study. *Pediatrics, 108*(3), 712–718.

Freedman, D. S., Mei, Z., Srinivasan, S. R., Berenson, G. S., & Dietz, W. H. (2007). Cardiovascular risk factors and excess adiposity among overweight children and adolescents: The Bogalusa Heart Study. *Journal of Pediatrics, 150*(1), 12–17.e2.

Freidson, E. (1961). *Patients' views of medical practice: A study of subscribers to a prepaid medical plan in the Bronx.* New York, NY: Russell Sage Foundation.

French, S. A., Story, M., & Jeffery, R. W. (2001). Environmental influences on eating and physical activity. *Annual Review of Public Health, 22,* 309–335.

Freud, S. (1920). *A general introduction to psychoanalysis.* New York, NY: Boni and Liveright.

Frey, S., Birchler-Pedross, A., Hofstetter, M., Brunner, P., Götz, T., Münch, M., … Cajochen, C. (2012). Young women with major depression live on higher homeostatic sleep pressure than healthy controls. *Chronobiology International, 29*(3), 278–294.

Fried, P. A., Watkinson, B., & Gray, R. (2005). Neurocognitive consequences of marihuana—A comparison with pre-drug performance. *Neurotoxicology and Teratology, 27*(2), 231–239.

Friedman, J. M. (2010). A tale of two hormones. *Nature Medicine, 16*(10), 1100–1106.

Friedman, M. A., & Brownell, K. D. (1995). Psychological correlates of obesity: Moving to the next research generation. *Psychological Bulletin, 117*(1), 3–20.

Friedman, B., Lyness, J. M., Delavan, R. L., Li, C., & Barker, W. H. (2008). Major depression and disability in older primary care patients with heart failure. *Journal of Geriatric Psychiatry and Neurology, 21*(2), 111–122.

Friedman, S. M., Mulhausen, P., Cleveland, M. L., Coll, P. P., Daniel, K. M., Hayward, A. D., … White, H. K. (2019). Healthy aging: American geriatrics society white paper executive summary. *Journal of the American Geriatrics Society, 67*(1), 17–20.

Friedman, M., & Rosenman, R. H. (1974). *Type A behavior and your heart.* New York, NY: Alfred A. Knopf.

Friedemann, C., Heneghan, C., Mahtani, K., Thompson, M., Perera, R., & Ward, A. M. (2012). Cardiovascular disease risk in healthy children and its association with body mass index: Systematic review and meta-analysis. *British Medical Journal, 345,* e4759.

Fryar, C. D., Hughes, J. P., Herrick, K. A., & Ahluwalia, N. (2018). *Fast food consumption among adults in the United States, 2013–2016.* NCHS Data Brief, no 322. Hyattsville, MD: National Center for Health Statistics.

FSNAU-FEWSNET. (2023). *Somalia food security outlook.* Retrieved from https://fsnau.org/downloads/ joint-fews-net-fsnau-somalia-food-security-out-look-report-jun-2022-jan-2023

Fuentes-Afflick, E., Hessol, N. A., & Pérez-Stable, E. J. (1999). Testing the epidemiologic paradox of low birth weight in Latinos. *Archives of Pediatrics and Adolescent Medicine, 153*(2), 147–153.

Furnham, A., Akande, D., & Baguma, P. (1999). Beliefs about health and illness in three countries: Britain, South Africa, and Uganda. *Psychology, Health and Medicine, 4,* 189–201.

Gahagan, J., & Subirana-Malaret, M. (2018). Improving pathways to primary health care among LGBTQ populations and health care providers: Key findings from Nova Scotia, Canada. *International Journal for Equity in Health, 17*(76). doi: 10.1186/s12939-018-0786-0

Gailliot, M. T., & Baumeister, R. F. (2018). The physiology of willpower: Linking blood glucose to self-control. In *Self-regulation and self-control* (pp. 137–180). Routledge.

Gaines, J., & Nguyen, D. B. (2014). Medical tourism. In *CDC health information for international travel, chapter 2: The pre-travel consultation.* Centers for Disease Control and Prevention. Retrieved from https://wwwnc.cdc.gov/travel/yellowbook/2016/the-pre-travel-consultation/medical-tourism

Galliher R. V., & Kerpelman, J. L. (2012). The intersection of identity development and peer relationship processes in adolescence and young adulthood: Contributions of the special issue. *Journal of Adolescence, 35*(6), 1409–1415.

Gallo, J. J., Bogner, H. R., Morales, K. H., Post, E. P., Lin, J. Y., & Bruce, M. L. (2007). The effect of a primary care practice–based depression intervention on mortality in older adults: A randomized trial. *Annals of Internal Medicine, 146*(10), 689–698.

Gallo, L. C., Bogart, L. M., Vranceanu, A. M., & Matthews, K. A. (2005). Socioeconomic status, resources, psychological experiences, and emotional responses: A test of the reserve capacity model. *Journal of Personality and Social Psychology, 88*(2), 386–399.

Gallus, S., Scala, M., Possenti, I., Jarach, C. M., Clancy, L., Fernandez, E., … Lugo, A. (2023). The role of smoking in COVID-19 progression: A comprehensive meta-analysis. *European Respiratory Review, 32*(167), 220191.

Galmiche, M., Déchelotte, P., Lambert, G., & Tavolacci, M. P. (2019). Prevalence of eating disorders over the 2000–2018 period: A systematic literature review. *The American Journal of Clinical Nutrition, 109*(5), 1402–1413.

Gao, C., & Scullin, M. K. (2023). Longitudinal trajectories of spectral power during sleep in middle-aged and older adults. *Aging Brain, 3*, 100058.

Gao, C., & Scullin, M. K. (2020). Sleep health early in the coronavirus disease 2019 (COVID-19) outbreak in the United States: integrating longitudinal, cross-sectional, and retrospective recall data. Sleep medicine, 73, 1–10.

Gardner, B., Richards, R., Lally, P., Rebar, A., Thwaite, T., & Beeken, R. J. (2021). Breaking habits or breaking habitual behaviours? Old habits as a neglected factor in weight loss maintenance. *Appetite, 162*, 105183.

Garland, E. L. (2012). Pain processing in the human nervous system: A selective review of nociceptive and biobehavioral pathways. *Primary Care: Clinics in Office Practice, 39*(3), 561–571.

Garmezy, N. (1991). Resiliency and vulnerability to adverse developmental outcomes associated with poverty. *American Behavioral Scientist, 34*(4), 416–430.

Garrett, M. T., Garrett, J. T., Rivera, E. T., & Roberts-Wilbur, J. (2005). Laughing it up: Native American humor as spiritual tradition. *Journal of Multicultural Counseling and Development, 33*(4), 194–204.

Gaskin, D. J., & Richard, P. (2012). The economic costs of pain in the United States. *Journal of Pain, 13*(8), 715–724. doi: 10.1016/j.jpain.2012.03.009

Gatchel, R. J., Peng, Y. B., Peters, M. L., Fuchs, P. N., & Turk, D. C. (2007). The biopsychosocial approach to chronic pain: Scientific advances and future directions. *Psychological Bulletin, 133*(4), 581–624.

Gawande, A. (2009). *The checklist manifesto: How to get things right.* New York, NY: Metropolitan Books.

GBD 2019 Mental Disorders Collaborators. (2022). Global, regional, and national burden of 12 mental disorders in 204 countries and territories, 1990–2019: A systematic analysis for the Global Burden of Disease Study 2019. *The Lancet Psychiatry, 9*(2), 137–150.

Geers, A. L., Wellman, J. A., Seligman, L. D., Wuyek, L. A., & Neff, L. A. (2010). Dispositional optimism, goals, and engagement in health treatment programs. *Journal of Behavioral Medicine, 33*(2), 123–134.

Geiker, N. R. W., Astrup, A., Hjorth, M. F., Sjödin, A., Pijls, L., & Markus, C. R. (2018). Does stress influence sleep patterns, food intake, weight gain, abdominal obesity and weight loss interventions and vice versa? *Obesity Reviews, 19*(1), 81–97.

Geller, S., Levy, S., Goldzweig, G., Hamdan, S., Manor, A., Dahan, S., … Abu-Abeid, S. (2019). Psychological distress among bariatric surgery candidates: The roles of body image and emotional eating. *Clinical Obesity, 9*(2), e12298.

Geller, S., & Yagil, Y. (2019). "SI VIS VITAM, PARA MORTEM" terror management theory and psychosocial health-care practice. *Social Work in Health Care, 58*(2), 182–200.

Gellert, E. (1958). Reducing the emotional stresses of hospitalization for children. *American Journal of Occupational Therapy, 12*(3), 125–129.

George, L. K., Larson, D. B., Koenig, H., & McCullough, M. E. (2000). Spirituality and health: What we know, what we need to know. *Journal of Social and Clinical Psychology, 19*(1), 102–116.

Gerber, M., Kellmann, M., Hartmann, T., & Pühse, U. (2010). Do exercise and fitness buffer against stress among Swiss police and emergency response service officers? *Psychology of Sport and Exercise, 11*(4), 286–294.

Gerlach, G., Herpertz, S., & Loeber, S. J. O. R. (2015). Personality traits and obesity: A systematic review. *Obesity Reviews, 16*(1), 32–63.

Gerrard, M., Stock, M. L., Roberts, M. E., Gibbons, F. X., O'Hara, R. E., Weng, C. Y., & Wills, T. A. (2012). Coping with racial discrimination: The role of substance use. *Psychology of Addictive Behaviors, 26*(3), 550–560.

Giedd, J. N. (2008) The teen brain: Insights from neuroimaging. *Journal of Adolescent Health, 42*(4), 335–343.

Giesler, R. B., Josephs, R. A., & Swann, W. B., Jr. (1996). Self-verification in clinical depression: The desire for negative evaluation. *Journal of Abnormal Psychology, 105*(3), 358–368.

Gilbert, D. G., & Spielberger, C. D. (1987). Effects of smoking on heart rate, anxiety, and feelings of success during social interaction. *Journal of Behavioral Medicine, 10*, 629–638.

Giletta, M., Slavich, G. M., Rudolph, K. D., Hastings, P. D., Nock, M. K., & Prinstein, M. J. (2018). Peer victimization predicts heightened inflammatory reactivity to social stress in cognitively vulnerable adolescents. *Journal of Child Psychology and Psychiatry, 59*(2), 129–139.

Glaser, R., & Kiecolt-Glaser, J. K. (2005). Stress-induced immune dysfunction: Implications for health. *Nature Reviews Immunology, 5*(3), 243–251.

Glaser, R., Thorn, B. E., Tarr, K. L., Kiecolt-Glaser, J. K., & D'Ambrosio, S. M. (1985). Effects of stress on methyltransferase synthesis: An important DNA repair enzyme. *Health Psychology, 4*, 403–412.

Glass, D. C., & Singer, J. E. (1972). *Urban stress: Experiments on noise and social stressors (social psychology).* New York, NY: Academic Press.

Global Burden of Disease Long COVID collaborators et al. (2022). Estimated global proportions of individuals with persistent fatigue, cognitive, and respiratory symptom clusters following symptomatic COVID-19 in 2020 and 2021. *JAMA*, *328*(16), 1604–1615. doi: 10.1001/jama.2022.18931

Global Burden of Disease (2019) Mental Disorders Collaborators. (2022). Global, regional, and national Burden of 12 mental disorders in 204 countries and territories, 1990–2019: A systematic analysis for the Global Burden of Disease Study 2019. *The Lancet Psychiatry*, *9(2)*, 137–150.

Glombiewski, J. A., Tersek, J., & Rief, W. (2008). Muscular reactivity and specificity in chronic back pain patients. *Psychosomatic Medicine*, *70*(1), 125–131.

Glover, L. M., Bass, M. A., Carithers, T., & Loprinzi, P. D. (2016). Association of kidney stones with atherosclerotic cardiovascular disease among adults in the United States: Considerations by race-ethnicity. *Physiology & Behavior*, *157*, 63–66.

Glynn, R. J., MacFadyen, J. G., & Ridker, P. M. (2009). Tracking of high-sensitivity C-reactive protein after an initially elevated concentration: The JUPITER Study. *Clinical Chemistry*, *55*(2), 305–312.

Goldberg, I. J., Mosca, L., Piano, M. R., & Fisher, E. A. (2001). Wine and your heart: A science advisory for health care professionals from the Nutrition Committee, Council on Epidemiology and Prevention, and Council on Cardiovascular Nursing of the American Heart Association. *Circulation*, *103*, 472–475. doi: 10.1161/01.CIR.103.3.472

Goldberg, L. R., & Strycker, L. A. (2002). Personality traits and eating habits: The assessment of food preferences in a large community sample. *Personality and Individual Differences*, *32*, 49–65.

Goldgruber, J., & Ahrens, D. (2010). Effectiveness of workplace health promotion and primary prevention interventions: A review. *Journal of Public Health*, *18*, 75–88.

Goldstein, G., & Shelly, C. (1980). Neuropsychological investigation of brain lesion localization in alcoholism. *Advances in Experimental Medicine and Biology*, *126*, 731–743.

Golub, S. A., Rendina, H. J., & Gamarel, K. E. (2013). Identity-related growth and loss in a sample of HIV-positive gay and bisexual men: Initial scale development and psychometric evaluation. *AIDS and Behavior*, *17*(2), 748–759.

Golub, S. A., Gamarel, K. E., Rendina, H. J., Surace, A., & Lelutiu-Weinberger, C. L. (2013). From efficacy to effectiveness: Facilitators and barriers to PrEP acceptability and motivations for adherence among MSM and transgender women in New York City. *AIDS Patient Care and STDs*, *27*(4), 248–254.

Golub, S. A., Gamarel, K. E., & Rendina, H. J. (2014). Loss and growth: Identity processes with distinct and complementary impacts on well-being among those living with chronic illness. *Psychology, Health & Medicine*, *19*(5), 572–579.

Go, A. S., Mozaffarian, D., Roger, V. L., Benjamin, E. J., Berry, J. D., Borden, W. B., … Turner, M. B. (2013). Heart disease and stroke statistics—2013 update. *Circulation*, *127*, e62–e245.

Gonzalez, R. (2007). Acute and non-acute effects of cannabis on brain functioning and neuropsychological performance. *Neuropsychological Review*, *17*(3), 347–361.

Gonzalez, A., Hogan, J., McLeish, A. C., & Zvolensky, M. J. (2010). An evaluation of pain-related anxiety among daily cigarette smokers in terms of negative and positive reinforcement smoking outcome expectancies. *Addictive Behaviors*, *35*(6), 553–557.

Gonzalez, J. S., Penedo, F. J., Antoni, M. H., Durán, R. E., McPherson-Baker, S., Ironson, G., … Schneiderman, N. (2004). Social support, positive states of mind, and HIV treatment adherence in men and women living with HIV/AIDS. *Health Psychology*, *23*(4), 413.

Goodin, B., Bier, S., & McGuire, L. (2009). Dispositional optimism buffers the negative influence of catastrophizing on pain response. *Journal of Pain*, *10*(4 Suppl.), S68.

Goodman, E., Daniels, S. R., Meigs, J. B., & Dolan, L. M. (2007). Instability in the diagnosis of metabolic syndrome in adolescents. *Circulation*, *115*(17), 2316–2322.

Gordon, A. R., Austin, S. B., Pantalone, D. W., Baker, A. M., Eiduson, R., & Rodgers, R. (2019). Appearance ideals and eating disorders risk among LGBTQ college students: The Being Ourselves Living in Diverse Bodies (BOLD) study. *Journal of Adolescent Health*, *64*(2), S43–S44.

Gordon, N. S., Merchant, J., Zanbaka, C., Hodges, L. F., & Goolkasian, P. (2011). Interactive gaming reduces experimental pain with or without a head mounted display. *Computers in Human Behavior*, *27*(6), 2123–2128.

Gorman, B. K., Denney, J. T., Dowdy, H., & Medeiros, R. A. (2015). A new piece of the puzzle: Sexual orientation, gender, and physical health status. *Demography*, *52*(4), 1357–1382.

Gortmaker, S. L., Eckenrode, J., & Gore, S. (1982). Stress and the utilization of health services: A time series and cross-sectional analysis. *Journal of Health and Social Behavior, 23*, 25–38.

Goto, V., Frange, C., Andersen, M. L., Júnior, J. M., Tufik, S., & Hachul, H. (2014). Chiropractic intervention in the treatment of postmenopausal climacteric symptoms and insomnia: A review. *Maturitas, 78*(1), 3–7.

Gottlieb, N. H., & Green, L. W. (1987). Ethnicity and lifestyle health risk: Some possible mechanisms. *American Journal of Health Promotion, 2*(1), 37–51.

Gouin, M. (2010). *Tibetan rituals of death: Buddhist funerary practices*. New York, NY: Routledge

Gould, J. B., Madan, A., Qin, C., & Chavez, G. (2003). Perinatal outcomes in two dissimilar immigrant populations in the United States: A dual epidemiologic paradox. *Pediatrics, 111*(6 Pt 1), e676–e682.

Grant, K. E., O'Koon, J. H., Davis, T. H., Roache, N. A., LaShaunda, M., Poindexter, M. L. A., … McIntosh, J. M. (2000). Protective factors affecting low-income urban African American youth exposed to stress. *Journal of Early Adolescence, 20*(4), 388–417.

Greaves, L., Poole, N., Okoli, T. C., Hemsing, N., Qu, A., Bialystok, L., & O'Leary, R. (2011). *Expecting to quit: A best-practices review of smoking cessation interventions for pregnant and postpartum girls and women* (2nd ed.). Vancouver, BC: British Columbia Centre of Excellence for Women's Health.

Gredig, D., Nideröst, S., & Parpan-Blaser, A. (2007). Explaining the condom use of heterosexual men in a high-income country: Adding somatic culture to the theory of planned behaviour. *Journal of Public Health, 15*(2), 129–140.

Green, C. R., Baker, T. A., Sato, Y., Washington, T. L., & Smith, E. M. (2003). Race and chronic pain: A comparative study of young black and white Americans presenting for management. *Journal of Pain, 4*(4), 176–183.

Greenberg, J., & Arndt, J. (2012). Terror management theory. In P. A. M. Van Lange, A. W. Kruglanski, & E. T. Higgins (Eds.), *Handbook of theories of social psychology* (Vol. 1, pp. 398–415). London, UK: SAGE Publications.

Greenberg, D. B., Braun, I. M., & Cassem, N. H. (2008). Functional somatic symptoms and somatoform disorders. In T. Stern, J. F. Rosenbam, M. Fava, J. Biederman, & S. L. Rauch (Eds.), *Massachusetts General Hospital comprehensive clinical psychiatry* (Chapter 24). Philadelphia, PA: Mosby Elsevier.

Greenberg, J., Pyszczynski, T., Solomon, S., Rosenblatt, A., Veeder, M., Kirkland, S., & Lyon, D. (1990). Evidence for terror management theory II: The effects of mortality salience on reactions to those who threaten or bolster the cultural worldview. *Journal of Personality and Social Psychology, 58*(2), 308–318.

Greenwood, P. M., & Parasuraman, R. (2010). Neuronal and cognitive plasticity: A neurocognitive framework for ameliorating cognitive aging. *Frontiers in Aging Neuroscience*. doi: 10.3389/fnagi.2010.00150

Greve, W., & Staudinger, U. M. (2006). Resilience in later adulthood and old age: Resources and potentials for successful aging. In D. Cicchetti & D. J. Cohen (Eds.), *Developmental psychopathology, Vol. 3. Risk, disorder, and adaptation* (2nd ed., pp. 796–840). Hoboken, NJ: Wiley.

Griffin, J. A., Umstattd, M. R., & Usdan, S. L. (2010). Alcohol use and high-risk sexual behavior among collegiate women: A review of research on alcohol myopia theory. *Journal of American College Health, 58*(6), 523–532. doi: 10.1080/07448481003621718

Grossarth-Maticek, R., & Eysenck, H. J. (1990). Personality, stress and disease: Description and validation of a new inventory. *Psychological Reports, 66*(2), 355–373.

Grotenhermen, F. (2003). Pharmacokinetics and pharmacodynamics of cannabinoids. *Clinical Pharmacokinetics, 42*(4), 327–360.

Grundman, M., Petersen, R. C., Ferris, S. H., Thomas, R. G., Aisen, P. S., Bennett, D. A., … Thal, L. J. (2004). Mild cognitive impairment can be distinguished from Alzheimer disease and normal aging for clinical trials. *Archives of Neurology, 61*(1), 59–66. doi: 10.1001/archneur.61.1.59

Gu, J., Wang, R., Chen, H., Lau, J. T., Zhang, L., Hu, X., … Tsui, H. (2009). Prevalence of needle sharing, commercial sex behaviors and associated factors in Chinese male and female injecting drug user populations. *AIDS Care: Psychological and Socio-Medical Aspects of HIV/AIDS, 21*(1), 31–41.

Gulliksson, M., Burell, G., Vessby, B., Lundin, L., Toss, H., & Svärdsudd, K. (2011). Randomized controlled trial of cognitive behavioral therapy vs standard treatment to prevent recurrent cardiovascular events in patients with coronary heart disease: Secondary Prevention in Uppsala Primary Health Care project (SUPRIM). *Archives of Internal Medicine, 171*(2), 134–140.

Guo, M., Gan, Y., & Tong, J. (2013). The role of meaning-focused coping in significant loss. *Anxiety, Stress and Coping, 26*(1), 87–102.

Guo, Y., Wang, Y., Sun, Y., & Wang, J. Y. (2016). A brain signature to differentiate acute and chronic pain in rats. *Frontiers in Computational Neuroscience, 10*, 41. doi: 10.3389/fncom.2016.00041

Gupta, N., & Jenkins, G. D., Jr. (1984). Substance use as an employee response to the work environment. *Journal of Vocational Behaviour, 24*, 84–93.

Gurung, R. A., Taylor, S. E., & Seeman, T. E. (2003). Accounting for changes in social support among married older adults: Insights from the MacArthur studies of successful aging. *Psychology and Aging, 18*(3), 487–496.

Gutierrez-Aguilar, R., Kim, D. H., Woods, S. C., & Seeley, R. J. (2012). Expression of new loci associated with obesity in diet-induced obese rats: From genetics to physiology. *Obesity (Silver Spring), 20*(2), 306–312. doi: 10.1038/oby.2011.236

Guyatt, G. H., Feeny, D. H., & Patrick, D. L. (1993). Measuring health-related quality of life. *Annals of Internal Medicine, 118*(8), 622–629.

Habibović, M., Broers, E., Piera-Jimenez, J., Wetzels, M., Ayoola, I., Denollet, J., & Widdershoven, J. (2018). Enhancing lifestyle change in cardiac patients through the do change system ("Do cardiac health: Advanced new generation ecosystem"): Randomized controlled trial protocol. *JMIR Research Protocols, 7*(2), e40. doi: 10.2196/resprot.8406

Hagger, M. S., & Orbell, S. (2003). A meta-analytic review of the common-sense model of illness representations. *Psychology & Health, 18*(2), 141–184.

Hair, E. C., Park, M. J., Ling, T. J., & Moore, K. A. (2009). Risky behaviors in late adolescence: Co-occurrence, predictors, and consequences. *Journal of Adolescent Health, 45*(3), 253–261.

Halbeisen, G., Brandt, G., & Paslakis, G. (2022). A plea for diversity in eating disorders research. *Frontiers in Psychiatry, 13*, 820043.

Hale, L., Troxel, W., Buysse, D. J. (2020). Sleep health: An opportunity for public health to address health equity. *Annual Review of Public Health, 41*, 81–99.

Halford, W. K., Cuddihy, S., & Mortimer, R. H. (1990). Psychological stress and blood glucose regulation in type I diabetic patients. *Health Psychology, 9*(5), 516–528.

Halim, M. L., Yoshikawa, H., & Amodio, D. M. (2013). Cross-generational effects of discrimination among immigrant mothers: Perceived discrimination predicts child's healthcare visits for illness. *Health Psychology, 32*(2), 203–211.

Hall, K. D., Farooqi, I. S., Friedman, J. M., Klein, S., Loos, R. J., Mangelsdorf, D. J., … Tobias, D. K. (2022). The energy balance model of obesity: Beyond calories in, calories out. *The American Journal of Clinical Nutrition, 115*(5), 1243–1254.

Hamer, M., Kivimaki, M., Stamatakis, E., & Batty, G. D. (2012). Psychological distress as a risk factor for death from cerebrovascular disease. *CMAJ, 184*(13), 1461–1466. doi: 10.1503/cmaj.111719

Hammen, C. (1991). Generation of stress in the course of unipolar depression. *Journal of Abnormal Psychology, 100*(4), 555.

Hammen, C. (2005). Stress and depression. *Annual Review of Clinical Psychology, 1*, 293–319.

Han, B. H., Sherman, S., Mauro, P. M., Martins, S. S., Rotenberg, J., & Palamar, J. J. (2017). Demographic trends among older cannabis users in the United States, 2006–13. *Addiction, 112*, 516–525. doi: 10.1111/add.13670

Hansen, T. B., Lindholt, J. S., Diederichsen, A. C. P., Bliemer, M. C., Lambrechtsen, J., Steffensen, F. H., & Søgaard, R. (2019). Individual preferences on the balancing of good and harm of cardiovascular disease screening. *Heart, 105*, 761–767. doi: 10.1136/heartjnl-2018-314103

Hansen, C. J., Stevens, L. C., & Coast, J. R. (2001). Exercise duration and mood state: How much is enough to feel better? *Health Psychology, 20*(4), 267–275.

Hanson, S. W., Abbafati, C., Aerts, J. G., Al-Aly, Z., Ashbaugh, C., Ballouz, T., … Global Burden of Disease Long COVID Collaborators. (2022). Estimated global proportions of individuals with persistent fatigue, cognitive, and respiratory symptom clusters following symptomatic COVID-19 in 2020 and 2021. *JAMA, 328*(16), 1604–1615.

Hanson, S., & Hanson, C. (2008, October 9). HIV control in low-income countries in sub-Saharan Africa: Are the right things done? *Global Health Action, 1*. doi: 10.3402/gha.v1i0.1837

Hantsoo, L., Jašarević, E., Criniti, S., McGeehan, B., Tanes, C., Sammel, M. D., … Epperson, C. N. (2019). Childhood adversity impact on gut microbiota and inflammatory response to stress during pregnancy. *Brain, Behavior, and Immunity, 75*, 240–250.

Harkness, K. L., Bruce, A. E., & Lumley, M. N. (2006). The role of childhood abuse and neglect in the sensitization to stressful life events in adolescent depression. *Journal of Abnormal Psychology, 115*, 730–741.

Harper, C. (2009). The neuropathology of alcohol-related brain damage. *Alcohol and Alcoholism, 44*(2), 136–140.

Harriger, J. A, & Thompson, J. K. (2012). Psychological consequences of obesity: Weight bias and body image in overweight and obese youth. *International Review of Psychiatry, 24*(3), 247–253. doi: 10.3109/09540261.2012.678817

Harris, J. L., Frazier, W., Romo-Palafox, M., Hyary, M., Fleming-Milici, F., Haraghey, K., ... Kalnova, S. (2017). *FACTS 2017: Food industry self-regulation after 10 years*. UConn Rudd Center. Retrieved from http://www.uconnruddcenter.org/files/Pdfs/FACTS-2017_Final.pdf

Harrist, A. W., Swindle, T. M., Hubbs-Tait, L., Topham, G. L., Shriver, L. H., & Page, M. C. (2016). The social and emotional lives of overweight, obese, and severely obese children. *Child Development, 87*(5), 1564–1580.

Hartley, H. (2007). An 'Exercise Snack' plan. *Newsweek*. Retrieved from https://www.newsweek.com/exercise-snack-plan-96095

Hartmann, E. (1996). Outline for a theory on the nature and functions of dreaming. *Dreaming, 6*(2), 147–170.

Hartmann, E. (2007). The nature and functions of dreaming. In D. Barrett & P. McNamara (Eds.), *The new science of dreaming, Vol. 3. Cultural and theoretical perspectives on dreaming* (pp. 171–192). Westport, CT: Praeger.

Hartmann-Boyce, J., Begh, R., & Aveyard, P. (2018). Electronic cigarettes for smoking cessation. *BMJ, 360*, j5543.

Hartmann-Boyce, J., McRobbie, H., Bullen, C., Begh, R., Stead, L. F., & Hajek, P. (2016). Electronic cigarettes for smoking cessation. *Cochrane Database of Systematic Reviews, 9*, CD010216.

Hart, C. L., Morrison, D. S., Batty, G. D., Mitchell, R. J., & Davey Smith, G. (2010). Effect of body mass index and alcohol consumption on liver disease: Analysis of data from two prospective cohort studies. *BMJ, 340*, c1240.

Harvard College. (2007, October). Sticking it to blood pressure? *Harvard Heart Letter*.

Harvard Health Publishing. (2018, April). *Reading the new blood pressure guidelines*. Retrieved from https://www.health.harvard.edu/heart-health/reading-the-new-blood-pressure-guidelines

Harvey, A. G., & Tang, N. K. (2012). (Mis)perception of sleep in insomnia: A puzzle and a resolution. *Psychological Bulletin, 138*(1), 77–101.

Hasin, D. S., Saha, T. D., Kerridge, B. T., Goldstein, R. B., Chou, S. P., Zhang, H., ... Grant, B. F. (2015). Prevalence of marijuana use disorders in the United States between 2001–2002 and 2012–2013. *JAMA Psychiatry, 72*(12), 1235–1242.

Haug, M. R., & Lavin, B. (1981). Practitioner or patient—who's in charge? *Journal of Health and Social Behavior, 22*(3), 212–229.

Hausmann, J. S., Touloumtzis, C., White, M. T., Colbert, J. A., & Gooding, H. C. (2017). Adolescent and young adult use of social media for health and its implications. *Journal of Adolescent Health, 60*(6), 714–719.

Havighurst, R. J. (1972). *Developmental tasks and education* (3rd ed.). New York, NY: David McKay.

Hay, P., Girosi, F., & Mond, J. (2015). Prevalence and sociodemographic correlates of DSM-5 eating disorders in the Australian population. *Journal of Eating Disorders, 3*, 1–7.

Haynes, R. B., McKibbon, K. A., & Kanani, R. (1996). Systematic review of randomised trials of interventions to assist patients to follow prescriptions for medications. *Lancet, 348*(9024), 383–386.

Haynos, A. F., Roberto, C. A., & Attia, E. (2015). Examining the associations between emotion regulation difficulties, anxiety, and eating disorder severity among inpatients with anorexia nervosa. *Comprehensive Psychiatry, 60*, 93–98.

Healy, Genevieve N., et al. (2008). Breaks in sedentary time: Beneficial associations with metabolic risk. *Diabetes Care, 31*(4), 661–666. doi: 10.2337/dc07-2046

Heaven, P. C., Mulligan, K., Merrilees, R., Woods, T., & Fairooz, Y. (2001). Neuroticism and conscientiousness as predictors of emotional, external, and restrained eating behaviors. *International Journal of Eating Disorders, 30*, 161–166. doi: 10.1002/eat.1068

Hechinger, P. (2011). Coroner: Winehouse's death was the result of alcohol poisoning. *BBC America*. Retrieved from http://www.bbcamerica.com/anglophenia/2011/10/coroner-winehouses-death-was-the-result-of-alcohol-poisoning

Hefferon, K., Grealy, M., & Mutrie, N. (2009). Post-traumatic growth and life threatening physical illness: A systematic review of the qualitative literature. *British Journal of Health Psychology, 14*(Pt 2), 343–378.

Heijmans, M. (1998). Coping and adaptive outcome in chronic fatigue syndrome: Importance of illness cognitions. *Journal of Psychosomatic Research, 45*, 39–51.

Heindel, J. J., Lustig, R. H., Howard, S., & Corkey, B. E. (2024). Obesogens: A unifying theory for the global rise in obesity. *International Journal of Obesity, 48*(4), 449–460.

Heitzeg, M. M., Hardee, J. E., & Beltz, A. M. (2018). Sex differences in the developmental neuroscience of adolescent substance use risk. *Current Opinion in Behavioral Sciences, 23*, 21–26.

Hekler, E. B., Lambert, J., Leventhal, E., Leventhal, H., Jahn, E., & Contrada, R. J. (2008). Commonsense illness beliefs, adherence behaviors, and hypertension control among African Americans. *Journal of Behavioral Medicine*, *31*(5), 391–400.

Helgeson, V. S., & Zajdel, M. (2017). Adjusting to chronic health conditions. *Annual Review of Psychology*, *68*, 545–571.

Helliwell, J. F. (2001). *Social capital, the economy and well-being. In The review of economic performance and social progress 2001: The longest decade: Canada in the 1990s* (pp. 43–60). Ottawa, ON: Centre for the Study of Living Standards, The Institute for Research on Public Policy.

Helliwell, J. F., Layard, R., & Sachs, J. (Eds.). (2015). World happiness report 2015.

Helliwell, J., Layard, R., & Sachs, J. (2019). *World happiness report 2019*. New York, NY: Sustainable Development Solutions Network.

Helman, C. G. (2001). *Culture, health and illness* (4th ed.). London, UK: Arnold.

Hendershot, C. S., Stoner, S. A., Pantalone, D. W., & Simoni, J. M. (2009). Alcohol use and antiretroviral adherence: Review and meta-analysis. *Journal of Acquired Immune Deficiency Syndromes*, *52*(2), 180–202.

Henderson, B. N., & Baum, A. (2004). Biological mechanisms of health and disease. In S. Sutton, A. Baum, & M. Johnston (Eds.), *The SAGE handbook of health psychology* (pp. 69–93). London, UK: Sage.

Henneghan, A. M., & Schnyer, R. N. (2013). Biofield therapies for symptom management in palliative and end-of-life care. *American Journal of Hospice and Palliative Medicine*, *32*(1), 90–100. doi: 10.1177/1049909113509400

Herman, C. P., Polivy, J., Lank, C. N., & Heatherton, T. F. (1987). Anxiety, hunger, and eating behavior. *Journal of Abnormal Psychology*, *96*, 264–269.

Hermon, D. A., & Hazler, R. J. (1999). Adherence to a wellness model and perceptions of psychological well-being. *Journal of Counseling and Development*, *77*(3), 339–343.

Hernández, R. J., & Villodas, M. (2019). Collectivistic coping responses to racial microaggressions associated with Latina/o college persistence attitudes. *Journal of Latinx Psychology*, *7*(1), 76.

Herold, D. M., & Conlon, E. J. (1981). Work factors as potential causal agents of alcohol abuse. *Journal of Drug Issues*, *11*, 337–356.

Heron, M. (2018). Deaths: Leading causes for 2016. *National Vital Statistics Report*, *67*(6). Retrieved from https://www.cdc.gov/nchs/data/nvsr/nvsr67/nvsr67_06.pdf

Herrald, M. M., & Tomaka, J. (2002). Patterns of emotion-specific appraisal, coping, and cardiovascular reactivity during an ongoing emotional episode. *Journal of Personality and Social Psychology*, *83*(2), 434–450.

Herrera, D., Sanz, M., Shapira, L., Brotons, C., Chapple, I., Frese, T., … Vinker, S. (2023). Association between periodontal diseases and cardiovascular diseases, diabetes and respiratory diseases: Consensus report of the Joint Workshop by the European Federation of Periodontology (EFP) and the European arm of the World Organization of Family Doctors (WONCA Europe). *Journal of Clinical Periodontology*, *50*(6), 819–841.

Herskind, A. M., McGue, M., Holm, N. V., Sorensen, T. I., Harvald, B., & Vaupel, J. W. (1996). The heritability of human longevity: A population-based study of 2872 Danish twin pairs born 1870–1900. *Human Genetics*, *97*, 319–323.

Herzog, T. A. (2008). Analyzing the transtheoretical model using the framework of Weinstein, Rothman, and Sutton (1998): The example of smoking cessation. *Health Psychology*, *27*(5), 548–556.

Heshka, S., Anderson, J. W., Atkinson, R. L., Greenway, F. L., Hill, J. O., Phinney, S. D., … Pi-Sunyer, F. X. (2003). Weight loss with self-help compared with a structured commercial program: A randomized trial. *JAMA*, *289*(14), 1792–1798.

Heshmati, H. M., Luzi, L., Greenway, F. L., & Rebello, C. J. (2023). Stress-induced weight changes. *Frontiers in Endocrinology*, *14*, 1209975.

Heslop, P., Smith, G. D., Carroll, D., Mcleod, J., Hyland, F., & Hart, C. (2001). Perceived stress and coronary heart disease risk factors: The contribution of socio-economic position. *British Journal of Health Psychology*, *6*, 167–178.

Heyse-Moore, L. H., & Johnson-Bell, V. E. (1987). Can doctors accurately predict the life expectancy of patients with terminal cancer? *Palliative Medicine*, *1*(2), 165–166.

Hildreth, C. J., Lynm, C., & Glass, R. M. (2009). Migraine headache. *Journal of the American Medical Association*, *301*(24), 2608.

Hilliard, M. E., Wu, Y. P., Rausch, J., Dolan, L. M., & Hood, K. K. (2013). Predictors of deteriorations in diabetes management and control in adolescents with type 1 diabetes. *Journal of Adolescent Health*, *52*(1), 28–34.

Hirayama, K., Miyaji, K., Kawamura, S., Itoh, K., Takahashi, E., & Mitsuoka, T. (1995). Development of intestinal flora of human-flora-associated (HFA) mice in the intestine of their offspring. *Experimental Animals*, *44*(3), 219–222.

Hobbs, M., Owen, S., & Gerber, L. (2017). Liquid love? Dating apps, sex, relationships and the digital transformation of intimacy. *Journal of Sociology, 53*(2), 271–284.

Hofmann, W., Dohle, S., & Diel, K. (2020). Changing behavior using integrative self-control theory. In M. S. Hagger, L. D. Cameron, K. Hamilton, N. Hankonen, & T. Lintunen (Eds.), *The Handbook of Behavior Change* (pp. 150–163). Cambridge University Press.

Hofstede, G. (1980). Motivation, leadership, and organization: Do American theories apply abroad? *Organizational Dynamics, 9*(1), 42–63.

Hoge, C. W., McGurk, D., Thomas, J., Cox, A. L., Engel, C. C., & Castro, C. A. (2008). Mild traumatic brain injury in U.S. soldiers returning from Iraq. *New England Journal of Medicine, 358*, 453–463.

Holahan, C. K., Holahan, C. J., & Belk, S. S. (1984). Adjustment in aging: The roles of life stress, hassles, and self-efficacy. *Health Psychology, 3*, 315–328.

Hollifield, M., Sinclair-Lian, N., Warner, T. D., & Hammerschlag, R. (2007). Acupuncture for posttraumatic stress disorder: A randomized controlled pilot trial. *Journal of Nervous and Mental Disease, 195*(6), 504–513.

Holmes, T. H., & Rahe, R. H. (1967). The social readjustment rating scale. *Journal of Psychosomatic Research, 11*(2), 213–218.

Holt, P. R., Altayar, O., & Alpers, D. H. (2023). Height with age affects body mass index (BMI) assessment of chronic disease risk. *Nutrients, 15*(21), 4694.

Hood, L., Sherrell, D., Pfeffer, C. A., & Mann, E. S. (2019). LGBTQ college students' experiences with university health services: An exploratory study. *Journal of Homosexuality, 66*(6), 797–814.

Hooker, K. (1992). Possible selves and perceived health in older adults and college students. *Journal of Gerontology, 47*(2), P85–P95.

Hooker, K., Frazier, L. D., & Monahan, D. J. (1994). Personality and coping among caregivers of spouses with dementia. *Gerontologist, 34*(3), 386–392.

Hooker, K., & Kaus, C. R. (1992). Possible selves and health behaviors in later life. *Journal of Aging and Health, 4*(3), 390–411.

Hooker, K., Manoogian-O'Dell, M., Monahan, D. J., Frazier, L. D., & Shifren, K. (2000). Does type of disease matter? Gender differences among Alzheimer's and Parkinson's disease spouse caregivers. *Gerontologist, 40*(5), 568–573.

Hooper, R., & Quincy, J. (1811). *Quincy's lexicon-medicum: A new medical dictionary, containing an explanation of the terms in anatomy, physiology, practice of physic, material medica, chemistry, pharmacy, surgery, midwifery, and the various branches of natural philosophy connected with medicine.* London, UK: Longman, Hurst, Rees, Orme.

Horgas, A. L. (2003). Assessing pain in older adults with dementia. In M. Boltz (Ed.), *Try this: Best practices in nursing care to older adults with dementia, D2.* Retrieved from https://consultgeri.org/try-this/dementia/issue-d2.pdf

Horton, S. E. (2015). Religion and health-promoting behaviors among emerging adults. *Journal of Religion and Health, 54*(1), 20–34.

Hospice Patients Alliance. (2019, February). *Signs and symptoms of approaching death.* Retrieved from https://hospicefoundation.org/when-death-is-near-signs-and-symptoms/

Houben, K., Nederkoorn, C., & Jansen, A. (2012) Too tempting to resist? Past success at weight control rather than dietary restraint determines exposure-induced disinhibited eating. *Appetite, 59*, 550–555.

Howren, M. B., & Suls, J. (2011). The symptom perception hypothesis revised: Depression and anxiety play different roles in concurrent and retrospective physical symptom reporting. *Journal of Personality and Social Psychology, 100*(1), 182–195.

Hoyt, C. L., Burnette, J. L., & Auster-Gussman, L. (2014). "Obesity is a disease": Examining the self-regulatory impact of this public-health message. *Psychological Science, 25*(4), 997–1002.

Hruschka, D. J., Brewis, A. A., Wutich, A., & Morin, B. (2011). Shared norms and their explanation for the social clustering of obesity. *American Journal of Public Health, 101*(S1), S295–S300. doi: 10.2105/AJPH.2010.300053

Huang, H. P., He, M., Wang, H. Y., & Zhou, M. (2016). A meta-analysis of the benefits of mindfulness-based stress reduction (MBSR) on psychological function among breast cancer (BC) survivors. *Breast Cancer, 23*(4), 568–576.

Huang, H. Y., Yang, W., & Omaye, S. T. (2011). Intimate partner violence, depression and overweight/obesity. *Aggression and Violent Behavior, 16*, 108–114.

Hudcova, J., McNicol, E., Quah, C. S., Lau, J., & Carr, D. B. (2006). Patient controlled opioid analgesia versus conventional opioid analgesia for postoperative pain. *Cochrane Database of Systematic Reviews, 4*, CD003348.

Hudson, D. L., Eaton, J., Lewis, P., Grant, P., Sewell, W., & Gilbert, K. (2016). "Racism?!?... just look at our neighborhoods": Views on racial discrimination and coping among African American men in Saint Louis. *Journal of Men's Studies, 24*(2), 130–150.

Hudson, J. I., Hiripi, E., Pope, H. G., Jr., & Kessler, R. C. (2007). The prevalence and correlates of eating disorders in the National Comorbidity Survey Replication. *Biological Psychiatry, 61,* 348–358.

Hudson, K. D., & Mehrotra, G. R. (2022). "That is when I changed and my whole life changed": Turning points in health perceptions among LGBTQ adults of color. *Journal of Ethnic & Cultural Diversity in Social Work, 31*(2), 84–95.

Hull, J. G., & Bond, C. F. (1986). Social and behavioral consequences of alcohol consumption and expectancy: A meta-analysis. *Psychological Bulletin, 99*(3), 347–360.

Hummer, R. A., Rogers, R. G., Nam, C. B., & Ellison, C. G. (1999). Religious involvement and U.S. adult mortality. *Demography, 36*(2), 273–285.

Hunter, A. (2022). *United Nations development programme: Human development report 2021–22: Uncertain times, unsettled lives: Shaping our future in a transforming world. Human development reports 272–275.* United Nations Development Programme (8 September 2022). Archived from the original on 8 September 2022. Retrieved on 8 September

Huta, V., Park, N., Peterson, C., & Seligman, M. (2003). *Pursuing pleasure versus eudaimonia: Which leads to greater satisfaction?* Poster presented at the 2nd International Positive Psychology Summit, Washington, DC.

Hyun, S. et al. (2021). Psychological correlates of poor sleep quality among U.S. young adults during the COVID-19 pandemic. *Sleep Medicine, 78,* 51–56.

Idler, E. L., & Benyamini, Y. (1997). Self-rated health and mortality: A review of twenty-seven community studies. *Journal of Health and Social Behavior, 38*(1), 21–37.

Ilgen, M. (2018). Pain, opioids, and suicide mortality in the United States. *Annals of Internal Medicine, 169*(7), 498–499.

Iliff, J. J., & Nedergaard, M. (2013). Is there a cerebral lymphatic system? *Stroke, 44*(6, Suppl. 1), S93–S95.

Illsley, R., & Baker, D. (1991). Contextual variations in the meaning of health inequality. *Social Science & Medicine, 32*(4), 359–365.

Indo, Y. (2012). Nerve growth factor and the physiology of pain: Lessons from congenital insensitivity to pain with anhidrosis. *Clinical Genetics, 82*(4), 341–350.

Ingersoll, K. S., & Cohen, J. (2008). The impact of medication regimen factors on adherence to chronic treatment: A review of literature. *Journal of Behavioral Medicine, 31*(3), 213–224.

Insel, K. C., Reminger, S. L., & Hsiao, C. P. (2006). The negative association of independent personality and medication adherence. *Journal of Aging and Health, 18*(3), 407–418.

Institute of Medicine. (2011). *The health of lesbian, gay, bisexual, and transgender people: Building a foundation for better understanding.* Washington, DC: Institute of Medicine of the National Academies. Retrieved from https://pubmed.ncbi.nlm.nih.gov/22013611/

International Agency for Research on Cancer. (2024). Retrieved from https://www.iarc.who.int/

International Association for the Study of Pain. (2017, December 14). *IASP terminology.* Retrieved from https://www.iasp-pain.org/terminology

International Diabetes Foundation. (2015). *IDF Diabetes Atlas* (7th ed.).

International Medical Travel Journal. (2019). *Medical travel and tourism global market report* (1st ed.). Berkhamsted, Herts: Youngman.

Inzlicht, M., Werner, K. M., Briskin, J. L., & Roberts, B. W. (2021). Integrating models of self-regulation. *Annual Review of Psychology, 72*(1), 319–345.

Iredale, J. (2013, July 28). Lady Gaga: "I'm every icon." *Women's Wear Daily.* Retrieved from https://wwd.com/eye/other/lady-gaga-im-every-icon-7068388/

Ireland, L. (2023). *Millenials are taking healthcare into their own hands with digital tools and social media.* Retrieved from https://hallandpartners.com/perspectives/millennials-are-taking-healthcare-into-their-own-hands

Ironson, G., O'Cleirigh, C., Fletcher, M. A., Laurenceau, J. P., Balbin, E., Klimas, N., … Solomon, G. (2005). Psychosocial factors predict CD4 and viral load change in men and women with human immunodeficiency virus in the era of highly active antiretroviral treatment. *Psychosomatic Medicine, 67*(6), 1013–1021.

Irwin, M., Mascovich, A., Gillin, J. C., & Willoughby, R. (1994). Partial sleep deprivation reduces natural killer cell activity in humans. *Psychosomatic Medicine, 56,* 493–498.

Islami, F., Kahn, A. R., Bickell, N. A., Schymura, M. J., & Boffetta, P. (2013). Disentangling the effects of race/ethnicity and socioeconomic status of neighborhood in cancer stage distribution in New York City. *Cancer Causes & Control, 24*(6), 1069–1078.

ISSP Research Group. (2015). *International Social Survey Programme: Health and health care—ISSP 2011.* GESIS Data Archive, Cologne. ZA5800 Data file Version 3.0.0. doi: 10.4232/1.12252

Jackson, J. S., Knight, K. M., & Rafferty, J. A. (2010). Race and unhealthy behaviors: Chronic stress, the HPA axis, and physical and mental health disparities over the life course. *American Journal of Public Health*, *100*(5), 933–939.

Jafarzadeh, S. R., & Felson, D. T. (2017). Updated estimates suggest a much higher prevalence of arthritis in US adults than previous ones. *Arthritis and Rheumatology*, *70*(2), 185–192. doi: 10.1002/art.40355

Jahrami, H., BaHammam, A. S., Bragazzi, N. L., Saif, Z., Faris, M., & Vitiello, M. V. (2021). Sleep problems during the COVID-19 pandemic by population: A systematic review and meta-analysis. *Journal of Clinical Sleep Medicine*, *17*(2), 299–313.

James, S. A. (1994). John Henryism and the health of African-Americans. *Culture, Medicine, and Psychiatry*, *18*(2), 163–182.

Janssen, I., Katzmarzyk, P. T., Boyce, W. F., King, M. A., & Pickett, W. (2004). Overweight and obesity in Canadian adolescents and their associations with dietary habits and physical activity patterns. *Journal of Adolescent Health*, *35*(5), 360–367.

Janz, N. K., & Becker, M. H. (1984). The Health Belief Model: A decade later. *Health Education Quarterly*, *11*(1), 1–47.

Jargon, J. (2019, August 6). Waiting-Room Anxiety Eased with Apps that Give Updates. *The Wall Street Journal*. Retrieved from https://www.wsj.com/articles/in-surgery-social-networks-aim-to-curb-waiting-room-anxiety-11565083801

Jaslow, R. (2013, November 29). *Magic Johnson's HIV activism hasn't slowed 22 years since historic announcement*. Retrieved from https://www.cbsnews.com/news/magic-johnsons-hiv-activism-hasnt-slowed-22-years-since-historic-announcement/

Jeffers, A. J., Benotsch, E. G., Green, B. A., Bannerman, D., Darby, M., Kelley, T., & Martin, A. M. (2015). Health anxiety and the non-medical use of prescription drugs in young adults: A cross-sectional study. *Addictive Behaviors*, *50*, 74–77.

Jemmott, J. B., & Magloire, K. (1988). Academic stress, social support, and secretory immunoglobulin A. *Journal of Personality and Social Psychology*, *55*(5), 803–810.

Jenkins, E. M., et al. (2019). Do stair climbing exercise "snacks" improve cardiorespiratory fitness?. *Applied Physiology, Nutrition, and Metabolism*, *44*(6), 681–684. doi: 10.1139/apnm-2018-0675

Jensen, T. K., Holt, T., Ormhaug, S. M., Egeland, K., Granly, L., Hoaas, L. C., … Wentzel-Larsen, T. (2014). A randomized effectiveness study comparing trauma-focused cognitive behavioral therapy with therapy as usual for youth. *Journal of Clinical Child and Adolescent Psychology*, *43*(3), 356–369. doi: 10.1080/15374416.2013.822307

Jensen, M. P., & Karoly, P. (1991). Motivation and expectancy factors in symptom perception: A laboratory study of the placebo effect. *Psychosomatic Medicine*, *53*(2), 144–152.

Jensen, C. B. F., Petersen, M. K., Larsen, J. E., Stopczynski, A., Stahlhut, C., Ivanova, M. G., … Hansen, L. K. (2013). *Spatio temporal media components for neurofeedback*. Presented at 2013 IEEE International Conference on Multimedia and Expo Workshops (ICMEW), San Jose, CA. Retrieved from http://ieeexplore.ieee.org/search/searchresult.jsp?queryText=media%20components&newsearch=true

Jessor, R. (1987). Problem-behavior theory, psychosocial development, and adolescent problem drinking. *British Journal of Addiction*, *82*, 331–342.

Jessor, R. (1992). Risk behavior in adolescence: A psychosocial framework for understanding and action. *Developmental Review*, *12*(4), 374–390.

Jessor, R., & Jessor, S. L. (1977). *Problem behavior and psychosocial development: A longitudinal study of youth*. New York, NY: Academic Press.

Jessor, R., Van Den Bos, J., Vanderryn, J., Costa, F. M., & Turbin, M. S. (1995). Protective factors in adolescent problem behavior: Moderator effects and developmental change. *Developmental Psychology*, *31*, 923–933.

Jha, P., Ramasundarahettige, C., Landsman, V., Rostron, B., Thun, M., Anderson, R. N., … Peto, R. (2013). 21st-century hazards of smoking and benefits of cessation in the United States. *New England Journal of Medicine*, *368*, 341–350.

Jia, X., Sheng, C., Han, X., Li, M., & Wang, K. (2024). Global burden of stomach cancer attributable to smoking from 1990 to 2019 and predictions to 2044. *Public Health*, *226*, 182–189.

Jiménez-Sánchez, S., Fernández-de-las-Peñas, C., Jiménez-García, R., Hernández-Barrera, V., Alonso-Blanco, C., Palacios-Ceña, D., & Carrasco-Garrido, P. (2013). Prevalence of migraine headaches in the Romany population in Spain: Sociodemographic factors, lifestyle and co-morbidity. *Journal of Transcultural Nursing*, *24*(1), 6–13.

Ji, R. R., Nackley, A., Huh, Y., Terrando, N., & Maixner, W. (2018). Neuroinflammation and central sensitization in chronic and widespread pain. *Anesthesiology*, *129*, 343–366.

Jobanputra, R., & Furnham, A. F. (2005). British Gujarati Indian immigrants' and British Caucasians' beliefs about health and illness. *International Journal of Social Psychiatry*, *51*(4), 350–364.

Johnson, J. H. (1986). *Life events as stressors in childhood and adolescence*. Newbury Park, CA: Sage.

Johnson, S. B. (1992). Methodological issues in diabetes research: Measuring adherence. *Diabetes Care*, *15*(11), 1658–1667.

Johnson, B. T., & Acabchuk, R. L. (2018). What are the keys to a longer, happier life? Answers from five decades of health psychology research. *Social Science and Medicine*, *196*, 218–226.

Johnson, S. L., Goodell, L. S., Williams, K., Power, T. G., & Hughes, S. O. (2015). Getting my child to eat the right amount: Mothers' considerations when deciding how much food to offer their child at a meal. *Appetite*, *88*, 24–32.

Johnson, J. E., Lauver, D. R., & Nail, L. M. (1989). Process of coping with radiation therapy. *Journal of Consulting and Clinical Psychology*, *57*(3), 358–364.

Johnson, S. B., Riley, A. W., Granger, D. A., & Riis, J. (2013). The science of early life toxic stress for pediatric practice and advocacy. *Pediatrics*, *131*(2), 319–327.

Johnson, D. K., Wilkins, C. H., & Morris, J. C. (2006). Accelerated weight loss may precede diagnosis in Alzheimer's disease. *Archives of Neurology*, *63*, 1312–1317.

Johnston, D. W., Tuomisto, M. T., & Patching, G. R. (2008). The relationship between cardiac reactivity in the laboratory and in real life. *Health Psychology*, *27*, 34–42.

Johnston-Brooks, C. H., Lewis, M. A., Evans, G. W., & Whalen, C. K. (1998). Chronic stress and illness in children: The role of allostatic load. *Psychosomatic Medicine*, *60*, 597–603.

Joiner, T. E., Jr., Conwell, Y., Fitzpatrick, K. K., Witte, T. K., Schmidt, N. B., Berlim, M. T., … Rudd, M. D. (2005). Four studies on how past and current suicidality relate even when "everything but the kitchen sink" is covaried. *Journal of Abnormal Psychology*, *114*(2), 291–303.

Joiner, T. E., Jr., & Metalsky, G. I. (2001). Excessive reassurance seeking: Delineating a risk factor involved in the development of depressive symptoms. *Psychological Science*, *12*(5), 371–378.

Jonas, W., Nissen, E., Ransjö-Arvidson, A. B., Wiklund, I., Henriksson, P., & Uvnas-Moberg, K. (2008). Short- and long-term decrease of blood pressure in women during breastfeeding. *Breastfeeding Medicine*, *3*, 103–109.

Jones, B. L. (2018). Making time for family meals: Parental influences, home eating environments, barriers and protective factors. *Physiology and Behavior*, *193*, 248–251.

Jones, C. M., et al. (2020). Prescription opioid misuse and use of alcohol and other substances among high school students—Youth Risk Behavior Survey, United States, 2019. *MMWR Supplements*, *69*(1), 38.

Jones, D. S., & Greene, J. A. (2016). Is dementia in decline? Historical trends and future trajectories. *New England Journal of Medicine*, *374*, 507–509.

Jones, L. J., Van Wassenhove-Paetzold, J., Thomas, K., Bancroft, C., Quinn Ziatyk, E., Kim, L. S. H., et al. (2020). Impact of a fruit and vegetable prescription program on health outcomes and behaviors in young navajo children. *Current Developments in Nutrition*, *4*(8), nzaa109.

Jopp, D., & Smith, J. (2006). Resources and life-management strategies as determinants of successful aging: On the protective effect of selection, optimization, and compensation. *Psychology and Aging*, *21*(2), 253–265.

Joseph, N. T., Kamarck, T. W., Muldoon, M. F., & Manuck, S. B. (2014). Daily marital interaction quality and carotid artery intima-medial thickness in healthy middle-aged adults. *Psychosomatic Medicine*, *76*(5), 347–354.

Joseph, J., & Kuo, B. C. H. (2009). Black Canadians' coping responses to racial discrimination. *Journal of Black Psychology*, *35*(1), 78–101.

Jozwiak, J. L. (2007). *The significance of religion on health factors related to aging among American adults using the National Survey of Midlife Development in the United States* (Doctoral dissertation). Retrieved from http://d-scholarship.pitt.edu/10151

Ju, H., Jones, M., & Mishra, G. (2013). The prevalence and risk factors of dysmenorrhea. *Epidemiologic Reviews*, *36*, 104–113.

Junger, M., & Van Kampen, M. (2010). Cognitive ability and self-control in relation to dietary habits, physical activity, and bodyweight in adolescents. *International Journal of Behavioral Nutrition and Physical Activity*, *7*(22), 1–12.

Juster, R. P., McEwen, B. S., & Lupien, S. J. (2010). Allostatic load biomarkers of chronic stress and impact on health and cognition. *Neuroscience and Biobehavioral Reviews*, *35*(1), 2–16.

Kahneman, D., & Tversky, A. (1973). On the psychology of prediction. *Psychological Review*, *80*(4), 237–251.

Kakizaki, M., Kuriyama, S., Sone, T., Ohmori-Matsuda, K., Hozawa, A., Nakaya, N., … Tsuji, I. (2008). Sleep duration and the risk of breast cancer: The Ohsaki Cohort Study. *British Journal of Cancer*, *99*(9), 1502–1505. doi: 10.1038/sj.bjc.6604684

Kaly, P. W., Heesacker, M., & Frost, H. M. (2002). Collegiate alcohol use and high-risk sexual behavior: A literature review. *Journal of College Student Development*, *43*(6), 838–850.

Kampmeier, R. H. (1974). Final report on the "Tuskegee syphilis study." *Southern Medical Journal*, *67*(11), 1349–1353.

Kann, L., McManus, T., Harris, W. A., Shanklin, S. L., Flint, K. H., Hawkins, J., & Zaza, S. (2016). Youth Risk Behavior Surveillance—United States, 2015. *Morbidity and Mortality Weekly Report. Surveillance Summaries*, *65*, 1–174.

Kann, L., McManus, T., Harris, W. A., Shanklin, S. L., Flint, K. H., Queens, B., ... Ethier, K. A. (2018). Youth risk behavior surveillance—United States, 2017. *Morbidity and Mortality Weekly Report Surveillance Summaries*, *67*(8), 1–113.

Kanna, B., Narang, T. K., Atwal, T., Paul, D., & Azeez, S. (2009). Ethnic disparity in mortality after diagnosis of colorectal cancer among inner city minority New Yorkers. *Cancer*, *115*(23), 5550–5555.

Kanner, A. D., Coyne, J. C., Schaeffer, C., & Lazarus, R. S. (1981). Comparison of two modes of stress measurement: Daily hassles and uplifts versus major life events. *Journal of Behavioral Medicine*, *4*, 1–39.

Kant, A. K., Block, G., Schatzkin, A., & Nestle, M. (1992). Association of fruit and vegetable intake with dietary fat intake. *Nutrition Research*, *12*(12), 1441–1454.

Kanu, M., Baker, E., & Brownson, R. C. (2008). Exploring associations between church-based social support and physical activity. *Journal of Physical Activity and Health*, *5*(4), 504–515.

Kao, S., Lai, K.-L., Lin, H.-C., Lee, H.-S., & Wen, H.-C. (2005). WHOQOL-BREF as predictors of mortality: A two-year follow-up study at veteran homes. *Quality of Life Research*, *14*(6), 1443–1454.

Kaplan, G. A., & Camacho, T. (1983). Perceived health and mortality: A nine-year follow-up of the human population laboratory. *American Journal of Epidemiology*, *117*, 292–304.

Karlamangla, A. S., Singer, B. H., & Seeman, T. E. (2006). Reduction in allostatic load in older adults is associated with lower all-cause mortality risk: MacArthur studies of successful aging. *Psychosomatic Medicine*, *68*, 500–507.

Kasdan, D. O., & Campbell, J. W. (2020). Dataveillant collectivism and the coronavirus in Korea: Values, biases, and socio-cultural foundations of containment efforts. *Administrative Theory & Praxis*, *42*(4), 604–613. doi: 10.1080/10841806.2020.1805272

Kashdan, T. B., Biswas-Diener, R., & King, L. A. (2008). Reconsidering happiness: The costs of distinguishing between hedonics and eudaimonia. *Journal of Positive Psychology*, *3*(4), 219–233.

Kasl, S. V., & Cobb, S. (1966). Health behavior, illness behavior, and sick role behavior. I. Health and illness behavior. *Archives of Environmental Health*, *12*, 246–266.

Kasparian, N. A., McLoone, J. K., & Meiser, B. (2009). Skin cancer-related prevention and screening behaviors: A review of the literature. *Journal of Behavioral Medicine*, *32*(5), 406–428.

Katsaridis, S., Grammatikopoulou, M. G., Gkiouras, K., Tzimos, C., Papageorgiou, S. T., Markaki, A. G., Exiara, T., Goulis, D. G., & Papamitsou, T. (2020). Low reported adherence to the 2019 American diabetes association nutrition recommendations among patients with type 2 diabetes mellitus, indicating the need for improved nutrition education and diet care. *Nutrients*, *12*(11), 3516. doi: 10.3390/nu12113516

Katz, D. L. (2009). School-based interventions for health promotion and weight control: Not just waiting on the world to change. *Annual Review of Public Health*, *30*, 253–272.

Katzmarzyk, P. T., Barreira, T. V., Broyles, S. T., Champagne, C. M., Chaput, J. P., Fogelholm, M., ... Lambert, E. V. (2013). The International Study of Childhood Obesity, Lifestyle and the Environment (ISCOLE): Design and methods. *BMC Public Health*, *13*, 900.

Kauppi, K., Vanhala, A., Roos, E., & Torkki, P. (2023). Assessing the structures and domains of wellness models: A systematic review. *International Journal of Wellbeing*, *13*(2), 1–19.

Kaye, W. H., Bailer, U. F., Frank, G., Wagner, A., & Henry, S. E. (2005). Brain imaging of serotonin after recovery from anorexia and bulimia nervosa. *Physiological Behavior*, *86*(1–2), 15–17.

Kaye, W. H., Wierenga, C. E., Bailer, U. F., Simmons, A. N., & Bischoff-Grethe, A. (2013). Nothing tastes as good as skinny feels: The neurobiology of anorexia nervosa. *Trends in Neurosciences*, *36*(2), 110–120.

Kazak, A. E., Bosch, J., & Klonoff, E. A. (2012). *Health Psychology* special series on health disparities. *Health Psychology*, *31*(1), 1–4.

Kazarian, S., & Evans, D. R. (2001). Health psychology and culture: Embracing the 21st century. In S. Kazarian & D. R. Evans (Eds.), *Handbook of cultural health psychology* (pp. 3–34). San Diego, CA: Academic Press.

Keating, N. L., Guadagnoli, E., Landrum, M. B., Borbas, C., & Weeks, J. C. (2002). Treatment decision making in early-stage breast cancer: Should surgeons match patients' desired level of involvement? *Journal of Clinical Oncology, 20*(6), 1473–1479.

Keith, K. D., & Schalock, R. L. (1994). The measurement of quality of life in adolescence: The quality of student life questionnaire. *American Journal of Family Therapy, 22*(1), 83–87.

Kelder, S. H., Perry, C. L., Klepp, K.-I., & Lytle, L. L. (1994). Longitudinal tracking of adolescent smoking, physical activity and food choice behaviors. *American Journal of Public Health, 84*, 1121–1126.

Kelley, A. E., Schochet, T., & Landry, C. F. (2004). Risk taking and novelty seeking in adolescence: Introduction to part I. *Annals of the New York Academy of Sciences, 1021*, 27–32.

Kelly, E. W., Jr. (1995). *Spirituality and religion in counseling and psychotherapy: Diversity in theory and practice.* Alexandria, VA: American Counseling Association.

Kelly, E. P., Agne, J. L., Meara, A., & Pawlik, T. M. (2019). Reciprocity within patient-physician and patient-spouse/caregiver dyads: Insights into patient-centered care. *Supportive Care in Cancer, 27*(4), 1237–1244.

Kelly, J. R., Kennedy, P. J., Cryan, J. F., Dinan, T. G., Clarke, G., & Hyland, N. P. (2015). Breaking down the barriers: The gut microbiome, intestinal permeability and stress-related psychiatric disorders. *Frontiers in Cellular Neuroscience, 9*, 392.

Kendrick, K. M., Lévy, F., & Keverne, E. B. (1992). Changes in the sensory processing of olfactory signals induced by birth in sheep. *Science, 256*, 833–836.

Kerin, J. L., Webb, H. J., & Zimmer-Gembeck, M. J. (2019). Intuitive, mindful, emotional, external and regulatory eating behaviours and beliefs: An investigation of the core components. *Appetite, 132*, 139–146.

Kerr, K. L., Moseman, S. E., Avery, J. A., Bodurka, J., Zucker, N. L., & Simmons, W. K. (2016). Altered insula activity during visceral interoception in weight-restored patients with anorexia nervosa. *Neurophsyopharmacology, 41*, 521–528.

Keverne, E. B., Nevison, C. M., & Martel, F. L. (1997). Early learning and the social bond. *Annals of the New York Academy of Sciences, 807*, 329–339.

Keyes, A., Brozek, J., Henschel, A., Mickelsen, O., & Taylor, H. L. (1950). *The biology of human starvation.* Minneapolis, MN: University of Minnesota Press.

Keyes, C. L., & Grzywacz, J. G. (2005). Health as a complete state: The added value in work performance and healthcare costs. *Journal of Occupational and Environmental Medicine, 47*(5), 523–532.

Kiecolt-Glaser, J. K., & Glaser, R. (1986). Psychological influences on immunity. *Psychosomatics, 27*, 621–624.

Kiecolt-Glaser, J. K., McGuire, L., Robles, T. F., & Glaser, R. (2002). Psychoneuroimmunology: Psychological influences on immune function and health. *Journal of Consulting and Clinical Psychology, 70*(3), 537–547.

Kiecolt-Glaser, J. K., Newton, T., Cacioppo, J. T., MacCallum, R. C., Glaser, R., & Malarkey, W. B. (1996). Marital conflict and endocrine function: Are men really more physiologically affected than women? *Journal of Consulting and Clinical Psychology, 64*(2), 324–332.

Kim, S., Kim, Y., & Park, S. M. (2016). Body mass index and decline of cognitive function. *PLoS One, 11*(2), e0148908.

Kim, K. H., & Sobal, J. (2004). Religion, social support, fat intake and physical activity. *Public Health Nutrition, 7*(6), 773–781.

Kim-Prieto, C. (Ed.). (2014). *Religion and spirituality across cultures.* Cross-cultural advancements in positive psychology (Vol. 9). New York, NY: Springer.

Kinder, L. S., Carnethon, M. R., Palaniappan, L. P., King, A. C., & Fortmann, S. P. (2004). Depression and the metabolic syndrome in young adults: Findings from the Third National Health and Nutrition Examination Survey. *Psychosomatic Medicine, 66*(3), 316–322.

King, P. S., Berg, C. A., Butner, J., Butler, J. M., & Wiebe, D. J. (2014). Longitudinal trajectories of parental involvement in type 1 diabetes and adolescents' adherence. *Health Psychology, 33*(5), 424–432.

King, N. B., & Fraser, V. (2013). Untreated pain, narcotics regulation, and global health ideologies. *PLoS Med, 10*(4), e1001411.

King Jones, T. C. (2010). "It drives us to do it": Pregnant adolescents identify drivers for sexual risk-taking. *Issues in Comprehensive Pediatric Nursing, 33*(2), 82–100. doi: 10.3109/01460861003663961

King-Meadows, T. D., & Agarwal, V. (2024). Mapping the spatial interdependence of adverse health outcomes and neighborhood socioeconomic conditions in Baltimore. *Journal of Maps, 20*(1), 2288855.

Kingston, J., Raggio, C., Spencer, K., Stalaker, K., & Tuchin, P. J. (2010). A review of the literature on chiropractic and insomnia. *Journal of Chiropractic Medicine, 9*(3), 121–126. doi: 10.1016/j.jcm.2010.03.003

Kirchner, T., Forns, M., Amador, J. A., & Muñoz, D. (2010). Stability and consistency of coping in adolescence: A longitudinal study. *Psicothema, 22*(3), 382–388.

Kirsch, I. (1999). *How expectancies shape experience.* Washington, DC: American Psychological Association.

Kirsch, I., & Sapirstein, G. (1998). Listening to Prozac but hearing placebo: A meta-analysis of antidepressant medication. *Prevention and Treatment, 1,* Article 2a. doi: 10.1037/1522-3736.1.1.12a

Kissen, D. M., & Eysenck, H. J. (1962). Personality in male lung cancer patients. *Journal of Psychosomatic Research, 6,* 123–127.

Kjaer, S. K., van den Brule, A. J., Paull, G., Svare, E. I., Sherman, M. E., Thomsen, B. L., … Meijer, C. J. (2002). Type specific persistence of high risk human papillomavirus (HPV) as indicator of high grade cervical squamous intraepithelial lesions in young women: Population based prospective follow up study. *BMJ, 325*(7364), 572–578.

Klabunde, T., Wendt, K. U., Kadereit, D., Brachvogel, V., Burger, H.-J., Herling, A. W., … Defossa, E. (2005). Acyl ureas as human liver glycogen phosphorylase inhibitors for the treatment of Type 2 diabetes. *Journal of Medicinal Chemistry, 48*(20), 6178–6193.

Kleftaras, G., & Psarra, E. (2012). Meaning in life, psychological well-being and depressive symptomatology: A comparative study. *Psychology, 3*(4), 337–345.

Klein, W. M., Chou, W. Y. S., & Vanderpool, R. C. (2023). Health information in 2023 (and beyond): Confronting emergent realities with health communication science. *JAMA, 330*(12), 1131–1132.

Klonoff, E. A., & Landrine, H. (1992). Sex roles, occupational roles, and symptom-reporting: A test of competing hypotheses on sex differences. *Journal of Behavioral Medicine, 15*(4), 355–364.

Knaapila, A., Tuorila, H., Silventoinen, K., Keskitalo, K., Kallela, M., Wessman, M., … Perola, M. (2007). Food neophobia shows heritable variation in humans. *Physiology & Behavior, 91,* 573–578.

Knutson, K. L. (2010). Sleep duration and cardiometabolic risk: A review of the epidemiologic evidence. *Journal of Clinical Endocrinology & Metabolism, 24*(5), 731–743. doi: 10.1016/j.beem.2010.07.001

Ko, C. H. (2014). Internet gaming disorder. *Current Addiction Reports, 1,* 177–185.

Kochanek, K. D., Murphy, S. L., Xu, J. Q., Arias, E. *Mortality in the United States, 2022. NCHS Data Brief, no 492.* Hyattsville, MD: National Center for Health Statistics. 2024. https://dx.doi.org/10.15620/cdc:135850

Koenen, K. C., Stellman, S. D., Dohrenwend, B. P., Sommer, J. F., & Stellman, J. M. (2007). The consistency of combat exposure reporting and course of PTSD in Vietnam War veterans. *Journal of Traumatic Stress, 20*(1), 3–13.

Koenig, H. G. (2018). *Religion and mental health: Research and clinical applications.* Cambridge, MA: Academic Press.

Koenig, H. G., Larson, D. B., & Larson, S. S. (2001). Religion and coping with serious medical illness. *Annals of Pharmacotherapy, 35*(3), 352–359.

Koenig, H. G., McCullough, M. E., & Larson, D. B. (Eds.). (2001). *Handbook of religion and health.* New York, NY: Oxford University Press.

Kohn, D. (2015, June 24). When gut bacteria changes brain function. *The Atlantic.* Retrieved from http://www.theatlantic.com/health/archive/2015/06/gut-bacteria-on-the-brain/395918/

Koivumaa-Honkanen, H., Honkanen, R., Viinamäki, H., Heikkilä, K., Kaprio, J., & Koskenvuo, M. (2000). Self-reported life satisfaction and 20-year mortality in healthy Finnish adults. *American Journal of Epidemiology, 152*(10), 983–991.

Kolata, G. (2016, July 8). A medical mystery of the best kind: Major diseases are in decline. *New York Times.* Retrieved from http://www.nytimes.com/2016/07/10/upshot/a-medical-mystery-of-the-best-kind-major-diseases-are-in-decline.html?_r=0

Koliaki, C., Dalamaga, M., & Liatis, S. (2023). Update on the obesity epidemic: After the sudden rise, is the upward trajectory beginning to flatten?. *Current Obesity Reports, 12,* 514–527. doi: 10.1007/s13679-023-00527-y

Koltyn, K. F. (2002). Exercise-induced hypoalgesia and intensity of exercise. *Sports Medicine, 32*(8), 477–487.

Konigsberg, R. D. (2011). *The truth about grief: The myth of its five stages and the new science of loss.* New York, NY: Simon & Schuster.

Konttinen, H., Haukkala, A., Sarlio-Lähteenkorva, S., Silventoinen, K., & Jousilahti, P. (2009). Eating styles, selfcontrol and obesity indicators: The moderating role of obesity status and dieting history on restrained eating. *Appetite, 53*(1), 131–134.

Koolhaas, J. M., De Boer, S. F., Buwalda, B., & Van Reenen, K. (2007). Individual variation in coping with stress: A multidimensional approach of ultimate and proximate mechanisms. *Brain, Behavior and Evolution, 70*(4), 218–226.

Koplan, J. P., Bond, T. C., Merson, M. H., Reddy, K. S., Rodriguez, M. H., Sewankambo, N. K., & Wasserheit, J. N., for the Consortium of Universities for Global Health Executive Board. (2009). Towards a common definition of global health. *Lancet, 373*(9679), 1993–1995.

Koplas, P. A., Gans, H. B., Wisely, M. P., Kuchibhatla, M., Cutson, T. M., Gold, D. T., … Schenkman, M. (1999). Quality of life and Parkinson's disease. *Journals of Gerontology Series A: Biological Sciences and Medical Sciences, 54*(4), M197–M202.

Kotabe, H. P., & Hofmann, W. (2015). On integrating the components of self-control *Perspectives on Psychological Science*, *10*, 618–638.

Koutsky, L. (1997). Epidemiology of genital human papillomavirus infection. *American Journal of Medicine*, *102*(5A), 3–8.

Koyama, T., McHaffie, J. G., Laurienti, P. J., & Coghill, R. C. (2005). The subjective experience of pain: Where expectations become reality. *Proceedings of the National Academy of Sciences of the United States of America*, *102*(36), 12950–12955.

Kral, T. V., & Rauh, E. M. (2010). Eating behaviors of children in the context of their family environment. *Physiology & Behavior*, *100*, 567–573.

Krause, N. M. (2008). *Aging in the church: How social relationships affect health*. West Conshohocken, PA: Templeton Foundation Press.

Kraut, R. (1979). Two conceptions of happiness. *Philosophical Review*, *88*(2), 167–197.

Krems, J. A., & Bock, J. E. (2023). The role of women's and men's body shapes in explicit and implicit fat stigma. *Obesities*, *3*(2), 97–118.

Kristoffersen, E. S., Lundqvist, C., & Russell, M. B. (2019). Illness perception in people with primary and secondary chronic headache in the general population. *Journal of Psychosomatic Research*, *116*, 83–92.

Kroenke, C. H., Kubzansky, L. D., Schernhammer, E. S., Holmes, M. D., & Kawachi, I. (2006). Social networks, social support, and survival after breast cancer diagnosis. *Journal of Clinical Oncology*, *24*(7), 1105–1111.

Kroenke, K., & Spitzer, R. L. (1998). Gender differences in the reporting of physical and somatoform symptoms. *Psychosomatic Medicine*, *60*(2), 150–155.

Krueger, A. B., & Stone, A. A. (2008). Assessment of pain: A community-based diary survey in the USA. *Lancet*, *371*(9623), 1519–1525.

Kruger, D. J., & Kruger, J. S. (2019). Medical cannabis users' comparisons between medical cannabis and mainstream medicine. *Journal of Psychoactive Drugs*, *51*(1), 31–36. doi: 10.1080/02791072.2018.1563314

Kruk, J. (2012). Self-reported psychological stress and the risk of breast cancer: A case-control study. *Stress*, *15*(2), 162–171.

Krupat, E., Hsu, J., Irish, J., Schmittdiel, J. A., & Selby, J. (2004). Matching patients and practitioners based on beliefs about care: Results of a randomized controlled trial. *American Journal of Managed Care*, *10*(11 Pt 1), 814–822.

Kübler-Ross, E. (1969). *On death and dying*. New York, NY: Macmillan.

Kuchibhatla, M., Hunter, J. C., Plassman, B. L., Lutz, M. W., Casanova, R., Saldana, S., & Hayden, K. M. (2019). The association between neighborhood socioeconomic status, cardiovascular and cerebrovascular risk factors, and cognitive decline in the health and retirement study (HRS). *Aging and Mental Health*. Advance online publication. doi: 10.1080/13607863.2019.1594169

Kuhrik, M., Seckman, C., Kuhrik, N., Ahearn, T., & Ercole, P. (2011). Bringing skin assessments to life using human patient simulation: An emphasis on cancer prevention and early detection. *Journal of Cancer Education*, *26*, 687–693. doi: 10.1007/s13187-011-0213-3

Kuiper, N. A., Martin, R. A., & Olinger, L. J. (1993). Coping humour, stress, and cognitive appraisals. *Canadian Journal of Behavioural Science*, *25*(1), 81–96.

Kuiper, N. A., & Nicholl, S. (2004). Thoughts of feeling better? Sense of humor and physical health. *Humor: International Journal of Humor Research*, *17*(1–2), 37–66.

Kulik, J. A., & Mahler, H. I. (1989). Social support and recovery from surgery. *Health Psychology*, *8*(2), 221.

Kundermann, B., Spernal, J., Huber, M. T., Krieg, J. C., & Lautenbacher, S. (2004). Sleep deprivation affects thermal pain thresholds but not somatosensory thresholds in healthy volunteers. *Psychosomatic Medicine*, *66*(6), 932–937.

Kunte, H., Rentzsch, J., & Kronenberg, G. (2015). A new role for nortriptyline in depression associated with vascular disease? *American Journal of Psychiatry*, *172*(2), 201.

Kuo, B. C. (2013). Collectivism and coping: Current theories, evidence, and measurements of collective coping. *International Journal of Psychology*, *48*(3), 374–388.

Kupper, N., & Denollet, J. (2007). Type D personality as a prognostic factor in heart disease: Assessment and mediating mechanisms. *Journal of Personality Assessment*, *89*(3), 265–276.

Kupper, N., Gidron, Y., Winter, J., & Denollet, J. (2009). Association between Type D personality, depression, and oxidative stress in patients with chronic heart failure. *Psychosomatic Medicine*, *71*(9), 973–980.

Kyrou, I., & Tsigos, C. (2009). Stress hormones: Physiological stress and regulation of metabolism. *Current Opinion in Pharmacology*, *9*, 787–793.

la Roi, C., Meyer, I. H., & Frost, D. M. (2019). Differences in sexual identity dimensions between bisexual and other sexual minority individuals: Implications for minority stress and mental health. *American Journal of Orthopsychiatry*, *89*(1), 40.

Lachance, P. A. (1992). Diet–health relationship. In J. W. Finley, S. F. Robinson, & D. J. Armstrong (Eds.), *Food safety assessment* (ACS Symposium Series, Vol. 484, pp. 278–296). Washington, DC: American Chemical Society.

Lachman, M. E., Röcke, C., Rosnick, C., & Ryff, C. D. (2008). Realism and illusion in Americans' temporal views of their life satisfaction: Age differences in reconstructing the past and anticipating the future. *Psychological Science, 19*(9), 889–897.

Lally, P., van Jaarsveld, C. H. M., Potts, H. W. W., & Wardle, J. (2010). How are habits formed: Modelling habit formation in the real world. *European Journal of Social Psychology, 40*, 998–1009.

Lally, P., Wardle, J., & Gardner, B. (2011). Experiences of habit formation: A qualitative study. *Psychology, Health & Medicine, 16*(4), 484–489.

Lamb, R., & Joshi, M. S. (1996). The stage model and processes of change in dietary fat reduction. *Journal of Human Nutrition and Dietetics, 9*(1), 43–53.

Lamprecht, F., & Sack, M. (2002). Posttraumatic stress disorder revisited. *Psychosomatic Medicine, 64*, 222–237.

Landro, L. (2013, February 14). The simple idea that is transforming health care. *Wall Street Journal.* Retrieved from http://www.wsj.com/articles/SB1000 142405270230445000457727591137055 1798

Lane, D. J., Gibbons, F. X., O'Hara, R. E., & Gerrard, M. (2011). Standing out from the crowd: How comparison to prototypes can decrease health-risk behavior in young adults. *Basic and Applied Social Psychology, 33*(3), 228–238.

Langer, E. J., & Rodin, J. (1976). The effects of enhanced personal responsibility for the aged. *Journal of Personality and Social Psychology, 34*(2), 191–198.

Lantz, P. M., House, J. S., Mero, R. P., & Williams, D. R. (2005). Stress, life events, and socioeconomic disparities in health: Results from the Americans' Changing Lives Study. *Journal of Health and Social Behavior, 46*(3), 274–288.

Lapp, H. E., Ahmed, S., Moore, C. L., & Hunter, R. G. (2019). Toxic stress history and hypothalamic-pituitary-adrenal axis function in a social stress task: Genetic and epigenetic factors. *Neurotoxicology and Teratology, 71*, 41–49.

Larimer, M. E., Palmer, R. S., & Marlatt, G. A. (1999). Relapse prevention: An overview of Marlatt's cognitive-behavioral model. *Alcohol Research and Health, 23*(2), 151–160.

Larson, E. B., & Yao, X. (2005). Clinical empathy as emotional labor in the patient-physician relationship. *JAMA, 293*(9), 1100–1106.

Lascaratou, C. (2007). *The language of pain: Expression or description?* Amsterdam, the Netherlands: John Benjamins.

Latané, B., & Wolf, S. (1981). The social impact of majorities and minorities. *Psychological Review, 88*(5), 438.

Latner, J. D., McLeod, G., O'Brien, K. S., & Johnston, L. (2013). The role of self-efficacy, coping, and lapses in weight maintenance. *Eating and Weight Disorders, 18*, 359–366.

Lau, R. R., & Hartman, K. A. (1983). Common sense representations of common illness. *Health Psychology, 2*, 167–185.

Laukens, D., Brinkman, B. M., Raes, J., De Vos, M., & Vandenabeele, P. (2015). Heterogeneity of the gut microbiome in mice: Guidelines for optimizing experimental design. *FEMS Microbiology Reviews, 40*(1), 117–132.

Lavee, Y., & Ben-Ari, A. (2008). The association of daily hassles and uplifts with family and life satisfaction: Does cultural orientation make a difference? *American Journal of Community Psychology, 41*(1–2), 89–98.

Lavin, D., & Groarke, A. (2005). Dental floss behaviour: A test of the predictive utility of the theory of planned behaviour and the effects of making implementation intentions. *Health & Medicine, 10*(3), 243–252.

Lawton, M. P. (1991). A multidimensional view of quality of life in frail elders. In J. Birren, J. Lubben, J. Rowe, & D. Deutchman (Eds.), *The concept and measurement of quality of life in the frail elderly* (pp. 3–27). Cambridge, MA: Academic Press.

Lazarus, R. S. (1993). From psychological stress to the emotions: A history of changing outlooks. *Annual Review of Psychology, 44*, 1–21.

Lazarus, R. S., & Folkman, S. (1984). *Stress, appraisal, and coping.* New York, NY: Springer.

Lazarus, R. S., & Launier, R. (1978). Stress-related transactions between person and environment. In L. A. Pervin & M. Lewis (Eds.), *Perspectives in interactional psychology* (pp. 287–327). New York, NY: Plenum.

Leary, K. A., & DeRosier, M. E. (2012). Factors promoting positive adaptation and resilience during the transition to college. *Psychology, 3*(12A), 1215–1222.

Leatherdale, S. T., & Papadakis, S. (2011). A multi-level examination of the association between older social models in the school environment and overweight and obesity among younger students. *Journal of Youth and Adolescence, 40*(3), 361–372. doi: 10.1007/s10964-009-9491-z

LeBlanc, A. (2014). "Feeling what happens": Full correspondence and the placebo effect. *Journal of Mind and Behavior, 35*(3), 167–184.

Lechuga, J., Swain, G. R., & Weinhardt, L. S. (2011). Impact of framing on intentions to vaccinate daughters against HPV: A cross-cultural perspective. *Annals of Behavioral Medicine, 42*(2), 221–226.

Lee, R. M. (2005). Resilience against discrimination: Ethnic identity and other-group orientation as protective factors for Korean Americans. *Journal of Counseling Psychology, 52*(1), 36–44.

Lee, H., Bahler, R., Chung, C., Alonzo, A., & Zeller, R. A. (2000). Prehospital delay with myocardial infarction: The interactive effect of clinical symptoms and race. *Applied Nursing Research, 13*(3), 125–133. doi: 10.1053/apnr.2000.7652

Lee, D. J., Elias, G. J., & Lozano, A. M. (2018). Neuromodulation for the treatment of eating disorders and obesity. *Therapeutic Advances in Psychopharmacology, 8*(2), 73–92.

Lee, T. H., Marcantonio, E. R., Mangione, C. M., Thomas, E. J., Polanczyk, C. A., Cook, E. F., … Goldman, L. (1999). Derivation and prospective validation of a simple index for prediction of cardiac risk of major noncardiac surgery. *Circulation, 100*(10), 1043–1049.

Lee, W. K., Milloy, M. J. S., Nosova, E., Walsh, J., & Kerr, T. (2019). Predictors of antiretroviral adherence self-efficacy among people living with HIV/AIDS in a Canadian setting. *Journal of Acquired Immune Deficiency Syndromes (1999), 80*(1), 103–109. doi: 10.1097/QAI.0000000000001878

Lee, S. E., & Neupert, S. D. (2024). The effect of control beliefs on the relationship between daily stressors and subjective age in younger adults. *Mental Health Science, 2*(2), e56. doi: 10.1002/mhs2.56

Lee, H., Park, J. H., Park, S., & Kim, H. C. (2019). Abstract P180: Combined effect of income and medication adherence on mortality in newly treated hypertension: A nationwide study of 16 million person-years. *Circulation, 139*(Suppl. 1), AP180.

Lee, J. J., Pedley, A., Hoffmann, U., Massaro, J. M., & Fox, C. S. (2016). Association of changes in abdominal fat quantity and quality with incident cardiovascular disease risk factors. *Journal of the American College of Cardiology, 68*(14), 1509–1521.

Lee, D. H., Rezende, L. F., Joh, H. K., Keum, N., Ferrari, G., Rey-Lopez, J. P., … Giovannucci, E. L. (2022). Long-term leisure-time physical activity intensity and all-cause and cause-specific mortality: A prospective cohort of US adults. *Circulation, 146*(7), 523–534.

Lehavot, K., Hoerster, K. D., Nelson, K. M., Jakupcak, M., & Simpson, T. L. (2012). Health indicators for military, veteran, and civilian women. *American Journal of Preventive Medicine, 42*(5), 473–480.

Leipold, B., Munz, M., & Michéle-Malkowsky, A. (2019). Coping and resilience in the transition to adulthood. *Emerging Adulthood, 7*(1), 12–20.

Lemogne, C., Consoli, S. M., Melchior, M., Nabi, H., Coeuret-Pellicer, M., Limosin, F., … Zins, M. (2013). Depression and the risk of cancer: A 15-year follow-up study of the GAZEL cohort. *American Journal of Epidemiology, 178*(12), 1712–1720.

Lennon, O., Hall, P., & Blake, C. (2021). Predictors of adherence to lifestyle recommendations in stroke secondary prevention. *International Journal of Environmental Research and Public Health, 18*(9), 4666.

Lerner, R. M. (2006). Developmental science, developmental systems, and contemporary theories of human development. In R. M. Lerner (Ed.), *Handbook of child psychology, vol. 1. Theoretical models of human development* (6th ed., pp. 1–17). Hoboken, NJ: Wiley.

Lerner, A., Jeremias, P., & Matthias, T. (2015). The world incidence and prevalence of autoimmune diseases is increasing. *International Journal of Celiac Disease, 3*(4), 151–155.

Lettieri, D. J., Sayers, M., & Pearson, H. W. (Eds.). (1980). *Theories on drug abuse: Selected contemporary perspectives.* NIDA Research Monograph 30. Rockville, MD: National Institute on Drug Abuse.

Leung, A. K., Wong, A. H., & Hon, K. L. (2024). Childhood obesity: An updated review. *Current Pediatric Reviews, 20*(1), 2–26.

Levenson, J. W., McCarthy, E. P., Lynn, J., Davis, R. B., & Phillips, R. S. (2000). The last six months of life for patients with congestive heart failure. *Journal of the American Geriatrics Society, 48*(5 Suppl.), S101–S109.

Levenstein, J. H., McCracken, E. C., McWhinney, I. R., Stewart, M. A., & Brown, J. B. (1986). The patient-centred clinical method. 1. A model for the doctor-patient interaction in family medicine. *Family Practice, 3*(1), 24–30.

Leventhal, H., Bodnar-Deren, S., Breland, J. Y., Hash-Converse, J., Phillips, L. A., Leventhal, E. A., & Cameron, L. D. (2011). *Modeling health and illness behavior: The approach of the commonsense model.* London, UK: Routledge.

Leventhal, H., Diefenbach, M., & Leventhal, E. A. (1992). Illness cognition: Using common sense to understand treatment adherence and affect cognition interactions. *Cognitive Therapy and Research, 16*(2), 143–163.

Leventhal, E. A., Hansell, S., Diefenbach, M., Leventhal, H., & Glass, D. C. (1996). Negative affect and self-report of physical symptoms: Two longitudinal studies of older adults. *Health Psychology, 15*(3), 193–199.

Leventhal, H., Leventhal, E. A., & Contrada, R. J. (1998). Self-regulation, health, and behavior: A perceptual-cognitive approach. *Psychology and Health, 13*(4), 717–733.

Leventhal, H., Meyer, D., & Nerenz, D. (1980). The common sense model of illness danger. In S. Rachman (Ed.), *Medical psychology* (Vol. 2, pp. 7–30). New York, NY: Pergamon.

Leventhal, H., Nerenz, D. R., & Steele, D. J. (1984). Illness representations and coping with health threats. In A. Baum, S. E. Taylor, & J. E. Singer (Eds.), *Handbook of psychology and health: Social psychological aspects of health* (Vol. 4, pp. 219–252). Hillsdale, NJ: Erlbaum.

Leventhal, H., Prochaska, T. R., & Hirschman, R. S. (1985). Preventive health behavior across the lifespan. In J. C. Rosen & L. J. Solomon (Eds.), *Prevention in health psychology* (Vol. 8, pp. 190–235). Hanover, NH: University Press of New England.

Levine, S. (1987). The changing terrain in medical sociology: Emergent concern with quality of life. *Journal of Health and Social Behavior, 28*, 1–6.

Levinsohn, J. A., McLaren, Z., Shisana, O., & Zuma, K. (2011). *HIV status and labor market participation in South Africa* (NBER Working Paper No. 16901). Cambridge, MA: National Bureau of Economic Research. Retrieved from http://www.nber.org/papers/w16901

Levinson, W., Kao, A., Kuby, A., & Thisted, R. A. (2005). Not all patients want to participate in decision making: A national study of public preferences. *Journal of General Internal Medicine, 20*(6), 531–535.

Lewis, S. J., Rodbard, H. W., Fox, K. M., & Grandy, S. (2008). Self-reported prevalence and awareness of metabolic syndrome: Findings from SHIELD. *International Journal of Clinical Practice, 62*(8), 1168–1176.

Lickliter, R., & Moore, D. S. (2023). Molecular and Systemic Epigenetic Inheritance: Integrating Development, Genetics, and Evolution, 67(5-6), 305–317.

Lickliter, R., & Moore, D. S. (2024). Molecular and systemic epigenetic inheritance: Integrating development, genetics, and evolution. *Human Development, 67*(5–6), 305–317.

Liew, H. P. (2012). Depression and chronic illness: A test of competing hypotheses. *Journal of Health Psychology, 17*(1), 100–109. doi: 10.1177/1359105311409788

Lilenfeld, L. R., Kaye, W. H., Greeno, C. G., Merikangas, K. R., Plotnicov, K., Pollice, C., ... Nagy, L. (1998). A controlled family study of anorexia nervosa and bulimia nervosa: Psychiatric disorders in first-degree relatives and effects of proband comorbidity. *Archives of General Psychiatry, 55*(7), 603–610.

Lilenfeld, L. R., Wonderlich, S., Riso, L. P., Crosby, R., & Mitchell, J. (2006). Eating disorders and personality: A methodological and empirical review. *Clinical Psychology Review, 26*(3), 299–320.

Lillberg, K., Verkasalo, P. K., Kaprio, J., Helenius, H., & Koskenvuo, M. (2002). Personality characteristics and the risk of breast cancer: A prospective cohort study. *International Journal of Cancer, 100*(3), 361–366.

Li, S. Y., Magrabi, F., & Coiera, E. (2012). A systematic review of the psychological literature on interruption and its patient safety implications. *Journal of the American Medical Informatics Association, 19*(1), 6–12.

Li, Y. H., Wang, F. Y., Feng, C. Q., Yang, X. F., & Sun, Y. H. (2014). Massage therapy for fibromyalgia: A systematic review and meta-analysis of randomized controlled trials. *PLoS One, 9*(2), e89304. doi: 10.1371/journal.pone.0089304

Linardon, J., Tylka, T. L., & Fuller-Tyszkiewicz, M. (2021). Intuitive eating and its psychological correlates: A meta-analysis. *International Journal of Eating Disorders, 54*(7), 1073–1098.

Lindberg, N. M., & Wellisch, D. K. (2004). Identification of traumatic stress reactions in women at increased risk for breast cancer. *Psychosomatics, 45*(1), 7–16.

Linden, G. J., Lyons, A., & Scannapieco, F. A. (2013). Periodontal systemic associations: Review of the evidence. *Journal of Periodontology, 84*, S8–S19.

Linden, W., Phillips, M. J., & Leclerc, J. (2007). Psychological treatment of cardiac patients: A meta-analysis. *European Heart Journal, 28*(24), 2972–2984.

Lindgren, E., Gray, K., Miller, G., Tyler, R., Wiers, C. E., Volkow, N. D., & Wang, G. J. (2018). Food addiction: A common neurobiological mechanism with drug abuse. *Frontiers in Bioscience (Landmark Edition), 23*, 811–836.

Lin, E. H., Katon, W., Von Korff, M., Rutter, C., Simon, G. E., Oliver, M., ... Young, B. (2004). Relationship of depression and diabetes self-care, medication adherence, and preventive care. *Diabetes Care, 27*(9), 2154–2160.

Lipman, A. G. (2005). Pain as a human right: The 2004 Global Day Against Pain. *Journal of Pain and Palliative Care Pharmacotherapy, 19*(3), 85–100.

Lippke, S., Nigg, C. R., & Maddock, J. E. (2012) Healthpromoting and health-risk behaviors: Theory-driven analyses of multiple health behavior change in three international samples. *International Journal of Behavioral Medicine, 19*(1), 1–13. doi: 10.1007/s12529-010-9135-4

Lissanu, L., Lopez, F., King, A., Robinson, E., Almazan, E., Metoyer, G., … Saunders, M. R. (2019). "I try not to even think about my health going bad": A qualitative study of chronic kidney disease knowledge and coping among a group of urban African-American patients with CKD. *Journal of Racial and Ethnic Health Disparities, 6*(3), 625–634. doi: 10.1007/s40615-019-00561-4

Little, M., Rosa, E., Heasley, C., Asif, A., Dodd, W., & Richter, A. (2022). Promoting healthy food access and nutrition in primary care: A systematic scoping review of food prescription programs. *American Journal of Health Promotion, 36*(3), 518–536.

Liu, M., Jiang, Y., Wedow, R., Li, Y., Brazel, D. M., Chen, F., … Zhan, X. (2019). Association studies of up to 1.2 million individuals yield new insights into the genetic etiology of tobacco and alcohol use. *Nature Genetics, 51*(2), 237–244. doi: 10.1038/s41588-018-0307-5

Liu, H., & Waite, L. (2014). Bad marriage, broken heart? Age and gender differences in the link between marital quality and cardiovascular risks among older adults. *Journal of Health and Social Behavior, 55*(4), 403–423.

Liu, Z., & Yang, J. (2023). Public support for COVID-19 responses: Cultural cognition, risk perception, and emotions. *Health Communication, 38*(4), 648–658.

Liu-Ambrose, T., Nagamatsu, L. S., Voss, M. W., Khan, K. M., & Handy, T. C. (2012). Resistance training and functional plasticity of the aging brain: A 12-month randomized controlled trial. *Neurobiology of Aging, 33*(8), 1690–1698.

Llewellyn, D. J. (2008). The psychology of risk taking: Toward the integration of psychometric and neuropsychological paradigms. *American Journal of Psychology, 121*(3), 363–376.

Lloyd, S. L., & Striley, C. W. (2018). Marijuana use among adults 50 years or older in the 21st century. *Gerontology and Geriatric Medicine, 4*, 2333721418781668.

Lloyd-Sherlock, P., Beard, J., Minicuci, N., Ebrahim, S., & Chatterji, S. (2014). Hypertension among older adults in low-and middle-income countries: Prevalence, awareness and control. *International Journal of Epidemiology, 43*(1), 116–128.

Lloyd-Williams, M., Shiels, C., Taylor, F., & Dennis, M. (2009). Depression—An independent predictor of early death in patients with advanced cancer. *Journal of Affective Disorders, 113*(1–2), 127–132.

Logg, J., et al. (2022). *Risk creep: A COVID-19 longitudinal field study (September 15, 2022)*. Georgetown McDonough School of Business Research Paper No. 4219931. Retrieved from SSRN: https://ssrn.com/abstract=4219931; http://dx.doi.org/10.2139/ssrn.4219931

Lohman, D., Schleifer, R., & Amon, J. J. (2010). Access to pain treatment as a human right. *BMC Medicine, 8*, 8. doi: 10.1186/1741-7015-8-8

Lomas, T., & Ivtzan, I. (2016). Second wave positive psychology: Exploring the positive–negative dialectics of wellbeing. *Journal of Happiness Studies, 17*, 1753–1768.

Lopez-Minguez, J., Saxena, R., Bandín, C., Scheer, F. A., & Garaulet, M. (2018). Late dinner impairs glucose tolerance in MTNR1B risk allele carriers: A randomized, cross-over study. *Clinical Nutrition, 37*(4), 1133–1140.

Lowe, M. R., Doshi, S. D., Katterman, S. N., & Feig, E. H. (2013). Dieting and restrained eating as prospective predictors of weight gain. *Frontiers in Psychology, 4*, 577. doi: 10.3389/fpsyg.2013.00577

Lox, C., Martin Ginis, K., & Petruzzello, S. (2010). *The psychology of exercise: Integrating theory and practice* (3rd ed.). Scottsdale, AZ: Holcomb Hathaway Publishers.

Lu, J. G., Jin, P., & English, A. S. (2021). Collectivism predicts mask use during COVID-19. *Proceedings of the National Academy of Sciences, 118*(23), e2021793118. https://doi.org/10.1073/pnas.2021793118

Lubbers, K., Cadwallader, J., Lin, Q., Clifford, C., & Frazier, L. D. (2023). Adult play and playfulness: A qualitative exploration of its meanings and importance. *The Journal of Play in Adulthood, 5*(2), 1–19.

Luby, S. P., Agboatwalla, M., Feikin, D. R., Painter, J., Billhimer, W., Altaf, A., & Hoekstra, R. M. (2005). Effect of handwashing on child health: A randomized controlled trial. *Lancet, 366*(9481), 225–233.

Luckow, A., Reifman, A., & McIntosh, D. N. (1998, August). *Gender differences in coping: A meta-analysis*. Poster presented at the 106th annual convention of the American Psychological Association, San Francisco.

Luders, E., Cherbuin, N., & Kurth, F. (2015). Forever young(er): Potential age-defying effects of long-term meditation on gray matter atrophy. *Frontiers in Psychology, 5*, 1551.

Ludwick-Rosenthal, R., & Neufeld, R. W. (1988). Stress management during noxious medical procedures: An evaluative review of outcome studies. *Psychological Bulletin, 104*(3), 326–342.

Ludyga, S., Pühse, U., Lucchi, S., Marti, J., & Gerber, M. (2019). Immediate and sustained effects of intermittent exercise on inhibitory control and task-related heart rate variability in adolescents. *Journal of Science and Medicine in Sport, 22*(1), 96–100.

Lumeng, J. C., Forrest, P., Appugliese, D. P., Kaciroti, N., Corwyn, R. F., & Bradley, R. H. (2010). Weight status as a predictor of being bullied in third through sixth grades. *Pediatrics, 125*(6), 31301–31307.

Lunney, J. R., Lynn, J., Foley, D. J., Lipson, S., & Guralnik, J. M. (2003). Patterns of functional decline at the end of life. *JAMA, 289*(18), 2387–2392.

Lynas, M., Houlton, B. Z., & Perry, S. (2021). Greater than 99% consensus on human caused climate change in the peer-reviewed scientific literature. *Environmental Research Letters, 16*(11), 114005.

Lynn, J., & Adamson, D. M. (2003). *Living well at the end of life: Adapting health care to serious chronic illness in old age*. Santa Monica, CA: RAND.

Lyon, M., Chatoor, I., Atkins, D., Silber, T., Mosimann, J., & Gray, J. (1997). Testing the hypothesis of the multidimensional model of anorexia nervosa in adolescents. *Adolescence, 32*(125), 101–111.

Lyubomirsky, S. (2008). *The how of happiness: A scientific approach to getting the life you want*. New York, NY: Penguin.

Lyubomirsky, S., Sheldon, K. M., & Schkade, D. (2005). Pursuing happiness: The architecture of sustainable change. *Review of General Psychology, 9*(2), 111–131.

Lyyra, T. M., Törmäkangas, T. M., Read, S., Rantanen, T., & Berg, S. (2006). Satisfaction with present life predicts survival in octogenarians. *Journals of Gerontology Series B: Psychological Sciences and Social Sciences, 61*(6), P319–P326.

Ma, Y., Ailawadi, K. L., & Grewal, D. (2013). Soda versus cereal and sugar versus fat: Drivers of healthful food intake and the impact of diabetes diagnosis. *Journal of Marketing, 77*(3), 101–120.

MacDorman, M. F., & Mathews, T. J. (2011, September). *Understanding racial and ethnic disparities in U.S. infant mortality rates* (NCHS Data Brief No. 74). Hyattsville, MD: National Center for Health Statistics.

MacGregor, D. G., & Fleming, R. (1996). Risk perception and symptom reporting. *Risk Analysis, 16*(6), 773–783.

Mackay, J., Eriksen, M., & Eriksen, M. P. (2002). *The tobacco atlas*. World Health Organization.

Maes, S., & Boersma, S. N. (2004). Applications in health psychology: How effective are interventions? In S. Sutton, A. Baum, & M. Johnston (Eds.), *The SAGE handbook of health psychology* (pp. 299–325). London, UK: Sage.

Magee, C. A., & Heaven, P. C. L. (2011). Big-five personality factors, obesity and 2-year weight gain in Australian adults. *Journal of Research in Personality, 45*(3), 332–335.

Mahler, H. I., & Kulik, J. A. (1998). Effects of preparatory videotapes on self-efficacy beliefs and recovery from coronary bypass surgery. *Annals of Behavioral Medicine, 20*(1), 39–46.

Maier, K. J., Waldstein, S. R., & Synowski, S. J. (2003). Relation of cognitive appraisal to cardiovascular reactivity, affect, and task engagement. *Annals of Behavioral Medicine, 26*, 32–41.

Maiman, L. A., & Becker, M. H. (1974). The health belief model: Origins and correlates in psychological theory. *Health Education & Behavior, 2*(4), 336–353. Retrieved from http://heb.sagepub.com/content/2/4/336.extract

Makarem, S. C., Hunt, J. M., Mudambi, S., & Aaronson, W. E. (2010). Emotions and cognitions in consumer health behaviors: A model of hope and control applied to chronic illnesses (Ph.D. dissertation, Temple University). Retrieved from http://digital.library.temple.edu/u?/p245801coll10,96030

Makin, T. R., Scholz, J., Filippini, N., Slater, D. H., Tracey, I., & Johansen-Berg, H. (2013). Phantom pain is associated with preserved structure and function in the former hand area. *Nature Communications, 4*, 1570.

Malouff, J. M., Thorsteinsson, E. B., Rooke, S. E., & Schutte, N. S. (2007). Alcohol involvement and the five-factor model of personality: A meta-analysis. *Journal of Drug Education, 37*(3), 277–294.

Maltoni, M., Nanni, O., Derni, S., Innocenti, M. P., Fabbri, L., Riva, N., … Amadori, D. (1994). Clinical prediction of survival is more accurate than the Karnofsky performance status in estimating life span of terminally ill cancer patients. *European Journal of Cancer, 30*(6), 764–766.

Maltz, M. (1960). *Psycho-cybernetics: A new way to get more living out of life*. New York, NY: Pocket Books.

Mandelblatt, J., Andrews, H., Kerner, J., Zauber, A., & Burnett, W. (1991). Determinants of late stage diagnosis of breast and cervical cancer: The impact of age, race, social class, and hospital type. *American Journal of Public Health, 81*(5), 646–649.

Mandolesi, L., Polverino, A., Montuori, S., Foti, F., Ferraioli, G., Sorrentino, P., & Sorrentino, G. (2018). Effects of physical exercise on cognitive functioning and wellbeing: Biological and psychological benefits. *Frontiers in Psychology*, *9*, 509.

Manuck, S. B. (1994). Cardiovascular reactivity in cardiovascular disease: "Once more unto the breach." *International Journal of Behavioral Medicine*, *1*, 4–31.

Marks, L. D., Kelley, H. H., Dollahite, D. C., Kimball, E. R., & James, S. (2023). Family dinners and family relationships following the initial onset of the COVID-19 pandemic. *Marriage & Family Review*, 59(2), 95–120.

Markus, H. R., & Kitayama, S. (1991). Culture and the self: Implications for cognition, emotion, and motivation. *Psychological Review*, *98*(2), 224–253.

Markus, H. R., & Kitayama, S. (1992). The what, why and how of cultural psychology: A review of Shweder's "Thinking Through Cultures." *Psychological Inquiry*, *3*(4), 357–364. Retrieved from https://www.jstor.org/stable/1448997

Marlatt, G. A., & Gordon, J. R. (1980). Determinants of relapse: Implications for the maintenance of behavior change. In P. O. Davidson & S. M. Davidson (Eds.), *Behavioral medicine: Changing health lifestyles* (pp. 410–452). New York, NY: Brunner/Mazel.

Marlatt, G. A., & Gordon, J. R. (1985). *Relapse prevention: A self-control strategy for the maintenance of behavior change* (2nd ed.). New York, NY: Guilford.

Marlatt, G. A., & Kaplan, B. E. (1972). Self-initiated attempts to change behavior: A study of New Year's resolutions. *Psychological Reports*, *30*, 123–131.

Martell, B. A., O'Connor, P. G., Kerns, R. D., Becker, W. C., Morales, K. H., & McCarthy, C. J. (1995). The relationship of cognitive appraisals and stress coping resources to emotioneliciting events. *Dissertation Abstracts International: Section B: The Sciences and Engineering*, *56*, 1746.

Martin, L. A., Doster, J. A., Critelli, J. W., Purdum, M., Powers, C., Lambert, P. L., & Miranda, V. (2011). The "distressed" personality, coping and cardiovascular risk. *Stress and Health*, *27*(1), 64–72.

Martin, R. A., Kuiper, N. A., Olinger, L. J., & Dance, K. A. (1993). Humor, coping with stress, self-concept, and psychological well-being. *Humor: International Journal of Humor Research*, *6*(1), 89–104.

Martin-Maria, N., Lara, E., Cabello, M., Olaya, B., Haro, J. M., Miret, M., & Ayuso-Mateos, J. L. (2023). To be happy and behave in a healthier way. A longitudinal study about gender differences in the older population. *Psychology & Health*, 38(3), 307–323.

Mason, P. B., Toney, M. B., & Cho, Y. (2011). Religious affiliation and Hispanic health in Utah. *Social Science Journal*, *48*(1), 175–192.

Masten, A. S. (2001). Ordinary magic: Resilience processes in development. *American Psychologist*, *56*(3), 227–238.

Mata, J., Frank, R., & Gigerenzer, G. (2014). Symptom recognition of heart attack and stroke in nine European countries: A representative survey. *Health Expectations*, *17*(3), 376–387. doi: 10.1111/j.1369-7625.2011.00764.x

Mata, J., Hogan, C. L., Joormann, J., Waugh, C. E., & Gotlib, I. H. (2013). Acute exercise attenuates negative affect following repeated sad mood inductions in persons who have recovered from depression. *Journal of Abnormal Psychology*, *122*(1), 45–50.

Matarazzo, J. D. (1979). President's column. *Health Psychologist*, *1*(1), 1.

Matthews, K. A., Croft, J. B, Liu, Y., Lu, H., Kanny, D., Wheaton, A. G., … Giles, W. H. (2017). Health-related behaviors by urban-rural county classifications—United States 2013. *Morbidity and Mortality Weekly Report Surveillance Summaries*, *66*(5), 1–8.

Matthews, K. A., Gump, B. B., & Owens, J. F. (2001). Chronic stress influences cardiovascular and neuroendocrine responses during acute stress and recovery, especially in men. *Health Psychology*, *20*(6), 403–410.

Maxfield, M., Pyszczynski, T., & Solomon, S. (2013). Finding meaning in death: Terror management among the terminally ill. In N. Straker (Ed.), *Facing cancer and the fear of death: A psychoanalytic perspective on treatment* (pp. 41–60). Lanham, MD: Rowman & Littlefield.

Maximova, K., McGrath, J. J., Barnett, T., O'Loughlin, J., Paradis, G., & Lambert, M. (2008). Do you see what I see? Weight status misperception and exposure to obesity among children and adolescents. *International Journal of Obesity (London)*, *32*(6), 1008–1015.

Mayer, J. D., Salovey, P. (1997). What is emotional intelligence? In P. Salovey, D. J. Sluyter (Eds.), *Emotional development and emotional intelligence: Educational implications* (pp. 3–31). New York, NY, USA: Basic Books.

MayoClinic.(2018,May).*Coronaryarterydisease*.Retrieved from https://www.mayoclinic.org/diseases-conditions/coronary-artery-disease/symptoms-causes/syc-20350613

Mazure, C. M. (1998). Life stressors as risk factors in depression. *Clinical Psychology: Science and Practice*, *5*, 291–313.

Mazzardo-Martins, L., Martins, D. F., Marcon, R., dos Santos, U. D., Speckhann, B., Gadotti, V. M., … Santos, A. R. (2010). High-intensity extended swimming exercise reduces pain-related behavior in mice: Involvement of endogenous opioids and the serotonergic system. *Journal of Pain, 11*(12), 1384–1393.

Mbonu, N. C., van den Borne, B., & De Vries, N. K. (2009). Stigma of people with HIV/AIDS in sub-Saharan Africa: A literature review. *Journal of Tropical Medicine, 2009,* 1–14. doi: 10.1155/2009/145891

McAndrew, F. T., Akande, A., Turner, S., & Sharma, Y. (1998). A cross-cultural ranking of stressful life events in Germany, India, South Africa, and the United States. *Journal of Cross-Cultural Psychology, 29*(6), 717–727.

McCaffery, M. (1972). *Nursing management of the patient with pain.* Philadelphia, PA: Lippincott, Williams & Wilkins.

McCarroll, J. E., Ursano, R. J., Fullerton, C. S., Liu, X., & Lundy, A. (2002). Somatic symptoms in Gulf War mortuary workers. *Psychosomatic Medicine, 64,* 29–33.

McCarthy, C. J. (1995). *The relationship of cognitive appraisals and stress coping resources to emotion-eliciting events* [Doctoral dissertation]. Retrieved from https://www.researchgate.net/publication/35046408_The_relationship_of_cognitive_appraisals_and_stress_coping_resources_to_emotion_eliciting_events

McClean, P., & Redmond, A. O. (1988). Hypothalamic tumour presenting as anorexia nervosa. *Ulster Medical Journal, 57,* 224–227.

McConnon, A., Raats, M., Astrup, A., Bajzová, M., Handjieva-Darlenska, T., Lindroos, A. K., … Shepherd, R. (2012). Application of the theory of planned behaviour to weight control in an overweight cohort: Results from a pan-European dietary intervention trial (DiOGenes). *Appetite, 58*(1), 313–318.

McCord, C., & Freeman, H. P. (1990). Excess mortality in Harlem. *New England Journal of Medicine, 322*(3), 173–177.

McCormick, C. M., Kuo, S. I.-C., & Masten, A. S. (2011). Developmental tasks across the life span. In K. L. Fingerman, C. A. Berg, J. Smith, & T. C. Antonucci (Eds.), *Handbook of life-span development* (pp. 117–140). New York, NY: Springer.

McCullough, M. E., Hoyt, W. T., Larson, D. B., Koenig, H. G., & Thoresen, C. (2000). Religious involvement and mortality: A meta-analytic review. *Health Psychology, 19*(3), 211–222.

McDougall, J., Bruce, B., Spiller, G., Westerdahl, J., & McDougall, M. (2002). Effects of a very low-fat, vegan diet in subjects with rheumatoid arthritis. *Journal of Alternative and Complementary Medicine, 8*(1), 71–75.

McEwen, B. S. (1998). Stress, adaptation, and disease: Allostasis and allostatic load. *Annals of the New York Academy of Sciences, 840*(1), 33–44.

McEwen, B. S. (2006). Sleep deprivation as a neurobiologic and physiologic stressor: Allostasis and allostatic load. *Metabolism, 55,* S20–S23.

McEwen, B. S., & Stellar, E. (1993). Stress and the individual: Mechanisms leading to disease. *Archives of Internal Medicine, 153*(18), 2093–2101.

McGlothlin, W. H., & West, L. J. (1968). The marihuana problem: An overview. *American Journal of Psychiatry, 125,* 126–134.

McGonagle, K. A., & Kessler, R. C. (1990). Chronic stress, acute stress, and depressive symptoms. *American Journal of Community Psychology, 18,* 681–706.

McGrady, M. E., Peugh, J. L., & Hood, K. K. (2014). Illness representations predict adherence in adolescents and young adults with type 1 diabetes. *Psychology & Health, 29*(9), 985–998.

McHale, S. M., Updegraff, K. A., & Whiteman, S. D. (2012). Sibling relationships and influences in childhood and adolescence. *Journal of Marriage and the Family, 74*(5), 913–930.

McIntosh, D. N., Silver, R. C., & Wortman, C. B. (1993). Religion's role in adjustment to a negative life event: Coping with the loss of a child. *Journal of Personality and Social Psychology, 65*(4), 812–821.

McIntyre, C. A., & Rhodes, R. E. (2009). Correlates of leisuretime physical activity during transitions to motherhood. *Women and Health, 49*(1), 66–83.

McKinley, N. M. (1999). Women and objectified body consciousness: Mothers' and daughters' body experience in cultural, developmental, and familial context. *Developmental Psychology, 35*(3), 760–769.

McKinley, N. M. (2006). The developmental and cultural contexts of objectified body consciousness: A longitudinal analysis of two cohorts of women. *Developmental Psychology, 42*(4), 679–687.

McLaughlin, K. A., Hatzenbuehler, M. L., & Keyes, K. M. (2010). Responses to discrimination and psychiatric disorders among black, Hispanic, female, and lesbian, gay, and bisexual individuals. *American Journal of Public Health, 100*(8), 1477–1484.

McLoughlin, E., et al. (2023). The tendency to appraise stressful situations as more of a threat is associated with poorer health and well-being. *Stress and Health.* doi: 10.1002/smi.3358

Meaney, M. J. (2001). Maternal care, gene expression, and the transmission of individual differences in stress reactivity across generations. *Annual Review of Neuroscience, 24*, 1161–1192.

Means-Christensen, A. J., Arnau, R. C., Tonidandel, A. M., Bramson, R., & Meagher, M. W. (2005). An efficient method of identifying major depression and panic disorder in primary care. *Journal of Behavioral Medicine, 28*(6), 565–572.

Mehta, N., & Atreja, A. (2018). Online social support networks. In *Social media in medicine* (pp. 36–41). Routledge.

Mehta, N. K., Lee, H., & Ylitalo, K. R. (2013). Child health in the United States: Recent trends in racial/ethnic disparities. *Social Science & Medicine, 95*, 6–15.

Meier, M. H., Caspi, A., Ambler, A., Harrington, H., Houts, R., Keefe, R. S. E., … Moffitt, T. E. (2012). Persistent cannabis users show neuropsychological decline from childhood to midlife. *Proceedings of the National Academy of Sciences of the United States of America, 109*(40), E2657–E2664.

Meier, D. E., Emmons, C. A., Wallenstein, S., Quill, T., Morrison, R. S., & Cassel, C. K. (1998). A national survey of physician-assisted suicide and euthanasia in the United States. *New England Journal of Medicine, 338*(17), 1193–1201.

Meier, M. H., & White, M. (2018). Do young-adult cannabis users show amotivation? An analysis of informant reports. *Translational Issues in Psychological Science, 4*(1), 99.

Melodia, F., Canale, N., & Griffiths, M. D. (2020). The role of avoidance coping and escape motives in problematic online gaming: A systematic literature review. *International Journal of Mental Health and Addiction, 20*, 996–1022.

Melzack, R. (1975). The McGill Pain Questionnaire: Major properties and scoring methods. *Pain, 1*(3), 277–299.

Melzack, R. (2001). Pain and the neuromatrix in the brain. *Journal of Dental Education, 65*(12), 1378–1382.

Melzack, R. (2005). Evolution of the neuromatrix theory of pain. The Prithvi Raj Lecture: Presented at the third World Congress of World Institute of Pain, Barcelona 2004. *Pain Practice, 5*(2), 85–94.

Melzack, R., & Katz, J. (2004). The gate control theory: Reaching for the brain. In T. Hadjistavropoulos & K. Craig (Eds.), *Pain: Psychological perspectives* (pp. 13–34). Mahwah, NJ: Erlbaum.

Melzack, R., & Torgerson, W. S. (1971). On the language of pain. *Anesthesiology, 34*, 50–59.

Melzack, R., & Wall, P. D. (1967). Pain mechanisms: A new theory. *Survey of Anesthesiology, 11*(2), 89–90.

Mennella, J. A., Kennedy, J. M., & Beauchamp, G. K. (2006). Vegetable acceptance by infants: Effects of formula flavors. *Early Human Development, 82*(7), 463–468.

Mensah, G. A., Stoney, C. M., Freemer, M. M., Smith, S., Engelgau, M. M., Hoots, K., … Goff, D. C. (2019). The national heart, lung, and blood institute strategic vision implementation for health equity research. *Ethnicity and Disease, 29*(Suppl. 1), 57–64.

Mercier, C., Peladeau, N., & Tempier, R. (1998). Age, gender and quality of life. *Community Mental Health Journal, 34*(5), 487–500.

Mereish, E. H., O'Cleirigh, C., & Bradford, J. B. (2014). Interrelationships between LGBT-based victimization, suicide, and substance use problems in a diverse sample of sexual and gender minorities. *Psychology, Health & Medicine, 19*(1), 1–13.

Merrill, R. M. (2004). Life expectancy among LDS and non-LDS in Utah. *Demographic Research, 10*, 61–82.

Mervosh, S., Lu, D., & Swales, V. (2020, April 20). See which states and cities have told residents to stay at home. *The New York Times.* https://www.nytimes.com/interactive/2020/us/coronavirus-stay-at-home-order.html

Metcalfe, K. A., Quan, M. L., Eisen, A., Cil, T., Sun, P., & Narod, S. A. (2013). The impact of having a sister diagnosed with breast cancer on cancer-related distress and breast cancer risk perception. *Cancer, 119*(9), 1722–1728.

Metcalfe, C., Smith, G. D., Wadsworth, E., Sterne, J. A., Heslop, P., Macleod, J., & Smith, A. (2003). A contemporary validation of the Reeder Stress Inventory. *British Journal of Health Psychology, 8*(Pt 1), 83–94.

Meule, A., Skirde, A. K., Freund, R., Vögele, C., & Kübler, A. (2012). High-calorie food-cues impair working memory performance in high and low food cravers. *Appetite, 59*(2), 264–269.

Micali, N., & Herle, M. (2023). Gone too soon: Studying mortality in eating disorders. *Acta Psychiatrica Scandinavica, 147*(2), 119–121.

Miech, R. A., Schulenberg, J. E., Johnston, L. D., Bachman, J. G., O'Malley, P. M., & Patrick, M. E. (2018, December 17). National adolescent drug trends in 2018. *Monitoring the Future.* Retrieved from http://www.monitoringthefuture.org

Migraine Research Foundation. (2016). *Migraine facts.* Retrieved from https://migraineresearchfoundation.org/about-migraine/migraine-facts/

Miles, J. L., Huber, K., Thompson, N. M., Davison, M., & Breier, B. H. (2009). Moderate daily exercise activates metabolic flexibility to prevent prenatally induced obesity. *Endocrinology, 150*(1), 179–186.

Miller, G. E., Chen, E., Fok, A. K., Walker, H., Lim, A., Nicholls, E. F., … Kobor, M. S. (2009). Low early-life social class leaves a biological residue manifested by decreased glucocorticoid and increased proinflammatory signaling. *Proceedings of the National Academy of Sciences of the USA, 106*(34), 14716–14721.

Miller, G. E., Cohen, S., & Ritchey, A. K. (2002). Chronic psychological stress and the regulation of pro-inflammatory cytokines: A glucocorticoid-resistance model. *Health Psychology, 21*(6), 531–541.

Miller, S. M., & Mangan, C. E. (1983). Interacting effects of information and coping style in adapting to gynecologic stress: Should the doctor tell all? *Journal of Personality and Social Psychology, 45*(1), 223–236.

Miller, P., Moore, R. H., & Kral, T. V. (2011). Children's daily fruit and vegetable intake: Associations with maternal intake and child weight status. *Journal of Nutrition Education and Behavior, 43*(5), 396–400. doi: 10.1016/j.jneb.2010.10.003

Miller, G. E., Rohleder, N., & Cole, S. W. (2009). Chronic interpersonal stress predicts activation of pro- and anti-inflammatory signaling pathways 6 months later. *Psychosomatic Medicine, 71*, 57–62.

Miller, P. M., Watkins, J. A., Sargent, R. G., & Rickert, E. J. (1999). Self-efficacy in overweight individuals with binge eating disorder. *Obesity Research, 7*, 552–555.

Milligan, R. A., Burke, V., Beilin, L. J., Richards, J., Dunbar, D., Spencer, M., … Gracey, M. P. (1997). Health-related behaviours and psycho-social characteristics of 18 year-old Australians. *Social Science and Medicine, 45*, 1549–1562.

Mishra, A., Baker-Eveleth, L., Gala, P., & Stachofsky, J. (2023). Factors influencing actual usage of fitness tracking devices: Empirical evidence from the UTAUT model. *Health Marketing Quarterly, 40*(1), 19–38.

Mitchell, A. J., Vaze, A., & Rao, S. (2009). Clinical diagnosis of depression in primary care: A meta-analysis. *Lancet, 374*(9690), 609–619.

Moerman, D. (2002). *Meaning, medicine and the "placebo effect."* Cambridge, UK: Cambridge University Press.

Mohr, D., Vedantham, K., Neylan, T., Metzler, T. J., Best, S., & Marmar, C. R. (2003). The mediating effects of sleep in the relationship between traumatic stress and health symptoms in urban police officers. *Psychosomatic Medicine, 65*, 485–489.

Mohseny, M., Amanpour, F., Mosavi-Jarrahi, A., et al. (2016). Application of Cox and parametric survival methods to assess social determinants of health affecting three-year survival of breast cancer patients. *Asian Pacific Journal of Cancer Prevention, 17*, 311–316.

Mokdad, A. H., Marks, J. S., Stroup, D. F., & Gerberding, J. L. (2004). Actual causes of death in the United States, 2000. *JAMA, 291*(10), 1238–1245.

Molla, M., Åstrøm, A. N., & Berhane, Y. (2007). Applicability of the theory of planned behavior to intended and self-reported condom use in a rural Ethiopian population. *AIDS Care, 19*(3), 425–431.

Mommersteeg, P. M., Kupper, N., & Denollet, J. (2010). Type D personality is associated with increased metabolic syndrome prevalence and an unhealthy lifestyle in a cross-sectional Dutch community sample. *BMC Public Health, 10*, 714.

Monroe, S. M., & Harkness, K. L. (2005). Life stress, the "kindling" hypothesis, and the recurrence of depression: Considerations from a life stress perspective. *Psychological Review, 112*, 417–445.

Monroe, S. M., & Simons, A. D. (1991). Diathesis-stress theories in the context of life stress research: Implications for the depressive disorders. *Psychological Bulletin, 110*, 406–425.

Montgomery, G., & Kirsch, I. (1996). Mechanisms of placebo pain reduction: An empirical investigation. *Psychological Science, 7*(3), 174–176.

Moore, K. J. (2019). Targeting inflammation in CVD: Advances and challenges. *Nature Reviews Cardiology, 16*(2), 74.

Moore D. R., et al. (2022). Walking or body weight squat "activity snacks" increase dietary amino acid utilization for myofibrillar protein synthesis during prolonged sitting. *Journal of Applied Physiology, 133*(3), 777–785.

Moore, J. L., & Constantine, M. G. (2005). Development and initial validation of the collectivistic coping styles measure with African, Asian, and Latin American international students. *Journal of Mental Health Counseling, 27*(4), 329–347.

Moos, R. H., & Schaefer, J. A. (1986). Life transitions and crises. In R. H. Moos (Ed.), *Coping with life crises* (pp. 3–28). Boston, MA: Springer.

Moos, R. H., & Schaefer, J. A. (1993). Coping resources and processes: Current concepts and measures. In L. Goldberger & S. Breznitz (Eds.), *Handbook of stress: Theoretical and clinical aspects* (2nd ed., pp. 234–257). New York, NY: Free Press.

Morelli, M., et al. (2024). Is Adolescents' cyber dating violence perpetration related to problematic pornography use? The moderating role of hostile sexism. *Health Communication, 39*(13), 3134–3144.

Morley, S., & Vlaeyen, J. W. (2010). 50 years on, Henry Beecher's "Measurement of subjective responses." *Pain*, *150*(2), 211–212.

Morreall, J. (1991). Humor and work. *Humor: International Journal of Humor Research*, *4*(3–4), 359–374.

Morris, K. L., Goldenberg, J. L., Arndt, J., & McCabe, S. (2018). The enduring influence of death on health: Insights from the terror management health model. *Self and Identity*, *18*(4), 378–404.

Mosconi, L., Nacmias, B., Sorbi, S., De Cristofaro, M. T. R., Fayazz, M., Tedde, A., … Pupi, A. (2004). Brain metabolic decreases related to the dose of the ApoE e4 allele in Alzheimer's disease. *Journal of Neurology, Neurosurgery & Psychiatry*, *75*(3), 370–376.

Moss-Morris, R., Petrie, K. J., & Weinman, J. (1996). Functioning in chronic fatigue syndrome: Do illness perceptions play a regulatory role? *British Journal of Health Psychology*, *1*, 15–25.

Mrus, J. M., Sherman, K. E., Leonard, A. C., Sherman, S. N., Mandell, K. L., & Tsevat, J. (2006). Health values of patients coinfected with HIV/hepatitis c: Are two viruses worse than one? *Medical Care*, *44*(2), 158–166.

Mubasshera, H. (2024). Pornography usage during adolescence: Does it lead to risky sexual behavior? *Health Economics*, *33*, 1682–1704.

Mullins, M., Cote, M. L., Abbott, S., Alberg, A. J., Bandera, E. V., Barnholtz-Sloan, J., … Peres, L. C. (2018). Abstract C24: Determinants of delays in care-seeking for ovarian cancer symptoms in African American women. *Cancer Epidemiology, Biomarkers and Prevention*, *27*(7 Suppl.), C24.

Muñoz-Silva, A., Sánchez-García, M., Nunes, C., & Martins, A. (2007). Gender differences in condom use prediction with theory of reasoned action and planned behavior: The role of self-efficacy and control. *AIDS Care*, *19*(9), 1177–1181.

Munro, S., Thomas, K. L., & Abu-Shaar, M. (1993). Molecular characterization of a peripheral receptor for cannabinoids. *Nature*, *365*(6441), 61–65.

Munro, L., Travers, R., & Woodford, M. R. (2019). Overlooked and invisible: Everyday experiences of microaggressions for LGBTQ adolescents. *Journal of Homosexuality*, *66*(10), 1439–1471. doi: 10.1080/00918369.2018.1542205

Murphy, H. (2019, March 28). At 71, she's never felt pain or anxiety. Now scientists know why. *New York Times*.

Murphy, S. T., Monahan, J. L., & Miller, L. C. (1998). Inference under the influence: The impact of alcohol and inhibition conflict on women's sexual decision making. *Personality and Social Psychology Bulletin*, *24*(5), 517–528.

Murphy, D. A., Stein, J. A., Schlenger, W., & Mailbach, E. (2001). Conceptualizing the multidimensional nature of self-efficacy: Assessment of situational context and level of behavioral challenge to maintain safer sex. *Health Psychology*, *20*, 281–290.

Murphy, S. L., Xu, J., Kochanek, K. D., & Arias, E. (2018). *Mortality in the United States, 2017*. Retrieved from https://www.cdc.gov/nchs/data/databriefs/db328-h.pdf

Myung, S. K., Ju, W., Jung, H. S., Park, C. H., Oh, S. W., Seo, H. G., & Kim, H. S. (2012). Efficacy and safety of pharmacotherapy for smoking cessation among pregnant smokers: A meta-analysis. *BJOG: An International Journal of Obstetrics and Gynaecology*, *111*(9) 1029–1039.

Najmi, S., & Wegner, D. (2008). The gravity of unwanted thoughts: Asymmetric priming effects in thought suppression. *Consciousness and Cognition*, *17*(1), 114–124.

Nakaya, N., Tsubono, Y., Hosokawa, T., Nishino, Y., Ohkubo, T., Hozawa, A., … Hisamichi, S. (2003). Personality and the risk of cancer. *Journal of the National Cancer Institute*, *95*(11), 799–805.

Namazi, H., Aramesh, K., & Larijani, B. (2016). The doctorpatient relationship: Toward a conceptual reexamination. *Journal of Medical Ethics and History of Medicine*, *9*, 10.

Narendorf, S. C., Fedoravicius, N., McMillen, J. C., McNelly, D., & Robinson, D. R. (2012). Stepping down and stepping in: Youth's perspectives on making the transition from residential treatment to treatment foster care. *Children and Youth Services Review*, *34*(1), 43–49.

Nasuti, G., Blanchard, C., Naylor, P. J., Levy-Milne, R., Warburton, D. E., Benoit, C., … Rhodes, R. E. (2014). Comparison of the dietary intakes of new parents, second-time parents, and nonparents: A longitudinal cohort study. *Journal of the Academy of Nutrition and Dietetics*, *114*(3), 450–456.

National Alliance for Eating Disorders. (2024). Retrieved from https://www.nationaleatingdisorders.org/resource-center/

National Association of Anorexia Nervosa and Associated Disorders. (2016). *Eating disorder statistics*. Retrieved from http://www.anad.org/get-information/about-eating-disorders/eating-disorders-statistics/

National Cancer Institute. (2024). *Cancer stats facts*. Retrieved from https://seer.cancer.gov/statfacts/html/common.html#:~:text=In%202024%2C%20an%20estimated%20611%2C720,to%20die%20from%20this%20disease

National Center for Complementary and Integrative Health. (2017). *Traditional Chinese medicine: In depth*. Retrieved from https://nccih.nih.gov/health/whati-scam/chinesemed.htm

National Center for Drug Abuse Statistics. (2024a). Alcohol Related Deaths. Retrieved from https://drugabusestatistics.org/alcohol-related-deaths/

National Center for Drug Abuse Statistics. (2024b). *Drug abuse statistics*. Retrieved from https://drugabusestatistics.org/

National Center for Health Statistics. (2010). *Health, United States, 2009: With special feature on medical technology*. Hyattsville, MD: U.S. Department of Health and Human Services. Retrieved from http://www.cdc.gov/nchs/data/hus/hus09.pdf

National Center for Health Statistics. (2017). Health, United States, 2016, with chartbook on long-term trends in health.

National Collaborating Centre for Mental Health (UK). (2010). Depression in adults with a chronic physical health problem: Treatment and management. *National clinical practice guideline 91*. Leicester, UK: British Psychological Society and Royal College of Psychiatrists.

National Conference of State Legislatures. (2019, January). *States with religious and philosophical exemptions from school immunization requirements*. Retrieved from http://www.ncsl.org/research/health/school-immunization-exemption-state-laws.aspx

National Council on Skin Cancer Prevention. (2016). Retrieved from http://www.skincancerprevention.org

National Eating Disorders Association. (2010). *National survey shows turning point in the war against eating disorders*. Retrieved from https://www.nationaleatingdisorders.org/press-rom/press-releases/2010-press-releases/national-survey-shows-turning-point-war-against-eating-disorders

National Eating Disorders Association. (2018, February 21). *Eating disorders in LGBTQ populations*. https://www.nationaleatingdisorders.org/learn/general-information/lgbtq

National Funeral Directors Association. (2017, June). *NFDA consumer survey: Funeral planning not a priority for Americans*. Retrieved from http://www.nfda.org/news/media-center/nfda-news-releases/id/2419

National Geographic. (2011). *Are you a risk taker?*

National Highway Traffic Safety Administration. (2018a). *Traffic safety facts: 2016 data: Occupant protection*. Publication no. DOT-HS-812-494. Retrieved from https://crashstats.nhtsa.dot.gov/Api/Public/ViewPublication/812494

National Highway Traffic Safety Administration. (2018b). *U.S. DOT announces 2017 roadway fatalities down*. Retrieved from https://www.nhtsa.gov/press-releases/us-dot-announces-2017-roadway-fatalities-down

National Highway Traffic Safety Administration. (2024). *Traffic Safety Facts Research Notes: Seatbelt Use 2023*. Retrieved from https://crashstats.nhtsa.dot.gov/Api/Public/ViewPublication/813543

National Hospice and Palliative Care Organization. (2019). *Hospice Care Overview for Professionals*. Retrieved from https://www.nhpco.org/hospice-care-overview/

National Institute on Drug Abuse. (2012). *Principles of drug addiction treatment: A research-based guide* (3rd ed.). Retrieved from https://www.drugabuse.gov/publications/principles-drug-addiction-treatment-research-based-guide-third-edition

National Institute on Drug Abuse. (2016a). *Drug facts*. Retrieved from https://www.drugabuse.gov/publications/finder/t/160/DrugFacts

National Institute on Drug Abuse. (2016b). *Drugs, brains, and behavior: The science of addiction*. Retrieved from https://www.drugabuse.gov/publications/drugs-brains-behavior-science-addiction/addiction-health

National Institute on Drug Abuse. (2018a, February 15). *College age & young adults*. Retrieved from https://www.drugabuse.gov/related-topics/college-age-young-adults

Nedergaard, M., Iliff, J. J., Benveniste, H., & Deane, R. (2018). *U.S. Patent No. 9,901,650*. Washington, DC: U.S. Patent and Trademark Office.

Negahban, H., Rezaie, S., & Goharpey, S. (2013). Massage therapy and exercise therapy in patients with multiple sclerosis: A randomized controlled pilot study. *Clinical Rehabilitation, 27*(12), 1126–1136. doi: 10.1177/0269215513491586

Nejad, L. M., Wertheim, E. H., & Greenwood, K. M. (2004). Predicting dieting behavior by using, modifying, and extending the theory of planned behavior. *Journal of Applied Social Psychology, 34*(10), 2099–2131.

Nekolaichuk, C. L. (2015). Hope in end-of-life care. In E. Bruera, I. Higginson, C. F. von Gunten, & T. Morita (Eds.), *Textbook of palliative medicine and supportive care* (2nd ed., pp. 743–749). Boca Raton, FL: CRC Press, Taylor & Francis.

Nelson, J. L., Furst, D. E., Maloney, S., Gooley, T., Evans, P. C., Smith, A., … Bianchi, D. W. (1998). Microchimerism and HLA-compatible relationships of pregnancy in scleroderma. *Lancet, 351*(9102), 559–562.

Nelson, D. R., Hammen, C., Daley, S. E., Burge, D., & Davila, J. (2001). Sociotropic and autonomous personality styles: Contributions to chronic life stress. *Cognitive Therapy and Research, 25*(1), 61–76.

Nelson, D. E., Jarman, D. W., Rehm, J., Greenfield, T. K., Rey, G., Kerr, W. C., … Naimi, T. S. (2013). Alcohol-attributable cancer deaths and years of potential life lost in the United States *American Journal of Public Health, 103*(4), 641–648. doi: 10.2105/AJPH.2012.301199

Neumark-Sztainer, D. (2005). Can we simultaneously work toward the prevention of obesity and eating disorders in children and adolescents? *International Journal of Eating Disorders, 38*(3), 220–227. doi: 10.1002/eat.20181

Neumark-Sztainer, D., Wall, M., Guo, J., Story, M., Haines, J., & Eisenberg, M. (2006). Obesity, disordered eating, and eating disorders in a longitudinal study of adolescents: How do dieters fare 5 years later? *Journal of the American Dietetic Association, 106*(4), 559–568.

Ng, D. M., & Jeffery, R. W. (2003). Relationships between perceived stress and health behaviors in a sample of working adults. *Health Psychology, 22*, 638–642.

Nguyen, L. T., Alexander, K., & Yates, P. (2018). Psychoeducational intervention for symptom management of fatigue, pain, and sleep disturbance cluster among cancer patients: A pilot quasi-experimental study. *Journal of Pain and Symptom Management, 55*(6), 1459–1472.

NHANES. (2018). *Childhood obesity trends.* Retrieved from https://www.cdc.gov/nchs/data/hestat/obesity-child-17-18/obesity-child.htm#:~:text=Results%20from%20the%202017%E2%80%932018,and%20another%2016.1%25%20are%20overweight.

Nicholson, A., Kuper, H., & Hemingway, H. (2006). Depression as an aetiologic and prognostic factor in coronary heart disease: A meta-analysis of 6362 events among 146 538 participants in 54 observational studies. *European Heart Journal, 27*(23), 2763–2774.

Nielsen, M. E. (2002). Religion's role in the terrorist attack of September 11, 2001. *North American Journal of Psychology, 3*(3), 377–383.

Nielsen-Bohlman, L., Panzer, A. M., & Kindig, D. A. (Eds.). (2004). *Health literacy: A prescription to end confusion.* Washington, DC: National Academies Press.

Nolen-Hoeksema, S., & Davis, C. G. (2002). Positive responses to loss: Perceiving benefits and growth. In C. R. Snyder & S. J. Lopez (Eds.), *Handbook of positive psychology* (pp. 598–606). New York, NY: Oxford University Press.

Norcross, J. C., Ratzin, A. C., & Payne, D. (1989). Ringing in the new year: The change processes and reported outcomes of resolutions. *Addictive Behaviors, 14*, 205–212.

North, R. B., Kidd, D. H., Farrokhi, F., & Piantadosi, S. A. (2005). Spinal cord stimulation versus repeated lumbosacral spine surgery for chronic pain: A randomized, controlled trial. *Neurosurgery, 56*(1), 98–106.

Nov, O, Singh, N., & Mann, D. (2023). Putting ChatGPT's medical advice to the (turing) test: Survey study. *JMIR Publications, 9*. Retrieved from https://mededu.jmir.org/2023/1/e46939

Nurius, P. S., Fleming, C. M., & Brindle, E. (2019). Life course pathways from adverse childhood experiences to adult physical health: A structural equation model. *Journal of Aging and Health, 31*(2), 211–230.

O'Connor, P. J. (2006). Improving medication adherence: Challenges for physicians, payers, and policy makers. *Archives of Internal Medicine, 166*(17), 1802–1804.

O'Donnell, M. J., Chin, S. L., Rangarajan, S., Xavier, D., Liu, L., Zhang, H., … Lopez-Jaramillo, P. (2016). Global and regional effects of potentially modifiable risk factors associated with acute stroke in 32 countries (INTERSTROKE): A case-control study. *The Lancet, 388*(10046), 761–775.

O'Donovan, G., Lee, I.-M., Hamer, M., & Stamatakis, E. (2017). Association of "weekend warrior" and other leisure time physical activity patterns with risks for all-cause, cardiovascular disease, and cancer mortality. *JAMA Internal Medicine, 177*(3), 335–342. doi: 10.1001/jamainternmed.2016.8014

O'Leary, K. J., Kulkarni, N., Landler, M. P., Jeon, J., Hahn, K. J., Englert, K. M., & Williams, M. V. (2010). Hospitalized patients' understanding of their plan of care. *Mayo Clinic Proceedings, 85*(1), 47–52.

O'Rourke, M. (2013, August 26). What's wrong with me? I had an autoimmune disease. Then the disease had me. *New Yorker.* Retrieved from http://www.newyorker.com/magazine/2013/08/26/whats-wrong-with-me

Oakes, K. (2018). Heart disease remains the leading cause of death in United States. *Clinician Reviews.* Retrieved from: https://www.mdedge.com/clinicianreviews/article/189878/cad-atherosclerosis/heart-disease-remains-leading-cause-death-us

Oberoi, D. V., Jiwa, M., McManus, A., & Hodder, R. (2015). Men's help-seeking behavior with regards to lower bowel symptoms. *American Journal of Health Behavior, 39*(2), 212–221.

Oddone, E. Z., Gierisch, J. M., Sanders, L. L., Fagerlin, A., Sparks, J., McCant, F., … Damschroder, L. J. (2018). A coaching by telephone intervention on engaging patients to address modifiable cardiovascular risk factors: A randomized controlled trial. *Journal of General Internal Medicine, 33*, 1487. doi: 10.1007/s11606-018-4398-6

Oerlemans, M. E., van den Akker, M., Schuurman, A. G., Kellen, E., & Buntinx, F. (2007). A meta-analysis on depression and subsequent cancer risk. *Clinical Practice and Epidemiology in Mental Health, 3*, 29.

Ogden, C. L. (2009). *Obesity and diet among U.S. adolescents.* Atlanta, GA: Centers for Disease Control and Prevention. Retrieved from http://www.cdc.gov/nchs/ppt/nchs2015/Ogden_Tuesday_WhiteFlint_CC1.pdf

Oikarinen, N., Jokelainen, T., Heikkilä, L., et al. (2023). Low eating self-efficacy is associated with unfavorable eating behavior tendencies among individuals with overweight and obesity. *Scientific Reports, 13*, 7730.

Oliveira, C. R., Paris, V. C., Pereira, R. A., & Lara, F. S. (2009). Anesthesia in a patient with congenital insensitivity to pain and anhidrosis. *Revista Brasileira de Anestesiologia, 59*(5), 602–609 [in Portuguese].

Olson, K. A., Patel, R. B., Ahmad, F. S., Ning, H., Bogle, B. M., Goldberger, J. J., & Lloyd-Jones, D. M. (2019). Sudden cardiac death risk distribution in the United States population (from NHANES, 2005–2012). *The American Journal of Cardiology, 123*(8), 1249–1254.

Olson, J. M., Roese, N. J., & Zanna, M. P. (1996). Expectancies. In E. T. Higgins & A. W. Kruglanski (Eds.), *Social psychology: Handbook of basic principles* (pp. 211–238). New York, NY: Guilford.

Oman, D. (2018). Elephant in the room: Why spirituality and religion matter for public health. In *Why religion and spirituality matter for public health* (pp. 1–16). New York, NY: Springer.

Oman, D., & Thoresen, C. E. (2007). How does one learn to be spiritual? The neglected role of spiritual modeling in health. In T. G. Plante & C. E. Thoresen (Eds.), *Spirit, science and health: How the spiritual mind fuels physical wellness* (pp. 39–54). Westport, CT: Praeger.

Onitilo, A. A., Nietert, P. J., & Egede, L. E. (2006). Effect of depression on all-cause mortality in adults with cancer and differential effects by cancer site. *General Hospital Psychiatry, 28*(5), 396–402.

Ormel, J. (1980). Do neuroticism inventories measure personality traits or psychosocial stress? *Acta Psychiatrica Scandinavica, 62*(S285), 196–203.

Orsak, G., Stevens, A. M., Brufsky, A., Kajumba, M., & Dougall, A. L. (2015). The effects of Reiki therapy and companionship on quality of life, mood, and symptom distress during chemotherapy. *Journal of Evidence-Based Complementary and Alternative Medicine, 20*(1), 20–27.

Orth-Gomér, K. (2012). Behavioral interventions for coronary heart disease patients. *BioPsychoSocial Medicine, 6*(1), 5.

Osterberg, L., & Blaschke, T. (2005). Adherence to medication. *New England Journal of Medicine, 353*(5), 487–497.

Oswald, A. J., & Powdthavee, N. (2008). Does happiness adapt? A longitudinal study of disability with implications for economists and judges. *Journal of Public Economics, 92*(5–6), 1061–1077.

Otto, M. W., Church, T. S., Craft, L. L., Greer, T. L., Smits, J. A., & Trivedi, M. H. (2007). Exercise for mood and anxiety disorders. *Primary Care Companion for DNS Disorders, 9*(4), 287–294.

Ouellette, J. A., Hessling, R., Gibbons, F. X., Reis-Bergan, M., & Gerrard, M. (2005). Using images to increase exercise behavior: Prototypes versus possible selves. *Personality and Social Psychology Bulletin, 31*(5), 610–620.

Owen, N., Healy, G. N., Matthews, C. E., & Dunstan, D. W. (2010). Too much sitting: The population health science of sedentary behavior. *Exercise and Sport Sciences Reviews, 38*(3), 105–113. doi: 10.1097/JES.0b013e3181e373a2

Owens, O. L., Beer, J. M., Reyes, L. I., Gallerani, D. G., Myhren-Bennett, A. R., & McDonnell, K. K. (2018). Mindfulness-based symptom and stress management apps for adults with chronic lung disease: Systematic search in app stores. *JMIR mHealth and uHealth, 6*(5), e9831.

Oz, M. (2011, March 11). The end of ouch? *Time.* Retrieved from http://content.time.com/time/specials/packages/article/0,28804,2053382_2053599,00.html

Ozer, E. J., Best, S. R., Lipsey, T. L., & Weiss, D. S. (2003). Predictors of posttraumatic stress disorder and symptoms in adults: A meta-analysis. *Psychological Bulletin, 129*, 52–73.

Pakenham, K. I., & Cox, S. (2009). The dimensional structure of benefit finding in multiple sclerosis and relations with positive and negative adjustment: A longitudinal study. *Psychology and Health, 24*(4), 373–393.

Palar, K., Frongillo, E. A., Escobar, J., Sheira, L. A., Wilson, T. E., Adedimeji, A., … Ofotokun, I. (2018). Food insecurity, internalized stigma, and depressive symptoms among women living with HIV in the United States. *AIDS and Behavior*, 1–10 22, 3869–3878.

Pandya, C., McHugh, M., & Batalova, J. (2011). *Limited English proficient individuals in the United States: Numbers, share, growth, and linguistic diversity*. Washington, DC: Migration Policy Institute. Retrieved from https://www.migrationpolicy.org/research/limited-english-proficient-individuals-united-states-number-share-growth-and-linguistic

Pangarkar, T. (2024). *Smart wearables statistics 2024 by devices, technology, usage*. Retrieved from https://scoop.market.us/smart-wearables-statistics/#:~:text=Global%20Smartwatch%20Market%20Size%20This%20upward%20trajectory,followed%20by%20USD%2073.6%20billion%20in%202028.

Panlilio, L. V., Zanettini, C., Barnes, C., Solinas, M., & Goldberg, S. R. (2013). Prior exposure to THC increases the addictive effects of nicotine in rats. *Neuropsychopharmacology*, 38(7), 1198–1208.

Panuganti, K. K., Tadi, P., & Lui, F. (2019). Transient ischemic attack. In *StatPearls [internet]*. StatPearls Publishing.

Pargament, K. I. (1997). *The psychology of religion and coping: Theory, research, practice*. New York, NY: Guilford.

Park, D. C. (1999). Aging and the controlled and automatic processing of medical information and medical intentions. In D. C. Park, R. W. Morrell, & K. Shifren (Eds.), *Processing of medical information in aging patients: Cognitive and human factors perspectives* (pp. 3–24). Mahwah, NJ: Erlbaum.

Park, C. L. (2005). Religion as a meaning-making framework in coping with life stress. *Journal of Social Issues*, 61(4), 707–729.

Park, C. L. (2007). Religiousness/spirituality and health: A meaning systems perspective. *Journal of Behavioral Medicine*, 30(4), 319–328.

Park, C. L. (2008). Testing the meaning making model of coping with loss. *Journal of Social and Clinical Psychology*, 27(9), 970–994.

Park, C. L., Armeli, S., & Tennen, H. (2004). The daily stress and coping process and alcohol use among college students. *Journal of Studies on Alcohol and Drugs*, 65(1), 126–135.

Park, C. L., Chmielewski, J., & Blank, T. O. (2010). Post-traumatic growth: Finding positive meaning in cancer survivorship moderates the impact of intrusive thoughts on adjustment in younger adults. *Psychooncology*, 19(11), 1139–1147.

Park, C. L., & Folkman, S. (1997). Stability and change in psychosocial resources during caregiving and bereavement in partners of men with AIDS. *Journal of Personality*, 65(2), 421–447.

Park, M. J., Scott, J. T., Adams, S. H., Brindis, C. D., & Irwin, C. E. (2014). Adolescent and young adult health in the United States in the past decade: Little improvement and young adults remain worse off than adolescents. *Journal of Adolescent Health*, 55(1), 3–16.

Park Lee, E., Ren, C., Cooper, M., Cornelius, M., Jamal, A., Cullen, K. A. (2022). Tobacco product use among middle and high school students – United States, 2022. *Morbidity and Mortality Weekly Report*, 71, 45.

Parker, L. L., & Harriger, J. A. (2020). Eating disorders and disordered eating behaviors in the LGBT population: A review of the literature. *Journal of Eating Disorders*, 8, 1–20.

Parks, G. A., Anderson, B. K., & Marlatt, G. A. (2003). Relapse prevention therapy. In N. Heather & T. Stockwell (Eds.), *The essential handbook of treatment and prevention of alcohol problems* (pp. 575–592). Sussex, England: John Wiley & Sons.

Párraga, J. P., & Castellanos, A. (2023). A manifesto in defense of pain complexity: A critical review of essential insights in pain neuroscience. *Journal of Clinical Medicine*, 12(22), 7080.

Parrish, J. (1986). Parent compliance with medical and behavioral recommendations. In N. A. Krasnegor, J. D. Arasteh, & M. F. Cataldo (Eds.), *Child health behavior* (pp. 453–501). New York, NY: Wiley.

Parrish, B. P., Zautra, A. J., & Davis, M. C. (2008). The role of positive and negative interpersonal events on daily fatigue in women with fibromyalgia, rheumatoid arthritis, and osteoarthritis. *Health Psychology*, 27, 694–702.

Parsons, O. A., & Prigatano, G. P. (1977). Memory functioning in alcoholics. In I. M. Birnbaum & E. S. Parker (Eds.), *Alcohol and human memory* (pp. 185–194). Hillsdale, NJ: Erlbaum.

Paschen-Wolff, M. M., Kelvin, E., Wells, B. E., Campbell, A. N., Grosskopf, N. A., & Grov, C. (2019). Changing trends in substance use and sexual risk disparities among sexual minority women as a function of sexual identity, behavior, and attraction: Findings from the National Survey of Family Growth, 2002–2015. *Archives of Sexual Behavior*, 48(4), 1137–1158. doi: 10.1007/s10508-018-1333-1

Pasquereau, A., Guignard, R., Andler, R., & Nguyen-Thanh, V. (2017). Electronic cigarettes, quit attempts and smoking cessation: A 6-month follow-up. *Addiction*, 112, 1620–1628.

Patanavanich, R., Siripoon, T., Amponnavarat, S., & Glantz, S. A. (2023). Active smokers are at higher risk of COVID-19 death: A systematic review and meta-analysis. *Nicotine and Tobacco Research, 25*(2), 177–184.

Patel, K., Tchanturia, K., & Harrison, A. (2016). An exploration of social functioning in young people with eating disorders: A qualitative study. *PLoS One, 11*(7), e0159910. doi: 10.1371/journal.pone.0159910

Patterson, P., & Gong, G. (2009). Addressing health disparities in immigrant populations in the United States. In S. Kosoko-Lasaki, C. T. Cook, & R. L. O'Brien (Eds.), *Cultural proficiency in addressing health disparities* (pp. 247–280). Sudbury, MA: Jones & Bartlett.

Pedersen, S. S., van Domburg, R. T., Theuns, D. A., Jordaens, L., & Erdman, R. A. (2004). Type D personality is associated with increased anxiety and depressive symptoms in patients with an implantable cardioverter defibrillator and their partners. *Psychosomatic Medicine, 66*(5), 714–719.

Pederson, L. L. (1982). Compliance with physician advice to quit smoking: A review of the literature. *Preventive Medicine, 11*(1), 71–84.

Pellizzer, M. L., & Wade, T. D. (2023). Developing a definition of body neutrality and strategies for an intervention. *Body Image, 46*, 434–442.

Peng, R., Guo, Y., Zhang, C., Li, X., Huang, J., Chen, X., & Feng, H. (2024). Internet-delivered psychological interventions for older adults with depression: A scoping review. *Geriatric Nursing, 55*, 97–104.

Penley, J. A., Tomaka, J., & Wiebe, J. S. (2002). The association of coping to physical and psychological health outcomes: A meta-analytic review. *Journal of Behavioral Medicine, 25*(6), 551–603.

Pennebaker, J. W. (1994). Psychological bases of symptom reporting: Perceptual and emotional aspects of chemical sensitivity. *Toxicology and Industrial Health, 10*(4–5), 497–511.

Pennebaker, J. W., & Epstein, D. (1983). Implicit psychophysiology: Effects of common beliefs and idiosyncratic physiological responses symptom reporting. *Journal of Personality, 51*(3), 468–496.

Penninx, B. W., van Tilburg, T., Deeg, D. J., Kriegsman, D. M., Boeke, A. J. P., & Van Eijk, J. T. (1997). Direct and buffer effects of social support and personal coping resources in individuals with arthritis. *Social Science and Medicine, 44*(3), 393–402.

Peralta-Ramírez, M. I., Jiménez-Alonso, J., Godoy-García, J. F., & Pérez-García, M. (2004). The effects of daily stress and stressful life events on the clinical symptomatology of patients with lupus erythematosus. *Psychosomatic Medicine, 66*, 788–794.

Pérez, A. E., Gamarel, K. E., van den Berg, J. J., & Operario, D. (2018). Sexual and behavioral health disparities among African American sexual minority men and women. *Ethnicity and Health*. Advance online publication. doi: 10.1080/13557858.2018.1444149

Pérez-Stable, E. J., & Collins, F. S. (2019). Science visioning in minority health and health disparities. *American Journal of Public Health, 109*(S1), S5. doi: 10.2105/AJPH.2019.304962

Person, A. I., & Frazier, P. A. (2024). Coping strategy-situation fit vs. present control: Relations with perceived stress in US college students. *Anxiety, Stress, & Coping, 37*(2), 219–232.

Pertl, M., Hevey, D., Thomas, K., Craig, A., Chuinneagáin, S. N., & Maher, L. (2010). Differential effects of self-efficacy and perceived control on intentions to perform skin cancer–related health behaviours. *Health Education Research, 25*(5), 769–779.

Pesa, J., & Lage, M. J. (2004). The medical costs of migraine and comorbid anxiety and depression. *Headache, 44*(6), 562–570.

Peters, M. L., Godaert, G. L., Ballieux, R. E., Brosschot, J. F., Sweep, F. C., Swinkels, L. M., … Heijnen, C. J. (1999). Immune responses to experimental stress: Effects of mental effort and uncontrollability. *Psychosomatic Medicine, 61*, 513–524.

Peters, A., & Laffel, L., American Diabetes Association Transitions Working Group. (2011). Diabetes care for emerging adults: Recommendations for transition from pediatric to adult diabetes care systems: A position statement of the American Diabetes Association, with representation by the American College of Osteopathic Family Physicians, the American Academy of Pediatrics, the American Association of Clinical Endocrinologists, the American Osteopathic Association, the Centers for Disease Control and Prevention, Children with Diabetes, the Endocrine Society, the International Society for Pediatric and Adolescent Diabetes, Juvenile Diabetes Research Foundation International, the National Diabetes Education Program, and the Pediatric Endocrine Society (formerly Lawson Wilkins Pediatric Endocrine Society). *Diabetes Care, 34*(11), 2477–2485.

Petersen, S., van den Berg, R. A., Janssens, T., & Van den Bergh, O. (2011). Illness and symptom perception: A theoretical approach towards an integrative measurement model. *Clinical Psychology Review, 31*(3), 428–439.

Peterson, C. (2006). *A primer in positive psychology*. New York, NY: Oxford University Press.

Peterson, C., Park, N., & Sweeney, P. J. (2008). Group well-being: Morale from a positive psychology perspective. *Applied Psychology*, *57*(s1), 19–36.

Petitti, D. B., Klingensmith, G. J., Bell, R. A., Andrews, J. S., Dabelea, D., Imperatore, G., … Mayer-Davis, E. (2009). Glycemic control in youth with diabetes: The SEARCH for diabetes in youth study. *Journal of Pediatrics*, *155*(5), 668–672.

Petraitis, J., Flay, B. R., & Miller, T. Q. (1995). Reviewing theories of adolescent substance use: Organizing pieces in the puzzle. *Psychological Bulletin*, *117*(1), 67–86.

Petrie, K. J., & Weinman, J. (2012). Patients' perceptions of their illness: The dynamo of volition in health care. *Current Directions in Psychological Science*, *21*(1), 60–65.

Peven, J. C., Grove, G. A., Jakicic, J. M., Alessi, M. G., & Erickson, K. I. (2018). Associations between short and long bouts of physical activity. *Journal of Cognitive Enhancement*, *2*(2), 137–145. doi: 10.1007/s41465-018-0080-5

Peyman, N., & Oakley, D. (2009). Effective contraceptive use: An exploration of theory-based influences. *Health Education Research*, *24*(4), 575–585.

Phillips, L. A., & Mullan, B. A. (2023). Ramifications of behavioural complexity for habit conceptualisation, promotion, and measurement. *Health Psychology Review*, *17*(3), 402–415.

Phinney, J. S., Lochner, B. T., & Murphy, R. (1990). Ethnic identity development and psychological adjustment in adolescence. In A. R. Stiffman & L. E. Davis (Eds.), *Ethnic issues in adolescent mental health* (pp. 53–72). Thousand Oaks, CA: Sage.

Piché, M., Arsenault, M., & Rainville, P. (2009). Cerebral and cerebrospinal processes underlying counterirritation analgesia. *Journal of Neuroscience*, *29*(45), 14236–14246.

Piercy, K. L., Troiano, R. P., Ballard, R. M., Carlson, S. A., Fulton, J. E., Galuska, D. A., … Olson, R. D. (2018). The physical activity guidelines for Americans. *Journal of the American Medical Association*, *320*(19), 2020–2028.

Pierewan, A. C., & Tampubolon, G. (2015). Happiness and health in Europe: A multivariate multilevel model. *Applied Research in Quality of Life*, *10*(2), 237–252.

Pignone, M., DeWalt, D. A., Sheridan, S., Berkman, N., & Lohr, K. N. (2005). Interventions to improve health outcomes for patients with low literacy: A systematic review. *Journal of General Internal Medicine*, *20*(2), 185–192.

Pila, E., Murray, S. B., Le Grange, D., Sawyer, S. M., & Hughes, E. K. (2019). Reciprocal relations between dietary restraint and negative affect in adolescents receiving treatment for anorexia nervosa. *Journal of Abnormal Psychology*, *128*(2), 129.

Pischon, T., Boeing, H., Hoffmann, K., Bergmann, M., Schulze, M. B., Overvad, K., … Riboli, E. (2008). General and abdominal adiposity and risk of death in Europe. *New England Journal of Medicine*, *359*(20), 2105–2120. doi: 10.1056/NEJMoa0801891

Plomin, R., DeFries, J. C., & McClearn, G. E. (1990). *Behavioral genetics: A primer*. (2nd rev. ed.). New York, NY: W. H. Freeman.

Pogue, D. (2015). You: By the numbers: Can personal fitness monitors whip us—and health research—Into shape? *Scientific American*, *312*(1), 31.

Polivy, J., & Herman, C. P. (2002). If at first you don't succeed: False hopes of self-change. *American Psychologist*, *57*(9), 677–689.

Polk, D. E., Cohen, S., Doyle, W. J., Skoner, D. P., & Kirschbaum, C. (2005). State and trait affect as predictors of salivary cortisol in healthy adults. *Psychoneuroendocrinology*, *30*(3), 261–272.

Poll, M. (2018). *12/20: Being a Better Person & Weight Loss Top 2018 New Year's Resolutions*. Retrieved from http://maristpoll.marist.edu/1220-being-a-better-person-weight-loss-top-2018-new-years-resolutions/#sthash.8OW7YCY4.dpbs

Pollack, A. (2013, June 18). A.M.A. recognizes obesity as a disease. *New York Times*. Retrieved from http://www.nytimes.com/2013/06/19/business/ama-recognizes-obesity-as-a-disease.html

Pollatos, O., Georgiou, E., Kobel, S., Schreiber, A., Dreyhaupt, J., & Steinacker, J. M. (2020). Trait-based emotional intelligence, body image dissatisfaction, and HRQoL in children. *Frontiers in Psychiatry*, *10*, 973.

Pollatos, O., & Herbert, B. M. (2018). Interoception: Definitions, dimensions, neural substrates. In *Embodiment in psychotherapy* (pp. 15–27). London, UK: Springer.

Polman, R., Borkoles, E., & Nicholls, A. R. (2010). Type D personality, stress, and symptoms of burnout: The influence of avoidance coping and social support. *British Journal of Health Psychology*, *15*(3), 681–696.

Pomery, E. A., Gibbons, F. X., Reis-Bergan, M., & Gerrard, M. (2009). From willingness to intention: Experience moderates the shift from reactive to reasoned behavior. *Personality and Social Psychology Bulletin*, *35*(7), 894–908.

Pompili, M., Girardi, P., Tatarelli, G., Ruberto, A., & Tatarelli, R. (2006). Suicide and attempted suicide in eating disorders, obesity and weight–image concern. *Eating Behaviors*, *7*(4), 384–394.

Poobalan, A. S., Bruce, J., Smith, W. C. S., King, P. M., Krukowski, Z. H., & Chambers, W. A. (2003). A review of chronic pain after inguinal herniorrhaphy. *Clinical Journal of Pain*, *19*(1), 48–54.

Pope, H. G., Jr., Gruber, A. J., Choi, P., Olivardia, R., & Phillips, K. A. (1997). Muscle dysmorphia: An under-recognized form of body dysmorphic disorder. *Psychosomatics*, *38*(6), 548–557.

Popescu, I., Duffy, E., Mendelsohn, J., Escarce, J. J. (2018). Racial residential segregation, socioeconomic disparities, and the White-Black survival gap. *PLoS ONE*, *13*(2): e0193222. https://doi.org/10.1371/journal.pone.0193222

Potente, S., Coppa, K., Williams, A., & Engels, R. (2011). Legally brown: Using ethnographic methods to understand sun protection attitudes and behaviours among young Australians "I didn't mean to get burnt—It just happened!" *Health Education Research*, *26*(1), 39–52.

Poulter, H., Eberhardt, J., Moore, H., & Windgassen, S. (2023). "Bottom of the Pile": Health behaviors within the context of in-work poverty in North East England. *Journal of Poverty*, *27*(3), 197–216.

Powell, D. J., Liossi, C., Moss-Morris, R., & Schlotz, W. (2013). Unstimulated cortisol secretory activity in everyday life and its relationship with fatigue and chronic fatigue syndrome: A systematic review and subset meta-analysis. *Psychoneuroendocrinology*, *38*(11), 2405–2422.

Powell, L. M., Szczypka, G., & Chaloupka, F. J. (2010). Trends in exposure to television food advertisements among children and adolescents in the United States. *Archives of Pediatrics & Adolescent Medicine*, *164*(9), 794–802.

Power, T. G. (2004). Stress and coping in childhood: The parents' role. *Parenting: Science and Practice, 4*(4), 271–317.

Power, M. L., & Schulkin, J. (2008). Sex differences in fat storage, fat metabolism, and the health risks from obesity: Possible evolutionary origins. *British Journal of Nutrition*, *99*(5), 931–940.

Pressman, S. D., & Cohen, S. (2005). Does positive affect influence health? *Psychological Bulletin*, *131*(6), 925.

Pressman, S. D., Jenkins, B. N., & Moskowitz, J. T. (2019). Positive affect and health: What do we know and where next should we go? *Annual Review of Psychology*, *70*, 627–650.

Prince, D. M., Epstein, M., Nurius, P. S., Gorman-Smith, D., & Henry, D. B. (2019). Reciprocal effects of positive future expectations, threats to safety, and risk behavior across adolescence. *Journal of Clinical Child and Adolescent Psychology*, *48*(1), 54–67.

Prochaska, J. O. (1994). Strong and weak principles for progressing from precontemplation to action on the basis of twelve problem behaviors. *Health Psychology*, *13*(1), 47–51.

Prochaska, J. O., DiClemente, C. C., & Norcross, J. C. (1992). In search of how people change: Applications to addictive behaviors. *American Psychologist*, *47*, 1102–1114.

Prochaska, J. O., Johnson, S., & Lee, P. (2009). The transtheoretical model of behavior change. In S. A. Shumaker, J. K. Ockene, & K. A. Riekert (Eds.), *The handbook of health behavior change* (3rd ed., pp. 59–83). New York, NY: Springer.

Prochaska, J. O., Velicer, W. F., Rossi, J. S., Goldstein, M. G., Marcus, B. H., Rakowski, W., … Rosenbloom, D. (1994). Stages of change and decisional balance for 12 problem behaviors. *Health Psychology*, *13*(1), 39–46.

Proyer, R. T., Gander, F., Bertenshaw, E. J., & Brauer, K. (2018). The positive relationships of playfulness with indicators of health, activity, and physical fitness. *Frontiers in Psychology*, *9*, 1440.

Pruitt, S. L., Lee, S. J., Tiro, J. A., Xuan, L., Ruiz, J. M., & Inrig, S. (2015). Residential racial segregation and mortality among black, white, and Hispanic urban breast cancer patients in Texas, 1995 to 2009. *Cancer*, *121*(11), 1845–1855.

Psarra, E., & Kleftaras, G. (2013). Adaptation to physical disabilities: The role of meaning in life and depression. *European Journal of Counselling Psychology*, *2*(1), 79–99.

PTSD: National Center for PTSD. (2016). How common is PTSD? Retrieved from https://www.ptsd.va.gov/understand/common/common_veterans.asp

Puhl, R. M., & Latner, J. D. (2007). Stigma, obesity, and the health of the nation's children. *Psychological Bulletin*, *133*(4), 557–580.

Pulice-Farrow, L., McNary, S. B., & Galupo, M. P. (2019). "Bigender is just a Tumblr thing": Microaggressions in the romantic relationships of gender non-conforming and agender transgender individuals. *Sexual and Relationship Therapy*. Advance online publication. doi: 10.1080/14681994.2018.1533245

Pulkki-Råback, L., Elovainio, M., Kivimäki, M., Mattsson, N., Raitakari, O. T., Puttonen, S., … Keltikangas-Järvinen,

L. (2009). Depressive symptoms and the metabolic syndrome in childhood and adulthood: A prospective cohort study. *Health Psychology, 28*(1), 108–116.

Purba, A. K., Thomson, R. M., Henery, P. M., Pearce, A., Henderson, M., Katikireddi, S. V., et al. (2023). Social media use and health risk behaviours in young people: Systematic review and meta-analysis. *BMJ, 383*, e073552. doi: 10.1136/bmj-2022-073552

Purchiaroni, F., Tortora, A., Gabrielli, M., Bertucci, F., Gigante, G., Ianiro, G., … Gasbarrini, A. (2013). The role of intestinal microbiota and the immune system. *European Review for Medical and Pharmacological Science, 17*(3), 323–333.

Qualls, S. H., & Kasl-Godley, J. E. (2011). *End-of-life issues, grief, and bereavement: What clinicians need to know.* Hoboken, NJ: Wiley.

Quick, J. C., Quick, J. D., Nelson, D. L., & Hurrell, J. J., Jr. (1997). *Preventive stress management in organizations.* Washington, DC: American Psychological Association.

Quigley, E. (2018). The gut-brain axis and the microbiome: Clues to pathophysiology and opportunities for novel management strategies in irritable bowel syndrome (IBS). *Journal of Clinical Medicine, 7*(1), 6.

Quinn, H. R., Matsumoto, I., Callaghan, P. D., Long, L. E., Arnold, J. C., Gunasekaran, N., … McGregor, I. S. (2008). Adolescent rats find repeated Delta(9)-THC less aversive than adult rats but display greater residual cognitive deficits and changes in hippocampal protein expression following exposure. *Neuropsychopharmacology, 33*(5), 1113–1126.

Quintanilla-Dieck, M. J., & Bichakjian, C. K. (2019). Management of early-stage melanoma. *Facial Plastic Surgery Clinics, 27*(1), 35–42.

Ragnarsson, A., Townsend, L., Thorson, A., Chopra, M., & Ekström, A. M. (2009). Social networks and concurrent sexual relationships–A qualitative study among men in an urban South African community. *AIDS Care, 21*(10), 1253–1258.

Räikkönen, K., Matthews, K. A., & Kuller, L. H. (2002). The relationship between psychological risk attributes and the metabolic syndrome in healthy women: Antecedent or consequence? *Metabolism, 51*(12), 1573–1577.

Räikkönen, K., Matthews, K. A., & Kuller, L. H. (2007). Depressive symptoms and stressful life events predict metabolic syndrome among middle-aged women: A comparison of World Health Organization, Adult Treatment Panel III, and International Diabetes Foundation definitions. *Diabetes Care, 30*(4), 872–877.

Raine, L. B., Kao, S. C., Pindus, D., Westfall, D. R., Shigeta, T. T., Logan, N., … Hillman, C. H. (2018). A large-scale reanalysis of childhood fitness and inhibitory control. *Journal of Cognitive Enhancement, 2*(2), 170–192. doi: 10.1007/s41465-018-0070-7

Raje, P., Ning, S., Branson, C., Saint-Hilaire, M., de Leon, M. P., & Hohler, A. D. (2019). Self-reported exercise trends in Parkinson's disease patients. *Complementary Therapies in Medicine, 42*, 37–41.

Rajkumar, R. P. (2021). The relationship between measures of individualism and collectivism and the impact of COVID-19 across nations. *Public Health in Practice, 2*, 100143. doi: 10.1016/j.puhip.2021.100143

Ramachandran, V. S., & Rogers-Ramachandran, D. (1996). Synaesthesia in phantom limbs induced with mirrors. *Proceedings of the Royal Society of London B: Biological Sciences, 263*(1369), 377–386.

Ramachandran, V. S., Rogers-Ramachandran, D., & Cobb, S. (1995). Touching the phantom limb. *Nature, 377*(6549), 489–490.

Ramana, R., Paykel, E. S., Cooper, Z., Hayhurst, H., Saxty, M., & Surtees, P. G. (1995). Remission and relapse in major depression: A two-year prospective follow-up study. *Psychological Medicine, 25*(6), 1161–1170.

Ramírez García, J. I. (2019). Integrating Latina/o ethnic determinants of health in research to promote population health and reduce health disparities. *Cultural Diversity and Ethnic Minority Psychology, 25*(1), 21.

Ramírez-Maestre, C., Esteve, R., & López, A. E. (2012). The role of optimism and pessimism in chronic pain patients adjustment. *Spanish Journal of Psychology, 15*(1), 286–294.

Rana, M. S., Asghar, R. J., Usman, M., Ikram, A., Salman, M., Umair, M., … Ullah, N. (2022). The resurgence of wild poliovirus in Pakistan and Afghanistan: A new setback for polio eradication. *The Journal of Infection, 85*(3), 334.

Rapoff, M. A., & Christophersen, E. R. (1982). Compliance of pediatric patients with medical regimens: A review and evaluation. In R. B. Stuart (Ed.), *Adherence, compliance, and generalization in behavioral medicine* (pp. 79–124). New York, NY: Brunner/Mazel.

Rasmussen, L. J. H., Moffitt, T. E., Eugen-Olsen, J., Belsky, D. W., Danese, A., Harrington, H., … Caspi, A. (2019). Cumulative childhood risk is associated with a new measure of chronic inflammation in adulthood. *Journal of Child Psychology and Psychiatry, 60*(2), 199–208.

Ravary, A., Baldwin, M. W., & Bartz, J. A. (2019). Shaping the body politic: Mass media fat-shaming affects implicit anti-fat attitudes. *Personality and Social Psychology Bulletin, 45*(11), 1580–1589.

Rebuffé-Scrive, M., Walsh, U. A., McEwen, B. S., & Rodin, J. (1992). Effect of chronic stress and exogenous glucocorticoids on regional fat distribution and metabolism. *Physiology and Behavior, 52*(3), 583–590.

Reifman, A., Luckow, A., & McIntosh, D. N. (1998, August). *Gender differences in coping: A meta-analysis.* Poster presented at the 106th annual convention of the American Psychological Association, San Francisco.

Reinarman, C., Nunberg, H., Lanthier, F., & Heddleston, T. (2011). Who are medical marijuana patients? Population characteristics from nine California assessment clinics. *Journal of Psychoactive Drugs, 43*(2), 128–135.

Reiss, S., Peterson, R. A., Gursky, D. M., & McNally, R. J. (1986). Anxiety sensitivity, anxiety frequency and the prediction of fearfulness. *Behaviour Research and Therapy, 24*(1), 1–8.

Reitsma, M. B., et al. (2021). Spatial, temporal, and demographic patterns in prevalence of smoking tobacco use and attributable disease burden in 204 countries and territories, 1990–2019: A systematic analysis from the Global Burden of Disease Study 2019. *Lancet, 397*, 2337–2360.

Reniers, G., & Watkins, S. (2010). Polygyny and the spread of HIV in sub-Saharan Africa: A case of benign concurrency. *AIDS, 24*(2), 299–307. doi: 10.1097/QAD.0b013e328333af03

Renner, M. J., & Mackin, R. S. (1998). A life stress instrument for classroom use. *Teaching of Psychology, 25*(1), 46–48.

Rew, L., Arheart, K. L., Horner, S. D., Thompson, S., & Johnson, K. E. (2015). Gender and ethnic differences in healthpromoting behaviors of rural adolescents. *Journal of School Nursing, 31*(3), 219–232.

Rhodes, R. E., Blanchard, C. M., Benoit, C., Levy-Milne, R., Naylor, P. J., Downs, D. S., & Warburton, D. E. (2014). Physical activity and sedentary behavior across 12 months in cohort samples of couples without children, expecting their first child, and expecting their second child. *Journal of Behavioral Medicine, 37*(3), 533–542.

Richman, J. (1995). The lifesaving function of humor with the depressed and suicidal elderly. *Gerontologist, 35*(2), 271–273.

Ridberg, R. A., Bell, J. F., Merritt, K. E., Harris, D. M., Young, H. M., Tancredi, D. J. (2019). Effect of a fruit and vegetable prescription program on children's fruit and vegetable consumption. *Preventing Chronic Disease, 16*(6), E73.

Ridley, N. J., Draper, B., & Withall, A. (2013). Alcohol-related dementia: An update of the evidence. *Alzheimer's Research and Therapy, 5*(1), 3. doi: 10.1186/alzrt157

Rietveld, S., & Brosschot, J. F. (1999). Current perspectives on symptom perception in asthma: A biomedical and psychological review. *International Journal of Behavioral Medicine, 6*(2), 120–134.

Rikard, S. M., Strahan, A. E., Schmit, K. M., Guy, G. P. Jr. (2023). Chronic pain among adults — United States, 2019–2021. *MMWR Morbidity and Mortality Weekly Report, 72*, 379–385. doi: 10.15585/mmwr.mm7215a1

Rios, R., & Zautra, A. J. (2011). Socioeconomic disparities in pain: The role of economic hardship and daily financial worry. *Health Psychology, 30*(1), 58–66.

Rippentrop, A. E. (2005). A review of the role of religion and spirituality in chronic pain populations. *Rehabilitation Psychology, 50*(3), 278–284.

Ritner, R. K. (2001). Medicine. In D. B. Redford (Ed.), *The Oxford encyclopedia of ancient Egypt.* New York, NY: Oxford University Press. Retrieved from http://www.oxfordreference.com/view/10.1093/acref/9780195102345.001.0001/acref-9780195102345-e-0437?rskey=nwsUYs&result=431

Robinson, M. E., Gagnon, C. M., Riley, J. L., & Price, D. D. (2003). Altering gender role expectations: Effects on pain tolerance, pain threshold, and pain ratings. *Journal of Pain, 4*(5), 284–288.

Roddenberry, A., & Renk, K. (2010). Locus of control and selfefficacy: Potential mediators of stress, illness, and utilization of health services in college students. *Child Psychiatry and Human Development, 41*, 353–370.

Rodin, J. (1981). Current status of the internal-external hypothesis for obesity. *American Psychologist, 36*, 361–372.

Rodin, J., Elias, M., Silberstein, L. R., & Wagner, A. (1988). Combined behavioral and pharmacologic treatment for obesity: Predictors of successful weight maintenance. *Journal of Consulting and Clinical Psychology, 56*(3), 399–404. doi: 10.1037/0022-006X.56.3.399

Rodriguez, L. M., Litt, D. M., & Stewart, S. H. (2020). Drinking to cope with the pandemic: The unique associations of COVID-19-related perceived threat and psychological distress to drinking behaviors in American men and women. *Addictive Behaviors, 110*, 106532.

Rodríguez-Alba, J. C., Abrego-Peredo, A., Gallardo-Hernández, C., Pérez-Lara, J., Santiago-Cruz, W., Jiang, W., & Espinosa, E. (2019). HIV disease progression: Overexpression of the ectoenzyme CD38 as a contributory factor? *BioEssays, 41*(1), 1800128.

Rodriguez-Miguelez, P., Heefner, A., & Carbone, S. (2023). Recognizing risk factors associated with poor outcomes among patients with COVID-19. *Progress in Cardiovascular Diseases, 76*, 3–11.

Roelofs, K. (2018). Neuro-endocrine control mechanisms in social motivational actions, relevance for social psychopathologies. *European Neuropsychopharmacology, 28*, S62.

Roesch, S. C., Wee, C., & Vaughn, A. A. (2006). Relations between the Big Five personality traits and dispositional coping in Korean Americans: Acculturation as a moderating factor. *International Journal of Psychology, 41*(2), 85–96.

Roland, A. (1989). *In search of self in India and Japan: Toward a cross-cultural psychology.* Princeton, NJ: Princeton University Press.

Rollins, B. Y., Loken, E., Savage, J. S., & Birch, L. L. (2014). Effects of restriction on children's intake differ by child temperament, food reinforcement, and parent's chronic use of restriction. *Appetite, 73*, 31–39.

Rollman, B. L., Belnap, B. H., LeMenager, M. S., Mazumdar, S., Houck, P. R., Counihan, P. J., … Reynolds, C. F., III. (2009). Telephone-delivered collaborative care for treating post-CABG depression: A randomized controlled trial. *JAMA, 302*(19), 2095–2103.

Romer, A. L., Kang, M. S., Nikolova, Y. S., Gearhardt, A. N., & Hariri, A. R. (2019). Dopamine genetic risk is related to food addiction and body mass through reduced reward-related ventral striatum activity. *Appetite, 133*, 24–31.

Rose, N. R. (2016). Prediction and prevention of autoimmune disease in the 21st century: A review and preview. *American Journal of Epidemiology, 183*(5), 403–406. doi: 10.1093/aje/kwv292

Rosenblatt, A., Greenberg, J., Solomon, S., Pyszczynski, T., & Lyon, D. (1989). Evidence for terror management theory: I. The effects of mortality salience on reactions to those who violate or uphold cultural values. *Journal of Personality and Social Psychology, 57*(4), 681–690.

Rosengard, C., Adler, N. E., Gurvey, J. E., Dunlop, M. B., Tschann, J. M., Millstein, S. G., & Ellen, J. M. (2001). Protective role of health values in adolescents' future intentions to use condoms. *Journal of Adolescent Health, 29*(3), 200–207.

Rosenstock, I. M. (1966). Why people use health services. *Milbank Memorial Fund Quarterly, 44*(3, Suppl.), 94–127.

Rosenthal, D. (1970). *Genetic theory and abnormal behavior.* New York: McGraw-Hill.

Rosenthal, T., Touyz, R. M., & Oparil, S. (2022). Migrating populations and health: risk factors for cardiovascular disease and metabolic syndrome. *Current Hypertension Reports, 24*(9), 325–340.

Rote, S., Angel, J. L., Markides, K. S., & Hill, T. D. (2019). Neighborhood cohesion and caregiver well-being among the Mexican-origin population. In *Contextualizing health and aging in the americas* (pp. 295–310). Springer, Cham.

Rotter, J. B. (1966). Generalized expectancies for internal versus external control of reinforcement. *Psychological Monographs: General and Applied, 80*(1), 1–28.

Rowe, J. W., & Kahn, R. L. (1997). Successful aging. *The Gerontologist, 37*(4), 433–440.

Roy, C., & Andrews, H. A. (1999). *The Roy adaptation model* (2nd ed.). Stamford, CT: Appleton & Lange.

Rubin, G. J., Cleare, A., & Hotopf, M. (2004). Psychological factors in postoperative fatigue. *Psychosomatic Medicine, 66*(6), 959–964.

Rubino, T., Realini, N., Braida, D., Guidi, S., Capurro, V., Viganò, D., … Parolaro, D. (2009). Changes in hippocampal morphology and neuroplasticity induced by adolescent THC treatment are associate with cognitive impairment in adulthood. *Hippocampus, 19*(8), 763–772.

Ruckenstein, M., & Pantzar, M. (2017). Beyond the quantified self: Thematic exploration of a dataistic paradigm. *New Media and Society, 19*(3), 401–418.

Rudd, R. E. (2007). Health literacy skills of US adults. *American Journal of Health Behavior, 31*(1), S8–S18.

Rudert, S. C., Reutner, L., Walker, M., & Greifeneder, R. (2015). An unscathed past in the face of death: Mortality salience reduces individuals' regrets. *Journal of Experimental Social Psychology, 58*, 34–41.

Ruini, C., & Fava, G. A. (2009). Well-being therapy for generalized anxiety disorder. *Journal of Clinical Psychology, 65*(5), 510–519.

Ruini, C., & Vescovelli, F. (2013). The role of gratitude in breast cancer: Its relationships with post-traumatic growth, psychological well-being and distress. *Journal of Happiness Studies, 14*(1), 263–274.

Ruiz-Gallardo, J. R., González-Geraldo, J. L., & Castaño, S. (2016). What are our students doing? Workload, time allocation and time management in PBL instruction: A case study in science education. *Teaching and Teacher Education, 53*, 51–62.

Rumsfeld, J. S., & Ho, P. M. (2005). Depression and cardiovascular disease: A call for recognition. *Circulation, 111*(3), 250–253.

Rumsfeld, J. S., Magid, D. J., Plomondon, M. E., Sales, A. E., Grunwald, G. K., Every, N. R., & Spertus, J. A. (2003). History of depression, angina, and quality of life after acute coronary syndromes. *American Heart Journal, 145*(3), 493–499.

Russell, J. (2014, June 17). "Pink slime" is making a comeback. Do you have a beef with that? *All Things Considered*, National Public Radio. Retrieved from http://www.npr.org/sections/thesalt/2014/06/17/322911060/pink-slime-is-making-a-comeback-do-you-have-a-beef-with-that

Russell, C. G., & Worsley, A. (2008). A population-based study of preschoolers' food neophobia and its associations with food preferences. *Journal of Nutrition Education and Behavior*, *40*(1), 11–19. doi: 10.1016/j.jneb.2007.03.007

Russo, E. B. (2004). Clinical endocannabinoid deficiency (CECD): Can this concept explain therapeutic benefits of cannabis in migraine, fibromyalgia, irritable bowel syndrome and other treatment-resistant conditions? *Neuroendocrinology Letters*, *25*(1–2), 31–39.

Ryan, R. M., & Deci, E. L. (2001). On happiness and human potentials: A review of research on hedonic and eudaimonic well-being. *Annual Review of Psychology*, *52*(1), 141–166.

Ryan, R., & Travis, J. W. (1981). *The wellness workbook*. Berkeley, CA: Ten Speed Press.

Ryff, C. D. (2013). Eudaimonic well-being and health: Mapping consequences of self-realization. In A. S. Waterman (Ed.), *The best within us: Positive psychology perspectives on eudaimonia* (pp. 77–98). Washington, DC: American Psychological Association.

Ryff, C. D. (2014). Psychological well-being revisited: Advances in the science and practice of eudaimonia. *Psychotherapy and Psychosomatics*, *83*(1), 10–28.

Rzeszutek, M., & Gruszczyń´ska, E. (2019). Positive and negative affect change among people living with HIV: A one-year prospective study. *International Journal of Behavioral Medicine*, *26*(1), 28–37. doi: 10.1007/s12529-018-9741-0

Saad, L. (2023). Grassroots Support for legalizing Marijuana hits Record 70%. Retrieved from https://news.gallup.com/poll/514007/grassroots-support-legalizing-marijuana-hits-record.aspx

Sachs, J. D. (2019). Introduction to the 2019 global happiness and wellbeing policy report. *Global happiness and wellbeing*. Global Happiness Council.

Sackett, D. L., Rosenberg, W. M., Gray, J. A., Haynes, R. B., & Richardson, W. S. (1996). Evidence based medicine: What it is and what it isn't. *BMJ*, *312*(7023), 71–72.

Safford, S. M., Alloy, L. B., Abramson, L. Y., & Crossfield, A. G. (2007). Negative cognitive style as a predictor of negative life events in depression-prone individuals: A test of the stress generation hypothesis. *Journal of Affective Disorders*, *99*(1–3), 147–154.

Sajjad, M., Bhatti, A., Hill, B., & Al-Omari, B. (2023). Using the theory of planned behavior to predict factors influencing fast-food consumption among college students. *BMC Public Health*, *23*(1), 987.

Saklayen, M. G. (2018). The global epidemic of the metabolic syndrome. *Current Hypertension Reports*, *20*(2), 12.

Saletin, J. M., Goldstein, A. N., & Walker, M. P. (2011). The role of sleep in directed forgetting and remembering of human memories. *Cerebral Cortex*, *21*(11), 2534–2541.

Sallis, J. F., Alcaraz, J. E., McKenzie, T. L., Hovell, M. F., Kolody, B., & Nader, P. R. (1992). Parental behavior in relation to physical activity and fitness in 9-year-old children. *American Journal of Diseases of Children*, *146*(11), 1383–1388.

Sallis, J. F., & Howell, M. F. (1990). Determinants of exercise behavior. *Exercise and Sport Sciences Review*, *18*, 307–330.

Salmon, J., Owen, N., Crawford, D., Bauman, A., & Sallis, J. F. (2003). Physical activity and sedentary behavior: A populationbased study of barriers, enjoyment, and preference. *Health Psychology*, *22*(2), 178–188.

Salovey, P., Mayer, J. D., Goldman, S. L., Turvey, C., Palfai, T. P. (1995). Emotional attention, clarity, and repair: Exploring emotional intelligence using the Trait Meta-Mood Scale. In J. W. Pennebaker, (Ed.), *Emotion, disclosure and health* (pp. 125–154). Washington, DC, USA: American Psychological Association.

Salvy, S.-J., de la Haye, K., Bowker, J. C., & Hermans, R. C. J. (2012). Influence of peers and friends on children's and adolescents' eating and activity behaviors. *Physiology & Behavior*, *106*(3), 369–378. doi: 10.1016/j.physbeh.2012.03.022

San, L., & Arranz, B. (2024). The night and day challenge of sleep disorders and insomnia: A narrative review. *Actas Españolas de Psiquiatría*, *52*(1), 45–56.

Sandroff, B. M., Pilutti, L. A., & Motl, R. W. (2019). Cardiorespiratory fitness and cognitive processing speed in multiple sclerosis: The possible roles of psychological symptoms. *Multiple Sclerosis and Related Disorders*, *27*, 23–29.

Sanz, M., Ceriello, A., Buysschaert, M., Chapple, I., Demmer, R. T., Graziani, F., … Vegh, D. (2018). Scientific evidence on the links between periodontal diseases and diabetes: Consensus report and guidelines of the joint workshop on periodontal diseases and diabetes by the International Diabetes Federation and the European Federation of Periodontology. *Diabetes Research and Clinical Practice*, *137*, 231–241.

Sanz, M., Marco del Castillo, A., Jepsen, S., Gonzalez-Juanatey, J. R., D'Aiuto, F., Bouchard, P., … Wimmer, G. (2020). Periodontitis and cardiovascular diseases: Consensus report. *Journal of Clinical Periodontology*, *47*(3), 268–288.

Sarafino, E. P., & Smith, T. W. (2011). *Health psychology: Biopsychosocial interactions* (7th ed.). New York, NY: Wiley.

Sarason, I. G., Johnson, J. H., & Siegel, J. M. (1978). Assessing the impact of life changes: Development of the Life Experiences Survey. *Journal of Consulting and Clinical Psychology*, *46*, 932–946.

Sarkar, S., & Mukhopadhyay, B. (2008). Perceived psychosocial stress and cardiovascular risk: Observations among the Bhutias of Sikkim, India. *Stress and Health*, *24*(1), 23–34.

Sata, F. (2019). Developmental origins of health and disease (DOHaD) cohorts and interventions: Status and perspective. In *Pre-emptive medicine: Public health aspects of developmental origins of health and disease* (pp. 53–70). Singapore: Springer.

Sato, F., Maeda, N., Yamada, T., Namazui, H., Fukuda, S., Natsukawa, T., … Obata, Y. (2018). Association of epicardial, visceral, and subcutaneous fat with cardiometabolic diseases. *Circulation Journal*, *82*(2), 502–508.

Sato, R., & von Haehling, S. (2023). Revisiting the obesity paradox in heart failure: What is the best anthropometric index to gauge obesity?. *European Heart Journal*, *44*(13), 1154–1156.

Saver, J. L. (2006). Time is brain—Quantified. *Stroke*, *37*(1), 263–266.

Sawyer, B., & Cox, C. (2018, December). How does health spending in the U.S. compare to other countries? *Peterson-Kaiser Health System Tracker*. Retrieved from https://www.healthsystemtracker.org/chart-collection/health-spending-u-s-compare-countries/#item-start

Saxe-Custack, A., LaChance, J., & Kerver, J. M. (2024). A fresh fruit and vegetable prescription program for prenatal patients in flint, Michigan: Baseline food security and dietary intake. *Nutrients*, *16*(8), 1234.

Saxena, S., & Orley, J. (1997). Quality of life assessment: The world health organization perspective. *European Psychiatry*, *12*(Suppl. 3), 263s–266s.

Scaglioni, S., Salvioni, M., & Galimberti, C. (2008). Influence of parental attitudes in the development of children's eating behaviour. *British Journal of Nutrition*, *99*(Suppl. 1), S22–S25.

Schachter, S., Goldman, R., & Gordon, A. (1968). Effects of fear, food deprivation, and obesity on eating. *Journal of Personality and Social Psychology*, *10*(2), 91–97.

Scheer, F. A., Morris, C. J., & Shea, S. A. (2013). The internal circadian clock increases hunger and appetite in the evening independent of food intake and other behaviors. *Obesity*, *21*(3), 421–423. doi: 10.1002/oby.20351

Scheier, M. F., & Carver, C. S. (1992). Effects of optimism on psychological and physical well-being: Theoretical overview and empirical update. *Cognitive Therapy and Research*, *16*(2), 201–228.

Scheier, M. F., Carver, C. S., & Bridges, M. W. (1994). Distinguishing optimism from neuroticism (and trait anxiety, self-mastery, and self-esteem): A reevaluation of the Life Orientation Test. *Journal of Personality and Social Psychology*, *67*(6), 1063–1078.

Scheier, M. F., Matthews, K. A., Owens, J. F., Magovern, G. J., Sr., Lefebvre, R. C., Abbott, R. A., & Carver, C. S. (1989). Dispositional optimism and recovery from coronary artery bypass surgery: The beneficial effects on physical and psychological well-being. *Journal of Personality and Social Psychology*, *57*(6), 1024–1040.

Schillinger, D., Bindman, A., Wang, F., Stewart, A., & Piette, J. (2004). Functional health literacy and the quality of physician–patient communication among diabetes patients. *Patient Education and Counseling*, *52*(3), 315–323.

Schmidt, R. A., Genois, R., Jin, J., Vigo, D., Rehm, J., & Rush, B. (2021). The early impact of COVID-19 on the incidence, prevalence, and severity of alcohol use and other drugs: A systematic review. *Drug and Alcohol Dependence*, *228*, 109065. doi: 10.1016/j.drugalcdep.2021.109065

Schneider, S., & Holzwarth, B. (2024). Approaches to eliminating obesogenic environments. In *Handbook of eating disorders and obesity* (pp. 559–565). Berlin, Heidelberg: Springer Berlin Heidelberg.

Schoenborn, C. A. (1986). Health habits of U.S. adults, 1985: The "Alameda 7" revisited. *Public Health Reports*, *101*(6), 571–580.

Schredl, M. (2018). Functions of dreaming. In *Researching dreams* (pp. 175–181). New York, NY: Palgrave Macmillan.

Schulz, R., & Decker, S. (1985). Long-term adjustment to physical disability: The role of social support, perceived control, and self-blame. *Journal of Personality and Social Psychology*, *48*(5), 1162–1172.

Schwartz, B. L., & Krantz, J. H. (2018). *Sensation and perception* (2nd ed.). London, UK: Sage.

Schwartz, J. E., Neale, J., Marco, C., Shiffman, S. S., & Stone, A. A. (1999). Does trait coping exist? A momentary assessment approach to the evaluation of traits. *Journal of Personality and Social Psychology, 77*(2), 360–369.

Scott, K. M., Von Korff, M., Alonso, J., Angermeyer, M. C., Benjet, C., Bruffaerts, R., ... Posada-Villa, J. (2008). Childhood adversity, early-onset depressive/anxiety disorders, and adult-onset asthma. *Psychosomatic Medicine, 70*, 1035–1043.

Scullin, M. K. (2019). The eight hour sleep challenge during final exams week. *Teaching of Psychology, 46(1)*, 55–63.

Seeman, T. E., Singer, B. H., Rowe, J. W., Horwitz, R. I., & McEwen, B. S. (1997). Price of adaptation—Allostatic load and its health consequences. *Archives of Internal Medicine, 157*, 2259–2268.

Segerstrom, S. C. (2007). Stress, energy, and immunity: An ecological view. *Current Directions in Psychological Science, 16*, 326–330.

Segerstrom, S. C., & Miller, G. E. (2004). Psychological stress and the human immune system: A meta-analytic study of 30 years of inquiry. *Psychological Bulletin, 130*(4), 601–630.

Segerstrom, S. C., & Sephton, S. E. (2010). Optimistic expectancies and cell-mediated immunity: The role of positive affect. *Psychological Science, 21*(3), 448–455.

Segrin, C. (2001). Social skills and negative life events: Testing the deficit stress generation hypothesis. *Current Psychology, 20*(1), 19–35.

Seligman, M. E., & Csikszentmihalyi, M. (2000). Positive psychology: An introduction. *American Psychologist, 55*(1), 5–14.

Seller, L., Bouthillier, M. È., & Fraser, V. (2019). Situating requests for medical aid in dying within the broader context of end-of-life care: Ethical considerations. *Journal of Medical Ethics, 45*(2), 106–111.

Selye, H. (1946). The general adaptation syndrome and the diseases of adaptation. *Journal of Clinical Endocrinology and Metabolism, 6*, 117–230.

Selye, H. (1956). *The stress of life.* New York, NY: McGraw-Hill.

Selye, H. (1974). *Stress without distress.* Philadelphia, PA: Lippincott.

Selye, H. (1976). *Stress in health and disease.* Reading, MA: Butterworth.

Selye, H. (1985). History and present status of the stress concept. In A. Monat & R. S. Lazarus (Eds.), *Stress and coping: An anthology* (2nd ed., pp. 17–29). New York, NY: Columbia University Press.

Seo, H. S., Lee, S. K., Nam, S. (2011). Factors influencing fast food consumption behaviors of middle-school students in Seoul: An application of theory of planned behaviors. *Nutrition Research and Practice, 5*(2):169–178.

Serido, J., Almeida, D. M., & Wethington, E. (2004). Chronic stressors and daily hassles: Unique and interactive relationships with psychological distress. *Journal of Health and Social Behavior, 45*, 17–33.

Severeijns, R., Vlaeyen, J. W., van den Hout, M. A., & Picavet, H. S. J. (2004). Pain catastrophizing is associated with health indices in musculoskeletal pain: A cross-sectional study in the Dutch community. *Health Psychology, 23*(1), 49–57.

Severino, A. L., Shadfar, A., Hakimian, J. K., Crane, O., Singh, G., Heinzerling, K., & Walwyn, W. M. (2018). Pain therapy guided by purpose and perspective in light of the opioid epidemic. *Frontiers in Psychiatry, 9*, 119. doi: 10.3389/fpsyt.2018.00119

Shahsavar, Y., Choudhury, A. (2023). User intentions to use ChatGPT for self-diagnosis and health-related purposes: Cross-sectional survey study. *JMIR Human Factors, 10*(1), e47564. Retrieved from https://humanfactors.jmir.org/2023//e47564/

Shaikh, S. S., Chen, Y. C., Halsall, S. A., Nahorski, M. S., Omoto, K., Young, G. T., ... Woods, C. G. (2017). A comprehensive functional analysis of NTRK1 missense mutations causing hereditary sensory and autonomic neuropathy Type IV (HSAN IV). *Human Mutation, 38*(1), 55–63.

Shankar, A., Koh, W. P., Yuan, J. M., Lee, H. P., & Yu, M. C. (2008). Sleep duration and coronary heart disease mortality among Chinese adults in Singapore: A population-based cohort study. *American Journal of Epidemiology, 168*, 1367–1373.

Shapiro, S. L., Lopez, A. M., Schwartz, G. E., Bootzin, R., Figueredo, A. J., Braden, C. J., & Kurker, S. F. (2001). Quality of life and breast cancer: Relationship to psychosocial variables. *Journal of Clinical Psychology, 57*(4), 501–519.

Shapiro, D. H., Jr., Schwartz, C. E., & Astin, J. A. (1996). Controlling ourselves, controlling our world: Psychology's role in understanding positive and negative consequences of seeking and gaining control. *American Psychologist, 51*(12), 1213–1230.

Sharma, R., & Rakshit, B. (2022). Global burden of cancers attributable to tobacco smoking, 1990–2019: An ecological study. *EPMA Journal, 14*, 167–182.

Shatnawi, A., Shafer, A., Ahmed, H., & Elbarbry, F. (2019). Complementary and alternative medicine use in hypertension: The good, the bad, and the ugly: Hypertension treatment from nature–myth or fact? In *Complementary and alternative medicine: Breakthroughs in research and practice* (pp. 61–93). IGI Global.

Shaw, B. A., & Agahi, N. (2012). A prospective cohort study of health behavior profiles after age 50 and mortality risk. *BMC Public Health, 12*, 803. doi: 10.1186/1471-2458-12-803

Shaw, L., Descarreaux, M., Bryans, R., Duranleau, M., Marcoux, H., Potter, B., … White, E. (2010). A systematic review of chiropractic management of adults with whiplash-associated disorders: Recommendations for advancing evidence-based practice and research. *Work, 35*(3), 369–394.

Shaw, L. H., & Gant, L. M. (2002). In defense of the Internet: The relationship between Internet communication and depression, loneliness, self-esteem, and perceived social support. *CyberPsychology and Behavior, 5*(2), 157–171.

Shea, J. L. (2006). Chinese women's symptoms: Relation to menopause, age and related attitudes. *Climacteric, 9*(1), 30–39.

Shearer, C., Rainham, D., Blanchard, C., Dummer, T., Lyons, R., & Kirk, S. (2015). Measuring food availability and accessibility among adolescents: Moving beyond the neighbourhood boundary. *Social Science and Medicine, 133*, 322–330.

Sheikh, A., Rudan, I., Cresswell, K., Dhingra-Kumar, N., Tan, M. L., Häkkinen, M. L., & Donaldson, L. (2019). Agreeing on global research priorities for medication safety: An international prioritization exercise. *Journal of Global Health, 9*(1) 010422.

Sheldon, K. M., Corcoran, M., & Prentice, M. (2019). Pursuing eudaimonic functioning versus pursuing hedonic well-being: The first goal succeeds in its aim, whereas the second does not. *Journal of Happiness Studies, 20*(3), 919–933.

Shen, X. (2020). Constructing an interactionist framework for playfulness research: Adding psychological situations and playful states. *Journal of Leisure Research, 51*(5), 536–558.

Sherman, R. A. (1994). What do we really know about phantom limb pain? *Pain Reviews, 1*(3), 261–274.

Sherman, J. J., LeResche, L., Huggins, K. H., Mancl, L. A., Sage, J. C., & Dworkin, S. F. (2004). The relationship of somatization and depression to experimental pain response in women with temporomandibular disorders. *Psychosomatic Medicine, 66*(6), 852–860.

Sherman, J. J., Turk, D. C., & Okifuji, A. (2000). Prevalence and impact of posttraumatic stress disorder-like symptoms on patients with fibromyalgia syndrome. *Clinical Journal of Pain, 16*(2), 127–134.

Sherwood, A., Smith, P. J., Hinderliter, A. L., Georgiades, A., & Blumenthal, J. A. (2017). Effects of exercise and stress management training on nighttime blood pressure dipping in patients with coronary heart disease: A randomized, controlled trial. *American Heart Journal, 183*, 85–90.

Shiels, M. S., Haque, A. T., Berrington de González, A., Freedman, N. D. (2022). Leading causes of death in the US during the COVID-19 pandemic, March 2020 to October 2021. *JAMA Internal Medicine, 182*(8), 883–886. doi: 10.1001/jamainternmed.2022.2476

Shih, J. H. (2006). Sex differences in stress generation: An examination of sociotropy/autonomy, stress, and depressive symptoms. *Personality and Social Psychology Bulletin, 32*(4), 434–446.

Shimoda, K., & Robinson, R. G. (1999). The relationship between poststroke depression and lesion location in long-term follow-up. *Biological Psychiatry, 45*(2), 187–192.

Shimura, A., Sugiura, K., Inoue, M., Misaki, S., Tanimoto, Y., Oshima, A., … Inoue, T. (2020). Which sleep hygiene factors are important? Comprehensive assessment of lifestyle habits and job environment on sleep among office workers. *Sleep Health, 6*(3), 288–298.

Shoamanesh, A., Preis, S. R., Beiser, A. S., Vasan, R. S., Benjamin, E. J., Kase, C. S., … Seshadri, S. (2015). Inflammatory biomarkers, cerebral microbleeds, and small vessel disease: Framingham Heart Study. *Neurology, 84*(8), 825–832.

Shrestha, S., & Zarit, S. H. (2012). Cultural and contextual analysis of quality of life among older Nepali women. *Journal of Cross-Cultural Gerontology, 27*(2), 163–182.

Shrout, P. E., & Rodgers, J. L. (2018). Psychology, science, and knowledge construction: Broadening perspectives from the replication crisis. *Annual Review of Psychology, 69*, 487–510.

Shumaker, S. A., Ockene, J. K., & Riekert, K. A. (Eds.). (2008). *The handbook of health behavior change* (4th ed.). New York, NY: Springer.

Siahpush, M., Spittal, M., & Singh, G. K. (2008). Happiness and life satisfaction prospectively predict self-rated health, physical health, and the presence of limiting, long-term health conditions. *American Journal of Health Promotion, 23*(1), 18–26.

Sibold, J. S., & Berg, K. M. (2010). Mood enhancement persists for up to 12 hours following aerobic exercise: A pilot study. *Perceptual and Motor Skills, 111*(2), 333–342.

Sibrava, N. J., Bjornsson, A. S., Pérez Benítez, A. C. I., Moitra, E., Weisberg, R. B., & Keller, M. B. (2019). Posttraumatic stress disorder in African American and Latinx adults: Clinical course and the role of racial and ethnic discrimination. *American Psychologist, 74*(1), 101.

Siegel, R. L., Miller, K. D., & Jemal, A. (2019). Cancer statistics, 2019. *CA: A Cancer Journal for Clinicians, 69*(1), 7–34.

Siegler, I. C., Bosworth, H. B., Davey, A., & Elias, M. F. (2012). Disease, health, and aging in the first decade of the 21st century. In R. M. Lerner, M. A. Easterbrooks, J. Mistry, & I. B. Weiner (Eds.), *Handbook of psychology, developmental psychology* (Vol. 6, pp. 437–449). Hoboken, NJ: Wiley.

Sieverding, M., Matterne, U., & Ciccarello, L. (2010). What role do social norms play in the context of men's cancer screening intention and behavior? Application of an extended theory of planned behavior. *Health Psychology, 29*(1), 72–81.

Simons, R. L., Lorenz, F. O., Wu, C., & Conger, R. D. (1993). Social network and marital support as mediators and moderators of the impact of stress and depression on parental behavior. *Developmental Psychology, 29*(2), 368–381.

Sinclair, K. A., Bogart, A., Buchwald, D., & Henderson, J. A. (2011). The prevalence of metabolic syndrome and associated risk factors in Northern Plains and Southwest American Indians. *Diabetes Care, 34*(1), 118–120.

Singh, D. (1993). Adaptive significance of female physical attractiveness: Role of waist-to-hip ratio. *Journal of Personality and Social Psychology, 65*(2), 293–307.

Sivertsen, B., Harvey, A. G., Pallesen, S., & Hysing, M. (2015). Mental health problems in adolescents with delayed sleep phase: Results from a large population-based study in Norway. *Journal of Sleep Research, 24*(1), 11–18.

Skinner, N., & Brewer, N. (2002). The dynamics of threat and challenge appraisals prior to stressful achievement events. *Journal of Personality and Social Psychology, 83*, 678–692.

Skinner, E. A., Edge, K., Altman, J., & Sherwood, H. (2003). Searching for the structure of coping: A review and critique of category systems for classifying ways of coping. *Psychological Bulletin, 129*, 216–269.

Skinner, E. A., & Zimmer-Gembeck, M. J. (2007). The development of coping. *Annual Review of Psychology, 58*, 119–144.

Skogstad, M., Skorstad, M., Lie, A., Conradi, H. S., Heir, T., & Weisæth, L. (2013). Work-related post-traumatic stress disorder. *Occupational Medicine, 63*(3), 175–182.

Slavich, G. M., & Cole, S. W. (2013). The emerging field of human social genomics. *Clinical Psychological Science, 1*(3), 331–348.

Slesnick, N., Kang, M. J., Bonomi, A. E., & Prestopnik, J. L. (2008). Six- and twelve-month outcomes among homeless youth accessing therapy and case management services through an urban drop-in center. *Health Services Research, 43*(1 Pt 1), 211–229.

Smalley, K. B., Warren, J. C., & Barefoot, K. N. (2016). Differences in health risk behaviors across understudied LGBT subgroups. *Health Psychology, 35*(2), 103–114.

Smith, B.W. et al., (2023). The effects of an online positive psychology course on happiness, health, and well-being. *Journal of Happiness Studies, 24*(3), 1145–1167.

Smith, A. A. (2003). Intimacy and family relationships of women with chronic pain. *Pain Management Nursing, 4*(3), 134–142.

Smith, A. W., & Baum, A. (2003). The influence of psychological factors on restorative function in health and illness. In J. Suls & K. A. Wallston (Eds.), *Social psychological foundations of health and illness* (pp. 432–457). Malden, MA: Blackwell.

Smith, M. T., Edwards, R. R., McCann, U. D., & Haythornthwaite, J. A. (2007). The effects of sleep deprivation on pain inhibition and spontaneous pain in women. *Sleep, 30*(4), 494–505.

Smith, A. D., Fildes, A., Cooke, L., Herle, M., Shakeshaaft, N., Plomin, R., & Llewellyn, C. (2016). Genetic and environmental influences on food preferences in adolescence. *American Journal of Clinical Nutrition, 104*(2), 446–453.

Smith, D. M., Loewenstein, G., Jankovic, A., & Ubel, P. A. (2009). Happily hopeless: Adaptation to a permanent, but not to a temporary, disability. *Health Psychology, 28*(6), 787–791.

Smith, T. W., Orleans, C. T., & Jenkins, C. D. (2004). Prevention and health promotion: Decades of progress, new challenges, and an emerging agenda. *Health Psychology, 23*(2), 126–131.

Smith, B. W., Papp, Z. Z., Tooley, E. M., Montague, E. Q., Robinson, A. E., & Cosper, C. J. (2010). Traumatic events, perceived stress and health in women with fibromyalgia and healthy controls. *Stress and Health, 26*(1), 83–93.

Smith, E. R., Perrin, P. B., & Rabinovitch, A. E. (2018). Sexual behavior in sexual minority women and connections with discrimination. *Sexuality Research and Social Policy, 15*(1), 1–11.

Smits, J. A., Berry, A. C., Rosenfield, D., Powers, M. B., Behar, E., & Otto, M. W. (2008). Reducing anxiety sensitivity with exercise. *Depression and Anxiety*, *25*(8), 689–699.

Smits, F., Schutter, D., van Honk, J., & Geuze, E. (2019). Feeling stressed: Are emotional reactions to stress affected by transcranial brain stimulation over the prefrontal cortex? A meta-analysis. *Brain Stimulation: Basic, Translational, and Clinical Research in Neuromodulation*, *12*(2), 456.

Smits, J. A., Tart, C. D., Rosenfield, D., & Zvolensky, M. J. (2011). The interplay between physical activity and anxiety sensitivity in fearful responding to carbon dioxide challenge. *Psychosomatic Medicine*, *73*(6), 498–503.

Snuggs, S., & Harvey, K. (2023). Family mealtimes: A systematic umbrella review of characteristics, correlates, outcomes and interventions. *Nutrients*, *15*(13), 2841.

Snyder, C. R. (2002). Hope theory: Rainbows in the mind. *Psychological Inquiry*, *13*(4), 249–275.

Snyder, F. J., & Flay, B. R. (2012). Brief introduction to the theory of triadic influence. Unpublished manuscript, Oregon State University.

Snyder, C. R., Rand, K. L., & Sigmon, D. R. (2002). Hope theory: A member of the positive psychology family. In C. R. Snyder & S. J. Lopez (Eds.), *Handbook of positive psychology* (pp. 257–276). New York, NY: Oxford University Press.

Södergren, M., Wang, W. C., Salmon, J., Ball, K., Crawford, D., & McNaughton, S. A. (2014). Predicting healthy lifestyle patterns among retirement age older adults in the WELL study: A latent class analysis of sex differences. *Maturitas*, *77*(1), 41–46.

Söderlund, J., Simonsen, J., Alanko, K., & Fagerlund, Å. (2024). Tweens: A positive psychology family intervention for adolescents with depression-or anxiety-related symptomatology. *International Journal of Applied Positive Psychology*, *9*(1), 137–163.

Solomon, J. C. (1996). Humor and aging well. *American Behavioral Scientist*, *39*(3), 249–271.

Solomon, S., & Greenberg, J. (2019). Existential meaning and terror management. In *Oxford Research Encyclopedia of Psychology*, 1–22.

Sompayrac, L. M. (2015). *How the immune system works*. Hoboken, NJ: John Wiley & Sons.

Sonnenberg, G. F., & Artis, D. (2012). Innate lymphoid cell interactions with microbiota: Implications for intestinal health and disease. *Immunity*, *37*(4), 601–610.

Sörensen, J., Rzeszutek, M., & Gasik, R. (2019). Social support and post-traumatic growth among a sample of arthritis patients: Analysis in light of conservation of resources theory. *Current Psychology*. Advance online publication. doi: 10.1007/s12144-019-0131-9

Sorkin, J. D., Muller, D. C., Andres, R. (1999). Longitudinal changes in height of men and women: Implications for interpretation of the Body Mass Index. The Baltimore longitudinal study of aging. *American Journal of Epidemiology*, *50*, 969–977.

Soucier, V. D., Doma, K. M., Farrell, E. L., Leith-Bailey, E. R., & Duncan, A. M. (2019). An examination of food neophobia in older adults. *Food Quality and Preference*, *72*, 143–146.

Southerland, J. L., Slawson, D. L., Pack, R., Sörensen, S., Lyness, J. M., & Hirsch, J. K. (2016). Trait hope and preparation for future care needs among older adult primary care patients. *Clinical Gerontologist*, *39*(2), 117–126.

Speisman, J., Lazarus, R. S., Mordkoff, A., & Davidson, L. (1964). Experimental reduction of stress based on ego-defense theory. *Journal of Abnormal Psychology*, *68*, 367–380.

Spencer, M. B., & Tinsley, B. (2008). Identity as coping: Assessing youths' challenges and opportunities for success. *Prevention Researcher*, *15*(4), 17–21.

Spiegel, K., Leproult, R., & Van Cauter, E. (1999). Impact of sleep debt on metabolic and endocrine function. *Lancet*, *354*(9188), 1435–1439.

Spina, M., Arndt, J., Landau, M. J., & Cameron, L. D. (2018). Enhancing health message framing with metaphor and cultural values: Impact on Latinas' cervical cancer screening, *Annals of Behavioral Medicine*, *52*(2), 106–115. doi: 10.1093/abm/kax009

Sponholtz, T. R., Palmer, J. R., Rosenberg, L., Hatch, E. E., Adams-Campbell, L. L., & Wise, L. A. (2016). Body size, metabolic factors, and risk of endometrial cancer in black women. *American Journal of Epidemiology*, *183*(4), 259–268.

Srinivasan, K., & Joseph, W. (2004). A study of lifetime prevalence of anxiety and depressive disorders in patients presenting with chest pain to emergency medicine. *General Hospital Psychiatry*, *26*(6), 470–474.

Staller, N., & Randler, C. (2021). Chronotype dependent choosiness and mate choice. *Personality and Individual Differences*, *168*, 110375.

Stamatakis, E., Hamer, M., & Dunstan, D. W. (2011). Screen-based entertainment time, all-cause mortality, and cardiovascular events: Population-based study with ongoing mortality and hospital events follow-up.

Journal of the American College of Cardiology, 57(3), 292–299. doi: 10.1016/j.jacc.2010.05.065

Stanton, A. L., & Revenson, T. A. (2011). Adjustment to chronic disease: Progress and promise in research. In H. S. Friedman (Ed.), *The Oxford handbook of health psychology* (pp. 241–268). New York, NY: Oxford University Press.

Stanton, A. L., Revenson, T. A., & Tennen, H. (2007). Health psychology: Psychological adjustment to chronic disease. *Annual Review of Psychology, 58*, 565–592.

Steele, E. M., et al. (2023). Identifying and estimating ultraprocessed food intake in the US NHANES according to the Nova classification system of food processing. *The Journal of Nutrition, 153*(1), 225–241.

Steele, C. M., & Josephs, R. A. (1990). Alcohol myopia: Its prized and dangerous effects. *American Psychologist, 45*(8), 921–933.

Steiger, H., & Bruce, K. R. (2007). Phenotypes, endophenotypes, and genotypes in bulimia spectrum eating disorders. *Canadian Journal of Psychiatry, 52*(4), 220–227.

Steinberg, L. (2008). A social neuroscience perspective on adolescent risk-taking. *Developmental Review, 28*(1), 78–106.

Steinberg, L. (2010). A dual systems model of adolescent risktaking. *Developmental Psychobiology, 52*(3), 216–224. doi: 10.1002/dev.20445

Steinbrook, R. (2006). Message from Toronto— Deliver AIDS treatment and prevention. *New England Journal of Medicine, 355*(11), 1081–1084.

Steingraber, S. (2007). *The falling age of puberty in U.S. girls: What we know, what we need to know.* San Francisco, CA: Breast Cancer Fund.

Steptoe, A. (2019). Happiness and health. *Annual Review of Public Health, 40*, 339–359.

Steptoe, A., & Ayers, S. (2004). Stress, health and illness. In S. Sutton, A. Baum, & M. Johnston (Eds.), *The SAGE handbook of health psychology* (pp. 169–196). Thousand Oaks, CA: Sage.

Steptoe, A., & Cox, S. (1988). Acute effects of aerobic exercise on mood. *Health Psychology, 7*(4), 329–340.

Steptoe, A., & Wardle, J. (2004). Health-related behavior: Prevalence and links with disease. In A. Kaptein & J. Weinmen (Eds.), *Health psychology* (pp. 21–51). Oxford, UK: British Psychological Society/Blackwell.

Steptoe, A., & Wardle, J. (2011). Positive affect measured using ecological momentary assessment and survival in older men and women. *Proceedings of the National Academy of Sciences, 108*(45), 18244–18248.

Sterling, P., & Eyer, J. (1988). Allostasis: A new paradigm to explain arousal pathology. In S. Fisher & J. Reason (Eds.), *Handbook of life stress, cognition, and health* (pp. 629–649). Oxford, UK: Wiley.

Stevens, B. S., Royal, K. D., Ferris, K., Taylor, A., & Snyder, A. M. (2019). Effect of a mindfulness exercise on stress in veterinary students performing surgery. *Veterinary Surgery, 48*(3), 360–366.

Stewart, T. (2023, April). Overview of motor vehicle traffic crashes in 2021 (Report No. DOT HS 813 435). National Highway Traffic Safety Administration.

Stewart, A. L., Hays, R. D., & Ware, J. E., Jr. (1988). The MOS short-form general health survey: Reliability and validity in a patient population. *Medical Care, 26*(7), 724–735.

Stewart, R., Masaki, K., Xue, Q. L., Peila, R., Petrovitch, H., White, L. R., & Launer, L. J. (2005). A 32-year prospective study of change in body weight and incident dementia: The Honolulu-Asia Aging Study. *Archives of Neurology, 62*, 55–60.

Stice, E. (1994). Review of the evidence for a sociocultural model of bulimia nervosa and an exploration of the mechanisms of action. *Clinical Psychology Review, 14*, 633–661.

Stice, E. (2001). A prospective test of the dual-pathway model of bulimic pathology: Mediating effects of dieting and negative affect. *Journal of Abnormal Psychology, 110*, 124–135.

Stice, E., South, K., & Shaw, H. (2012). Future directions in etiologic, prevention, and treatment research for eating disorders. *Journal of Clinical Child & Adolescent Psychology, 41*(6), 845–855.

Stice, E., & Van Ryzin, M. J. (2019). A prospective test of the temporal sequencing of risk factor emergence in the dual pathway model of eating disorders. *Journal of Abnormal Psychology, 128*(2), 119.

Stice, E., Yokum, S., Blum, K., & Bohon, C. (2010). Weight gain is associated with reduced striatal response to palatable food. *Journal of Neuroscience, 30*(39), 13105–13109.

Stich, C., Knauper, B., & Tint, A. (2009). A scenario-based dieting self-efficacy scale: The DIET-SE. *Assessment, 16*(1), 16–30.

Stilley, C. S., Bender, C. M., Dunbar-Jacob, J., Sereika, S., & Ryan, C. M. (2010). The impact of cognitive function on medication management: Three studies. *Health Psychology, 29*(1), 50–55.

Stone, A. A., & Neale, J. M. (1984). New measure of daily coping: Development and preliminary results. *Journal of Personality and Social Psychology, 46*(4), 892–906.

Stoner, L., & Cornwall, J. (2014). Did the American Medical Association make the correct decision classifying obesity as a disease? *Australasian Medical Journal*, *7*(11), 462–464. doi: 10.4066/AMJ.2014.2281

Stoppelbein, L. A., Greening, L., & Elkin, T. D. (2006). Risk of posttraumatic stress symptoms: A comparison of child survivors of pediatric cancer and parental bereavement. *Journal of Pediatric Psychology*, *31*(4), 367–376.

Strachan, S. M., Marcotte, M. M. E., Giller, T. M. T., Brunet, J., & Schellenberg, B. J. I. (2017). An online intervention to increase physical activity: Self-regulatory possible selves and the moderating role of task self-efficacy. *Psychology of Sport and Exercise*, *31*, 158–165.

Strine, T. W., Kroenke, K., Dhingra, S., Balluz, L. S., Gonzalez, O., Berry, J. T., & Mokdad, A. H. (2009). The associations between depression, health-related quality of life, social support, life satisfaction, and disability in community-dwelling US adults. *Journal of Nervous and Mental Disease*, *197*(1), 61–64.

Stunkard, A. J., & Messick, S. (1985). The three-factor eating questionnaire to measure dietary restraint, disinhibition and hunger. *Journal of Psychosomatic Research*, *29*(1), 71–83.

Subar, A. F., Heimendinger, J., Patterson, B. H., Krebs-Smith, S. M., Pivonka, E., & Kessler, R. (1995). Fruit and vegetable intake in the United States: The baseline survey of the Five A Day for Better Health Program. *American Journal of Health Promotion*, *9*(5), 352–360.

Substance Abuse and Mental Health Services Administration. (2021). *2021 National Survey on Drug Use and Health (NSDUH) Release*. Retrieved from https://www.samhsa.gov/data/release/2021-national-survey-drug-use-and-health-nsduh-releases

Sue, D. W., Alsaidi, S., Awad, M. N., Glaeser, E., Calle, C. Z., & Mendez, N. (2019). Disarming racial microaggressions: Microintervention strategies for targets, white allies, and bystanders. *American Psychologist*, *74*(1), 128.

Sun, W., Matsuoka, T., Imai, A., & Narumoto, J. (2023). Relationship between eating problems and the risk of dementia: A retrospective study. Psychogeriatrics, 23(6), 1043–1050.

Susan G. Komen. (2019, March). *Breast Cancer in Men*. Retrieved from https://ww5.komen.org/BreastCancer/BreastCancerinMen.html

Sutaria, S., Devakumar, D., Yasuda, S. S., Das, S., & Saxena, S. (2019). Is obesity associated with depression in children? Systematic review and meta-analysis. *Archives of Disease in Childhood*, *104*(1), 64–74.

Sutton, S., McVey, D., & Glanz, A. (1999). A comparative test of the theory of reasoned action and the theory of planned behavior in the prediction of condom use intentions in a national sample of English young people. *Health Psychology*, *18*, 72–81.

Swayden, K. J., Anderson, K. K., Connelly, L. M., Moran, J. S., McMahon, J. K., & Arnold, P. M. (2012). Effect of sitting vs. standing on perception of provider time at bedside: A pilot study. *Patient Education and Counseling*, *86*(2), 166–171.

Swazey, K. (2015). *Life that doesn't end with death*. Retrieved from https://www.ted.com/talks/kelli_swazey_life_that_doesn_t_end_with_death

Sweeney, T. J., & Witmer, J. M. (1991). Beyond social interest: Striving toward optimum health and wellness. *Individual Psychology: Journal of Adlerian Theory, Research and Practice*, *47*(4), 527–540.

Swinburn, B., Egger, G., & Raza, F. (1999). Dissecting obesogenic environments: The development and application of a framework for identifying and prioritizing environmental interventions for obesity. *Preventive Medicine*, *29*(6), 563–570.

Syed, M., & Seiffge-Krenke, I. J. (2013). Personality development from adolescence to emerging adulthood: Linking trajectories of ego development to the family context and identity formation. *Journal of Personality and Social Psychology*, *104*(2), 371–384.

Taber, J. M., Klein, W. M., Ferrer, R. A., Kent, E. E., & Harris, P. R. (2016). Optimism and spontaneous self-affirmation are associated with lower likelihood of cognitive impairment and greater positive affect among cancer survivors. *Annals of Behavioral Medicine*, *50*(2), 198–209. doi: 10.1007/s12160-015-9745-9

Taghizadeh, S., Hashemi, M. G., Zarnag, R. K., Fayyazishishavan, E., Gholami, M., Farhangi, M. A., & Gojani, L. J. (2023). Barriers and facilitators of childhood obesity prevention policies: A systematic review and meta-synthesis. *Frontiers in Pediatrics*, 10, 1054133.

Taillard, J., Sagaspe, P., Berthomier, C., Brandewinder, M., Amieva, H., Dartigues, J. F., … Philip, P. (2019). Non-REM sleep characteristics predict early cognitive impairment in an aging population. *Frontiers in Neurology*, *10*, 197.

Tam, V., Turcotte, M., & Meyre, D. (2019). Established and emerging strategies to crack the genetic code of obesity. *Obesity Reviews*, *20*(2), 212–240.

Tamashiro, K. L., Sakai, R. R., Shively, C. A., Karatsoreos, I. N., & Reagan, L. P. (2011). Chronic stress, metabolism, and metabolic syndrome. *Stress*, *14*(5), 468–474.

Tamminen, J., Lambon Ralph, M. A., & Lewis, P. A. (2013). The role of sleep spindles and slow-wave activity in integrating new information in semantic memory. *Journal of Neuroscience, 33*(39), 15376–15381. doi: 10.1523/JNEUROSCI.5093-12.2013

Tamres, L., Janicki, D., & Helgeson, V. S. (2002). Sex differences in coping behavior: A meta-analytic review and an examination of relative coping. *Personality and Social Psychology Review, 6*, 2–30.

Tan, C. C., & Holub, S. C. (2012). Maternal feeding practices associated with food neophobia. *Appetite, 59*(2), 483–487.

Tan, S. T., Quek, R. Y. C., Haldane, V., Koh, J. J. K., Han, E. K. L., Ong, S. E., … Legido-Quigley, H. (2019). The social determinants of chronic disease management: Perspectives of elderly patients with hypertension from low socio-economic background in Singapore. *International Journal for Equity in Health, 18*(1), 1.

Tanaka, R., Ozawa, J., Kito, N., & Moriyama, H. (2013). Efficacy of strengthening or aerobic exercise on pain relief in people with knee osteoarthritis: A systematic review and meta-analysis of randomized controlled trials. *Clinical Rehabilitation, 27*(12), 1059–1071. doi: 10.1177/0269215513488898

Tandler, N., & Proyer, R. T. (2022). Deriving information on play and playfulness of 3–5-year-olds from short written descriptions: Analyzing the frequency of usage of indicators of playfulness and their associations with maternal playfulness. *Behavioral Sciences, 12*(10), 385.

Tandler, N., Schilling-Friedemann, S., Frazier, L. D., Sendatzki, R., & Proyer, R. T. (2024). New insights into the contributions of playfulness to dealing with stress at work: Correlates of self-and peer-rated playfulness and coping strategies. *New Ideas in Psychology, 75*, 101109.

Tang, A. T., Choi, J. P., Kotzin, J. J., Yang, Y., Hong, C. C., Hobson, N., … Kahn, M. L. (2017). Endothelial TLR4 and the microbiome drive cerebral cavernous malformations. *Nature, 545*, 305. doi: 10.1038/nature22075

Tangney, J. P., Baumeister, R. F., & Boone, A. L. (2004). High self-control predicts good adjustment, less pathology, better grades, and interpersonal success. *Journal of Personality, 72*(2), 271–324.

Taveras, E. M., Gillman, M. W., Kleinman, K. P., Rich-Edwards, J. W., & Rifas-Shiman, S. L. (2013). Reducing racial/ethnic disparities in childhood obesity: The role of early life risk factors. *JAMA Pediatrics, 167*(8), 731–738. doi: 10.1001/jamapediatrics.2013.85

Taveras, E. M., McDonald, J., O'Brien, A., Haines, J., Sherry, B., Bottino, C. J., … Koziol, R. (2012). Healthy habits, happy homes: Methods and baseline data of a randomized controlled trial to improve household routines for obesity prevention. *Preventive Medicine, 55*(5), 418–426.

Taylor, S. E. (1983). Adjustment to threatening events: A theory of cognitive adaptation. *American Psychologist, 38*(11), 1161–1173.

Taylor, S. E. (2002). *The tending instinct: How nurturing is essential to who we are and how we live.* New York, NY: Holt.

Taylor, A. L. (2007). Addressing the global tragedy of needless pain: Rethinking the United nations single convention on narcotic drugs. *Journal of Law, Medicine and Ethics, 35*(4), 556–570, 511.

Taylor, P. (2009). *Growing old in America: Expectations vs. reality.* Pew Research Center. Retrieved from https://www.pewsocialtrends.org/2009/06/29/growing-old-in-america-expectations-vs-reality/

Taylor, R. J., & Chatters, L. M. (1991). Extended family networks of older black adults. *Journal of Gerontology, 46*(4), S210–S217.

Taylor, S. E., Gonzaga, G. C., Klein, L. C., Hu, P., Greendale, G. A., & Seeman, T. E. (2006). Relation of oxytocin to psychological stress responses and hypothalamic-pituitary-adrenocortical axis activity in older women. *Psychosomatic Medicine, 68*, 238–245.

Taylor, S. E., Klein, L. C., Lewis, B. P., Gruenewald, T. L., Gurung, R. A. R., & Updegraff, J. A. (2000). Biobehavioral responses to stress in females: Tend-and-befriend, not fight-or-flight. *Psychological Review, 107*, 411–429.

Taylor, S. E., & Master, S. L. (2011). Social response to stress: The tend-and-befriend model. In R. J. Contrada & A. Baum (Eds.), *The handbook of stress science: Biology, psychology and health* (pp. 101–110). New York, NY: Springer.

Taylor, S. E., Way, B. M., & Seeman, T. E. (2011). Early adversity and adult health outcomes. *Development and Psychopathology, 23*(3), 939–954.

Telazzi, I., & Colombo, B. (2024). Health disparities among LGBTQ+ older adults: Challenges and resources. *A systematic review. Behavioral Neuroscience, 1*, 9929–3349.

Temoshok, L. (1987). Personality, coping style, emotion and cancer: Towards an integrative model. *Cancer Surveys, 6*(3), 545–567.

ten Brinke, L. F., Hsu, C. L., Best, J. R., Barha, C. K., & Liu-Ambrose, T. (2018). Increased aerobic fitness is associated with cortical thickness in older adults with mild vascular cognitive impairment. *Journal of Cognitive Enhancement.* doi: 10.1007/s41465-018-0077-0

Tennen, H., Affleck, G., Armeli, S., & Carney, M. A. (2000). A daily process approach to coping: Linking theory, research, and practice. *American Psychologist, 55*(6), 626–636.

Tennen, H., Affleck, G., & Zautra, A. (2006). Depression history and coping with chronic pain: A daily process analysis. *Health Psychology, 25*(3), 370–379.

Teoh, A. N., Chong, L. X., Yip, C. C. E., Lee, P. S. H., & Wong, J. W. K. (2015). Gender as moderator of the effects of online social support from friends and strangers: A study of Singaporean college students. *International Perspectives in Psychology: Research, Practice, Consultation, 4*(4), 254–256.

Terracciano, A., Sutin, A. R., McCrae, R. R., Deiana, B., Ferrucci, L., Schlessinger, D., … Costa, P. T., Jr. (2009). Facets of personality linked to underweight and overweight. *Psychosomatic Medicine, 71*(6), 682–689.

Tetel, M. J., De Vries, G. J., Melcangi, R. C., Panzica, G., & O'Mahony, S. M. (2018). Steroids, stress and the gut microbiome- brain axis. *Journal of Neuroendocrinology, 30*(2), e12548.

Theeke, L., Carpenter, R. D., Mallow, J., & Theeke, E. (2019). Gender differences in loneliness, anger, depression, selfmanagement ability and biomarkers of chronic illness in chronically ill mid-life adults in Appalachia. *Applied Nursing Research, 45,* 55–62.

Theorell, T. (2019). A long-term perspective on cardiovascular job stress research. *Journal of Occupational Health, 61*(1), 3–9.

Thoits, P. A. (2010). Stress and health: Major findings and policy implications. *Journal of Health and Social Behavior, 51*(Suppl.), S41–S53.

Thompson, S. C. (1981). Will it hurt less if i can control it? A complex answer to a simple question. *Psychological Bulletin, 90,* 89–101.

Thompson, M. (1995). *Gay soul: Finding the heart of gay spirit and nature.* San Francisco, CA: HarperCollins.

Thompson, B., Coronado, G., Snipes, S. A., & Puschel, K. (2003). Methodologic advances and ongoing challenges in designing community-based health promotion programs. *Annual Review of Public Health, 24,* 315–340.

Thompson, J. K., Shroff, H., Herbozo, S., Cafri, G., Rodriguez, J., & Rodriguez, M. (2007). Relations among multiple peer influences, body dissatisfaction, eating disturbance, and selfesteem: A comparison of average weight, at risk of overweight, and overweight adolescent girls. *Journal of Pediatric Psychology, 32*(1), 24–29.

Thompson, J. K., & Stice, E. (2001). Thin-ideal internalization: Mounting evidence for a new risk factor for body-image disturbance and eating pathology. *Current Directions in Psychological Science, 10*(5), 181–183.

Thomson, S., Osborn, R., Squires, D., & Reed, S. J. (2011). International profiles of health care systems 2011: Australia, Canada, Denmark, England, France, Germany, Iceland, Italy, Japan, the Netherlands, New Zealand, Norway, Sweden, Switzerland, and the United States.

Thornton, L. E., Pearce, J. R., & Kavanagh, A. M. (2011). Using Geographic Information Systems (GIS) to assess the role of the built environment in influencing obesity: A glossary. *International Journal of Behavioral Nutrition and Physical Activity, 8,* 71. doi: 10.1186/1479-5868-8-71

Todd, M., Tennen, H., Carney, M. A., Armeli, S., & Affleck, G. (2004). Do we know how we cope? Relating daily coping reports to global and time-limited retrospective assessments. *Journal of Personality and Social Psychology, 86*(2), 310–319.

Tolma, E. L., Reininger, B. M., Evans, A., & Ureda, J. (2006). Examining the theory of planned behavior and the construct of self-efficacy to predict mammography intention. *Health Education & Behavior, 33*(2), 233–251.

Torrecillas-Martínez, L., Catena, A., O'Valle, F., Padial-Molina, M., & Galindo-Moreno, P. (2019). Does experienced pain affects local brain volumes? Insights from a clinical acute pain model. *International Journal of Clinical and Health Psychology, 19*(2), 115–123. doi: 10.1016/j.ijchp.2019.01.001

Torres, L. (2010). Predicting levels of Latino depression: Acculturation, acculturative stress, and coping. *Cultural Diversity and Ethnic Minority Psychology, 16*(2), 256–263.

Torres, X., Arroyo, S., Araya, S., & Pablo, J. (1999). The Spanish version of the Quality-of-Life in Epilepsy Inventory (QOLIE-31): Translation, validity, and reliability. *Epilepsia, 40*(9), 1299–1304.

Torres, L., & Rollock, D. (2004). Acculturative distress among Hispanics: The role of acculturation, coping, and intercultural competence. *Journal of Multicultural Counseling and Development, 32*(3), 155–167.

Tourula, M., Fukazawa, T., Isola, A., Hassi, J., Tochihara, Y., & Rintamäki, H. (2011). Evaluation of the thermal insulation of clothing of infants sleeping outdoors in Northern winter. *European Journal of Applied Physiology, 111*(4), 633–640.

Tourula, M., Isola, A., & Hassi, J. (2008). Children sleeping outdoors in winter: Parents' experiences of a culturally bound childcare practice. *International Journal of Circumpolar Health, 67,* 269–278.

Tourula, M., Pölkki, T., & Isola, A. (2013). The cultural meaning of children sleeping outdoors in Finnish winter: A qualitative study from the viewpoint of mothers. *Journal of Transcultural Nursing, 24*(2), 171–179.

Tov, W., & Diener, E. (2009). Culture and subjective well-being. In E. Diener (Ed.), *Culture and well-being* (pp. 9–41). Dordrecht, the Netherlands: Springer.

Towers, E. B., Kilgore, M., Bakhti-Suroosh, A., Pidaparthi, L., Williams, I. L., Abel, J. M., & Lynch, W. J. (2023). Sex differences in the neuroadaptations associated with incubated cocaine-craving: A focus on the dorsomedial prefrontal cortex. *Frontiers in Behavioral Neuroscience, 16,* 1027310.

Trammell, PhD, J. P., Joseph, PhD, N. T., & Harriger, PhD, J. A. (2023). Racial and ethnic minority disparities in COVID-19 related health, health beliefs and behaviors, and well-being among students. *Journal of American College Health, 71*(1), 242–248.

Trapl, E. S., Joshi, K., Taggart, M., Patrick, A., Meschkat, E., Freedman, D. A. (2017). Mixed methods evaluation of a produce prescription program for pregnant women. *Journal of Hunger & Environmental Nutrition 12(4), 529–543.*

Trapl, E. S., Smith, S., Joshi, K., Osborne. A, Matos AT, Bolen S. Dietary impact of produce prescriptions for patients with hypertension. *Preventing Chronic Disease 15, E138.*

Triandis, H. C. (1995). *Individualism & collectivism.* Boulder, CO: Westview Press.

Triandis, H. C. (2001). Individualism-collectivism and personality. *Journal of Personality, 69*(6), 907–924.

Tribole, E., & Resch, E. (2003). *Intuitive eating: A revolutionary program that works.* (2nd ed.). New York, NY: St. Martin's Press.

Troutman-Jordan, M., & Staples, J. (2014). Successful aging from the viewpoint of older adults. *Research and Theory for Nursing Practice, 28*(1), 87–104.

Truth Initiative. (2019, July 3). *New Research from Truth Initiative® Illustrates Dramatic Increase in Smoking Imagery in Shows Popular with Young People [Press release].* Retrieved from https://truthinitiative.org/press/press-release/new-research-truth-initiativer-illustrates-dramatic-increase-smoking-imagery

Tsao, C. W., Aday, A. W., Almarzooq, Z. I., Anderson, C. A., Arora, P., Avery, C. L., … American Heart Association Council on Epidemiology and Prevention Statistics Committee and Stroke Statistics Subcommittee. (2023). Heart disease and stroke statistics—2023 update: A report from the American Heart Association. *Circulation, 147*(8), e93–e621.

Tsui, P., & Leung, M. C. (2002). Comparison of the effectiveness between manual acupuncture and electro-acupuncture on patients with tennis elbow. *Acupuncture and Electrotherapeutics Research, 27*(2), 107–117.

Tulloch, P. (2016). *Men break their silence on eating disorders and distorted body image. STV News.*

Turcios, Y. (2023). *Digital Access: A Super Determinant of Health. Substance Abuse and Mental Health Services Administration.* Retrieved from https://www.samhsa.gov/blog/digital-access-super-determinant-health#1

Turiano, N. A., Chapman, B. P., Agrigoroaei, S., Infurna, F. J., & Lachman, M. (2014). Perceived control reduces mortality risk at low, not high, education levels. *Health Psychology, 33*(8), 883–890.

Turk, D. C., & Meichenbaum, D. (1991). Adherence to selfcare regimens: The patient's perspective. In J. J. Sweet, R. H. Rozensky, & S. M. Tovan (Eds.), *Handbook of clinical psychology in medical settings* (pp. 249–266). New York, NY: Springer.

Turk, D. C., & Winter, F. (2005). *The pain survival guide: How to reclaim your life.* Washington, DC: American Psychological Association.

Turk-Charles, S., Meyerowitz, B. E., & Gatz, M. (1997). Age differences in information-seeking among cancer patients. *International Journal of Aging and Human Development, 45*(2), 85–98.

Turner, S. G., & Hooker, K. (2022). Are thoughts about the future associated with perceptions in the present?: Optimism, possible selves, and self-perceptions of aging. *The International Journal of Aging and Human Development, 94*(2), 123–137.

Turner, C., McClure, R., & Pirozzo, S. (2004). Injury and risktaking behavior—A systematic review. *Accident Analysis and Prevention, 36*(1), 93–101.

Turpin, R., Brotman, R. M., Miller, R. S., Klebanoff, M. A., He, X., & Slopen, N. (2019). Perceived stress and incident sexually transmitted infections in a prospective cohort. *Annals of Epidemiology, 32,* 20–27.

Turvey, C. L., & Klein, D. M. (2008). Remission from depression comorbid with chronic illness and physical impairment. *American Journal of Psychiatry, 165*(5), 569–574.

Tuschl, R. J. (1990). From dietary restraint to binge eating: Some theoretical considerations. *Appetite, 14*(2), 105–109.

Tyler, D. C. (1990). Patient-controlled analgesia in adolescents. *Journal of Adolescent Health Care, 11*(2), 154–158.

Tylka, T. L. (2006). Development and psychometric evaluation of a measure of intuitive eating. *Journal of Counseling Psychology*, *53*(2), 226–240.

U.S. Bureau of Labor Statistics, Department of Labor. (2019, February 27). *Access to paid and unpaid family leave in 2018*. Retrieved from https://www.bls.gov/opub/ted/2019/access-to-paid-and-unpaid-family-leave-in-2018.htm

U.S. Department of Health and Human Services. (2000a). Effects on well-being and quality of life. In *Oral health in America: A report of the surgeon general*. Rockville, MD: National Institute of Dental and Craniofacial Research. Retrieved from http://www.nidcr.nih.gov/DataStatistics/SurgeonGeneral/sgr/chap6.htm

U.S. Department of Health and Human Services. (2000b). *Oral health in America: A report of the surgeon general*. Rockville, MD: National Institute of Dental and Craniofacial Research.

U.S. Department of Health and Human Services. (2018). *Physical activity guidelines for Americans* (2nd ed.). Retrieved from https://health.gov/paguidelines/second-edition/pdf/Physical_Activity_Guidelines_2nd_edition.pdf

U.S. Department of Health and Human Services. (2024). *Opioid facts and statistics*. Retrieved from https://www.hhs.gov/opioids/statistics/index.html

U.S. Department of Veterans Affairs. (2024a). *PTSD: National Center for PTSD*. Retrieved from https://www.ptsd.va.gov/understand/common/common_veterans.asp

U.S. Department of Veterans Affairs. (2024b). *Understanding veterans and PTSD*. Retrieved from https://nvhs.org/veterans-and-ptsd/?gad_source=1&gclid=Cj0KCQiAy8K8BhCZARIsAKJ8sfRvUzbw1ygJLg63rNGToJH66DL1GLXaqYJ-_HKvUhVNyPtOogC1vUUaAmTHEALw_wcB

U.S. Government Accountability Office. (2018). *Health insurance exchanges: HHS should enhance its management of open enrollment performance*. Washington, DC. Retrieved from https://www.gao.gov/assets/700/693362.pdf

Ubel, P. A., Loewenstein, G., & Jepson, C. (2003). Whose quality of life? A commentary exploring discrepancies between health state evaluations of patients and the general public. *Quality of Life Research*, *12*(6), 599–607.

Ubel, P. A., Loewenstein, G., Schwarz, N., & Smith, D. (2005). Misimagining the unimaginable: The disability paradox and health care decision making. *Health Psychology*, *24*(4S), S57–S62.

Uchino, B. N., de Grey, R. G. K., Cronan, S., Smith, T. W., Diener, E., Joel, S., & Bosch, J. (2018). Life satisfaction and inflammation in couples: An actor-partner analysis. *Journal of Behavioral Medicine*, *41*, 22. doi: 10.1007/s10865-017-9880-9

Uchino, B. N., Smith, T. W., Holt-Lunstead, J., Campo, R., & Reblin, M. (2007). Stress and illness. In J. T. Cacioppo, L. G. Tassinary, & G. C. Berntson (Eds.), *Handbook of psychophysiology* (pp. 608–632). New York, NY: Cambridge University Press.

Uhlenbusch, N., Löwe, B., Härter, M., Schramm, C., Weiler-Normann, C., & Depping, M. K. (2019). Depression and anxiety in patients with different rare chronic diseases: A crosssectional study. *PloS ONE*, *14*(2), e0211343.

Umaña-Taylor, A. J., Vargas-Chanes, D., Garcia, C. D., & Gonzales-Backen, M. (2008). A longitudinal examination of Latino adolescents' ethnic identity, coping with discrimination, and self-esteem. *Journal of Early Adolescence*, *28*(1), 16–50.

Umuco, et al., (2024). Evaluating optimism, hope, resilience, coping flexibility, secure attachment, and PERMA as a well-being model for college life adjustment of student veterans: A hierarchical regression analysis. *Rehabilitation Counseling Bulletin*, *67*(2), 94–110.

UNAIDS. (2012). *Global report: UNAIDS report on the global AIDS epidemic*. Geneva: Joint United Nations Programme on HIV/AIDS (UNAIDS). Retrieved from http://www.unaids.org/sites/default/files/media_asset/20121120_UNAIDS_Global_Report_2012_with_annexes_en_1.pdf

UNAIDS. (2018a). *Global HIV & AIDS statistics—2018 fact sheet*. Retrieved from http://www.unaids.org/en/resources/fact-sheet

UNAIDS. (2018b). *UNAIDS Data 2018*. Retrieved from http://www.unaids.org/sites/default/files/media_asset/unaids-data-2018_en.pdf

UNAIDS. (2024). *2024 global AIDS report — The Urgency of Now: AIDS at a Crossroads*. Retrieved from https://www.unaids.org/en/resources/documents/2024/global-aids-update-2024

UNICEF. (2018). *Annual report on Somalia*. Retrieved from https://www.unicef.org/somalia/media/191/file/Somalia-annual-report-2018-eng.pdf

United Nations, Department of Economic and Social Affairs, Population Division. (2017). *World population ageing 2017—highlights* (ST/ESA/SER.A/397).

United Nations High Commissioner for Refugees (UNHCR). (2016). *Missing out: Refugee education in crisis*. Retrieved from http://www.unhcr.org/57d9d01d0

University of Michigan Institute for Social Research. (2018, December 17). *National Adolescent Drug Trends in 2018* [Press release]. Retrieved from http://monitoringthefuture.org/pressreleases/18drugpr.pdf

Uppal, S. (2006). Impact of the timing, type and severity of disability on the subjective well-being of individuals with disabilities. *Social Science & Medicine, 63*(2), 525–539.

Uzogara, E. E. (2019). Dark and sick, light and healthy: Black women's complexion-based health disparities. *Ethnicity and Health, 24*(2), 125–146.

Vaegter, H. B., Handberg, G., & Graven-Nielsen, T. (2014). Similarities between exercise-induced hypoalgesia and conditioned pain modulation in humans. *Pain, 155*(1), 158–167.

van Achterberg, T., Huisman-De Waal, G. G., Ketelaar, N. A., Oostendorp, R. A., Jacobs, J. E., & Wollersheim, H. C. (2011). How to promote healthy behaviours in patients? An overview of evidence for behavioural change techniques. *Health Promotion International, 26*(2), 148–162.

van den Bree, M. B., Przybeck, T. R., & Cloninger, R. C. (2006). Diet and personality: Associations in a population-based sample. *Appetite, 46*(2), 177–188.

van den Heuvel, E., Newbury, A., & Appleton, K. M. (2019). The psychology of nutrition with advancing age: Focus on food neophobia. *Nutrients, 11*(1), 151.

van Doren, T. P., Zajdman, D., Brown, R. A., Gandhi, P., Heintz, R., Busch, L., … Paddock, R. (2023). Risk perception, adaptation, and resilience during the COVID-19 pandemic in Southeast Alaska natives. *Social Science & Medicine, 317*, 115609.

van Strien, T. (2000). Ice-cream consumption, tendency toward overeating, and personality. *International Journal of Eating Disorders, 28*, 460–464.

van Strien, T., Frijters, J. E. R., Bergers, G. P. A., & Defares, P. B. (1986). The Dutch eating behavior questionnaire (DEBQ) for assessment of restrained, emotional, and external eating behavior. *International Journal of Eating Disorders, 5*, 295–315.

Van Tongeren, D. R., Green, J. D., Davis, D. E., Worthington, E. L., Jr., & Reid, C. A. (2013). Till death do us part: Terror management and forgiveness in close relationships. *Personal Relationships, 20*, 755–768. doi: 10.1111/pere.12013

van Willigen, J., & Chadha, N. K. (1999). *Social aging in a Delhi neighborhood*. Westport, CT: Bergin & Garvey.

Van Zyl, L. E. et al. (2024). The critiques and criticisms of positive psychology: A systematic review. *The Journal of Positive Psychology, 19*(2), 206–235. doi: 10.1080/17439760.2023.2178956

Vanderbilt, A. A., & Wright, M. S. (2013). Infant mortality: A call to action overcoming health disparities in the United States. *Medical Education Online, 18*, 22503. doi: 10.3402/meo.v18i0.22503

Varkevisser, R. D. M., van Stralen, M. M., Kroeze, W., Ket, J. C. F., & Steenhuis, I. H. M. (2019). Determinants of weight loss maintenance: A systematic review. *Obesity Reviews, 20*, 171–211. doi: 10.1111/obr.12772

Vaughan, A. S., Quick, H., Schieb, L., Kramer, M. R., Taylor, H. A., & Casper, M. (2019). Changing rate orders of race-gender heart disease death rates: An exploration of county-level racegender disparities. *SSM-Population Health, 7*, 100334.

Vedhara, K., Cox, N. K., Wilcock, G. K., Perks, P., Hunt, M., Anderson, S., … Shanks, N. M. (1999). Chronic stress in elderly carers of dementia patients and antibody response to influenza vaccination. *Lancet, 353*(9153), 627–631.

Veenhoven, R. (2008). Healthy happiness: Effects of happiness on physical health and the consequences for preventive health care. *Journal of Happiness Studies, 9*(3), 449–469.

Veenhoven, R., & Hagerty, M. (2006). Rising happiness in nations 1946–2004: A reply to Easterlin. *Social Indicators Research, 79*(3), 421–436.

Vega, W. A., Sribney, W. M., Aguilar-Gaxiola, S., & Kolody, B. (2004). 12-month prevalence of DSM-III-R psychiatric disorders among Mexican Americans: Nativity, social assimilation, and age determinants. *Journal of Nervous and Mental Disease, 192*(8), 532–541.

Vélez, C. E., Krause, E. D., Brunwasser, S. M., Freres, D. R., Abenavoli, R. M., & Gillham, J. E. (2014). Parent predictors of adolescents' explanatory style. *Journal of Early Adolescence, 35*(7), 931–946.

Vente, T., Daley, M., Killmeyer, E., & Grubb, L. K. (2020). Association of social media use and high-risk behaviors in adolescents: Cross-sectional study. *JMIR Pediatrics and Parenting, 3*(1), e18043.

Ventola, C. L. (2010). Current issues regarding complementary and alternative medicine (CAM) in the United States: Part 1: The widespread use of CAM and the need for better-informed health care professionals to provide patient counseling. *Pharmacy and Therapeutics, 35*(8), 461–468.

Vera, E., Vacek, K., Coyle, L. D., Stinson, J., Mull, M., Doud, K., … Langrehr, K. J. (2011). An examination of culturally relevant stressors, coping, ethnic identity, and subjective well-being in urban, ethnic minority adolescents. *Professional School Counseling, 15*(2), 55–66.

Verbrugge, L. M. (1985). Gender and health: An update on hypotheses and evidence. *Journal of Health and Social Behavior, 26*, 156–182.

Vereen, R. N., Kurtzman, R., & Noar, S. M. (2023). Are social media interventions for health behavior change efficacious among populations with health disparities?: A meta-analytic review. *Health Communication, 38*(1), 133–140.

Verkuyten, M. (2010). Assimilation ideology and situational well-being among ethnic minority members. *Journal of Experimental Social Psychology, 46*(2), 269–275.

Vickers, A. J., Cronin, A. M., Maschino, A. C., Lewith, G., MacPherson, H., Foster, N. E., … Acupuncture Trialists' Collaboration. (2012). Acupuncture for chronic pain: Individual patient data meta-analysis. *Archives of Internal Medicine, 172*(19), 1444–1453.

Vilhjalmsson, R., & Thorlindsson, T. (1998). Factors related to physical activity: A study of adolescents. *Social Science & Medicine, 47*(5), 665–675.

Violanti, J., Marshall, J., & Howe, B. (1983) Police occupational demands, psychological distress and the coping function of alcohol. *Journal of Occupational Medicine, 25*, 455–458.

Vittersø, J. (2004). Subjective well-being versus self-actualization: Using the flow-simplex to promote a conceptual clarification of subjective quality of life. *Social Indicators Research, 65*(3), 299–331.

Vogels, E. A. (2020). About one-in-five Americans use a smart watch or fitness tracker. *Pew Research Center.* Retrieved from https://www.pewresearch.org/short-reads/2020/01/09/about-one-in-five-americans-use-a-smart-watch-or-fitness-tracker/

Vogels, E. A., Gelles-Watnick, R., & Massarat, N. (2022, August 10). Teens, social media and technology 2022. *Pew Research Center.*

Vohra, S., Zorzela, L., Kemper, K., Vlieger, A., & Pintov, S. (2019). Setting a research agenda for pediatric complementary and integrative medicine: A consensus approach. *Complementary Therapies in Medicine, 42*, 27–32.

Vohs, K. D., & Baumeister, R. F. (Eds.). (2011). *Handbook of selfregulation: Research, theory, and applications* (2nd ed.). New York, NY: Guilford Press.

Volkow, N. D., Koob, G. F., & McLellan, A. T. (2016). Neurobiologic advances from the brain disease model of addiction. *The New England Journal of Medicine, 374*(4), 363–371.

Vollrath, M., Torgersen, S., & Alnæs, R. (1995). Personality as long-term predictor of coping. *Personality and Individual Differences, 18*(1), 117–125.

von Dawans, B., Ditzen, B., Trueg, A., Fischbacher, U., & Heinrichs, M. (2019). Effects of acute stress on social behavior in women. *Psychoneuroendocrinology, 99*, 137–144.

von Dawans, B., Fischbacher, U., Kirschbaum, C., Fehr, E., & Heinrichs, M. (2012). The social dimension of stress reactivity: Acute stress increases prosocial behavior in humans. *Psychological Science, 23*, 651–660.

Voss, M. W., Prakash, R. S., Erickson, K. I., Basak, C., Chaddock, L., Kim, J. S., … Kramer, A. F. (2010). Plasticity of brain networks in a randomized intervention trial of exercise training in older adults. *Frontiers in Aging Neuroscience, 2*, 32.

Wade, T. D., Keski-Rahkonen, A., & Hudson, J. (2011). Epidemiology of eating disorders. In M. Tsuang, M. Tohen, & P. Jones (Eds.), *Textbook in psychiatric epidemiology* (3rd ed., pp. 343–360). New York, NY: Wiley.

Waheed, Y. (2018). Polio eradication challenges in Pakistan. *Clinical Microbiology and Infection, 24*(1), 6–7.

Waid, L. D., & Frazier, L. D. (2003). Cultural differences in possible selves during later life. *Journal of Aging Studies, 17*(3), 251–268.

Waldinger, R. J., & Schulz, M. S. (2010). What's love got to do with it? Social functioning, perceived health, and daily happiness in married octogenarians. *Psychology and Aging, 25*(2), 422–431.

Waldorf, M., Vocks, S., Düsing, R., Bauer, A., & Cordes, M. (2019). Body-oriented gaze behaviors in men with muscle dysmorphia diagnoses. *Journal of Abnormal Psychology, 128*(2), 140.

Walinski, A., Sander, J., Gerlinger, G., Clemens, V., Meyer-Lindenberg, A., & Heinz, A. (2023). The effects of climate change on mental health. *Deutsches Ärzteblatt International, 120*(8), 117.

Walker, J. G., Jackson, H. J., & Littlejohn, G. O. (2004). Models of adjustment to chronic illness: Using the example of rheumatoid arthritis. *Clinical Psychology Review, 24*(4), 461–488.

Wall, P. D. (1978). The gate control theory of pain mechanisms. A re-examination and re-statement. *Brain: A Journal of Neurology, 101*(1), 1–18.

Wallace, J. M., Jr., Forman, T. A., Caldwell, C. H., & Willis, D. S. (2003). Religion and U.S. secondary school students: Current patterns, recent trends, and sociodemographic correlates. *Youth & Society, 35*(1), 98–125.

Wallston, K. A. (1996). Healthy, wealthy, and weiss: A history of division 38 (Health psychology). In D. A. Dewsbury (Ed.), *Histories of the APA divisions*. Washington, DC: American Psychological Association. doi: 10.1037/10234-009

Wallston, K. A., Wallston, B. S., & DeVellis, R. (1978). Development of the Multidimensional Health Locus of Control (MHLC) scales. *Health Education Monographs, 6*, 160–170.

Walsh, D. (2012, October 9). Taliban gun down girl who spoke up for rights. *New York Times.*

Wang, Y. C., Bleich, S. N., & Gortmaker, S. L. (2008). Increasing caloric contribution from sugar-sweetened beverages and 100% fruit juices among US children and adolescents, 1988–2004. *Pediatrics, 121*, e1604–e1614.

Wang, C., & Coups, E. J. (2010). Causal beliefs about obesity and associated health behaviors: Results from a population-based survey. *International Journal of Behavioral Nutrition and Physical Activity, 7*, 19. doi: 10.1186/1479-5868-7-19

Wang, Y., Lopez, J. M., Bolge, S. C., Zhu, V. J., & Stang, P. E. (2016). Depression among people with type 2 diabetes mellitus, US National Health and Nutrition Examination Survey (NHANES), 2005–2012. *BMC Psychiatry, 16*(1), 88.

Wang, Y., Xiao, H., Zhang, X., & Wang, L. (2020). The role of active coping in the relationship between learning burnout and sleep quality among college students in China. *Frontiers in Psychology, 11*, 647.

Ward, R. A. (2010). How old am i? Perceived age in middle and later life. *International Journal of Aging and Human Development, 71*(3), 167–184.

Warren-Findlow, J. (2019). Stress and heart disease in African American women living in Chicago. *Community Health Equity: A Chicago Reader, 325.*

Watanabe, J. H., McInnis, T., & Hirsch, J. D. (2018). Cost of prescription drug–related morbidity and mortality. *Annals of Pharmacotherapy, 52*(9), 829–837.

Watson, R. J., Grossman, A. H., & Russell, S. T. (2019). Sources of social support and mental health among LGB youth. *Youth and Society, 51*(1), 30–48.

Watson, H. J., Joyce, T., French, E., Willan, V., Kane, R. T., Tanner-Smith, E. E., … Egan, S. J. (2016). Prevention of eating disorders: A systematic review of randomized, controlled trials. *International Journal of Eating Disorders, 49*(9), 833–862.

Watson, J., & Nesdale, D. (2012). Rejection sensitivity, social withdrawal, and loneliness in young adults. *Journal of Applied Social Psychology, 42*, 1984–2005. doi: 10.1111/j.1559-1816.2012.00927.x

Webb, J. R. (2019). Overview of disability. In *Dental care for children with special needs* (pp. 1–26). New York, NY: Springer.

Weber, K., Rockstroh, B., Borgelt, J., Awiszus, B., Popov, T., Hoffmann, K., … Pröpster, K. (2008). Stress load during childhood affects psychopathology in psychiatric patients. *BMC Psychiatry, 8*, 63.

Weber, L., & Seetharaman, D. (2017, December 27). The worst job in technology: Staring at human depravity to keep it off Facebook. *Wall Street Journal.* Retrieved from https://www.wsj.com/articles/the-worst-job-in-technology-staring-at-human-depravity-to-keep-it-off-facebook-1514398398

WebMD.com. (2017). *Drugs & medications search: Pain.* Retrieved from http://www.webmd.com/drugs/condition-3079-Pain.aspx

Wei, M., Heppner, P. P., & Mallinckrodt, B. (2003). Perceived coping as a mediator between attachment and psychological distress: A structural equation modeling approach. *Journal of Counseling Psychology, 50*(4), 438–447.

Wei, M., Liao, K. Y. H., Heppner, P. P., Chao, R. C. L., & Ku, T. Y. (2012). Forbearance coping, identification with heritage culture, acculturative stress, and psychological distress among Chinese international students. *Journal of Counseling Psychology, 59*(1), 97.

Weidner, G., Kohlmann, C. W., Dotzauer, E., & Burns, L. R. (1996). The effect of academic stress on health behaviors in young adults. *Anxiety, Stress, and Coping, 9*, 123–133.

Weierstall-Pust, R., Schnell, T., Heßmann, P., Feld, M., Höfer, M., Plate, A., & Müller, M. J. (2022). Stressors related to the Covid-19 pandemic, climate change, and the Ukraine crisis, and their impact on stress symptoms in Germany: Analysis of cross-sectional survey data. *BMC Public Health, 22*(1), 2233.

Weiland, N. (2018, March 24). At rallies, students with a different view of gun violence: As urban reality. *New York Times.* Retrieved from https://www.nytimes.com/2018/03/24/us/gun-rally-urban.html

Weinert, C., Cudney, S., & Spring, A. (2008). Evolution of a conceptual model for adaptation to chronic illness. *Journal of Nursing Scholarship, 40*(4), 364–372.

Weinman, J., Petrie, K. J., Moss-Morris, R., & Horne, R. (1996). The illness perception questionnaire: A new method for assessing the cognitive representation of illness. *Psychology and Health, 11*(3), 431–445.

Weinstein, A. M., Voss, M. W., Prakash, R. S., Chaddock, L., Szabo, A., White, S. M., … Erickson, K. I. (2012). The association between aerobic fitness and executive function is mediated by prefrontal cortex volume. *Brain, Behavior, and Immunity, 26*(5), 811–819.

Weir, K. (2016). New insights on eating disorders. *Monitor on Psychology, 47*(4), 36. Retrieved from http://www.apa.org/monitor/2016/04/eating-disorders.aspx

Weiss, T. (2004). Correlates of posttraumatic growth in husbands of breast cancer survivors. *Psychooncology, 13*(4), 260–268.

Wells, P. M., Williams, F. M., Matey-Hernandez, M. L., Menni, C., & Steves, C. J. (2019). RA and the microbiome: Do host genetic factors provide the link? *Journal of Autoimmunity, 99*, 104–115.

Werner, K. M., & Ford, B. Q. (2023). Self-control: An integrative framework. *Social and Personality Psychology Compass, 17*(5), e12738.

Wesseldijk, L. W., Tybur, J. M., Boomsma, D. I., Willemsen, G., & Vink, J. M. (2023). The heritability of pescetarianism and vegetarianism. *Food Quality and Preference, 103*, 104705.

West, L. M., & Cordina, M. (2019). Educational intervention to enhance adherence to short-term use of antibiotics. *Research in Social and Administrative Pharmacy, 15*(2), 193–201.

Whitbourne, S. K., & Ebmeyer, J. B. (2013). *Identity and intimacy in marriage: A study of couples.* New York, NY: Springer Science & Business Media.

White, A. M., Castle, I. P., Powell, P. A., Hingson, R. W., & Koob, G. F. (2022). Alcohol-related deaths during the COVID-19 pandemic. *JAMA, 327*(17), 1704–1706. doi: 10.1001/jama.2022.4308

Whitmer, R. A., Gustafson, D. R., Barrett-Connor, E., Haan, M. N., Gunderson, E. P., & Yaffe, K. (2008). Central obesity and increased risk of dementia more than three decades later. *Neurology, 71*(14), 1057–1064. doi: 10.1212/01.wnl.0000306313.89165.ef

WHO Expert Consultation. (2004). Appropriate body-mass index for Asian populations and its implications for policy and intervention strategies. *Lancet, 363*(9403), 157–163.

Wiebe, D. J., & McCallum, D. M. (1986). Health practices and hardiness as mediators in the stress-illness relationship. *Health Psychology, 5*, 425–438.

Williams, R. D., Jr., Housman, J. M., Woolsey, C. L., & Sather, T. E. (2018). High-risk driving behaviors among 12th grade students: Differences between alcohol-only and alcohol mixed with energy drink users. *Substance Use and Misuse, 53*(1), 137–142.

Williams, P. G., Smith, T. W., Gunn, H. E., & Uchino, B. N. (2011). Personality and stress: Individual differences in exposure, reactivity, recovery, and restoration. In R. J. Contrada & A. Baum (Eds.), *Handbook of stress science* (pp. 231–245). New York, NY: Springer.

Williams, P. G., Suchy, Y., & Rau, H. K. (2009). Individual differences in executive functioning: Implications for stress regulation. *Annals of Behavioral Medicine, 37*, 126–140.

Williams, M., Teasdale, J., Segal, Z., & Kabat-Zinn, J. (2007). *The mindful way through depression: Freeing yourself from chronic unhappiness.* New York, NY: Guilford Press.

Williams, L., & Wingate, A. (2012). Type D personality, physical symptoms and subjective stress: The mediating effects of coping and social support. *Psychology and Health, 27*(9), 1075–1085.

Wills, T. A. (1985). Supportive functions of interpersonal relationships. In S. Cohen & S. I. Syme (Eds.), *Social support and health* (pp. 61–82). San Diego, CA: Academic.

Wills, T. A., Isasi, C. R., Mendoza, D., & Ainette, M. G. (2007). Self-control constructs related to measures of dietary intake and physical activity in adolescents. *Journal of Adolescent Health, 41*(6), 551–558.

Wilson, S. J., Barrineau, M. J., Butner, J., & Berg, C. A. (2014). Shared possible selves, other-focus, and perceived wellness of couples with prostate cancer. *Journal of Family Psychology, 28*(5), 684–691.

Wimberly, A. E. S. (2001). The role of black faith communities in fostering health. In R. L. Braithwaite & S. E. Taylor (Eds.), *Health issues in the black community* (pp. 129–150). San Francisco, CA: Jossey-Bass.

Wingard, D. L., Berkman, L. F., & Brand, R. J. (1982). A multivariate analysis of health-related practices: A nine-year mortality follow-up of the Alameda County Study. *American Journal of Epidemiology, 116*, 765–775.

Wirtz, P. H., Ehlert, U., Emini, L., Rüdisüli, K., Groessbauer, S., Gaab, J., … von Känel, R. (2006). Anticipatory cognitive stress appraisal and the acute procoagulant stress response in men. *Psychosomatic Medicine, 68*, 851–858.

Witkiewitz, K., & Marlatt, G. A. (2007). Modeling the complexity of post-treatment drinking: It's a rocky road to relapse. *Clinical Psychology Review*, *27*(6), 724–738.

Witmer, J. M., & Sweeney, T. J. (1992). A holistic model for wellness and prevention over the life span. *Journal of Counseling and Development*, *71*(2), 140–148.

Witmer, J. M., Sweeney, T. J., & Myers, J. E. (1998). *The wheel of wellness*. Greensboro, NC: Authors.

Wittig, R. M., Crockford, C., Weltring, A., Langergraber, K. E., Deschner, T., & Zuberbühler, K. (2016). Social support reduces stress hormone levels in wild chimpanzees across stressful events and everyday affiliations. *Nature Communications*, *7*, 13361.

Wittman, C., & Swigris, J. J. (2019). The role of pulmonary rehabilitation and supplemental oxygen therapy in the treatment of patients with idiopathic pulmonary fibrosis. In K. C. Meyer & S. D. Nathan (Eds.), *Idiopathic pulmonary fibrosis* (pp. 389–399). New York, NY: Humana Press.

Wium-Andersen, M. K., Ørsted, D. D., Nielsen, S. F., & Nordestgaard, B. G. (2013). Elevated C-reactive protein levels, psychological distress, and depression in 73,131 individuals. *JAMA Psychiatry*, *70*(2), 176–184.

Wojcicki, S. (2014, December 16). Paid maternity leave is good for business. *Wall Street Journal*. Retrieved from https://www.wsj.com/articles/susan-wojcicki-paid-maternity-leave-is-good-for-business-1418773756

Wong, C. W., Kwok, C. S., Narain, A., Gulati, M., Mihalidou, A. S., Wu, P., … Mamas, M. A. (2018). Marital status and risk of cardiovascular diseases: A systematic review and metaanalysis. *Heart*, *104*(23), 1937–1948.

Wong, J. M., Sin, N. L., & Whooley, M. A. (2014). A comparison of cook-medley hostility subscales and mortality in patients with coronary heart disease: Data from the heart and soul study. *Psychosomatic Medicine*, *76*(4), 311–317.

Wong-Baker FACES Foundation. (2009). Wong-Baker FACES® Pain Rating Scale. Retrieved from http://wongbakerfaces.org/

Wood, A. M., Kaptoge, S., Butterworth, A. S., Willeit, P., Warnakula, S., Bolton, T., … Bell, S. (2018). Risk thresholds for alcohol consumption: Combined analysis of individual participant data for 599 912 current drinkers in 83 prospective studies. *The Lancet*, *391*(10129), 1513–1523.

Wood, J. V., Taylor, S. E., & Lichtman, R. R. (1985). Social comparison in adjustment to breast cancer. *Journal of Personality and Social Psychology*, *49*(5), 1169–1183.

Woon, T.-H., Masuda, M., Wagner, N. N., & Holmes, T. H. (1971). The social readjustment rating scale: A cross-cultural study of Malaysians and Americans. *Journal of Cross-Cultural Psychology*, *2*(4), 373–386.

World Economic Forum. (2023a). *Trends shaping global health care*. Retrieved from https://www.gavi.org/vaccineswork/world-health-day-8-trends-shaping-global-healthcare?gclid=CjwKCAjwo7iiBhAEEiwAsIxQEbziirMk1k9ChJJsyvrWNTSIrLjmIA3TRdJzo0ae-QonL4x0fOAUnwhoC-HAQAvD_BwE

World Economic Forum. (2023b). *World Health Day: 8 trends shaping global healthcare*. Retrieved from: https://www.gavi.org/vaccineswork/world-health-day-8-trends-shaping-global-healthcare?gclid=CjwKCAjwo7iiBhAEEiwAsIxQEbziirMk1k9ChJJsyvrWNTSIrLjmIA3TRdJzo0aeQonL4x0fOAUnwhoC-HAQAvD_BwE

World Health Organization. (1946). *Preamble to the Constitution of the World Health Organization as adopted by the International Health Conference, New York, 19–22 June, 1946; signed on 22 July 1946 by the representatives of 61 States (Official Records of the World Health Organization, no. 2, p. 100) and entered into force on 7 April 1948*. Retrieved from http://apps.who.int/gb/bd/PDF/bd47/EN/constitution-en.pdf?ua=1

World Health Organization. (1997). *WHOQOL: Measuring Quality of Life*.

World Health Organization. (2005). *World alliance for patient safety—Global patient safety challenge 2005–2006: Clean care is safer care*.

World Health Organization. (2009a). *World health report: World Health Organization assesses the world's health systems*. Retrieved from http://www.who.int/whr/2000/media_centre/press_release/en/

World Health Organization. (2009b). *World health statistics 2009*.

World Health Organization. (2011). *World health statistics 2011*.

World Health Organization. (2015b). *World health statistics 2015*. Geneva: World Health Organization. Retrieved from http://www.who.int/gho/publications/world_health_statistics/2015/en/

World Health Organization. (2016a). *Global database on body mass index*. Retrieved from http://apps.who.int/bmi/index.jsp

World Health Organization. (2016b). *Life expectancy increased by 5 years since 2000, but health inequalities persist*. Retrieved from http://www.who.int/mediacentre/news/releases/2016/health-inequalities-persist/en/

World Health Organization. (2017a). *Human rights and health.* Retrieved from http://www.who.int/news-room/fact-sheets/detail/human-rights-and-health

World Health Organization. (2017e). *WHO model lists of essential medicines.* Retrieved from https://www.who.int/medicines/publications/essentialmedicines/en/

World Health Organization. (2017f). *WHO report finds dramatic increase in life-saving tobacco control policies in last decade.* Retrieved from https://www.who.int/en/news-room/detail/19-07-2017-who-report-finds-dramatic-increase-in-life-saving-tobacco-control-policies-in-last-decade

World Health Organization. (2018d). *WHE Situation Report #6: Somalia (June 2018).* http://www.emro.who.int/images/stories/somalia/documents/Somalia_Emergency_Health_Update_June_2018.pdf?ua=1&ua=1

World Health Organization. (2020). *Top ten causes of death.* Retrieved from https://www.who.int/news-room/fact-sheets/detail/the-top-10-causes-of-death

World Health Organization. (2021). *WHO global report on trends in prevalence of tobacco use 2000–2025* (4th ed.). Retrieved from https://www.who.int/publications/i/item/9789240039322

World Health Organization. (2022). *Refugee and migrant health.* Retrieved from https://www.who.int/health-topics/refugee-and-migrant-health#tab=tab_1

World Health Organization. (2023a). *Health Emergency Programme Update: Somalia.* Retrieved from https://www.emro.who.int/images/stories/somalia/Health-Emergency-Programme-February-2023.pdf

World Health Organization. (2023b). *WHO global report on trends in prevalence of tobacco use 2000-2025* (4th ed.). Geneva: WHO. Retrieved from https://www.who.int/news-room/fact-sheets/detail/tobacco

World Health Organization. (2023c). *Climate Change.* Retrieved from https://www.who.int/news-room/fact-sheets/detail/climate-change-and-health

World Health Organization. (2023d). *Tobacco.* Retrieved from https://www.who.int/news-room/fact-sheets/detail/tobacco

World Health Organization. (2024a). *Number of Covid-19 cases reported to WHO.* Retrieved from https://covid19.who.int/

World Health Organization. (2024b). *Snakebite envenoming.* Retrieved from http://www.who.int/news-room/fact-sheets/detail/snakebite-envenoming

World Health Organization. (2024c). *The top 10 causes of death.* Retrieved from http://www.who.int/news-room/fact-sheets/detail/the-top-10-causes-of-death

World Health Organization. (2024d). *Cardiovascular disease.* Retrieved from https://www.who.int/health-topics/cardiovascular-diseases#tab=tab_1

World Health Organization. (2024e) *Healthy diet.* Retrieved from https://www.who.int/health-topics/healthy-diet#tab=tab_1

World Health Organization. (2024f). *Global status report on physical activity 2022.* Retrieved from https://www.who.int/teams/health-promotion/physical-activity/global-status-report-on-physical-activity-2022#:~:text=Let's%20get%20moving!&text=Regular%20physical%20activity%20promotes%20both,recommended%20levels%20of%20physical%20activity

World Health Organization. (2024g). *Alcohol.* Retrieved from https://www.who.int/news-room/fact-sheets/detail/alcohol

World Health Organization. (2024h). *Global information systems on alcohol.* Retrieved from https://www.who.int/data/gho/data/themes/global-information-system-on-alcohol-and-health

World Health Organization. (2024i). *Obesity and overweight.* Retrieved from https://www.who.int/news-room/fact-sheets/detail/obesity-and-overweight

World Health Organization. (2024j). *Stroke, cerebral accident.* Retrieved from https://www.emro.who.int/health-topics/stroke-cerebrovascular-accident/index.html

World Health Organization Expert Consultation. (2024). Appropriate body-mass index for Asian populations and its implications for policy and intervention strategies. *Lancet, 363*(9403), 157–163. Retrieved from http://www.who.int/nutrition/publications/bmi_asia_strategies.pdf

World Population Review. (2023). *Population by country.* Retrieved from https://worldpopulationreview.com/

Wright, A. A., Zhang, B., Ray, A., Mack, J. W., Trice, E., Balboni, T., ... Prigerson, H. G. (2008). Associations between end-of-life discussions, patient mental health, medical care near death, and caregiver bereavement adjustment. *JAMA, 300*(14), 1665–1673.

Würtzen, H., Clausen, L. H., Andersen, P. B., Santini, Z. I., Erkmen, J., & Pedersen, H. F. (2022). Mental well-being, health, and locus of control in Danish adults before and during COVID-19. *Acta Neuropsychiatrica, 34*(2), 93–98.

Xiao, D., Dasgupta, C., Li, Y., Huang, X., & Zhang, L. (2014). Perinatal nicotine exposure increases angiotensin II receptor-mediated vascular contractility in adult offspring. *PLoS One, 9*(9), e108161.

Xie, L., Kang, H., Xu, Q., Chen, M. J., Liao, Y., Thiyagarajan, M., O'Donnell, J., Christensen, D. J., Nicholson, C., Iliff, J. J., et al. (2013). Sleep drives metabolite clearance from the adult brain. *Science, 342*(6156), 373–377.

Xie, J., Price, A., Curran, N., Ostbye, T. (2021). The impact of a produce prescription programme on healthy food purchasing and diabetes-related health outcomes. *Public Health Nutrition, 24*(12), 3945–3955.

Xu, W., Atti, A. R., Gatz, M., & Fratiglioni, L. (2011). Midlife overweight and obesity increases late-life dementia risk: A population-based twin study. *Neurology, 76*(18), 1568–1574.

Xu, Z., Hou, B., Gao, Y., He, F., & Zhang, C. (2007). Effects of enriched environment on morphine-induced reward in mice. *Experimental Neurology, 204*(2), 714–719.

Xu, J., Murphy, S. L., Kochanek, K. D., & Arias, E. (2016). *Mortality in the United States, 2015* (NCHS data brief no. 267). Hyattsville, MD: National Center for Health Statistics. Retrieved from https://www.cdc.gov/nchs/data/databriefs/db267.pdf

Xu, J., & Roberts, R. E. (2010). The power of positive emotions: It's a matter of life or death—Subjective well-being and longevity over 28 years in a general population. *Health Psychology, 29*(1), 9–19.

Yaden, D. B., Claydon, J., Bathgate, M., Platt, B., Santos, L. R. (2021). Teaching well-being at scale: An intervention study. *PLoS ONE, 16*(4), e0249193.

Yang, C., Fang, X., Zhan, G., Huang, N., Ll, S., Bi, J., ... Luo, A. (2019). Key role of gut microbiota in anhedonia-like phenotype in rodents with neuropathic pain. *Translational Psychiatry, 9*(1), 57.

Yawn, B. P., Wollan, P. C., Weingarten, T. N., Watson, J. C., Hooten, W. M., & Melton, L. J. III. (2009). The prevalence of neuropathic pain: Clinical evaluation compared with screening tools in a community population. *Pain Medicine, 10*(3), 586–593.

Yeh, C. J., Arora, A. K., & Wu, K. A. (2006). A new theoretical model of collectivistic coping. In *Handbook of multicultural perspectives on stress and coping* (pp. 55–72). Boston, MA: Springer.

Yeh, C., & Inose, M. (2002). Difficulties and coping strategies of Chinese, Japanese, and Korean immigrant students. *Adolescence, 37*(145), 69–82.

Yeo, H., Mendenhall, R., Harwood, S., & Huntt, M. (2019). Asian international student and Asian American student: Mistaken identity and racial microaggressions. *Journal of International Students, 9*(1), 39–65.

Yildirim, S., Onder, N., & Avci, A. G. (2020). Examination of sleep quality and factors affecting sleep quality of a group of university students. *International Journal of Caring Sciences, 13*(2), 1431–1439.

Young, C. M. (1985). Aristotle's eudemian ethics. *Teaching Philosophy, 8*(1), 55–58.

Young, S. K. (2010). *Promoting healthy eating among college women: Effectiveness of an intuitive eating intervention* (Doctoral dissertation, Iowa State University). Retrieved from Iowa State University Digital Repository. Paper 11308.

Young, J. D., Abdel-Massih, R., Herchline, T., McCurdy, L., Moyer, K. J., Scott, J. D., ... Siddiqui, J. (2019). Infectious Diseases Society of America position statement on telehealth and telemedicine as applied to the practice of infectious diseases. *Clinical Infectious Diseases, 64*(3), 237–242.

Youngstedt, S. D., & Kripke, D. F. (2004). Long sleep and mortality: Rationale for sleep restriction. *Sleep Medicine Reviews, 8*(3), 159–174.

Yousafzai, M., & Lamb, C. (2013). *I am Malala: The girl who stood up for education and was shot by the Taliban.* London, UK: Weidenfeld & Nicolson.

Yu, X. N., Chen, Z., Zhang, J., & Liu, X. (2011). Coping mediates the association between type D personality and perceived health in Chinese patients with coronary heart disease. *International Journal of Behavioral Medicine, 18*(3), 277–284.

Yu, M. A., Sánchez-Lozada, L. G., Johnson, R. J., & Kang, D. H. (2010). Oxidative stress with an activation of the renin–angiotensin system in human vascular endothelial cells as a novel mechanism of uric acid-induced endothelial dysfunction. *Journal of Hypertension, 28*(6), 1234–1242.

Yun, K., Kim, S. H., & Awasu, C. R. (2019). Stress and impact of spirituality as a mediator of coping methods among social work college students. *Journal of Human Behavior in the Social Environment, 29*(1), 125–136.

Zakrzewska, J. M. (2002). Diagnosis and differential diagnosis of trigeminal neuralgia. *Clinical Journal of Pain, 18*(1), 14–21.

Zarski, J. J. (1984). Hassles and health: A replication. *Health Psychology, 3*, 243–251.

Zautra, A. J. (2003). *Emotions, stress, and health.* New York, NY: Oxford University Press.

Zautra, A. J., Arewasikporn, A., & Davis, M. C. (2010). Resilience: Promoting well-being through recovery, sustainability, and growth. *Research in Human Development, 7*(3), 221–238.

Zautra, A. J., Burleson, M. H., Matt, K. S., Roth, S., & Burrows, L. (1994). Interpersonal stress, depression, and disease activity in rheumatoid arthritis and osteoarthritis patients. *Health Psychology, 13*(2), 139–148.

Zautra, A. J., Hall, J. S., & Murray, K. E. (2010). Resilience: A new definition of health for people and communities. In J. R. Reich, A. J. Zautra, & J. S. Hall (Eds.), *Handbook of adult resilience* (pp. 3–29). New York, NY: Guilford Press.

Zautra, A. J., & Smith, B. W. (2001). Depression and reactivity to stress in older women with rheumatoid arthritis and osteoarthritis. *Psychosomatic Medicine, 63*(4), 687–696.

Zeidan, F., Martucci, K. T., Kraft, R. A., Gordon, N. S., McHaffie, J. G., & Coghill, R. C. (2011). Brain mechanisms supporting the modulation of pain by mindfulness meditation. *Journal of Neuroscience, 31*(14), 5540–5548.

Zeidan, F., Salomons, T., Farris, S. R., Emerson, N. M., Adler-Neal, A., Jung, Y., & Coghill, R. C. (2018). Neural mechanisms supporting the relationship between dispositional mindfulness and pain. *Pain, 159*(12), 2477–2485.

Zhang, W., Hashemi, M. M., Kaldewaij, R., Koch, S. B., Beckmann, C., Klumpers, F., & Roelofs, K. (2019). Acute stress alters the "default" brain processing. *NeuroImage, 189*, 870–877.

Zhang, X., Li, Y., & Liu, D. (2019). Effects of exercise on the quality of life in breast cancer patients: A systematic review of randomized controlled trials. *Supportive Care in Cancer, 27*(1), 9–21.

Zhang, H., Wang, Z., Wang, G., Song, X., Qian, Y., Liao, Z., ... Xia, Y. (2023). Understanding the connection between gut homeostasis and psychological stress. *The Journal of Nutrition, 153*(4), 924–939.

Zhu, H., Luo, X., Cai, T., Li, Z., & Liu, W. (2014). Self-control and parental control mediate the relationship between negative emotions and emotional eating among adolescents. *Appetite, 82*, 202–207.

Zias, J., Stark, H., Seligman, J., Levy, R., Werker, E., Breuer, A., & Mechoulam, R. (1993). Early medical use of cannabis. *Nature, 363*(6426), 215.

Ziemssen, T. (2012). Psychoneuroimmunology—Psyche and autoimmunity. *Current Pharmaceutical Design, 18*(29), 4485–4488.

Ziemssen, T., & Kern, S. (2007). Psychoneuroimmunology—Cross-talk between the immune and nervous systems. *Journal of Neurology, 254*(Suppl. 2), II8–II11.

Zietsch, B. P., Verweij, K. J., Bailey, J. M., Wright, M. J., & Martin, N. G. (2010). Genetic and environmental influences on risky sexual behaviour and its relationship with personality. *Behavior Genetics, 40*(1), 12–21.

Zimmer-Gembeck, M. J., & Skinner, E. A. (2011). The development of coping across childhood and adolescence: An integrative review and critique of research. *International Journal of Behavioral Development, 35*, 1–17.

Zitting, K. M., Vujovic, N., Yuan, R. K., Isherwood, C. M., Medina, J. E., Wang, W., ... Duffy, J. F. (2018). Human resting energy expenditure varies with circadian phase. *Current Biology, 28*(22), 3685–3690.e3.

Zorrilla, E. P., McKay, J. R., Luborsky, L., & Schmidt, K. (1996). Relation of stressors and depressive symptoms to clinical progression of viral illness. *American Journal of Psychiatry, 153*(5), 626–635.

Zucker, D. J. (2009). Book review and note: ABCs of healthy grieving: A companion for everyday coping. *Journal of Pastoral Care & Counseling, 63*(1–2), 1. doi: 10.1177/154230500906300127

Zunker, C., Mitchell, J. E., & Wonderlich, S. A. (2011). Exercise interventions for women with anorexia nervosa: A review of the literature. *International Journal of Eating Disorders, 44*(7), 579–584. doi: 10.1002/eat.20862

Zupanc, M. (2015, June 25). Sharing my story with patients. *New York Times*. Retrieved from http://well.blogs.nytimes.com/2015/06/25/sharing-my-story-with-patients/

Zwahr, M. D., Park, D. C., & Shifren, K. (1999). Judgments about estrogen replacement therapy: The role of age, cognitive abilities, and beliefs. *Psychology and Aging, 14*(2), 179–191.

Zweig, J. M., Lindberg, L. D., & McGinley, K. A. (2001). Adolescent health risk profiles: The co-occurrence of health risks among females and males. *Journal of Youth and Adolescence, 30*(6), 707–728.

Zyriax, B. C., & Windler, E. (2023). Lifestyle changes to prevent cardio-and cerebrovascular disease at midlife: A systematic review. *Maturitas, 167*, 60–65.

Index

Note: Page references in *italics* denote figures and in **bold** tables.